Autoimmune Diseases in Endocrinology

CONTEMPORARY ENDOCRINOLOGY

P. Michael Conn, SERIES EDITOR

AUTOIMMUNE DISEASES IN ENDOCRINOLOGY

Edited by

ANTHONY P. WEETMAN, MD, DSc

School of Medicine and Biomedical Sciences
University of Sheffield,
Sheffield, United Kingdom

HUMANA PRESS ✳ TOTOWA, NEW JERSEY

For additional copies, pricing for bulk purchases, and/or information about other Humana titles, contact Humana at the above address or at any of the following numbers: Tel: 973-256-1699; Fax: 973-256-8341; E-mail: humana@humanapr.com or visit our website at http://humanapress.com

Photocopy Authorization Policy:
Authorization to photocopy items for internal or personal use, or the internal or personal use of specific clients, is granted by Humana Press, provided that the base fee of US $30 per copy is paid directly to the Copyright Clearance Center at 222 Rosewood Drive, Danvers, MA 01923. For those organizations that have been granted a photocopy license from the CCC, a separate system of payment has been arranged and is acceptable to Humana Press. The fee code for users of the Transactional Reporting Service is: [978-1-58829-733-4/08 $30].

Printed in the United States of America. 10 9 8 7 6 5 4 3 2 1

eISBN: 978-1-59745-517-6

Library of Congress Control Number: 2007928339

PREFACE

It was a real pleasure to be asked to edit *Autoimmune Diseases in Endocrinology* by the Series Editor, P. Michael Conn. As a contributor to the last volume in this series that addressed the subject, *Autoimmune Endocrinopathies*, edited by Bob Volpé and published in 1999, I was proud to be asked to write a chapter in an outstanding volume of essays on the important topic of autoimmunity and endocrine disease. The present volume will, I hope, be a useful update on what has happened in the intervening eight years. Sadly Bob Volpé died two years ago and I would like to join the many others who have mourned his passing. I remember as a medical student in Newcastle-upon-Tyne this renowned figure in the field visiting us and giving the most impressive lecture I had then heard. Bob's ability to enthuse people and to challenge dogma have been as important as his scientific contributions, and we all owe him a great deal in the development in this field.

Another reason I was delighted to undertake this task was the fact that last year saw the 50th anniversary of the discovery of autoimmunity, with the initial description by Rose & Witebsky of thyroglobulin antibodies and thyroiditis in rabbits immunized with thyroid extract (1), followed in the same year by the description of thyroglobulin antibodies in Hashimoto's thyroiditis (2). This was indeed an annus mirabilis because at the same time Adams and Purves described a substance in the serum of Graves' disease patients, which turned out to stimulate the thyroid in a fashion totally different to TSH (3). This long acting thyroid stimulator was later shown independently by Kriss and McKenzie to be an IgG and of course this was a thyroid-stimulating antibody, directed against the TSH receptor, which is the cause of Graves' disease. The initial description of this stimulator appeared in the local medical school journal, something I think that would be unlikely in these days of impact factors and citation indices, but reminds us that highly significant developments can start from simple and apparently modest origins. So I hope that this volume is a celebration of the first half century of discoveries in the field of autoimmunity, and I am particularly pleased that Noel Rose, who has done so much in the discovery and elucidation of autoimmune phenomena, is a contributor to the present volume.

I have grouped the chapters in a somewhat different way to *Autoimmune Endocrinopathies*, and I have also asked an (almost) entirely different group of colleagues to contribute. This is not merely to provide a different perspective but also to give an introduction to what is an increasingly complex field. It is impossible in a book of this size to cover the complexities of modern immunology, but I felt that a set of introductory chapters would provide sufficient information to understand the developments in the field for those without a background in recent immunology, together with suitable references for further reading. The authors of these three introductory chapters are ideally placed to bridge the gap that can exist between theoretical immunology and its application to clinical disease, and have produced an excellent start to the book.

The next section concerns autoimmune thyroid disease and this is unashamedly the largest section. Not only are there diverse mechanisms that lie at the heart of these different autoimmune diseases, but also as a group they constitute the exemplar still of autoimmunity. I have asked the authors of each of the clinical chapters to follow a similar structure, taking the reader through the basic epidemiology, genetic and environmental risk factors, immunopathogenesis and then detailing the diagnostic and management aspects of the disease. Hopefully this will give the reader easy access to the information he or she needs, and this layout will allow comparisons between the different autoimmune disorders under each of these broad headings.

The third section of the book consists of three chapters on type 1 diabetes mellitus. Despite the frequency of thyroid disease and the often neglected fact that many of these patients are less than happy with current treatment, nonetheless type 1 diabetes must be the most severe of the autoimmune endocrinopathies. The autoimmune origin of type 1 diabetes was only suspected in the early 1970s when Bottazzo and colleagues found islet cell autoantibodies at the onset of disease (4). Since then the field has made major progress, particularly with the identification of key islet cell autoantigens and the development of increasingly innovative and complex animal models. If any disease deserves an immunological solution, it is this, given both its frequency and the young population that is affected.

The last section concerns the other autoimmune endocrinopathies, which range in frequency from common to rare, but the immunological changes in each have important clinical and therapeutic implications. Our understanding of these is even more recent than that of type 1 diabetes, and it is salutary to compare the chapters in this volume and *Autoimmune Endocrinopathies* to see really how far we have come. The cloning of the *AIRE* gene has been a major triumph and allowed new insights into type 1 autoimmune polyglandular syndrome, key autoantigens have been identified in Addison's disease and we have a much greater understanding of the tempo of disease evolution, and many more clinical studies have been done in autoimmune hypophysitis. Questions still remain over the role of autoimmunity in many cases of premature ovarian failure, but slowly this condition is becoming disaggregated and better understood, and we also have fresh insights into the mechanisms in autoimmune polyglandular syndrome type 2.

Finally, and most importantly, I want to thank all of the chapter editors who have contributed so diligently and enthusiastically to this project. Their scholarship is evident in each of the chapters and I am deeply grateful to them for all of their hard work. I am also indebted to the Series Editor, Dr. P. Michael Conn, for the invitation to contribute to this series and to Richard Lansing and Saundra Bunton for seeing the project through to completion. Last but certainly not least I need to thank Mrs. Kathryn Watson for her excellent secretarial assistance and help in ensuring the deadlines have been met.

REFERENCES

1. Rose NR, Witebsky E. Studies in organ specificity. V. Changes in the thyroid glands of rabbits following active immunisation with rabbit thyroid extracts. J Immunol 1956;**76**:417-427.
2. Roit IM, Doniach D, Campbell PN, Vaughan Hudson R. Autoantibodies in Hashimoto's disease (lymphadenoid goitre). Lancet 1956;ii 820-821.

3. Adams DD & Purves HD. Abnormal responses in the assay of thyrotrophin. Proceedings of the University of Otago Medical School. 1956;**34**:11-12.

4. Bottazzo GF, Florin-Christensen A, Doniach D. Islet cell antibodies in diabetes mellitus with autoimmune polyendocrine deficiencies. Lancet 1974;**2**:1279-1283.

Tony Weetman, MD, DSc.

CONTENTS

PART IV: OTHER AUTOIMMUNE ENDOCRINOPATHIES

Contributors

SOPHIE BENSING, MD, PhD, *Department of Molecular Medicine and Surgery, Karolinska Institutet, Karolinska University Hospital, Stockholm, Sweden*

CORRADO BETTERLE, MD, *Department of Medical and Surgical Sciences, Unit of Endocrinology, University of Padua, Padua, Italy*

HURIYA BEYAN, PhD, *Institute of Cell and Molecular Science, Queen Mary College, University of London, London, UK*

C. LYNNE BUREK, PhD, *Department of Pathology, Johns Hopkins Medical Institutions, Baltimore, MD*

CHRISTINE BURNS, BSc, GRAD. DIP. MED. LAB. SCI., *Department of Immunology, Hunter Area Pathology Service, John Hunter Hospital, Newcastle, Australia*

EDUARDO H. CHARREAU, PhD, *Instituto de Biología y Medicina Experimental-CONICET, Buenos Aires, Argentina*

LUCIENNE CHATENOUD, MD, PhD, *Université René Descartes Paris 5, Institut National de la Santé et de la Recherche Médicale U580, Hôpital Necker-Enfants Malades, Paris, France*

VIOLETA A. CHIAUZZI, PhD, *Instituto de Biología y Medicina Experimental-CONICET, Buenos Aires, Argentina*

DANIELA CIHÁKOVA, MD, PhD, *Department of Pathology, Johns Hopkins Medical Institutions, Baltimore, MD*

PATRICIAN ANNE CROCK, MBBS, FRACP, *Department of Paediatric Endocrinology, John Hunter Children's Hospital, Newcastle, Australia*

MANUELA DITTMAR, PROF, *Department of Biology, Gutenberg University, Mainz, Germany*

STEPHEN GOUGH, MD, *Department of Medicine, Division of Medical Science, Institute of Biomedical Research, University of Birmingham, Birmingham, UK*

JOANNE HEWARD, PhD, *Department of Medicine, Institute of Biomedical Research, University of Birmingham, Birmingham, UK*

BARBRO HOLM, MD, *Department of Clinical Sciences, Diabetes and Celiac Disease Unit, Lund University/CRC, University Hospital MAS, Malmo, Sweden*

GEORGE J. KAHALY, PROF, *Department of Medicine, Gutenberg University, Mainz, Germany*

ANASTASIA KATSAROU, MD, *Department of Clinical Sciences, Diabetes and Celiac Disease Unit, Lund University/CRS, University Hospital MAS, Malmo, Sweden*

FRANCESCO LATROFA, MD, *Department of Endocrinology and Metabolism, University Hospital of Pisa, Pisa, Italy*

JOHN H. LAZARUS, MA, MD, FRCP, FACE, FRCOG, *Centre for Endocrine and Diabetes Sciences, Cardiff University, University Hospital of Wales, Cardiff, UK*

ÅKE LERNMARK, PhD, *Department of Medicine, University of Washington, R.H. Williams Laboratory, Seattle, WA*

R. DAVID G. LESLIE, FRCP, *Department of Diabetes, St. Bartholomew's Hospital, London, UK*

MARIAN LUDGATE, BSc, PhD, *Centre for Endocrine and Diabetes Sciences, School of Medicine, Cardiff University, Cardiff, UK*

KRISTIAN LYNCH, MSc, *Department of Clinical Sciences, Diabetes and Celiac Disease Unit, Lund University/CRC, University Hospital MAS, Malmo, Sweden*

DOLORES B. NJOKU, MD, *Departments of Anesthesiology and Critical Care Medicine, Johns Hopkins Medical Institutions, Baltimore, MD*

SIMON H. S. PEARCE, MD, FRCP, *Department of Endocrinology, University of Newcastle and Royal Victoria Infirmary, Newcastle upon Tyne, UK*

PÄRT PETERSON, PhD, *Molecular Pathology, University of Tartu, Tartu, Estonia*

ALDO PINCHERA, MD, *Department of Endocrinology and Metabolism, University Hospital of Pisa, Pisa, Italy*

L. D. K. E. PREMAWARDHANA, MBBS, FRCP, *Centre for Endocrine and Diabetes Sciences, Cardiff University, University Hospital of Wales, Cardiff, UK*

FABIO PRESOTTO, MD, PhD, *Department of Medical and Surgical Sciences, Third Unit of Internal Medicine, University of Padua, Padua, Italy*

SONIA QUARATINO, MD, PhD, *Cancer Research UK Clinical Centre, Cancer Sciences Division, University of Southampton, Southampton, UK*

PHILLIP J. ROBINSON, BSc, PhD, *Cell Signalling Unit, Children's Medical Research Institute, Sydney, Australia*

NOEL R. ROSE, MD, PhD, *Departments of Pathology, School of Medicine and Molecular Microbiology and Immunology, Bloomberg School of Public Health, Johns Hopkins Medical Institutions, Baltimore, MD*

NAGAT SAEED, PhD, *Section of Human Metabolism and Endocrinology, School of Medicine and Biomedical Sciences, University of Sheffield, Sheffield, UK*

RAJNI B. SHARMA, PhD, *Department of Pathology, Johns Hopkins Medical Institutions, Baltimore, MD*

CASEY JO ANNE SMITH, BBIomedSc (HONS), *Department of Paediatric Endocrinology, John Hunter Children's Hospital, Newcastle, Australia*

VICTORIA SUNDBLAD, PhD, *Instituto de Biología y Medicina Experimental-CONICET, Buenos Aires, Argentina*

PHILIP F. WATSON, PhD, *Section of Human Metabolism and Endocrinology, School of Medicine and Biomedical Sciences, University of Sheffield, Sheffield, UK*

ANTHONY P. WEETMAN, MD, DSc, *School of Medicine and Biomedical Sciences, University of Sheffield, Sheffield, UK*

WILMAR M. WIERSINGA, MD, PhD, *Department of Endocrinology and Metabolism, Academic Medical Center, University of Amsterdam, Amsterdam, The Netherlands*

RENATO ZANCHETTA, MD, *Department of Medical and Surgical Sciences, Unit of Endocrinology, University of Padua, Padua, Italy*

I INTRODUCTORY CHAPTERS

1 Basic Mechanisms in Autoimmunity

Sonia Quaratino, MD, PhD

CONTENTS

Summary

Activation of self-reactive T cells is a critical step in the pathogenesis of autoimmune diseases. The mechanisms underpinning this remain elusive and difficult to prove in the complex human system. The most intriguing hypotheses and the mechanisms that control T-cell activation and regulation, which have been studied in vitro and in experimental animal models, will be discussed in this chapter together with their relevance to human diseases.

Key Words: Autoimmune diseases, molecular mimicry, disease mechanisms, T cells, cryptic epitopes, T-cell activation, T-cell tolerance, animal models.

INTRODUCTION

The underlying basic mechanisms of autoimmune reactivity have been puzzling immunologists for decades. What makes the immune system, which has evolved over the millennia to combat the assaults of invading microorganisms, turn against the organism itself? It now seems clear that avoiding autoreactivity while maintaining immunocompetence is a complex assignment that can sometimes go wrong. Although the innate and adaptive branches of the immune system have been involved in the induction and evolution of autoimmunity, it is well accepted that adaptive (T and B cells) responses are the main initiators and regulators of autoimmunity.

From: *Contemporary Endocrinology: Autoimmune Diseases in Endocrinology*
Edited by: A. P. Weetman © Humana Press, Totowa, NJ

Because T and B cells have predetermined specificities, some will be self-reactive and have the potential to cause damage. Several mechanisms must therefore exist to neutralize self-reactive lymphocytes and maintain self-tolerance.

Self-tolerance is imposed in the bone marrow at the B-cell level to prevent the production of potentially damaging autoantibodies (1). Although complex mechanisms are involved in the regulation and activation of self-reactive B cells (1,2), major interest has recently focused on T cells. Indeed, T cells are not only powerful effector cells but have also established themselves as the main regulators of autoimmune responses (3). In this chapter, I will therefore focus on basic mechanisms of T-cell-related initiation of autoimmunity.

At the T-cell level, the first and most important step to generate the tolerant status takes place in the thymus, where autoreactive T cells with high affinity for self-antigens are deleted (4). Potentially self-reactive T cells that escape thymus censorship are also subjected to a further regulation. In peripheral tissues, regulatory mechanisms of the immune system may hold autoreactive lymphocytes in check, for example, through the operation of specialized cells with suppressor activity (5). Although the mechanisms that silence self-reactive lymphocytes are very efficient, self-tolerance can however break down, and autoimmunity will thus ensue. It is indeed likely that autoimmune diseases are initiated in response to a single antigen, which may be restricted to a single organ. The evidence that autoimmunity in animal models can be initiated with a single autoreactive T cell supports this notion (6–11).

The most tantalizing mechanisms responsible for break of tolerance and peripheral activation of self-reactive T cells are briefly described in this chapter.

ESCAPE OF SELF-REACTIVE T CELLS FROM THE THYMUS

Studies from the autoimmune regulator (AIRE) have shown that self-antigens expressed in the thymus play an important role in promoting deletion of self-reactive T cells (12,13). Indeed, both human and mice deficient for AIRE develop extensive autoimmune diseases in endocrine organs (14–16). Tissue-specific antigens are expressed in the thymus and contribute to shape the mature T-cell repertoire. They usually mediate deletion of high-affinity self-reactive T cells, whereas low-affinity T cells are positively selected to migrate to the periphery (17).

Thymic Expression of Splice Variants of Tissue-Specific Self-Antigens

A mechanism that allows self-reactive T cells to escape negative selection is when the cognate antigen expressed in the thymus differs from that expressed in the target organ. This is best illustrated by studies in autoimmune thyroiditis and experimental autoimmune encephalomyelitis (EAE). In the first case, only a truncated isoform of the thyroglobulin has been detected in the thymus (18), whereas in the second case, the predominant forms of myelin basic protein (MBP) and the proteolipid antigen expressed in the thymus are splice variants (19–21). The lack of tolerance to these epitopes offers an explanation for the remarkable susceptibility of SJL/J mice to EAE.

Self-Peptides with Low Affinity for Major Histocompatibility Complex Molecules

Another mechanism that has been proposed to explain the thymic escape of the self-reactive T cells foresees an inefficient antigen presentation of thymically expressed self-antigens. The immunogenic MBP(Ac1-9) epitope that is expressed in the thymus displays low affinity for H2-Au, enabling autoreactive T cells to escape self-tolerance *(22)*. In contrast, peptide analogs displaying a higher affinity for H2-Au mediated thymic deletion of the specific T cells *(22)*.

Similarly, in nonobese diabetic (NOD) mice, the type-1 diabetes (T1D)-associated H2-Ag *(7)* molecule has also been shown to be structurally unstable and to be a poor peptide binder *(17,23,24)*.

Altogether, these studies demonstrate that thymic deletion may not be complete or may not occur because of the limited affinity of the major histocompatibility complex (MHC) molecule for the self-antigen or because of the expression of a splice variant or isoform of the self-antigen.

GENETIC EFFECTS ON AUTOIMMUNITY

Of the many genes involved in autoimmunity, none can be considered a real triggering factor but rather an influence to the susceptibility to a particular disease. Indeed, the concordance rate for autoimmune diseases among monozygotic twins is well below 1, suggesting that other factors, possibly environmental, must play an important role *(25,26)*.

MHC Genes

MHC class II alleles have been linked to several autoimmune conditions in human and mouse, but the mechanism by which they might mediate susceptibility to a given autoimmune disease remains still elusive *(27,28)*. The increased susceptibility seems to be associated with the polymorphic regions unique to these predisposing MHC alleles. These may influence disease susceptibility by selecting potential autoreactive T cells during thymic education, as shown in animal models *(28)*. Alternatively, these alleles might have different abilities to present peptides from target tissues to self-reactive T cells *(29)*. In T1D, probably the most intensively studied autoimmune disease and the best paradigm of MHC-associated disease, MHC susceptibility for T1D is recessive, with susceptibility alleles more common than protective alleles *(30)*. Approximately 30% of T1D patients are heterozygous for HLA-DQA1*0501-DQB1*0201 and DQA1*0301-DQB1*0302 alleles (usually shortened to HLA-DQ2/DQ8), whereas HLA-DQA1*0102-DQB1*0602 is associated with dominant protection from the disease *(31,32)*. In autoimmune thyroiditis, a more refined linkage analysis has confirmed the contribution of the MHC, but the effects are modest and not disease-specific *(33)*.

Non-MHC Genes

Because the influence of MHC seems insufficient to account for the entire genetic contribution to the majority of autoimmune diseases, the hunt has shifted on to identify new non-MHC susceptibility genes *(34)*.

Because of its inhibitory role, a polymorphism in the cytotoxic T-lymphocyte-associated antigen (*CTLA*)-4 gene is associated to several autoimmune diseases such as T1D, lupus, celiac disease, and autoimmune thyroid disease *(34–40)*.

Likewise, the majority of the polymorphisms in the *AIRE* gene decrease its trans-activation activity, leading to autoimmune polyendocrinopathy-candidiasis ectodermal dystrophy (APECED), a syndrome characterized by a variable combination of autoimmune diseases of endocrine origin *(41–43)*. So far, at least 50 different mutations within putative DNA binding and transactivation domains of the *AIRE* gene have been identified, suggesting the importance of each of these domains in the function of AIRE *(16)*.

Polymorphisms of FAS have also been linked to the pathogenesis of autoimmune diseases; in particular, this has been recently documented in systemic lupus erythematosus (SLE) *(44)*. Although inherited deficiencies in tolerogenic costimulatory pathways such as FAS predisposes humans and mice toward systemic autoimmunity *(45)*, Fas–FasL interactions can also facilitate organ-specific autoimmune diseases, as highlighted for autoimmune thyroiditis *(46,47)*.

Can Epigenetic be the Answer to the Question?

In the last couple of years, another explanation for the low concordancy rate in identical twins has been proposed, based on the existence of epigenetic differences. Indeed, locus-specific differences in DNA methylation and histone acetylation exist between monozygotic twins, affecting their gene-expression portrait *(48)*. These findings may explain how different phenotypes can still originate from the same genotype and reassess the role of genetics in the pathogenesis of autoimmune diseases *(49–51)*.

MOLECULAR MIMICRY: AUTOIMMUNITY PROVOKED BY INFECTIONS

One of the most intriguing hypotheses is that autoimmunity is the by-product of the immune response fighting infections. The initial demonstration that a virus-specific cytotoxic T lymphocyte (CTL) response can lead to selective damage of pancreatic β cells resulting in diabetes *(52)* has opened a new axis of research. For two decades, the known associations between infectious agents and autoimmunity, such as β-hemolytic streptococci and rheumatic fever *(53)*, cytomegalovirus and T1D *(54)*, viruses and multiple sclerosis (MS) *(55)*, and so on, have fueled speculation that infectious agents can activate self-reactive T cells *(56,57)* (Fig. 1). The basis for molecular mimicry lies on the intrinsic flexibility of the T-cell receptor (TCR), a molecule capable to interact with multiple ligands with a certain degree of degeneracy *(58,59)*. As a result, T cells can be triggered by peptides, which often have minimal homology to the primary immunogenic peptide, as long as they present a similar antigenic conformation *(60)*. This is an important feature of T cells, which permits effective T-cell responses to the largest number of potential foreign peptide sequences complexed to MHC molecules. Furthermore, even a shift in the binding register can cause a dramatic change in the appearance of a peptide:MHC complex *(60,61)*. By changing the MHC-binding residues into TCR contact residues, the TCR antigenic surface can be highly altered, converting two different peptide:MHC complexes into a cross-reactive pair. The observation that a single TCR can recognize quite distinct but structurally related peptides from multiple pathogens has important implications for understanding the pathogenesis of autoimmunity. Evidence for a role of molecular mimicry in autoimmunity has been reported in mouse and human. In a murine model of autoimmune herpes stromal keratitis, an epitope of herpes simplex virus-type 1 has been shown to be recognized by autoreactive T cells that target corneal antigens *(62)*. In human, both viral and bacterial

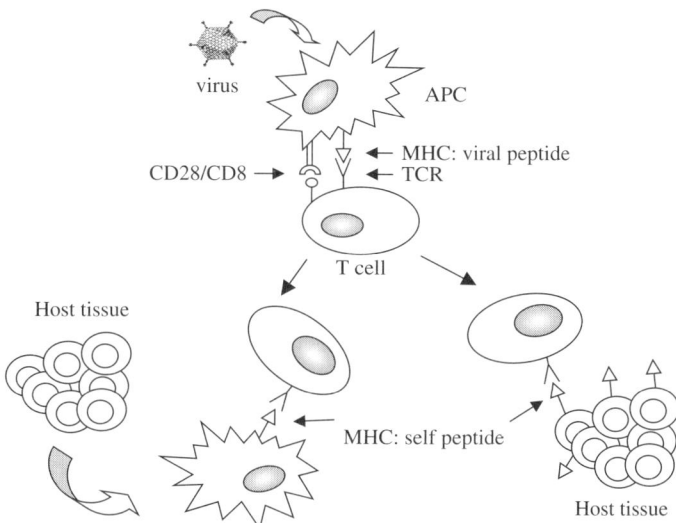

Fig. 1. Molecular mimicry. A T cell expressing a TCR specific for a foreign (viral) peptide and a self-peptide, is activated by a virus-derived peptide presented by fully mature dendritic cells. The resulting activated T cell, with less stringent costimulatory requirements, will also be able to recognize a similar self-peptide and mediate a self-reactive response.

peptides can efficiently activate MBP-specific T cells isolated from MS patients *(63)*. Also in MS, a particular human T-cell clone can recognize peptide MBP(85–99) and an Epstein-Barr virus (EBV) DNA polymerase epitope (627–641) presented by DRB1*1501 and DRB5*0101, respectively, two MHC molecules contained in the MS-associated DR2 haplotype *(64)*. Viral infections play a role in shaping the peripheral T-cell repertoire and also in the initiation of autoimmunity through molecular mimicry. This hypothesis is strengthened by a recent report, where a hemagglutinin (Flu-HA)-specific T-cell clone derived from an MS patient is cross-reactive against 14 Flu-HA variants, 11 viral, 15 human, and 3 myelin-derived peptides *(65)*.

Thus, autoimmune responses provoked by molecular mimicry should occur when the foreign and self-determinants are similar enough to cross-react yet different enough to break immunological tolerance.

Does the Theory Mirror Reality?

In recent years, computational analysis and in vitro experimental screenings have identified several candidate epitopes *(66)*. This leads to a compelling issue that needs to be addressed: according to this fascinating hypothesis, autoimmunity should be very common, as there are too many examples of cross-reactivity or degeneracy of the TCR. However, there is no definite proof of molecular mimicry in humans, and evidence is frequently circumstantial *(57)*. It is possible that to avoid an uncontrolled induction of autoimmunity, infection-induced molecular mimicry must satisfy some criteria: (1) it must be able to stimulate the innate immune system toward a Th1-type of response, (2) the mimic epitope must be processed from its native form and presented onto MHC molecules, (3) infection of the target organ might be required to sustain the self-reactive response, and (4) the infection must be persistent with continuous presentation of the mimic epitope to sustain activation of the self-reactive T cells. So far, it has been difficult to prove or disprove this suggestive hypothesis in the difficult human system. Adequate mouse models will be instrumental for understanding how and when mimicry could be involved in the pathogenesis of autoimmunity.

DUAL RECEPTOR T CELLS: ANOTHER TYPE OF CROSS-REACTIVITY

T cells expressing two TCR with different specificities follow into a different category of cross-recognition and the potential involvement of such T cells in autoimmunity has been suggested. Described in human *(67)* and in mouse *(68)*, T cells with two TCR-α chains paired to a single TCR-β chain make up to 30 % of the peripheral T-cell repertoire *(69)*. T cells that express two TCRs are the result of the incomplete allelic exclusion at the TCR-α chain locus. The expression of a second TCR can rescue T cells with a self-reactive TCR from thymic deletion and allow their exit into the periphery *(70)*. Indeed, positive selection of one foreign-specific TCR may allow the second TCR (potentially self-reactive) to escape negative selection. In the periphery, this T cell will have an allo-reactive and self-reactive function: it will be activated upon encountering the foreign antigen that engages the pathogen-specific TCR, at the same time leading to autoimmunity (Fig. 2).

BYSTANDER ACTIVATION

An antigen-nonspecific theory has also been evoked to explain the surge of autoimmunity. This theory comprehends several variants under the term "bystander activation." Bystander activation occurs during viral infections, and no particular microbial determinant is implicated *(71,72)*. As a result of an infection, large quantities of normally sequestered antigens might be released following the host cell destruction. These antigens could be presented on site or be trafficked to the draining lymph

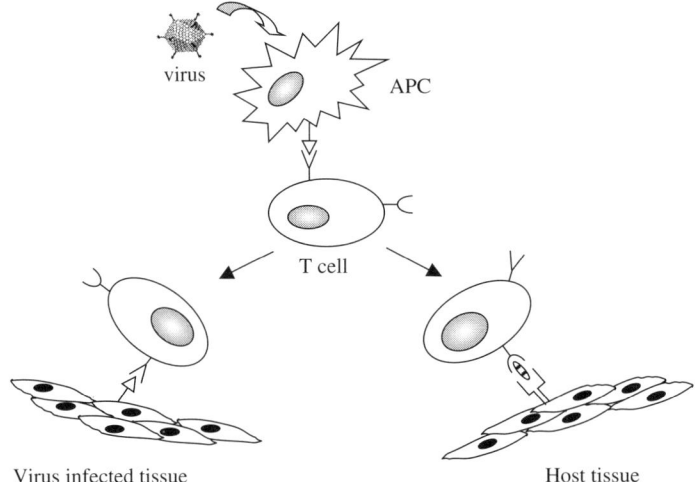

Fig. 2. Expression of dual T-cell receptor (TCR) can mediate autoimmunity. T-cell activation can be mediated by the first TCR recognizing the foreign antigen (virus). Once the T cell is activated, the second TCR (specific for self) can attack the host tissue.

nodes *(73)*. Owing to the local production of cytokines such as tumor necrosis factor (TNF)-α, interferon (IFN)-γ, interleukin (IL)-1, and the "danger" signal induced by the viral infection, the phenotype and the maturation status of professional and nonprofessional antigen-presenting cells (APC) might be changed by boosting the antigen-processing machinery, upregulating the surface expression of MHC class II molecules and the expression of costimulatory molecules *(71,72)*. Under these conditions, it might be envisaged that an uncontrolled polyclonal activation of the immune system may contribute to the autoimmune pathogenesis.

CRYPTIC EPITOPES

The concept that recognition of self-antigens in the thymic environment is a pivotal event in shaping T-cell tolerance has brought to life another challenging hypothesis for the pathogenesis of autoimmune diseases. Sercarz and colleagues *(74)* originally speculated that self-epitopes that are cryptic (hidden), because they are not generated at all or are generated at subthreshold levels, may not be involved in thymic education and allow the specific T cells to migrate to the periphery. There are multiple reasons for crypticity: they are related to antigen processing, hindrance, and competition *(75,76)*. The processing may be too indolent or excessive, leading to destruction of the epitope *(77)*; or flanking determinants might compete for the MHC binding *(76,78–80)*. As a result, T cells specific for cryptic self-epitopes are present in the normal repertoire and might become activated and autoaggressive if the epitopes are presented at higher concentrations.

The key question is how epitopes that are usually cryptic may become visible enough to trigger the specific T cells. Plausible mechanisms for an upregulation of cryptic epitopes have been demonstrated. Cytokines can increase synthesis of MHC class II molecules and proteases *(78)*. Thus, this process can become self-sustaining through the reciprocal stimulation of T and B cells, antibodies and cytokines, contributing to the spreading of the autoimmune response *(81,82)*. Another possibility is that, under inflammatory conditions, upregulation of antigen processing can lead to enhanced presentation of the previously cryptic epitope *(77,78)*. This might lead to priming of the cryptic epitope-specific T cells. A third possibility, the cryptic epitopes may be presented on nonprofessional APC, such as epithelial cells. An upregulation of MHC class II molecules on these cells could favor sudden presentation of the cryptic epitope by the nonprofessional APC with relative trigger of the T cells, even in the absence of a second signal. This situation might not be totally remote, as may occur at inflammatory sites or in the lymph node where costimulation could be provided in a bystander fashion *(83)*.

Role of Cryptic Epitopes in Experimental Models

Studies in different animal models have shown that T cells specific for dominant self-epitopes are made tolerant in the thymus, whereas those specific for cryptic epitopes escape tolerance induction *(74,76)*. In these models, the cryptic epitope-specific T cells can be activated by a synthetic peptide but not by the native antigen *(84,85)*. Once activated, these T cells can then lead to the induction of autoimmunity. Indeed, it has been documented that epitope spreading observed during the course of EAE targets various cryptic epitopes of MBP *(76,81)*. Presentation of the HLA-DR2-restricted

MBP *(85–99)* epitope is greatly enhanced by inhibition of the cysteine protease asparagine endopeptidase (AEP), whereas overexpression of AEP diminishes presentation of this epitope *(77)*. AEP is therefore able to unmask cryptic epitopes, leading to the activation of pathogenic T cells *(86)*. There is an enhanced processing and presentation of previously cryptic epitopes of MBP, which are then revealed to the T cells as the disease progresses.

Nondominant cryptic pathogenic epitopes of thyroglobulin have also been described in autoimmune thyroiditis *(87)*. These epitopes can become dominant following posttranscriptional modifications or formation of antigen–antibody complexes *(87,88)*.

The significance of cryptic epitopes in human autoimmunity, however, has been more difficult to establish.

Role of Cryptic Epitopes in Human Autoimmunity

The most compelling description of cryptic epitopes in human autoimmune diseases is in autoimmune thyroiditis. A panel of thyroid peroxidase (TPO)-specific T cells isolated from a patient could be stimulated by the autologous thyroid epithelial cells (MHC class II$^+$) but not by dendritic cells (DC) pulsed with the native TPO *(89)*. Because thyroid epithelial cells are normally MHC class II$^-$, the cryptic TPO epitope (536–547) may be usually not available for the specific T cells. Detailed studies have identified that only endogenous processing of TPO, usually operated by thyroid epithelial cells, can upregulate presentation of this cryptic epitope, whereas exogenous processing operated by DC does not *(90)*. In vitro presentation of this TPO cryptic epitope cannot be enhanced by bound antibodies that are on the contrary very efficient in modulating presentation of other dominant epitopes *(91)*. The generation of a humanized mouse model that expresses the human TCR specific for the cryptic TPO epitope (536–547) has further strengthened the importance of this cryptic TPO epitope in autoimmune thyroiditis *(7,11)*. In this humanized model, the TPO-specific TCR not only does not get deleted, but it induces spontaneous autoimmune thyroiditis in all animals, confirming the pathogenic role of the cryptic epitope-specific T cells *(7,11)*.

Failure of Peripheral Regulation

We have just appreciated that there are several mechanisms that may trigger self-reactive T cells in the periphery, leading to a transient autoimmunity that may (or may not) develop into a frank autoimmune disease. It is now accepted that peripheral suppression of self-reactive T cells is another essential mechanism to maintain self-tolerance *(3)*. Indeed, abnormality in the number or function of these regulatory cells can lead to autoimmune diseases in animals and humans *(92)*. This specialized subset of regulatory T cells (Treg) that maintain immunological homeostasis originates in the thymus has the CD4+CD25+ phenotype and expresses the transcription factor *Foxp3* (or *FOXP3* in human) *(93)*. CD4+CD25+ Treg can act locally in tissues and draining lymph nodes; they can suppress APC and effector T cell through a cell–cell interaction or through soluble mediators such as cytokines (mainly IL-10 and TGF-β) or chemokines *(3,93)* (Fig. 3).

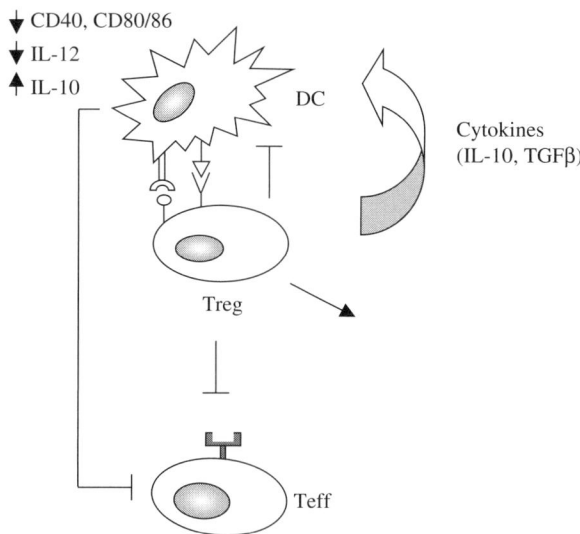

Fig. 3. Regulatory T cells (Treg) can maintain immunological tolerance. Treg cells can directly suppress dendritic cells (DC) through cell–cell interactions or indirectly through soluble mediators such as cytokines. The result is a modulated antigen-presenting cell (APC) that is incapable of triggering self-reactive T effector cells. Alternatively, Treg cells can directly inhibit self-reactive T effector cells.

Role of Treg in Autoimmune Diseases

Removal of Treg from the normal immune system inevitably results in break of T-cell tolerance and development of several autoimmune diseases, such as autoimmune gastritis and pernicious anemia, Hashimoto thyroiditis, adrenalitis and Addison's disease, insulitis and T1D, and inflammatory bowel disease *(93)*. On the contrary, injection of Treg has been shown to prevent or ameliorate several experimental autoimmune diseases *(94–96)*. Furthermore, retroviral gene transfer of *Foxp3* converts naive T cells toward a Treg phenotype similar to that of naturally occurring Treg *(97)*.

Interestingly, Treg constitutively express CTLA-4, and administration of anti-CTLA-4 antibodies to normal young naive mice elicits autoimmune diseases similar to that produced by the depletion of CD4+CD25+ Treg cells, without reducing their number *(98)*. It is likely that CTLA-4 blockade prevents Treg activation and hence attenuates suppression, causing autoimmune diseases. Of note, even in this case, polymorphisms of the *CTLA-4* gene have also been shown to affect autoimmunity in humans and rodents *(99)*.

The dominant regulatory effect of Treg is also broken by ligation of glucocorticoid-induced TNF receptor (GITR) family-related gene, which is preferentially expressed by these cells *(92)*. This implies that expression of the ligand for GITR at sites of inflammation might also be crucial for Treg activity. This suggests that autoimmune diseases may be not only the result of the activation of effectors but also the failure of Treg cells.

Evidence for Treg in Humans

A disruption of *Foxp3* is responsible for an X-linked recessive inflammatory disease in scurfy mutant mice and subsequently for immune dysregulation, polyendocrinopathy, enteropathy, X-linked (IPEX) syndrome in human *(100)*. The disruption of *FOXP3* abrogates the development of Treg cells or alters their function, leading to hyperactivation of self-reactive T cells, intestinal bacteria, or innocuous environmental substances. This causes the X-linked immunodeficiency syndrome IPEX, which is associated with autoimmune disease in multiple endocrine organs (such as T1D and thyroiditis), inflammatory bowel disease, atopic dermatitis, and fatal infection *(92)*.

Further studies on these patients and the molecular basis of Treg development and function might shed some light on the pathogenic mechanism of autoimmune diseases in general.

CONCLUSIONS

Despite our understanding of the immunological mechanisms that has progressed tremendously in the last 20 years, much confusion still remains on the pathogenesis of autoimmune diseases. All the hypotheses drawn in this chapter are not just plausible but always substantiated by a cohort of experimental data and often demonstrated in animal models. However, they are not yet conclusive, and what we need at this point are new approaches to fully understand the difficult human system.

REFERENCES

1. Eisenberg R. Mechanisms of autoimmunity. *Immunol Res* 2003;27(2–3):203–18.
2. Grimaldi CM, Hicks R, Diamond B. B cell selection and susceptibility to autoimmunity. *J Immunol* 2005;174(4):1775–81.
3. Shevach EM. Regulatory T cells in autoimmmunity*. *Annu Rev Immunol* 2000;18:423–49.
4. Hogquist KA, Baldwin TA, Jameson SC. Central tolerance: learning self-control in the thymus. *Nat Rev Immunol* 2005;5(10):772–82.
5. Sakaguchi S, Takahashi T, Yamazaki S, et al. Immunologic self tolerance maintained by T-cell-mediated control of self-reactive T cells: implications for autoimmunity and tumor immunity. *Microbes Infect* 2001;3(11):911–8.
6. Goverman J, Woods A, Larson L, Weiner L, Hood L, Zaller D. Transgenic mice that express a myelin basic protein-specific T cell receptor develop spontaneous autoimmunity. *Cell* 1993;72:551–60.
7. Quaratino S, Badami E, Pang YY, et al. Degenerate self-reactive human T-cell receptor causes spontaneous autoimmune disease in mice. *Nat Med* 2004;10(9):920–6.
8. Candon S, McHugh RS, Foucras G, Natarajan K, Shevach EM, Margulies DH. Spontaneous organ-specific Th2-mediated autoimmunity in TCR transgenic mice. *J Immunol* 2004;172(5):2917–24.
9. Waldner H, Whitters MJ, Sobel RA, Collins M, Kuchroo VK. Fulminant spontaneous autoimmunity of the central nervous system in mice transgenic for the myelin proteolipid protein-specific T cell receptor. *Proc Natl Acad Sci USA* 2000;97(7):3412–7.
10. Kouskoff V, Korganow AS, Duchatelle V, Degott C, Benoist C, Mathis D. Organ-specific disease provoked by systemic autoimmunity. *Cell* 1996;87(5):811–22.
11. Badami E, Maiuri L, Quaratino S. High incidence of spontaneous autoimmune thyroiditis in immunocompetent self-reactive human T cell receptor transgenic mice. *J Autoimmun* 2005;24(2):85–91.
12. Anderson MS, Venanzi ES, Chen Z, Berzins SP, Benoist C, Mathis D. The cellular mechanism of Aire control of T cell tolerance. *Immunity* 2005;23(2):227–39.
13. Derbinski J, Schulte A, Kyewski B, Klein L. Promiscuous gene expression in medullary thymic epithelial cells mirrors the peripheral self. *Nat Immunol* 2001;2(11):1032–9.

14. Peterson P, Nagamine K, Scott H, et al. APECED: a monogenic autoimmune disease providing new clues to self-tolerance. *Immunol Today* 1998;19(9):384–6.

15. Anderson MS, Venanzi ES, Klein L, et al. Projection of an immunological self shadow within the thymus by the aire protein. *Science* 2002;298(5597):1395–401.

16. Villasenor J, Benoist C, Mathis D. AIRE and APECED: molecular insights into an autoimmune disease. *Immunol Rev* 2005;204:156–64.

17. Anderson AC, Kuchroo VK. Expression of self-antigen in the thymus: a little goes a long way. *J Exp Med* 2003;198(11):1627–9.

18. Li HS, Carayanniotis G. Detection of thyroglobulin mRNA as truncated isoform(s) in mouse thymus. *Immunology* 2005;115(1):85–9.

19. Kuchroo VK, Anderson AC, Waldner H, Munder M, Bettelli E, Nicholson LB. T cell response in experimental autoimmune encephalomyelitis (EAE): role of self and cross-reactive antigens in shaping, tuning, and regulating the autopathogenic T cell repertoire. *Annu Rev Immunol* 2002;20(1):101–23.

20. Klein L, Klugmann M, Nave K-A, Tuohy VK, Kyewski B. Shaping of the autoreactive T-cell repertoire by a splice variant of self protein expressed in thymic epithelial cells. *Nat Med* 2000;6(1):56–61.

21. Mathisen PM, Pease S, Garvey J, Hood L, Readhead C. Identification of an embryonic isoform of myelin basic protein that is expressed widely in the mouse embryo. *PNAS* 1993;90(21):10125–9.

22. Liu GY, Fairchild PJ, Smith RM, Prowle JR, Kioussis D, Wraith DC. Low avidity recognition of self-antigen by T cells permits escape from central tolerance. *Immunity* 1995;3:407–15.

23. Carrasco-Marin E, Shimizu J, Kanagawa O, Unanue ER. The class II MHC I-Ag7 molecules from non-obese diabetic mice are poor peptide binders. *J Immunol* 1996;156(2):450–8.

24. Peterson M, Sant AJ. The inability of the nonobese diabetic class II molecule to form stable peptide complexes does not reflect a failure to interact productively with DM. *J Immunol* 1998;161(6):2961–7.

25. Larsen CE, Alper CA. The genetics of HLA-associated disease. *Curr Opin Immunol* 2004;16(5):660–7.

26. Prummel MF, Strieder T, Wiersinga WM. The environment and autoimmune thyroid diseases. *Eur J Endocrinol* 2004;150(5):605–18.

27. McDevitt HO. The role of MHC class II molecules in susceptibility and resistance to autoimmunity. *Curr Opin Immunol* 1998;10(6):677–81.

28. Das P, Abraham R, David C. HLA transgenic mice as models of human autoimmune diseases. *Rev Immunogenet* 2000;2(1):105–14.

29. Stratmann T, Apostolopoulos V, Mallet-Designe V, et al. The I-Ag7 MHC class II molecule linked to murine diabetes is a promiscuous peptide binder. *J Immunol* 2000;165(6):3214–25.

30. Pociot F, McDermott MF. Genetics of type 1 diabetes mellitus. *Genes Immun* 2002;3(5):235–49.

31. Cucca F, Lampis R, Congia M, et al. A correlation between the relative predisposition of MHC class II alleles to type 1 diabetes and the structure of their proteins. *Hum Mol Genet* 2001;10(19):2025–37.

32. Lee KH, Wucherpfennig KW, Wiley DC. Structure of a human insulin peptide-HLA-DQ8 complex and susceptibility to type 1 diabetes. *Nat Immunol* 2001;2(6):501–7.

33. Weetman AP. Determinants of autoimmune thyroid disease. *Nat Immunol* 2001;2(9):769–70.

34. Steck AK, Bugawan TL, Valdes AM, et al. Association of non-HLA genes with type 1 diabetes autoimmunity. *Diabetes* 2005;54(8):2482–6.

35. Gough SC, Walker LS, Sansom DM. CTLA4 gene polymorphism and autoimmunity. *Immunol Rev* 2005;204:102–15.

36. Haller K, Kisand K, Nemvalts V, Laine AP, Ilonen J, Uibo R. Type 1 diabetes is insulin-2221 MspI and CTLA-4 +49 A/G polymorphism dependent. *Eur J Clin Invest* 2004;34(8):543–8.

37. Barreto M, Santos E, Ferreira R, et al. Evidence for CTLA4 as a susceptibility gene for systemic lupus erythematosus. *Eur J Hum Genet* 2004;12(8):620–6.

38. Badenhoop K, Seidl C. Fine-tuning of T lymphocytes in autoimmunity: genetic association of CTLA-4 variants and Graves' disease revisited. *Clin Endocrinol (Oxf)* 2003;59(5):555–7.

39. Chistiakov DA, Turakulov RI. CTLA-4 and its role in autoimmune thyroid disease. *J Mol Endocrinol* 2003;31(1):21–36.

40. Kristiansen OP, Larsen ZM, Pociot F. CTLA-4 in autoimmune diseases – a general susceptibility gene to autoimmunity? *Genes Immun* 2000;1(3):170–84.

41. Nagamine K, Peterson P, Scott HS, et al. Positional cloning of the APECED gene. *Nat Genet* 1997;17(4):393–8.

42. Kudoh J, Nagamine K, Asakawa S, et al. Localization of 16 exons to a 450-kb region involved in the autoimmune polyglandular disease type I (APECED) on human chromosome 21q22.3. *DNA Res* 1997;4(1):45–52.

43. Halonen M, Kangas H, Rüppell T, et al. APECED-causing mutations in AIRE reveal the functional domains of the protein. *Hum Mutat* 2004;23(3):245–57.

44. Nolsoe RL, Kelly JA, Pociot F, et al. Functional promoter haplotypes of the human FAS gene are associated with the phenotype of SLE characterized by thrombocytopenia. *Genes Immun* 2005;6(8):699–706.

45. Siegel RM, Ka-Ming Chan F, Chun HJ, Lenardo MJ. The multifaceted role of Fas signaling in immune cell homeostasis and autoimmunity. *Nat Immunol* 2000;1(6):469–74.

46. Giordano C, Stassi G, De Maria R, et al. Potential involvement of Fas and its ligand in the pathogenesis of Hashimoto's thyroiditis. *Science* 1997;275(5302):960–3.

47. Stassi G, De Maria R. Autoimmune thyroid disease: new models of cell death in autoimmunity. *Nat Rev Immunol* 2002;2(3):195–204.

48. Fraga MF, Ballestar E, Paz MF, et al. From the cover: epigenetic differences arise during the lifetime of monozygotic twins. *PNAS* 2005;102(30):10604–9.

49. Brooks WH. Autoimmune disorders result from loss of epigenetic control following chromosome damage. *Med Hypotheses* 2005;64(3):590–8.

50. Januchowski R, Prokop J, Jagodzinski PP. Role of epigenetic DNA alterations in the pathogenesis of systemic lupus erythematosus. *J Appl Genet* 2004;45(2):237–48.

51. Sekigawa I, Okada M, Ogasawara H, Kaneko H, Hishikawa T, Hashimoto H. DNA methylation in systemic lupus erythematosus. *Lupus* 2003;12(2):79–85.

52. Oldstone MB, Nerenberg M, Southern P, Price J, Lewicki H. Virus infection triggers insulin-dependent diabetes mellitus in a transgenic model: role of anti-self (virus) immune response. *Cell* 1991;65(2):319–31.

53. Rose NR. The role of infection in the pathogenesis of autoimmune disease. Semin Immunol 1998;10(1):5–13.

54. von Herrath MG, Holz A, Homann D, Oldstone MB. Role of viruses in type I diabetes. *Semin Immunol* 1998;10(1):87–100.

55. Oldstone MB. Molecular mimicry and immune-mediated diseases. *FASEB J* 1998;12(13):1255–65.

56. Oldstone MBA. Molecular mimicry and autimmune disease. *Cell* 1987;50:819–20.

57. Rose NR, Mackay IR. Molecular mimicry: a critical look at exemplary instances in human diseases. *Cell Mol Life Sci* 2000;57(4):542–51.

58. Evavold BD, Sloan-Lancaster J, Wilson KJ, Rothbard JB, Allen PM. Specific T cell recognition of minimally homologous peptides: evidence for multiple endogenous ligands. *Immunity* 1995;2(6):655–63.

59. Ford ML, Evavold BD. Degenerate recognition of T cell epitopes: impact of T cell receptor reserve and stability of peptide:MHC complexes. *Mol Immunol* 2004;40(14–15):1019–25.

60. Quaratino S, Thorpe CJ, Travers PJ, Londei M. Similar antigenic surfaces, rather than sequence homology, dictate T-cell epitope molecular mimicry. *Proc Natl Acad Sci USA* 1995;92(22):10398–402.

61. Bankovich AJ, Girvin AT, Moesta AK, Garcia KC. Peptide register shifting within the MHC groove: theory becomes reality. *Mol Immunol* 2004;40(14–15):1033–9.

62. Zhao ZS, Granucci F, Yeh L, Schaffer PA, Cantor H. Molecular mimicry by herpes simplex virus-type 1: autoimmune disease after viral infection. *Science* 1998;279(5355):1344–7.

63. Wucherpfennig KW, Strominger JL. Molecular mimicry in T cell-mediated autoimmunity: viral peptides activate human T cell clones specific for myelin basic protein. *Cell* 1995;80(5):695–705.

64. Lang HL, Jacobsen H, Ikemizu S, et al. A functional and structural basis for TCR cross-reactivity in multiple sclerosis. *Nat Immunol* 2002;3(10):940–3.

65. Markovic-Plese S, Hemmer B, Zhao Y, Simon R, Pinilla C, Martin R. High level of cross-reactivity in influenza virus hemagglutinin-specific CD4+ T-cell response: implications for the initiation of autoimmune response in multiple sclerosis. *J Neuroimmunol* 2005;169(1–2):31–8.

66. Reiser JB, Darnault C, Gregoire C, et al. CDR3 loop flexibility contributes to the degeneracy of TCR recognition. *Nat Immunol* 2003;4(3):241–7.

67. Padovan E, Casorati G, Dellabona P, Meyer S, Brockhaus M, Lanzavecchia A. Expression of two T cell receptor a chains: dual receptor T cells. *Science* 1993;262:422–4.

68. Heath WR, Miller JF. Expression of two alpha chains on the surface of T cells in T cell receptor transgenic mice. *J Exp Med* 1993;178(5):1807–11.

69. Padovan E, Casorati G, Dellabona P, Giachino C, Lanzavecchia A. Dual receptor T-cells. Implications for alloreactivity and autoimmunity. *Ann NY Acad Sci* 1995;756:66–70.

70. Zal T, Weiss S, Mellor A, Stockinger B. Expression of a second receptor rescues self-specific T cells from thymic deletion and allows activation of autoreactive effector function. *Proc Natl Acad Sci USA* 1996;93(17):9102–7.

71. Benoist C, Mathis D. Autoimmunity provoked by infection: how good is the case for T cell epitope mimicry? *Nat Immunol* 2001;2(9):797–801.

72. Wucherpfennig KW. Mechanisms for the induction of autoimmunity by infectious agents. *J Clin Invest* 2001;108(8):1097–104.

73. Horwitz MS, Sarvetnick N. Viruses, host responses, and autoimmunity. *Immunol Rev* 1999;169:241 –53.

74. Sercarz EE, Lehmann PV, Ametani A, Benichou G, Miller A, Moudgil K. Dominance and crypticity of T cell antigenic determinants. *Annu Rev Immunol* 1993;11:729–66.

75. Moudgil KD, Ametani A, Grewal IS, Kumar V, Sercarz EE. Processing of self-proteins and its impact on shaping the T cell repertoire, autoimmunity and immune regulation. *Int Rev Immunol* 1993;10(4):365–77.

76. Moudgil KD, Sercarz EE. Understanding crypticity is the key to revealing the pathogenesis of autoimmunity. *Trends Immunol* 2005;26(7):355–9.

77. Manoury B, Mazzeo D, Fugger L, et al. Destructive processing by asparagine endopeptidase limits presentation of a dominant T cell epitope in MBP. *Nat Immunol* 2002;3(2):169–74.

78. Moss CX, Matthews SP, Lamont DJ, Watts C. Asparagine deamidation perturbs antigen presentation on class II major histocompatibility complex molecules. *J Biol Chem* 2005;280(18):18498–503.

79. Moudgil KD, Deng H, Nanda NK, Grewal IS, Ametani A, Sercarz EE. Antigen processing and T cell repertoires as crucial aleatory features in induction of autoimmunity. *J Autoimmun* 1996;9(2):227–34.

80. Soares L, Deng H, Grewal IS, et al. Determinant flanking regions and the design of appropriate vaccines. *Ann NY Acad Sci* 1995;754:48–56.

81. Lehmann PV, Forsthuber T, Miller A, Sercarz EE. Spreading of T-cell autoimmunity to cryptic determinants of an autoantigen. *Nature* 1992;358(6382):155–7.

82. Lanzavecchia A. How can cryptic epitopes trigger autoimmunity. *J Exp Med* 1995;181:1945–8.

83. Ding L, Shevach EM. Activation of CD4+ T cells by delivery of the B7 costimulatory signal on bystander antigen-presenting cells (trans-costimulation). *Eur J Immunol* 1994;24(4):859–66.

84. Gammon G, Sercarz E. How some T cells escape tolerance induction. *Nature* 1989;342 (6246):183–5.

85. Fairchild PJ, Pope H, Wraith DC. The nature of cryptic epitopes within the self-antigen myelin basic protein. *Int Immunol* 1996;8(7):1035–43.

86. Anderton SM, Viner NJ, Matharu P, Lowrey PA, Wraith DC. Influence of a dominant cryptic epitope on autoimmune T cell tolerance. *Nat Immunol* 2002;3(2):175–81.

87. Carayanniotis G. The cryptic self in thyroid autoimmunity: the paradigm of thyroglobulin. *Autoimmunity* 2003;36(6–7):423–8.

88. Dai YD, Eliades P, Carayanniotis KA, et al. Thyroxine-binding antibodies inhibit T cell recognition of a pathogenic thyroglobulin epitope. *J Immunol* 2005;174(5):3105–10.

89. Quaratino S, Feldmann M, Dayan CM, Acuto O, Londei M. Human self-reactive T cell clones expressing identical T cell receptor beta chains differ in their ability to recognize a cryptic self-epitope. *J Exp Med* 1996;183(2):349–58.

90. Quaratino S, Duddy LP, Londei M. Fully competent dendritic cells as inducers of T cell anergy in autoimmunity. *Proc Natl Acad Sci USA* 2000;97(20):10911–6.

91. Quaratino S, Ruf J, Osman M, et al. Human autoantibodies modulate the T cell epitope repertoire but fail to unmask a pathogenic cryptic epitope. *J Immunol* 2005;174(1):557–63.

92. Sakaguchi S. Naturally arising Foxp3-expressing CD25+CD4+ regulatory T cells in immunological tolerance to self and non-self. *Nat Immunol* 2005;6(4):345–52.

93. Sakaguchi S. Naturally arising CD4+ regulatory T cells for immunologic self-tolerance and negative control of immune responses. *Annu Rev Immunol* 2004;22:531–62.

94. Walker LS. Antigen-dependent proliferation of CD4+ CD25+ regulatory T cells in vivo. *J Exp Med* 2003;198:249–58.

95. Green EA, Choi Y, Flavell RA. Pancreatic lymph node-derived CD4(+)CD25(+) Treg cells: highly potent regulators of diabetes that require TRANCE-RANK signals. *Immunity* 2002;16(2):183–91.

96. Eggena MP, Walker LSK, Nagabhushanam V, Barron L, Chodos A, Abbas AK. Cooperative roles of CTLA-4 and regulatory T cells in tolerance to an islet cell antigen. *J Exp Med* 2004;199(12):1725–30.

97. Hori S, Nomura T, Sakaguchi S. Control of regulatory T cell development by the transcription factor foxp3. *Science* 2003;299(5609):1057–61.

98. Takahashi T. Immunologic self-tolerance maintained by CD25+CD4+ regulatory T cells constitutively expressing cytotoxic T lymphocyte-associated antigen 4. *J Exp Med* 2000;192:303–10.

99. Ueda H. Association of the T-cell regulatory gene CTLA4 with susceptibility to autoimmune disease. *Nature* 2003;423:506–11.

100. Brunkow ME. Disruption of a new forkhead/winged-helix protein, scurfin, results in the fatal lymphoproliferative disorder of the scurfy mouse. *Nat Genet* 2001;27:68–73.

2

Immunogenetic Factors in Autoimmunity

Joanne Heward, PhD, and Stephen Gough, MD

Contents

Summary

Many genetic loci are likely to contribute to the genetic susceptibility to autoimmune diseases. To date, however, only three genes/gene regions have been consistently associated with multiple autoimmune diseases, namely the human leukocyte antigen class II region on chromosome 6p21, the cytotoxic T-lymphocyte-associated antigen-4 gene on chromosome 2q33, and the *PTPN22* encoding lymphoid tyrosine phosphatase on chromosome 1p13. Further genes have been identified that contribute specifically to a particular disease, and many putative genes are awaiting replication in further data sets. Identification of susceptibility loci is confounded by the involvement of environmental factors in many of these conditions and by their complex polygenic nature requiring large data sets to detect genes of small effect. To identify genes that may increase susceptibility to these diseases, it is necessary to understand the role that the immune response plays in such disorders. This chapter aims to provide an overview of this role and how breakdown of complex immune mechanisms may lead to disease presentation. The role of the three common autoimmunity genes above is also discussed along with new developments in the field.

Key Words: Autoimmune disease, HLA, CTLA-4, *PTPN22*, LYP, single-nucleotide polymorphism.

INTRODUCTION

Autoimmune diseases are common polygenic disorders affecting between 5 and 10% of the population *(1)*. They include a wide spectrum of diseases such as type 1 diabetes ([T1D]; also known as insulin-dependent diabetes mellitus [IDDM]), Graves' disease

From: *Contemporary Endocrinology: Autoimmune Diseases in Endocrinology*
Edited by: A. P. Weetman © Humana Press, Totowa, NJ

(GD), autoimmune hypothyroidism ([AIH]; also known as Hashimoto's thyroiditis [HT]), systemic lupus erythematosus (SLE), multiple sclerosis (MS), inflammatory bowel disease (IBD), autoimmune Addison's disease (AAD), rheumatoid arthritis (RA), celiac disease (CD), and psoriasis. They are of unknown etiology but are thought to be caused by both genetic and environmental factors where disease onset can be triggered in a genetically susceptible individual by a permissive environment. Research to date on environmental triggers of such diseases in humans is inconclusive with the exception of CD, which is known to be caused by the presence of gluten in the diet *(2,3)*, although many factors have been postulated as playing a role in these disorders including smoking, diet, stress, and viral or bacterial infections.

In contrast, evidence for a genetic basis for these diseases is strong with studies showing higher disease concordance rates in monozygotic twins (ranging from 30 to 70%) compared with dizygotic twins *(4)*. The lack of complete concordance in monozygotic twins has largely been attributed to the influence of environmental factors on disease manifestation. However, a recent study has suggested that this could be owing to epigenetic differences that have an impact on gene expression *(5)*. It was observed that, as monozygotic twins got older, they exhibited marked differences in DNA methylation and histone modification, which could affect gene expression *(5)*. These modifications could be influenced by external factors such as diet and lifestyle but equally could be attributed to defects in transmitting or maintaining epigenetic information in cells *(5)*. Whatever the cause of these differences, they could go some way to explain why subjects with the same genotype can exhibit different disease phenotypes. Further evidence for a strong genetic link to these diseases comes from the observation that individual diseases tend to cluster within families *(1,6,7)* and that multiple autoimmune diseases are also seen to cluster within families *(8)*, suggesting that not only are these disorders genetically based but some of the genes that contribute to their development are shared between the diseases.

Autoimmune diseases occur because of a breakdown in the tightly regulated immune cascade (*see* Chap. 1). This system is designed to recognize foreign antigens within the body and to eliminate them with minimum disruption to normal function. This is an extremely complex process involving many components. Defects in any of these components may cause failure to distinguish between foreign and "self"-antigens, resulting in an immune attack being mounted against one or more systems or organs within the body. The mechanisms that the body uses to prevent such an attack are known as central and peripheral tolerances.

TOLERANCE MECHANISMS

Central Tolerance – Regulation and Breakdown

The prevention of autoimmunity begins in the thymus with the process of central tolerance, whereby self-reactive T cells are deleted through positive and negative selection. Immature thymocytes undergo gene rearrangement of their T-cell receptor (TCR) in the thymus such that each thymocyte displays a unique TCR capable of binding self-peptides from the periphery bound to the major histocompatibility complex (MHC) molecules. The strength of this interaction will determine the fate of the thymocyte. Those that fail to interact with MHC–peptide complexes undergo apoptosis in the positive selection process, whereas those that exhibit high affinity for such complexes are deleted in the negative selection process *(9)*. The remaining population of the mature thymocytes are then released into the periphery.

Expression of peripheral genes in the thymus is known to be controlled by the autoimmune regulator (AIRE) protein, although the mode of action by which this occurs is currently unknown *(10)*. Evidence of the importance of AIRE in central tolerance can be seen from studies in both mice *(11)* and humans *(9)* where deficiency of this molecule causes a reduction in gene expression in the thymus, leading to the production of autoantibodies to multiple organs, and results in a phenotype in mice, which is similar to the human disease autoimmune polyglandular syndrome type (APS)-1 described in Chap. 16. It clearly demonstrates an important mechanism by which central tolerance can be broken. Loss of function of AIRE causes a decrease of AIRE-dependent thymic antigens resulting in an increased incidence of autoreactive T cells escaping control of central tolerance and entering the periphery where they are too numerous to contain leading to the onset of autoimmunity *(12)*.

A further mechanism by which central tolerance can be broken can be shown by studies into the non-obese diabetic (NOD) mouse, the animal model of T1D. It has been observed that thymocytes within these mice exhibit a reduction in thymic deletion when present on the NOD.H-2^k background that leads to diabetes onset *(13)*. Further analysis has indicated that the genes responsible for apoptosis of these self-reactive thymocytes are poorly induced in these mice *(12,14)* and that additional loci that contribute to this trait are present within regions identified as diabetes susceptibility loci *(Idd* regions) *(14)*. Such studies have important implications for research into the role that defects in central tolerance regulation may have in the onset of human autoimmune disease.

An inherent problem of the central tolerance system is that not all peripheral self-peptides are expressed in the thymus. It is estimated that medullary thymic epithelial cells express 10% of all known genes in addition to those basally expressed on such cells *(15)*. It is, therefore, necessary to have a second-line of defence against the onset of autoimmunity, namely peripheral tolerance.

Peripheral Tolerance – Regulation and Breakdown

Mature T cells that enter the periphery from the thymus have low to intermediate affinity for self-antigens presented in the thymus. However, a small subset of T cells released will be autoreactive to self-antigens because of the absence of their expression in the thymus. Control and/or deletion of such T cells is essential if the autoimmune state is to be prevented. Peripheral tolerance mechanisms that perform this role can act directly on the T cell and include ignorance and anergy, phenotype skewing, and apoptosis *(16)*, or they can act by activating other cells such as dendritic cells (DCs) and regulatory T cells (Treg).

Ignorance is probably the simplest mechanism of peripheral tolerance whereby a T-cell response to self-antigen does not occur because the antigens are either located in sites that are not accessible to the T cell *(17)* or present in insufficient numbers to trigger a T-cell response *(18)*. However, if the T cell does interact with self-antigens, this can lead to anergy, which is a functional inactivation of the T cell itself. Two molecules that have been proposed as contributing to the anergic state are the costimulatory molecule, cytotoxic T-lymphocyte-associated antigen (CTLA)-4 and the programmed cell death (PD)-1 molecule. Although the mechanisms by which they contribute to anergy are unknown, it has been noted that the absence of CTLA-4 results in a fatal lymphoproliferative disorder (19), suggesting that this molecule is essential for control of the T-cell response to self-antigen. PD-1 may act by inhibiting cytokine secretion or by causing cell-cycle arrest (20,21).

Phenotypic skewing is also thought to be partially mediated by costimulatory molecules and involves alteration of the Th1/Th2 cytokine response by T cells in response to signals from these molecules received when the TCR is activated (22,23). This can result in the development of a non-pathogenic phenotype, thus preventing autoimmune damage (16).

Apoptosis is probably the most effective direct-acting mechanism to prevent autoimmunity from developing, as it involves deletion of the autoreactive T cell through interaction between Fas ligand and its receptor (16). However, in most cases, not all T cells are deleted but remain in the periphery in an anergic state, suggesting that apoptosis only occurs until the levels of autoreactive T cells are such that they can be controlled by the process of anergy (16).

In addition to these direct-acting mechanisms, activation of other cells can also aid peripheral tolerance. The major cells involved in this process are DCs and T regs. DCs have been proposed to aid tolerance by two mechanisms. The first hypothesizes that DCs have receptors that recognize pathogen-associated molecules and initiate an immune response upon encountering such a molecule (24,25). In the absence of such an encounter, any interaction with a T cell will lead to anergy or apoptosis. The second theory suggests that immune responses to pathogens only occur when the pathogen causes damage to the body. This is detected by the release of intracellular components of the cell and provides a signal to DCs to initiate an immune response (25). Absence of these "danger" signals would result in induction of tolerance upon interaction with a T cell.

Regulatory T cells are either naturally expressed in the thymus and express CD25 or are induced in the periphery (16). Absence of CD25+ T cells in mice has been shown to lead to multiple autoimmune diseases (26), indicating their importance in regulating peripheral tolerance. They represent 10% of CD4+ T cells in humans (27) and are thought to function by preventing T-cell proliferation to self-antigen (28) through cell–cell contact (29). These cells have been shown to express CTLA-4 (30) along with other members of the B7/CD28 family, suggesting that these molecules play important roles in T reg maturation and function and, therefore, in preventing autoimmunity (9). They also express the forkhead/winged helix transcription factor Foxp3, with loss of function mutations of this gene leading to the absence of CD25+ T regs and the development of autoimmune endocrinopathy, T1D, and thyroiditis in both humans and mice (31). Other factors that impact on the ability of T regs to regulate autoreactive T cells are the numbers of these cells produced in the thymus and their functional capacity (12). Lack of regulatory CD25+ T cells has been shown to increase autoimmunity (32), and, although the molecules required to enable T regs to function are unknown, it can be hypothesized that downregulation of such molecules would affect the ability of T regs to inactivate autoreactive T cells (12,33).

Induced T regs are termed T_R1 cells (33) and rely on interleukin 10 (IL)-10 and transforming growth factor (TGF)-β to function. They have been shown to inhibit T-cell proliferation in vitro, suppress autoimmune disease that has been experimentally induced and control CD4+ and CD8+ numbers in vivo *(33–35)*. It is unclear how these derived T regs relate to naturally occurring T regs in respect to function and control of peripheral tolerance *(27)*.

As can be seen, both central and peripheral tolerances are complex processes, involving the interaction of many components, defects of which could cause a breakdown in tolerance as previously illustrated. However, other mechanisms that could cause tolerance breakdown and lead to autoimmunity have been postulated. These include molecular mimicry, exposure of cryptic epitopes, or microbial superantigens.

OTHER FACTORS CAUSING TOLERANCE BREAKDOWN

Molecular Mimicry

Molecular mimicry is based on the concept that sufficient similarity exists between foreign antigen and self-antigens such that the immune system cannot distinguish between them *(36)*. It has been postulated that this can lead to autoimmunity because of inappropriate responses to self-antigens. The presence of cross-reactive T cells and autoantibodies in certain autoimmune conditions such as ankylosing spondylitis *(37)*, MS *(38)*, and T1D *(39)* has increased favor for this hypothesis. However, no direct evidence for this hypothesis exists to date because of its complex nature. The presence of similar epitopes on both foreign and self-antigens does not ensure that they will elicit the same immune response *(36)*. Also, a microbial epitope may display different avidity to the self-epitope such that an additional immune event may be required to activate the T cell and cause disease *(36)*. It seems unlikely that molecular mimicry alone can account for onset of autoimmune disease as these disorders would be far more common if this was the case. A more likely scenario is that this process may enhance clinical presentation of disease in a genetically susceptible individual through activation of other mechanisms of innate immunity *(40)*. This may lead to an amplification of the autoimmune process, thus leading to disease presentation.

Cryptic Epitopes

T cells can only be tolerized to epitopes that are presented to them in sufficient levels to be recognized. However, epitopes exist that are not recognized by T cells as they are either present at very low levels or inaccessible to the T cell. They are known as cryptic epitopes, and it has been proposed that they may play a major role in the autoimmune response if they increase in number or become visible to the immune system *(41)*. Several mechanisms have been proposed as to how this may occur. First, increased antigen may be processed, leading to levels of the epitope increasing above the threshold for recognition *(42)*. Second, the antigen may be processed in a different manner, thus revealing cryptic epitopes to the immune system *(43)*, and, third, there may be an increase in human leukocyte antigen (HLA) class II or costimulatory molecule expression, leading to increased levels of the epitope being present to activate T cells *(41)*. These mechanisms may act together or independently to initiate an autoimmune response. These mechanisms could be triggered by presentation of self-antigen containing cryptic epitopes on DCs, presentation of these epitopes by non-professional APCs such as B cells, or activation of autoreactive B cells by these epitopes *(41)*—possibilities that all warrant further investigation.

Superantigens

Superantigens, of either viral or bacterial origin, activate T cells through the variable domain of the beta chain of the TCR. They are capable of binding to a large number of MHC class II molecules, thus activating a large population of T cells with a wide variety of MHC/peptide specificities *(44)*. It has been shown that they are capable of causing relapse and exacerbation of experimental autoimmune encephalomyelitis (EAE) in mice *(45)* but cannot induce this disease in previously unaffected animals. However, in a similar scenario to molecular mimicry, it is difficult to prove a causative role for superantigens in autoimmune disease. The pathogen needs to be identified in patients with autoimmune disease and be isolated at the time of infection. This relies on the diagnosis of the autoimmune disease at the time of infection—an impossible task for most autoimmune disorders that do not exhibit an acute onset following infection *(44)*, therefore, although the hypothesis of microbial superantigens triggering autoimmunity is attractive, it remains to be proven for the majority of such disorders.

GENETIC REGIONS ASSOCIATED WITH AUTOIMMUNE DISEASE

Owing to the observation that multiple autoimmune diseases can cluster within families, it has been postulated that such disorders will be caused by a combination of common and specific genes. Specific genes will largely depend on the disease studied, for example, the insulin gene region (designated *IDDM2*) is involved in T1D and the thyrotropin-stimulating hormone receptor (*TSHR*) gene is involved in GD. To date, only three genes/gene regions have been consistently associated with multiple autoimmune conditions namely the HLA class II region on chromosome 6p21 *(46–48)*, the *CTLA-4* gene on chromosome 2q33 *(49,50)*, and the *PTPN22* gene encoding lymphoid tyrosine phosphatase (LYP) on chromosome 1p13 *(51,52)*.

HLA Class II Region

The HLA class II region contains many genes including those that encode the DRB1, DQB1, and DQA1 molecules. These molecules are involved in processing and presentation of exogenous antigens. The region is highly polymorphic, with many different alleles of the DR and DQ genes being associated with various autoimmune diseases. The presence of strong linkage disequilibrium (LD) within this region makes the analysis and identification of primary etiological variants difficult, and for this reason, it remains unclear whether association of the HLA region is restricted to class II genes or, as seems increasingly likely from tag single-nucleotide polymorphism (SNP) LD-mapping studies of the MHC *(53)*, that other loci outside the class II region are also exerting primary disease-causing effects.

Alleles and haplotypes of the *DRB1*, *DQB1*, and *DQA1* genes have been consistently shown to confer both predisposition and protection to many autoimmune diseases *(54–59)* (Table 1). There is increasing evidence to suggest that the ability of HLA class II molecules to bind antigens, present them at the immunological synapse and allow correct TCR interaction could be determined, at least in part, by DNA polymorphisms causing amino acid substitutions in these molecules. This in turn could lead to the development of the autoimmune phenotype.

Table 1
HLA Class II Haplotype Associations with Autoimmune Disease

Disease	Predisposing haplotypes/alleles	Protective haplotypes/alleles
Type 1 diabetes	DR3, DR4	DR2
Multiple sclerosis	DR2	DRB1*01, *07, *11
Rheumatoid arthritis	DRB1*0401,*0404, *0405, *0408, *0102, *0101, *1402, *09, *1001	DRB1*07, *1201, *1301, *0103, *1501
Graves' disease	DR3	DR7
Autoimmune Addison's disease	DR3	
Autoimmune hypothyroidism	DR3, DR4	
Systemic lupus erythematosus	DR3, DR2, DR8	

DR3, DRB1*03-DQB1*02-DQA1*05; DR4, DRB1*04-DQB1*0302-DQA1*0301; DR7, DRB1*07-DQB1*02/03032-DQA1*02; DR2, DRB1*1501-DQB1*0602-DQA1*0102; DR8, DRB1*08-DQB1*04-DQA1*04.

This hypothesis was first examined in T1D where it was observed that association of the *DQB1* gene with disease appeared to be stronger than that of the *DRB1* gene, and this could be explained largely by the specific residue present at position 57 of the DQβ chain. Neutrally or negatively associated DQβ alleles possessed Asp at position 57, whereas positively associated DQβ alleles contained Ala, Val, or Ser at this position *(60)*. Substitution of Asp at β57 has been shown to adversely affect the interaction of the DQβ chain with the DQα chain, thus affecting the heterodimeric structure and, therefore, antigen-binding ability and TCR interaction. However, this association with T1D is incomplete, suggesting that other residues in this and other binding pockets might contribute to disease susceptibility.

More recent studies *(48,61)* have focused on the role played by position 74 of the DRB1 chain (β74). A study of patients with GD noted a significant increase in Arg at position 74 in GD patients compared with that in healthy controls *(61)*. Structural modelling indicated that the presence of a positively charged Arg in the peptide-binding pocket can alter the three-dimensional structure thereby potentially affecting antigen binding *(61)*. An in-depth study performed by Simmonds and colleagues identified nine amino acids in the DRB1 chain that conferred susceptibility to GD. Analysis by two-locus stepwise logistic regression showed that β74 was the most strongly associated position. Encouragingly, the DRB1*03 allele found to confer susceptibility in this study contained arginine at β74, whereas the DRB1*07 allele seen at a reduced frequency in GD patients encodes glutamine at β74. Simmonds also noted association between DRB1*08 alleles and GD, which encode either Leu or Ala at β74, suggesting that association cannot entirely be explained by a simple association between Glu and Arg at β74 disrupting the three-dimensional structure in the binding pocket. Further support for position 74 in autoimmune disease comes from studies in T1D *(62,63)*, RA *(56,64)*, and MS *(65)*.

Structural changes in the binding pockets of HLA molecules caused by amino acids of different size and charge may alter T-cell recognition owing to changes in conformation of the peptide–MHC complex *(66,67)*. It has been shown that different

TCRs can interact with the same peptide–MHC complex but that different residues of the peptide can bind to the TCR to elicit different responses (68,69). Such differences might, for example, explain the association of MS with DR15-containing haplotypes, which confer protection to T1D (55,70). The observation that a single T cell can recognize different peptides bound to the same MHC molecule (71) might also go some way to explain why the same HLA molecules are involved in many different autoimmune diseases that are triggered by different auto-antigen binding.

HLA-associated autoimmunity could result from activation of either peripheral T cells that have escaped immune tolerance and have high affinity for self-antigens or those with low affinity but with the ability to cross-react with external stimuli (such as viruses or bacteria) that mimic self-antigens (72). HLA molecules could play a role in the autoimmune disease process with the particular HLA type of an individual controlling the level of amplification of the T-cell response following activation (72). The HLA molecule could also influence the autoimmune disease process through its stability when complexed with peptide. For example, the DQ3.2 molecule (encoding DQB1*0302/DQA1*0301) is the HLA molecule most associated with T1D and is also extremely unstable when complexed with peptide. Molecules such as this could escape the negative selection process, as interaction between the peptide and the HLA molecule is too short to be detected in the thymus, and therefore, even T cells with high affinity for self-peptide displayed on these molecules will escape tolerance (72). This scenario could also apply to other autoimmune diseases in which the DR3 haplotype is predisposing (Table 1) as the DQA1*0501/DQB1*0201 molecule is also highly unstable (72). However, as shown in Table 1, some HLA haplotypes provide protection from disease, and it is thought that they confer protection by binding to the same peptides as susceptibility haplotypes, thus preventing the threshold for an autoimmune response being reached (73).

CTLA-4 Gene

CTLA-4 is an important negative regulator of T-cell activation (74). Owing to this role in the regulation of T-cell activation and its potential to affect the autoimmune disease process, numerous association studies have been performed, with SNPs within this gene being associated with GD (50,75,76), T1D (50,77), AIH (78), AAD (79,80), SLE (81), and MS (82). A fine-mapping study of the CTLA-4 gene and surrounding region located the etiological variant/s within a 6.1-kb region in the 3′-untranslated region (50). Owing to strong LD between the four most associated SNPs within this region, it was impossible to determine which of CT60, JO30, JO31, and JO27_1 is/are the primary etiological variant(s). Differences in the relative amounts of the two isoforms of CTLA-4 were seen, depending on CT60 genotype, with increased levels of the soluble isoform seen in protective genotypes (50), suggesting that the 6.1-kb region might determine the efficiency of CTLA-4 splicing and therefore the control of T-cell activation. This result, however, was not replicated in a more recent study by Anjos et al. (83), which found no significant difference in the levels of either mRNA transcript in heterozygous individuals. Further studies in mice have identified an additional ligand-independent isoform (liCTLA-4), which lacks the ligand-binding domain (MYPPPY) but can associate independently with the TCR-ζ chain to be a more potent inhibitor of T-cell proliferation and cytokine production compared with full-length CTLA-4 (flCTLA4) (84). The expression of liCTLA-4 in T reg cells of diabetes-resistant NOD congenic mice has been shown to be enhanced in comparison with flCTLA-4, illustrating an important regulatory role for liCTLA-4 in the activation of mouse T reg cells (84).

Although the mechanism by which CTLA-4 inhibits T-cell activation is currently unknown, various theories have been proposed (Fig. 1). First, CTLA-4 might successfully compete with CD28 for the CD80/86 ligands owing to its greater affinity for these molecules and thereby inhibit the costimulatory effect of CD28 (Fig. 1A). Evidence in support of this model comes from differences observed in the expression kinetics exhibited between CD28 and CTLA-4 (74). Second, CTLA-4 might apply its inhibitory effect by acting on downstream signaling pathways at activation (Fig. 1B). It is well known

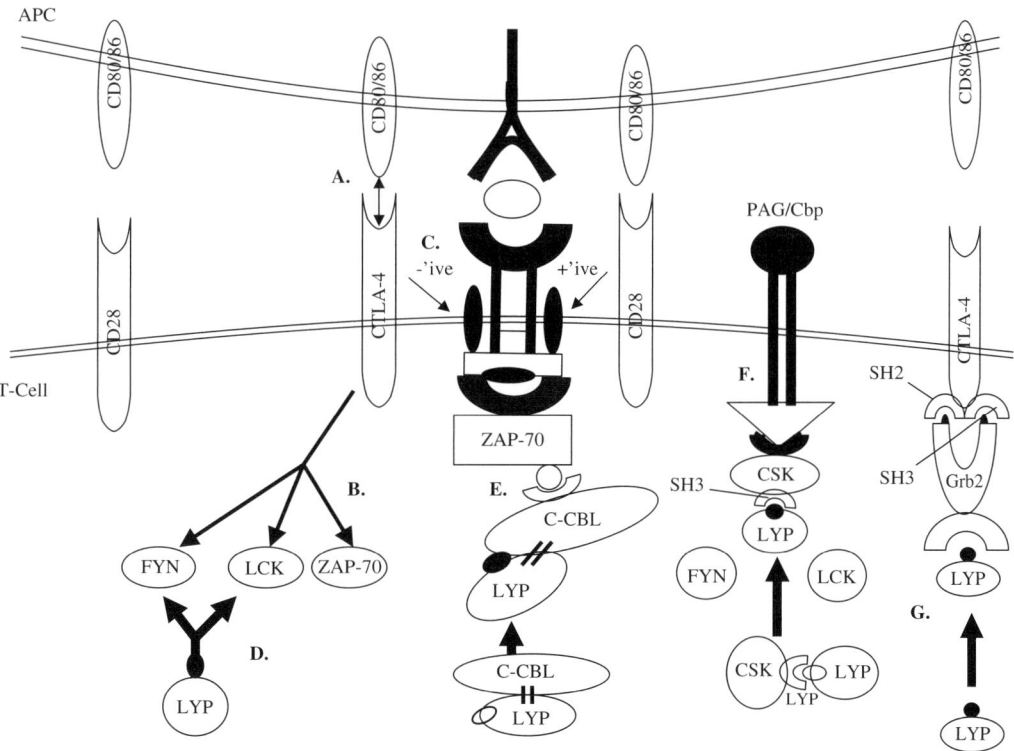

Fig. 1. Potential mechanisms of action of cytotoxic T-lymphocyte-associated antigen (CTLA)-4 and lymphoid tyrosine phosphatase (LYP). (**A**) CTLA-4 might successfully compete with CD28 for the CD80/86 ligands owing to its greater affinity for these molecules and thereby inhibit the costimulatory effect of CD28. (**B**) CTLA-4 might apply its inhibitory effect by acting on downstream signaling pathways at activation. (**C**) CTLA-4 directly interacts with TCR-ζ at the immunological synapse. (**D**) LYP might associate with PTK without the aid of adaptor molecules. (**E**) LYP bound to c-Cbl might target ZAP-70 through the SH2 domain on c-Cbl binding to the phosphorylated Tyr292 of the ZAP-70 molecule. (**F**) It is known that the SH2 domain of Csk can bind to PAG/Cbp molecules present in the lipid rafts of the cell membrane. If LYP and Csk were bound through the SH3 domain of Csk and the P1 domain of LYP, and Csk was bound to PAG/Cbp, this would bring LYP closer to Lck and Fyn and might enable dephosphorylation. (**G**) It has been well established that Grb2 plays a role in the downstream signaling pathway for CD28-mediated T-cell activation, and the presence of similar binding domains between CTLA-4 and CD28 has raised the possibility that CTLA-4 might bind to Grb2 through one of these domains and use its association with LYP to regulate T cells negatively.

that Lck, Fyn, and ZAP-70 protein kinases are instrumental in phosphorylating protein tyrosines of the TCR–CD3 complex during downstream cell signaling pathways at T-cell activation. Studies have shown that T cells in CTLA-4$^{-/-}$ mutant mice displayed constitutive activity of Fyn, Lck, and ZAP-70, as well as the Ras pathway, thus suggesting that CTLA-4 interacts with these molecules through SHP1 phosphatases to prevent constitutive expression *(85,86)*. A third possibility is that CTLA-4 directly interacts with TCR-ζ at the immunological synapse (Fig. 1C). This would essentially disrupt the cascade of biochemical signals that lead to activation of the T cell *(87)*.

A more recent study implicates a role for CTLA-4 in the regulation of the Cbl-b molecule as a possible mechanism for aberrant T-cell activation that might lead to autoimmunity *(88)*. The Cbl family of ubiquitin ligases regulates the threshold of signaling for T-cell activation by negative regulation of activated tyrosine kinase-coupled receptors *(89)*. Loss or impairment of Cbl-b can result in the development of autoimmunity *(90)*; indeed, a nonsense mutation in the gene encoding Cbl-b has been associated with the development of T1D in the Komeda diabetes prone rat *(91)*. A recent study in T1D in humans found association of an SNP in exon 12 of the *Cbl-b* gene with T1D, and, when stratified with the CT60 SNP of the *CTLA-4* gene, significant genetic interaction was observed *(92)*. Cbl-b protein expression appears to correlate with rates of T-cell activation leading to the hypothesis that CTLA-4/CD28 might control T-cell activation by regulating Cbl-b expression *(88)*.

PTPN22 Encoding LYP

Some protein tyrosine phosphatases (PTPs) play a negative role in TCR signaling by dephosphorylation of protein tyrosine kinases *(93)*. These PTPs include LYP encoded by the *PTPN22 (94)*. It is a strong negative regulator of T-cell activation through binding to various adaptor molecules including Csk kinase *(95)*, c-Cbl *(94)*, and Grb2 *(96)*. Owing to this function, many recent studies have focused on the role that this PTP may play in the development of autoimmune disease.

An SNP within the *PTPN22* at position 1858 in codon 620 (R620W) has been identified that results in an arginine to tryptophan (C to T) shift *(97)*. The T allele has been associated with T1D *(51,98–100)*, RA *(52,100– 103)*, SLE *(52,104)*, AIH *(52)*, and GD *(51,105,106)*, although no such association has been observed with MS *(107,108)*. A recent fine mapping study in patients with RA *(109)* identified 37 SNPs within the coding region of the *PTPN22* which formed 10 common haplotypes. Stratification by R620W revealed that association of this gene with RA could not be fully explained by the R620W SNP with a further two SNPs being identified that seemed to exert an independent disease-causing effect. Further studies in other autoimmune disease are needed to replicate these findings.

It is known that the presence of tryptophan at position 620 (Trp620) can disrupt the ability of LYP to bind to at least one of its adaptor molecules, namely Csk kinase *(97)*. Csk kinase has been documented as being a negative regulator of TCR signaling through phosphorylation of Lck and Fyn *(110)*. Inhibition of T-cell activation requires the physical association of Csk and LYP to dephosphorylate the Src kinases and ZAP-70 that facilitate activation of the T cell *(95)*. This physical association is achieved by the Arg620 residue of LYP interacting with Trp 47 of Csk *(111)*. Replacement of Arg620 with Trp620 would be expected to prevent this interaction, as Trp is a larger molecule that would not be able to fit into the binding pocket on the Csk molecule. Indeed, this has been demonstrated experimentally by Bottini et al. *(97)* in both *Escherichia coli* and COS cells where only the construct containing Arg620 was precipitated by Csk. These data strongly suggest that LYP containing Trp at this position cannot form a complex with Csk and therefore abrogates inhibition of T-cell activation. Murine LYP has been shown to inhibit T-cell activation in a synergistic manner with Csk *(112)*, leading to the hypothesis that those individuals heterozygous for the T allele of this SNP will have reduced LYP–Csk complexes, and those homozygous for this allele will have none *(97)*. Absence of these complexes would lead to massive T-cell proliferation and ultimately an autoimmune phenotype that could be potentially fatal. However, the fact that homozygous individuals exist indicates that the LYP–Csk interaction is not the only pathway leading to negative regulation of T-cell activation.

Studies have shown that LYP can also associate with other adaptor molecules to inhibit T-cell activation, namely c-Cbl *(94)* and Grb2 *(96)*. c-Cbl is a proto-oncogene that is associated with LYP in thymocytes, and phosphorylation of c-Cbl is reduced when LYP is overexpressed *(94)*. These data suggest that LYP might regulate the activity of c-Cbl by controlling its phosphorylation status, although the precise mechanism by which LYP and c-Cbl associate is currently unknown. A recent study has shown that Grb2 binds to LYP through its SH3 domain, leading to formation of a functional complex resulting in negative regulation of T cells *(96)*.

The previously described data strongly support the role of LYP in inhibition of T-cell activation, and, although the exact mechanisms by which this occurs have yet to be confirmed, three mechanisms have been postulated as to how LYP may perform this function (Fig. 1). First, LYP might associate with PTK without the aid of adaptor molecules *(93)* (Fig. 1D). Second, LYP bound to c-Cbl might target ZAP-70 through the SH2 domain on c-Cbl binding to the phosphorylated Tyr292 of the ZAP-70 molecule (Fig. 1E). This residue is phosphorylated when ZAP-70 is activated in the T-cell activation pathway; so this might be the mechanism by which targeting between these two molecules occurs to dephosphorylate ZAP-70 and inhibit further T-cell activation *(93)*. Third, it is known that the SH2 domain of Csk can bind to PAG/Cbp molecules present in the lipid rafts of the cell membrane (Fig. 1F). If LYP and Csk were bound through the SH3 domain of Csk and the P1 domain of LYP and Csk was bound to PAG/Cbp, this would bring LYP closer to Lck and Fyn and might enable dephosphorylation *(93)*.

The role of Grb2 is particularly interesting as it has been postulated that CTLA-4 could use LYP complexed with Grb2 to aid inhibition of T-cell activation *(96)*. CTLA-4 and CD28 contain both SH2- and SH3-binding sites *(96)*. It has been well established that Grb2 plays a role in the downstream signaling pathway for CD28-mediated T-cell activation, and the presence of similar binding domains between CTLA-4 and CD28 has raised the possibility that CTLA-4 might bind to Grb2 through one of these domains and use its association with LYP to regulate T cells negatively (Fig. 1G).

IDENTIFICATION OF NEW GENES AND PRIMARY ETIOLOGICAL VARIANTS

With the exception of the three genes previously mentioned, identification of novel susceptibility loci has been a slow process largely because of such loci only contributing small effects to disease susceptibility. To detect such effects, large data sets are needed to provide sufficient power to ensure that any association seen is a true association and not a false-positive result because of a small data set. A further confounding problem in this search is that some genes appear to confer susceptibility only to specific diseases or in specific populations, making replication studies difficult. Candidates that fall into this category include the *FCRL3* gene, associated with RA, SLE, and autoimmune thyroid disease in Japanese populations *(113)* but awaiting replication in Caucasian populations; the *SLC22A4 (114)* and *PADI4 (115)* genes, associated in Japanese RA patients but not in Caucasian RA patients; the *SUMO4* gene, initially associated with T1D in a multiethnic data set *(116)* but not replicated in a number of large follow-up studies *(117,118)* and the *CD25* gene, associated with T1D in Caucasians *(119)* but awaiting replication in further populations.

Despite consistent associations of some genes with disease, the identification of the primary etiological variant within these genes has also been difficult largely as a result of the strong LD present in the human genome. To successfully identify such variants, large-scale genotyping studies of all DNA variants in the associated region need to be undertaken in adequately powered data sets.

CONCLUSIONS

The pathways leading to the development of autoimmune disease are complex, involving defects in the immune system leading to the release of autoreactive T cells into the periphery, which can trigger disease. Many genes and gene products are involved in this process with a combination of both common and specific genes leading to the development of specific disorders. The recent advances in genotyping technology have vastly improved the ability of the geneticist to narrow down the search for primary etiological variants within these genes; however, further advances are necessary to identify rare variants that may contribute to these disorders and to elucidate the functional role that susceptibility loci play in disease development.

REFERENCES

1. Vyse TJ, Todd JA. Genetic analysis of autoimmune disease. *Cell* 1996;85(3):311–8.
2. Sollid LM, McAdam SN, Molberg O, et al. Genes and environment in celiac disease. *Acta Odontol Scand* 2001;59(3):183–6.
3. Koning F, Gilissen L, Wijmenga C. Gluten: a two-edged sword. Immunopathogenesis of celiac disease. *Springer Semin Immunopathol* 2005;27(2):217–32.
4. Heward J, Gough SC. Genetic susceptibility to the development of autoimmune disease. *Clin Sci (Lond)* 1997;93(6):479–91.
5. Fraga MF, Ballestar E, Paz MF, et al. Epigenetic differences arise during the lifetime of monozygotic twins. *Proc Natl Acad Sci USA* 2005;102(30):10604–9.
6. Vyse TJ, Kotzin BL. Genetic susceptibility to systemic lupus erythematosus. *Annu Rev Immunol* 1998;16:261–92.
7. Becker KG. Comparative genetics of type 1 diabetes and autoimmune disease: common loci, common pathways? *Diabetes* 1999;48(7):1353–8.
8. Tait KF, Marshall T, Berman J, et al. Clustering of autoimmune disease in parents of siblings from the Type 1 diabetes Warren repository. *Diabet Med* 2004;21(4):358–62.
9. Keir ME, Sharpe AH. The B7/CD28 costimulatory family in autoimmunity. *Immunol Rev* 2005;204:128–43.

10. Pitkanen J, Peterson P. Autoimmune regulator: from loss of function to autoimmunity. *Genes Immun* 2003;4(1):12–21.

11. Anderson MS, Venanzi ES, Klein L, et al. Projection of an immunological self shadow within the thymus by the aire protein. *Science* 2002;298(5597):1395–401.

12. Liston A, Lesage S, Gray DH, Boyd RL, Goodnow CC. Genetic lesions in T-cell tolerance and thresholds for autoimmunity. *Immunol Rev* 2005;204:87–101.

13. Lesage S, Hartley SB, Akkaraju S, Wilson J, Townsend M, Goodnow CC. Failure to censor forbidden clones of CD4 T cells in autoimmune diabetes. *J Exp Med* 2002;196(9):1175–88.

14. Ghosh S, Palmer SM, Rodrigues NR, et al. Polygenic control of autoimmune diabetes in nonobese diabetic mice. *Nat Genet* 1993;4(4):404–9.

15. Kyewski B, Derbinski J. Self-representation in the thymus: an extended view. *Nat Rev Immunol* 2004;4(9):688–98.

16. Walker LS, Abbas AK. The enemy within: keeping self-reactive T cells at bay in the periphery. *Nat Rev Immunol* 2002;2(1):11–9.

17. Alferink J, Tafuri A, Vestweber D, Hallmann R, Hammerling GJ, Arnold B. Control of neonatal tolerance to tissue antigens by peripheral T cell trafficking. *Science* 1998;282(5392):1338–41.

18. Kurts C, Miller JF, Subramaniam RM, Carbone FR, Heath WR. Major histocompatibility complex class I-restricted cross-presentation is biased towards high dose antigens and those released during cellular destruction. *J Exp Med* 1998;188(2):409–14.

19. Waterhouse P, Penninger JM, Timms E, et al. Lymphoproliferative disorders with early lethality in mice deficient in Ctla-4. *Science* 1995;270(5238):985–8.

20. Freeman GJ, Long AJ, Iwai Y, et al. Engagement of the PD-1 immunoinhibitory receptor by a novel B7 family member leads to negative regulation of lymphocyte activation. *J Exp Med* 2000;192(7):1027–34.

21. Latchman Y, Wood CR, Chernova T, et al. PD-L2 is a second ligand for PD-1 and inhibits T cell activation. *Nat Immunol* 2001;2(3):261–8.

22. Kuchroo VK, Das MP, Brown JA, et al. B7-1 and B7-2 costimulatory molecules activate differentially the Th1/Th2 developmental pathways: application to autoimmune disease therapy. *Cell* 1995;80(5):707–18.

23. Dong C, Juedes AE, Temann UA, et al. ICOS co-stimulatory receptor is essential for T-cell activation and function. *Nature* 2001;409(6816):97–101.

24. Janeway CA, Jr. The immune system evolved to discriminate infectious nonself from noninfectious self. *Immunol Today* 1992;13(1):11–6.

25. Matzinger P. Tolerance, danger, and the extended family. *Annu Rev Immunol* 1994;12:991–1045.

26. Asano M, Toda M, Sakaguchi N, Sakaguchi S. Autoimmune disease as a consequence of developmental abnormality of a T cell subpopulation. *J Exp Med* 1996;184(2):387–96.

27. O'Garra A, Vieira P. Regulatory T cells and mechanisms of immune system control. *Nat Med* 2004;10(8):801–5.

28. Thornton AM, Shevach EM. Suppressor effector function of CD4+CD25+ immunoregulatory T cells is antigen nonspecific. *J Immunol* 2000;164(1):183–90.

29. Kuniyasu Y, Takahashi T, Itoh M, Shimizu J, Toda G, Sakaguchi S. Naturally anergic and suppressive CD25(+)CD4(+) T cells as a functionally and phenotypically distinct immunoregulatory T cell subpopulation. *Int Immunol* 2000;12(8):1145–55.

30. Salomon B, Lenschow DJ, Rhee L, et al. B7/CD28 costimulation is essential for the homeostasis of the CD4+CD25+ immunoregulatory T cells that control autoimmune diabetes. *Immunity* 2000;12(4):431–40.

31. Ramsdell F. Foxp3 and natural regulatory T cells: key to a cell lineage? *Immunity* 2003;19(2):165–8.

32. McHugh RS, Shevach EM. Cutting edge: depletion of CD4+CD25+ regulatory T cells is necessary, but not sufficient, for induction of organ-specific autoimmune disease. *J Immunol* 2002;168(12):5979–83.

33. Groux H, O'Garra A, Bigler M, et al. A CD4+ T-cell subset inhibits antigen-specific T-cell responses and prevents colitis. *Nature* 1997;389(6652):737–42.

34. Sundstedt A, O'Neill EJ, Nicolson KS, Wraith DC. Role for IL-10 in suppression mediated by peptide-induced regulatory T cells in vivo. *J Immunol* 2003;170(3):1240–8.

35. Oida T, Zhang X, Goto M, et al. CD4+CD25− T cells that express latency-associated peptide on the surface suppress CD4+CD45RB high-induced colitis by a TGF-beta-dependent mechanism. *J Immunol* 2003;170(5):2516–22.

36. Christen U, von Herrath MG. Induction, acceleration or prevention of autoimmunity by molecular mimicry. *Mol Immunol* 2004;40(14–15):1113–20.

37. Schwimmbeck PL, Oldstone MB. Klebsiella pneumoniae and HLA B27-associated diseases of Reiter's syndrome and ankylosing spondylitis. *Curr Top Microbiol Immunol* 1989;145:45–56.

38. Panitch HS. Influence of infection on exacerbations of multiple sclerosis. *Ann Neurol* 1994;36(Suppl):S25–8.

39. Yoon JW, Morishima T, McClintock PR, Austin M, Notkins AL. Virus-induced diabetes mellitus: mengovirus infects pancreatic beta cells in strains of mice resistant to the diabetogenic effect of encephalomyocarditis virus. *J Virol* 1984;50(3):684–90.

40. Fourneau JM, Bach JM, van Endert PM, Bach JF. The elusive case for a role of mimicry in autoimmune diseases. *Mol Immunol* 2004;40(14–15):1095–102.

41. Lanzavecchia A. How can cryptic epitopes trigger autoimmunity? *J Exp Med* 1995;181(6): 1945–8.

42. Salemi S, Caporossi AP, Boffa L, Longobardi MG, Barnaba V. HIVgp120 activates autoreactive CD4-specific T cell responses by unveiling of hidden CD4 peptides during processing. *J Exp Med* 1995;181(6):2253–7.

43. Simitsek PD, Campbell DG, Lanzavecchia A, Fairweather N, Watts C. Modulation of antigen processing by bound antibodies can boost or suppress class II major histocompatibility complex presentation of different T cell determinants. *J Exp Med* 1995;181(6):1957–63.

44. Wucherpfennig KW. Mechanisms for the induction of autoimmunity by infectious agents. *J Clin Invest* 2001;108(8):1097–104.

45. Brocke S, Gaur A, Piercy C, et al. Induction of relapsing paralysis in experimental autoimmune encephalomyelitis by bacterial superantigen. *Nature* 1993;365(6447):642–4.

46. Awata T, Kuzuya T, Matsuda A, Iwamoto Y, Kanazawa Y. Genetic analysis of HLA class II alleles and susceptibility to type 1 (insulin-dependent) diabetes mellitus in Japanese subjects. *Diabetologia* 1992;35(5):419–24.

47. Badenhoop K, Walfish PG, Rau H, et al. Susceptibility and resistance alleles of human leukocyte antigen (HLA) DQA1 and HLA DQB1 are shared in endocrine autoimmune disease. *J Clin Endocrinol Metab* 1995;80(7):2112–7.

48. Simmonds MJ, Howson JM, Heward JM, et al. Regression mapping of association between the human leukocyte antigen region and Graves disease. *Am J Hum Genet* 2005;76(1):157–63.

49. Vaidya B, Imrie H, Perros P, et al. The cytotoxic T lymphocyte antigen-4 is a major Graves' disease locus. *Hum Mol Genet* 1999;8(7):1195–9.

50. Ueda H, Howson JM, Esposito L, et al. Association of the T-cell regulatory gene CTLA4 with susceptibility to autoimmune disease. *Nature* 2003;423(6939):506–11.

51. Smyth D, Cooper JD, Collins JE, et al. Replication of an association between the lymphoid tyrosine phosphatase locus (LYP/*PTPN22*) with type 1 diabetes, and evidence for its role as a general autoimmunity locus. *Diabetes* 2004;53(11):3020–3.

52. Criswell LA, Pfeiffer KA, Lum RF, et al. Analysis of families in the multiple autoimmune disease genetics consortium (MADGC) collection: the *PTPN22* 620W allele associates with multiple autoimmune phenotypes. *Am J Hum Genet* 2005;76(4):561–71.

53. Miretti MM, Walsh EC, Ke X, et al. A high-resolution linkage-disequilibrium map of the human major histocompatibility complex and first generation of tag single-nucleotide polymorphisms. *Am J Hum Genet* 2005;76(4):634–46.

54. Nerup J, Platz P, Andersen OO, et al. HL-A antigens and diabetes mellitus. *Lancet* 1974;2(7885):864–6.

55. Giordano M, D'Alfonso S, Momigliano-Richiardi P. Genetics of multiple sclerosis: linkage and association studies. *Am J Pharmacogenomics* 2002;2(1):37–58.

56. Newton JL, Harney SM, Wordsworth BP, Brown MA. A review of the MHC genetics of rheumatoid arthritis. *Genes Immun* 2004;5(3):151–7.

57. Heward JM, Allahabadia A, Daykin J, et al. Linkage disequilibrium between the human leukocyte antigen class II region of the major histocompatibility complex and Graves' disease: replication using a population case control and family-based study. *J Clin Endocrinol Metab* 1998;83(10): 3394–7.

58. Weetman AP, Zhang L, Tandon N, Edwards OM. HLA associations with autoimmune Addison's disease. *Tissue Antigens* 1991;38(1):31–3.

59. Graham RR, Ortmann WA, Langefeld CD, et al. Visualizing human leukocyte antigen class II risk haplotypes in human systemic lupus erythematosus. *Am J Hum Genet* 2002;71(3):543–53.

60. Todd JA, Bell JI, McDevitt HO. HLA-DQ beta gene contributes to susceptibility and resistance to insulin-dependent diabetes mellitus. *Nature* 1987;329(6140):599–604.

61. Ban Y, Davies TF, Greenberg DA, et al. Arginine at position 74 of the HLA-DR beta1 chain is associated with Graves' disease. *Genes Immun* 2004;5(3):203–8.

62. Cucca F, Muntoni F, Lampis R, et al. Combinations of specific DRB1, DQA1, DQB1 haplotypes are associated with insulin-dependent diabetes mellitus in Sardinia. *Hum Immunol* 1993;37(2):85–94.

63. Cucca F, Lampis R, Frau F, et al. The distribution of DR4 haplotypes in Sardinia suggests a primary association of type I diabetes with DRB1 and DQB1 loci. *Hum Immunol* 1995;43(4):301–8.

64. du Montcel ST, Michou L, Petit-Teixeira E, et al. New classification of HLA-DRB1 alleles supports the shared epitope hypothesis of rheumatoid arthritis susceptibility. *Arthritis Rheum* 2005;52(4):1063–8.

65. Greer JM, Pender MP. The presence of glutamic acid at positions 71 or 74 in pocket 4 of the HLA-DRbeta1 chain is associated with the clinical course of multiple sclerosis. *J Neurol Neurosurg Psychiatry* 2005;76(5):656–62.

66. Kwok WW, Mickelson E, Masewicz S, Milner EC, Hansen J, Nepom GT. Polymorphic DQ alpha and DQ beta interactions dictate HLA class II determinants of allo-recognition. *J Exp Med* 1990;171(1):85–95.

67. Stern LJ, Brown JH, Jardetzky TS, et al. Crystal structure of the human class II MHC protein HLA-DR1 complexed with an influenza virus peptide. *Nature* 1994;368(6468):215–21.

68. Jorgensen JL, Esser U, Fazekas de St Groth B, Reay PA, Davis MM. Mapping T-cell receptor-peptide contacts by variant peptide immunization of single-chain transgenics. *Nature* 1992;355(6357):224–30.

69. Bhayani H, Paterson Y. Analysis of peptide binding patterns in different major histocompatibility complex/T cell receptor complexes using pigeon cytochrome c-specific T cell hybridomas. Evidence that a single peptide binds major histocompatibility complex in different conformations. *J Exp Med* 1989;170(5):1609–25.

70. Cucca F, Lampis R, Congia M, et al. A correlation between the relative predisposition of MHC class II alleles to type 1 diabetes and the structure of their proteins. *Hum Mol Genet* 2001;10(19):2025–37.

71. Nanda NK, Arzoo KK, Geysen HM, Sette A, Sercarz EE. Recognition of multiple peptide cores by a single T cell receptor. *J Exp Med* 1995;182(2):531–9.

72. Nepom GT, Kwok WW. Molecular basis for HLA-DQ associations with IDDM. *Diabetes* 1998;47(8):1177–84.

73. Nepom GT. A unified hypothesis for the complex genetics of HLA associations with IDDM. *Diabetes* 1990;39(10):1153–7.

74. Egen JG, Allison JP. Cytotoxic T lymphocyte antigen-4 accumulation in the immunological synapse is regulated by TCR signal strength. *Immunity* 2002;16(1):23–35.

75. Furugaki K, Shirasawa S, Ishikawa N, et al. Association of the T-cell regulatory gene CTLA4 with Graves' disease and autoimmune thyroid disease in the Japanese. *J Hum Genet* 2004;49(3):166–8.

76. Heward JM, Allahabadia A, Armitage M, et al. The development of Graves' disease and the CTLA-4 gene on chromosome 2q33. *J Clin Endocrinol Meta*b 1999;84(7):2398–401.

77. Nistico L, Buzzetti R, Pritchard LE, et al. The CTLA-4 gene region of chromosome 2q33 is linked to, and associated with, type 1 diabetes. Belgian Diabetes Registry. *Hum Mol Genet* 1996;5(7):1075–80.

78. Nithiyananthan R, Heward JM, Allahabadia A, Franklyn JA, Gough SC. Polymorphism of the CTLA-4 gene is associated with autoimmune hypothyroidism in the United Kingdom. *Thyroid* 2002;12(1):3–6.

79. Vaidya B, Imrie H, Geatch DR, et al. Association analysis of the cytotoxic T lymphocyte antigen-4 (CTLA-4) and autoimmune regulator-1 (AIRE-1) genes in sporadic autoimmune Addison's disease. *J Clin Endocrinol Metab* 2000;85(2):688–91.

80. Blomhoff A, Lie BA, Myhre AG, et al. Polymorphisms in the cytotoxic T lymphocyte antigen-4 gene region confer susceptibility to Addison's disease. *J Clin Endocrinol Metab* 2004;89(7):3474–6.

81. Torres B, Aguilar F, Franco E, et al. Association of the CT60 marker of the CTLA4 gene with systemic lupus erythematosus. *Arthritis Rheum* 2004;50(7):2211–5.

82. Suppiah V, Alloza I, Heggarty S, et al. The CTLA4 +49 A/G*G-CT60*G haplotype is associated with susceptibility to multiple sclerosis in Flanders. *J Neuroimmunol* 2005;164(1–2):148–53.

83. Anjos SM, Shao W, Marchand L, Polychronakos C. Allelic effects on gene regulation at the autoimmunity-predisposing CTLA4 locus: a re-evaluation of the 3′ +6230G>A polymorphism. *Genes Immun* 2005;6(4):305–11.

84. Vijayakrishnan L, Slavik JM, Illes Z, et al. An autoimmune disease-associated CTLA-4 splice variant lacking the B7 binding domain signals negatively in T cells. *Immunity* 2004;20(5):563–75.

85. Marengere LE, Waterhouse P, Duncan GS, Mittrucker HW, Feng GS, Mak TW. Regulation of T cell receptor signaling by tyrosine phosphatase SYP association with CTLA-4. *Science* 1996;272(5265):1170–3.

86. Masteller EL, Chuang E, Mullen AC, Reiner SL, Thompson CB. Structural analysis of CTLA-4 function in vivo. *J Immunol* 2000;164(10):5319–27.

87. Lee KM, Chuang E, Griffin M, et al. Molecular basis of T cell inactivation by CTLA-4. *Science* 1998;282(5397):2263–6.

88. Li D, Gal I, Vermes C, et al. Cutting edge: Cbl-b: one of the key molecules tuning CD28- and CTLA-4-mediated T cell costimulation. J Immunol 2004;173(12):7135–9.

89. Duan L, Reddi AL, Ghosh A, Dimri M, Band H. The Cbl family and other ubiquitin ligases: destructive forces in control of antigen receptor signaling. *Immunity* 2004;21(1):7–17.

90. Bachmaier K, Krawczyk C, Kozieradzki I, et al. Negative regulation of lymphocyte activation and autoimmunity by the molecular adaptor Cbl-b. *Nature* 2000;403(6766):211–6.

91. Yokoi N, Komeda K, Wang HY, et al. Cblb is a major susceptibility gene for rat type 1 diabetes mellitus. *Nat Genet* 2002;31(4):391–4.

92. Bergholdt R, Taxvig C, Eising S, Nerup J, Pociot F. CBLB variants in type 1 diabetes and their genetic interaction with CTLA4. *J Leukoc Biol* 2005;77(4):579–85.

93. Mustelin T, Alonso A, Bottini N, et al. Protein tyrosine phosphatases in T cell physiology. *Mol Immunol* 2004;41(6–7):687–700.

94. Cohen S, Dadi H, Shaoul E, Sharfe N, Roifman CM. Cloning and characterization of a lymphoid-specific, inducible human protein tyrosine phosphatase, Lyp. *Blood* 1999;93(6):2013–24.

95. Cloutier JF, Veillette A. Cooperative inhibition of T-cell antigen receptor signaling by a complex between a kinase and a phosphatase. *J Exp Med* 1999;189(1):111–21.

96. Hill RJ, Zozulya S, Lu YL, Ward K, Gishizky M, Jallal B. The lymphoid protein tyrosine phosphatase Lyp interacts with the adaptor molecule Grb2 and functions as a negative regulator of T-cell activation. *Exp Hematol* 2002;30(3):237–44.

97. Bottini N, Musumeci L, Alonso A, et al. A functional variant of lymphoid tyrosine phosphatase is associated with type I diabetes. *Nat Genet* 2004;36(4):337–8.

98. Qu H, Tessier MC, Hudson TJ, Polychronakos C. Confirmation of the association of the R620W polymorphism in the protein tyrosine phosphatase *PTPN22* with type 1 diabetes in a family based study. *J Med Genet* 2005;42(3):266–70.

99. Zheng W, She JX. Genetic association between a lymphoid tyrosine phosphatase (*PTPN22*) and type 1 diabetes. *Diabetes* 2005;54(3):906–8.

100. Zhernakova A, Eerligh P, Wijmenga C, Barrera P, Roep BO, Koeleman BP. Differential association of the *PTPN22* coding variant with autoimmune diseases in a Dutch population. *Genes Immun* 2005;6(6):459–61.

101. Steer S, Lad B, Grumley JA, Kingsley GH, Fisher SA. Association of R602W in a protein tyrosine phosphatase gene with a high risk of rheumatoid arthritis in a British population: evidence for an early onset/disease severity effect. *Arthritis Rheum* 2005;52(1):358–60.

102. Simkins HM, Merriman ME, Highton J, et al. Association of the *PTPN22* locus with rheumatoid arthritis in a New Zealand Caucasian cohort. *Arthritis Rheum* 2005;52(7):2222–5.

103. van Oene M, Wintle RF, Liu X, et al. Association of the lymphoid tyrosine phosphatase R620W variant with rheumatoid arthritis, but not Crohn's disease, in Canadian populations. *Arthritis Rheum* 2005;52(7):1993–8.

104. Kyogoku C, Langefeld CD, Ortmann WA, et al. Genetic association of the R620W polymorphism of protein tyrosine phosphatase *PTPN22* with human SLE. *Am J Hum Genet* 2004;75(3):504–7.

105. Velaga MR, Wilson V, Jennings CE, et al. The codon 620 tryptophan allele of the lymphoid tyrosine phosphatase (LYP) gene is a major determinant of Graves' disease. *J Clin Endocrinol Metab* 2004;89(11):5862–5.

106. Skorka A, Bednarczuk T, Bar-Andziak E, Nauman J, Ploski R. Lymphoid tyrosine phosphatase (*PTPN22*/LYP) variant and Graves' disease in a Polish population: association and gene dose-dependent correlation with age of onset. *Clin Endocrinol (Oxf)* 2005;62(6):679–82.

107. Begovich AB, Caillier SJ, Alexander HC, et al. The R620W polymorphism of the protein tyrosine phosphatase *PTPN22* is not associated with multiple sclerosis. *Am J Hum Genet* 2005;76(1):184–7.

108. Matesanz F, Rueda B, Orozco G, et al. Protein tyrosine phosphatase gene (*PTPN22*) polymorphism in multiple sclerosis. *J Neurol* 2005;252(8):994–5.

109. Carlton VE, Hu X, Chokkalingam AP, et al. *PTPN22* genetic variation: evidence for multiple variants associated with rheumatoid arthritis. *Am J Hum Genet* 2005;77(4):567–81.

110. Chow LM, Fournel M, Davidson D, Veillette A. Negative regulation of T-cell receptor signalling by tyrosine protein kinase p50csk. *Nature* 1993;365(6442):156–60.

111. Ghose R, Shekhtman A, Goger MJ, Ji H, Cowburn D. A novel, specific interaction involving the Csk SH3 domain and its natural ligand. *Nat Struct Biol* 2001;8(11):998–1004.

112. Gjorloff-Wingren A, Saxena M, Williams S, Hammi D, Mustelin T. Characterization of TCR-induced receptor-proximal signaling events negatively regulated by the protein tyrosine phosphatase PEP. *Eur J Immunol* 1999;29(12):3845–54.

113. Kochi Y, Yamada R, Suzuki A, et al. A functional variant in FCRL3, encoding Fc receptor-like 3, is associated with rheumatoid arthritis and several autoimmunities. *Nat Genet* 2005;37(5):478–85.

114. Tokuhiro S, Yamada R, Chang X, et al. An intronic SNP in a RUNX1 binding site of SLC22A4, encoding an organic cation transporter, is associated with rheumatoid arthritis. *Nat Genet* 2003;35(4):341–8.

115. Suzuki A, Yamada R, Chang X, et al. Functional haplotypes of PADI4, encoding citrullinating enzyme peptidylarginine deiminase 4, are associated with rheumatoid arthritis. *Nat Genet* 2003;34(4):395–402.

116. Guo D, Li M, Zhang Y, et al. A functional variant of SUMO4, a new I kappa B alpha modifier, is associated with type 1 diabetes. *Nat Genet* 2004;36(8):837–41.

117. Smyth DJ, Howson JM, Lowe CE, et al. Assessing the validity of the association between the SUMO4 M55V variant and risk of type 1 diabetes. *Nat Genet* 2005;37(2):110–1; author reply 2–3.

118. Kosoy R, Concannon P. Functional variants in SUMO4, TAB2, and NFkappaB and the risk of type 1 diabetes. *Genes Immun* 2005;6(3):231–5.

119. Vella A, Cooper JD, Lowe CE, et al. Localization of a type 1 diabetes locus in the IL2RA/CD25 region by use of tag single-nucleotide polymorphisms. *Am J Hum Genet* 2005;76(5):773–9.

3 Environmental Factors in Autoimmune Endocrinopathies

Rajni B. Sharma, PhD, C. Lynne Burek, PhD, Daniela Cihákova, MD, PhD, Dolores B. Njoku, MD, and Noel R. Rose, MD, PhD

Contents

Summary

The autoimmune endocrinopathies include a wide range of diseases affecting one or more endocrine glands. While a strong genetic predisposition underlies their development, environmental factors are also involved in their pathogenesis. These environmental agents include infections, therapeutic drugs, chemicals, and radiation. A firm relationship between these environmental agents and autoimmune diseases is difficult to establish as exposure to these agents often precedes onset of disease by a considerable margin. Animal models have helped considerably to establish a cause/effect relationship. The mechanisms by which autoimmunity may be initiated include changes in autologous antigens, alterations in immune regulation, or altered gene expression. Environmental factors alter the immune responses depending on the genetic susceptibility of the host and may be regulated by the quality, quantity, and duration of exposure.

Key Words: Environmental factors, diabetes, thyroid diseases.

From: *Contemporary Endocrinology: Autoimmune Diseases in Endocrinology*
Edited by: A. P. Weetman © Humana Press, Totowa, NJ

INTRODUCTION

The autoimmune endocrinopathies encompass a wide range of diseases affecting one or more endocrine glands. Like most autoimmune diseases, a strong genetic predisposition underlies their development. The first hint that there is a genetic component in these diseases arose from the observations of astute clinicians who noticed a clustering of diseases of the thyroid and other endocrine organs in certain families *(1)*. Similarly, siblings and offspring of patients with type 1 diabetes mellitus (T1DM) showed a higher prevalence of disease than that found in the general population *(2)*. These observations were strengthened by large-scale studies showing that relatives of patients with autoimmune endocrine disease often have antibodies to the same or other endocrine organs *(3)*. Finally, a large body of investigations has clearly implicated the major histocompatibility complex (MHC) as a prominent genetic risk factor in the development of autoimmune endocrinopathy (*see* Chap. 2). More recently, a number of immunoregulatory genes that contribute to a heightened susceptibility to particular autoimmune diseases of the endocrine organs have been identified, such as the cytotoxic T-lymphocyte-associated antigen (CTLA)-4 and lymphoid tyrosine phosphatase locus LYP/PTPN22 loci *(4–7)*. In addition, genetic traits that heighten the vulnerability of the target organ have been described. Thus, at least three major categories of genes seem to participate in determining inherited susceptibility to autoimmune disease: (1) genes that determine recognition of immunodominant, pathogenic epitopes (MHC and autoimmune regulator [AIRE]); (2) traits that modify the immune response (CTLA-4); and (3) inherited characteristics that predispose to damaging inflammation in the target organ (e.g., adhesion molecules) *(8)*. A number of years ago, one of us (NRR) predicted that the accumulation of a number of unrelated genetic traits contributing to susceptibility to autoimmune-mediated tissue injury by different pathways represents the most appropriate model for describing the genetic predisposition to autoimmune disease *(9)*. Termed the "3 gene hypothesis," experimental evidence accumulating since the original proposal seems to have justified that prediction.

In experimental animals, the aggregation of disease susceptibility genes by artificial breeding has produced models of autoimmune endocrinopathy that occur spontaneously. They include, for example, the non-obese diabetic (NOD) mouse model of T1DM or the obese strain (OS) chicken and NOD.H2^{h4} mouse model of Hashimoto's thyroiditis. Among humans, in contrast, it appears that genetic predisposition in total accounts for less than half of the susceptibility to autoimmune disease *(10–12)*. Concurrence rates of 5–50% for T1DM and for autoimmune thyroid disease in genetically identical twins indicates that environmental agents as well as genetic factors are involved in the etiology of autoimmune endocrinopathies.

A note of caution is needed. Not all non-inherited differences are due to external factors. During their generation of diversity, the lymphocyte receptors of the immune system undergo extensive, post-germline recombination. Immune recognition even in genetically identical mice or monozygotic twins may vary greatly. In addition, the immune response is influenced over time by other regulatory activities of the endocrine and nervous systems. Thus, many autoimmune diseases, especially autoimmune diseases of the thyroid, are much more prevalent in females than in males *(13,14)*. Those diseases may remit during pregnancy but recur and exacerbate post-partum *(15)*. Nervous stimuli including stress also influence the immune response *(16)*. Thus, the relatively low concordance rates in monozygotic twins may be due in part to immunologic randomness and physiologic changes and not solely because of environmental factors.

Yet, an increasing number of epidemiologic studies support the view that the environment does play a significant role in triggering autoimmune diseases in humans. As examples, the onset of clinical T1DM is less in the summer than in the winter months in both the northern and the southern hemispheres *(17)*. Incidence or prevalence of T1DM tends to be higher in northern European countries compared with the southern ones and greater in the southern states of Australia than the northern ones with no clear association with genetic differences *(17)*. The incidence of T1DM in a number of countries has risen rapidly over the past three to five decades accompanied by a decreasing age of onset and a broadening of the human leucocyte antigen (HLA)-risk profile. These results suggest increasing environmental influence in a constant proportion of genetically susceptible individuals.

The previously listed examples clearly demonstrate that environmental factors participate in the etiology of the autoimmune diseases, including those that affect endocrine organs. In this chapter, we will discuss the role of environmental agents such as infections, therapeutic drugs, chemicals, and radiation, which have been associated with the most common autoimmune endocrinopathies in humans and animal models.

AUTOIMMUNE ENDOCRINOPATHIES AND INFECTIOUS AGENTS

The onset of autoimmune diseases following infection has given rise to conjectures that infection plays a direct or indirect role in disease etiology. It is well recognized that infections modulate immune responsiveness and may prepare the ground for the seed, which later germinates into autoimmune disease. Infections may provide the inflammatory milieu that increases the potency of self-antigens, a phenomenon that we have termed the "adjuvant effect" of infection *(18)*. An infectious agent can upregulate costimulatory molecules and increase production of proinflammatory cytokines. As a result, autoreactive T cells can be easily activated and can start an autoimmune reaction. Sometimes, infections produce a shift in the Th1/Th2 balance, favoring the induction of pathogenic rather than benign autoimmunity. In other instances, infection may alter self-antigens or express them in a setting that heightens their immunogenic potency. Finally, epitopes represented by particular pathogens may mimic epitopes present on self-antigens leading to a subsequent autoimmune response, a phenomenon termed "molecular mimicry."

It is difficult to establish a firm relationship between infectious agents and autoimmune diseases. The problem can be attributed to the following issues:

1. The onset of autoimmune disease may occur much later than the infection. Once set into motion, an autoimmune response often requires months or years before reaching a clinically apparent state. Therefore, an infection acquired in childhood may not be expressed until adolescence or early adulthood as an autoimmune disease.
2. Different infectious agents can cause the same or a virtually similar clinical outcome.
3. An infectious agent may trigger autoimmune disease only in genetically more susceptible individuals as determined by non-HLA and HLA genes.
4. An infection might not add to the risk of developing an autoimmune disease in patients with highly susceptible genetic backgrounds. The additive effect of infection may increase the chance for developing autoimmune disease in patients with lower genetic

predisposition. For example, Weets et al. *(19)* showed that a seasonal increase of T1DM occurred only in the genetically low-risk population without the high-risk HLA background.

It is very likely that many infections can lead to harmless autoimmune responses in the form of autoantibodies. It remains unknown what factors trigger a full-blown autoimmune disease in some patients.

Diabetes and Viral Infections

The incidence of some autoimmune diseases has increased over the past decades. In particular, it is well documented that the incidence of T1DM increased in Finland between 1965 and 1996 of 0.67 per year on average *(20)*. This increase is probably caused by environmental factors, because no important genetic changes occur in the population in such a short period of time. Viral infections are the first candidate among the environmental factors. Many studies looked at different viruses to explain the increase in T1DM incidence. One of the main suspects in triggering T1DM is enterovirus infection. However, it is known that frequency of enterovirus infections decreased in Finland in the 1980s and 1990s *(21)*. In addition, although the incidence of T1DM increased in Finland, it remained stable in the genetically similar populations of Estonia and Russian Karelia.

Many studies show only presence of autoantibodies following the onset of an infectious disease, which is far from indicating causality. Only longitudinal, HLA-matched studies can answer the question whether a single virus infection can increase the incidence of an autoimmune disease. If a viral infection acts as an adjuvant in autoimmune disease development, as we have shown in mice, the same autoimmune disease in humans might be triggered by many different viruses.

DIABETES AND RUBELLA

Increased incidence of T1DM and thyroid disease has long been recognized as part of the congenital rubella syndrome (CRS). Patients can also develop other endocrine tribulations such as Addison's disease and growth hormone deficiency *(22,23)*. Rubella virus can be isolated from the pancreas as well as other fetal tissues. Up to 20% of children infected with rubella *in utero* develop T1DM *(24)*. It was originally thought that rubella initiates the autoimmune destruction of islet cells. An association with the HLA haplotype DR3 has been reported along with the recognition of glutamic acid decarboxylase (GAD) 65/67 determinants by T cells of the CRS patients *(25)*. Also, 20% of CRS patients tested positive for diabetes-associated autoantibodies *(26,27)*. However, the autoantibody assays used in these studies had serious problems *(28,29)*. No diabetes-associated autoantibodies such as GAD, islet cell antibodies (ICA), insulin autoantibodies (IAA), or IA-2a were detected in any of 37 CRS patients from Finland and Poland in study in 2003 *(30)*.

The incidence of rubella infection in fetus has decreased by 99% since the introduction of the rubella vaccine in the United States in 1969. This decrease in the fetal exposure to rubella did not reverse the increase in diabetes incidence in the population, showing that rubella is not responsible for the majority of the diabetes cases. Therefore, it seems that diabetes in CRS might develop mainly after destruction of the pancreatic beta cells by the virus rather than by an autoimmune process.

DIABETES AND MUMPS

Several clinical reports have associated mumps with diabetes for many years. In 1927, a report suggested possible association between increased incidence of T1DM 2–4 years of following mumps infection *(31)*. Numerous case reports since that time have linked mumps and autoimmune diabetes. In one report, 127 children who developed natural mumps infection and 7 children who developed active mumps infection after vaccination produced antibodies to islet cells, but no clinical disease *(32)*. Infection of the human beta cells with mumps virus in vitro leads to their upregulated HLA class I expression and increased production of proinflammatory cytokines *(33–35)*. In Finland, the introduction of mumps measles/rubella (MMR) vaccination in 1982 was followed by a brief pause in the rising incidence of T1DM, but the pause was only temporary *(36)*. In general, the introduction of mumps vaccine did not cause a decrease in the incidence of T1DM. Therefore, the association of mumps virus infection with T1DM remains unproven.

DIABETES AND ENTEROVIRUSES

Of the large family of enteroviruses, some are pancreotropic with a potential to damage the islet cells. A case of neonatal diabetes was described in which the mother had an Echovirus 6 infection diagnosed by neutralizing antibodies at 14-weeks gestation. Antibodies to insulin and GAD were present in the infant but not in the mother *(37)*. Coxsackievirus B (CB) 4 was isolated from the pancreas of a patient who died shortly after the onset of acute T1DM *(38)*. The autopsy showed lymphocytic infiltration of the pancreas islet cells with beta cell necrosis. Serologic data revealed a rise in titer from less than 4 on day 2 to 32 on the day of death. Transfer of the virus associated with this patient to mice induced severe diabetes within a few days. In other experiments, CB4-specific antigens were demonstrated in the islets in association with beta cell damage *(39)*. Coxsackievirus can replicate in human beta cells as demonstrated by RNA hybridization in beta cells of infants who died of fulminant infection *(40)*. Cocultivation of virus with pancreatic beta cells impaired the metabolism of islets, showing a decreased insulin secretion as early as 24 hours after infection *(39)*. These data show that enteroviruses have great potential to damage the pancreas and may cause a person or an animal to become diabetic. They do not, however, show that the disease is caused by an autoimmune response.

There are numerous epidemiologic studies indicating that, at the onset of diabetes, patients are more likely to also have antienterovirus (mainly CB3) immunoglobulin (Ig)M antibodies than healthy controls *(41,42)*.

Blood spots taken routinely on days 2–4 of life from 600 children with early diabetes in Sweden were analyzed for enterovirus RNA. It was found that 4.5% of children, who later develop diabetes, had enterovirus RNA in their blood compared with 2.3% controls ($p < 0.04$) *(43)*. In another study, T-cell responses to enterovirus were detected at the time of onset of T1DM *(44,45)*. Enteroviral RNA has been also detected in T1DM patients' sera *(46,47)*. Using a molecular approach with PCR of peripheral blood mononuclear cells, a study of diabetics in Sweden showed evidence of CB4, CB5, and CB6 in 50% of the subjects compared with 26% of normal siblings with no evidence of infection in age- and sex-matched normal controls *(48)*. Another study on patients from England, Austria, and Australia provides evidence for the virus-specific

IgM responses to CB4 and CB5 during the juvenile onset of T1DM *(49)*. Jones and Crosby *(50)* assessed the proliferation of T cells to viral proteins and showed an association among T1DM, MHC II (DRB 1*04), and CB infection.

These studies consistently show that enterovirus infection can precede the onset of diabetes. However, they do not exclude possibilities that prediabetic patients with ongoing yet clinically silent diabetes are more prone to CB3 infection or that their genetic makeup predisposes them independently to both diabetes and enterovirus infection. Indeed, the diabetic patients with anti-CB3 IgM antibodies are also more likely to be HLA-DR3 or HLA-DR4 positive than controls *(42,51)*. In a longitudinal diabetes prevention study carried out in Finland, enterovirus infections were diagnosed in 51% of cases and 28% of controls in the 6 months before the development of ICA *(52)*. On the contrary, other longitudinal studies in the United States (DAISY Study) and Australia (Baby Diab Study) did not confirm any association of enteroviral infection with the onset of islet cell autoimmunity or symptoms of diabetes *(49)*. The results may reflect differences in geographic distribution of disease, differing genetic backgrounds of the populations, variations in the viruses that are involved, or different ages of the population studied.

The possibility that the CB3 infection is able to accelerate an already ongoing autoimmune process can be found in animal models. In the NOD mouse model of autoimmune diabetes, it has been reported that the infection 8 weeks after the development of insulitis accelerates the onset of disease, whereas pre-insulitis CB infection protects against the development of diabetes *(53)*.

The main question of whether the CB3 infection is able to initiate autoimmune destruction of the pancreas by itself still remains to be answered.

THYROID DISEASE AND VIRAL INFECTIONS

Viruses are suspected to be a cause of subacute thyroiditis, which usually lasts several weeks and resolves itself, although the thyroid gland destruction can lead to hypothyroidism. Subacute thyroiditis clinically manifests itself as painful enlargement of the thyroid gland, destruction of follicular epithelium, dysphagia and hoarseness, and symptoms of thyrotoxicosis. Mumps infection is a notorious suspect in subacute thyroiditis. Other viruses that are suspected to cause subacute thyroiditis are measles virus, influenza, adenovirus, Epstein-Barr virus (EBV), and enteroviruses. EBV DNA was detected in the thyroid gland of a 3-year-old girl with subacute thyroiditis *(54)*. An early study reported changes in antibody titers against some viruses such as influenza and mumps, in half of the tested patients with subacute thyroiditis *(55)*. However, these findings were not supported by more recent studies. No changes in antiviral antibody titers against measles, rubella, mumps, type I herpes, chicken pox, parvovirus B19, and cytomegalovirus (CMV) were observed in 10 patients with subacute thyroiditis *(56)*. Also, there was no EBV or CMV DNA detected in thyroid of these patients. Thus, it seems that many different viruses can cause subacute thyroiditis.

However, the role of autoimmunity in the disease pathology is uncertain. This is supported by the finding of thyroid autoantibodies in some cases *(55)*. The autoimmune part of the process may represent non-specific response to inflammation and release of thyroid antigens. The majorities of subacute thyroiditis cases resolve spontaneously and do not evolve into typical autoimmune thyroiditis.

Autoimmune thyroid disease (both Hashimoto's and Graves' disease) is sometimes associated with several viral infections. The data on association of chronic hepatitis

C virus (HCV) infection of the liver with several autoimmune diseases including autoimmune thyroiditis have thus far been mixed. Several studies found an increase in antithyroid antibodies and hypothyroidism in HCV patients before interferon treatment *(57–60)*. An Italian study showed a high frequency of hypothyroidism (13%) and antithyroid antibodies positivity (27%) in 630 untreated HCV patients. About 657 healthy controls had a 3.8% incidence of hypothyroidism and 16% were positive for at least one of the anti-thyroid antibodies *(61)*. However, other investigations did not find such an association. A UK study on 111 hepatitis C patients *(62)* and a Spanish study on 107 patients *(63)* did not report a significant increase of hypothyroidism or anti-thyroid antibodies. Differences in the genetic background of the populations and environmental cofactors, such as iodine, are usually cited as reasons for the different results. Thus, it is unknown whether HCV can interact with other environmental factors or whether the risk of thyroiditis is increased only in part of the HCV population such as older females as some studies would suggest.

Retroviruses have been also implicated in the induction of autoimmune thyroid disease. Human T-cell leukemia virus type I (HTLV-I) is a human retrovirus highly endemic in southern Japan, tropical Africa, Melanesia, Latin America, and the Caribbean and is suspected of causing T-cell leukemia. It is also suspected to have a role in Hashimoto's as well as Graves' disease. It was shown that there is a larger percentage of patients with Hashimoto's with HTLV-1 positivity than expected (6.3–2.2%) *(64)*. Also HTLV-1 carriers have higher prevalence of anti-thyroid antibodies than the general population *(65,66)*. HTLV-I envelope protein and DNA were detected in follicular epithelial cells of the thyroid gland of a patient with Hashimoto's thyroiditis *(67)* and Graves' disease *(68)*.

Thyroid Disease and Bacterial Infections

Chronic infection by *Yersinia enterocolitica* has been suspected to be a cause or trigger of autoimmune thyroid disease for a number of years. A study in 1970 reported a high incidence of *Yersinia* antibodies in thyroid disease patients *(69)*. Among the patients, 66% had Graves' disease and 83% Hashimoto's thyroiditis. All subjects were positive for antibodies to *Yersinia* compared with 8% of controls *(69)*. This result was attributed to cross-reaction between thyroid antibodies and *Yersinia* antigens. An association of Graves' disease with *Yersinia* infection was further suggested in a study of 30 twins where there was an increased frequency of antibodies to *Yersinia* serotype 3 in the thyroid patients *(70)*. Leukocytes from Graves' disease patients are also able to recognize *Yersinia* antigens, as was demonstrated in leukocyte migration inhibition assays *(71)*. With respect to a possible mechanism linking *Yersinia* infection with Graves' disease, a binding site for thyroid-stimulating hormone (TSH) has been found on *Y. enterocolitica (72,73)*. Purified antibody to *Y. enterocolitica* envelop proteins have shown to bind with human thyrotropin receptor *(74,75)*. Mice produced anti-thyrotropin receptor antibodies after immunization with *Yersinia (76)*. The cross-reaction between epitopes of *Y. enterocolitica* and human thyrotropin receptor might be an example of molecular mimicry *(77)*. However, it is still unclear whether infection with *Yersinia* can induce autoimmune thyroid disease in susceptible individuals or whether it just induces transient anti-TSH-R antibodies.

Correlation of infection with *Helicobacter pylori* and autoimmune thyroid disease has been also proposed. In one investigation, four women with autoimmune thyroid disease and 33 euthyroid-matched controls were compared for serologic evidence of *H. pylori* infection *(78)*. The prevalence of antibodies to *H. pylori* was 78.0% in the patients compared with 48.4% in controls. A more recent study evaluated 90 children with autoimmune thyroid disease, 70 age- and sex-matched healthy controls as well as 65 patients with Turner syndrome *(79)*. The prevalence of positive *H. pylori* antibodies was significantly higher in the thyroid disease patients than in the control group. No association was found between individual HLA haplotypes and helicobacter serology. The evidence is not strong enough to establish that *H. pylori* plays any causative role in thyroiditis pathogenesis or whether the increased *H. pylori* infection is because of same genetic susceptibility factors.

Thyroid Disease and Parasitic Infections

Autoantibodies developed as the result of parasitic infections are often polyreactive, binding to a number of self-antigen as well as foreign antigens. Although several instances of the association of parasitic infections with other autoimmune diseases are cited in the literature, only a few examples have been reported for the autoimmune endocrinopathies. One study reported no correlation between 17 schistosomiasis-infected men and abnormal serum thyroxin (T4) or serum tri-iodothyronine (T3) levels *(80)*. Infectious pathogens may also influence the disease pathology by altering the Th1/Th2 responses. Environmental factors may further alter these responses as explained by the hygiene hypothesis *(81)*. Another study describes immune polarization induced by schistosomiasis infection in a mouse model of Graves' disease. A synthetic glycolipid α-galactosylceramide was used as it is known to skew immunity toward Th2 responses *(82)*. Helminth infection is Th1-dominant and not a Th2 disease as believed previously. Furthermore, once the thyrotropin receptor response was fully induced neither infection nor α-galactosylceramide could suppress disease, suggesting that the time of antigen priming is crucial in relation to infection. Once antigen priming is initiated, inhibition of pathogenic responses becomes difficult *(82)*. Moreover, all autoimmune endocrinopathies display mixed Th1/Th2 responses. It is, therefore, difficult to relate these responses to a specific autoimmune disease.

Thyroid Disease and Vaccination

A study of 386 school children in the age group of 11–13 years found an inhibitory effect of IgG antibodies against measles, mumps, or both on the prevalence of thyroperoxidase antibodies (5%) as compared with seronegative controls (15%) *(83)*. No such correlation was found for rubella antibodies. There were no changes in the prevalence of islet cell antibody in the seropositive group for measles, mumps, or rubella. None of the children had thyroid disease. It is unknown whether any of the children with thyroid antibodies will develop autoimmune thyroiditis in the future and whether the measles or mumps infection or immunization will have any protective effect against thyroid disease *(83)*. There are a few case reports of development of a subacute thyroiditis after hepatitis B vaccination, which resolved themselves and one case following streptococcal vaccination *(84,85)*.

AUTOIMMUNE ENDOCRINOPATHIES AND DRUGS

Concurrent or recent exposures to drugs such as beta blockers, thiazide diuretics, and antipsychotics have been associated with glucose intolerance in some patients *(86,87)*, whereas thyroid dysfunction associated with lithium carbonate, aminoglutethimide, thalidomide, betaroxine, stavudine, and amiodarone is well known *(88)*. In contrast, drugs that have been clinically associated with the autoimmune endocrinopathies, T1DM, and autoimmune thyroiditis are rarer. In this respect, streptozotocin (STZ) *(89)*, Vacor *(90,91)*, cyclosporine *(92)*, and tacrolimus *(93,94)* have been associated with an acute onset of diabetes with features resembling T1DM. Additionally, amiodarone *(95,96)*, interferon (IFN)-α *(88)*, and interleukin (IL)-2 *(97)* have been associated with hypothyroidism with autoimmune features. The development of autoimmune endocrinopathies in these patients has left clinicians wondering whether the primary inciting agent is the drug or whether the patient has some previously unrecognized tendency for the development of autoimmune endocrinopathy.

Fortunately, some drugs associated with autoimmune endocrinopathies in patients have also been associated with the induction of diabetes and autoimmune thyroiditis in animal models of these diseases. These drug-induced animal models of diabetes or autoimmune thyroiditis have provided some insights into mechanisms that may be associated with the development of autoimmune endocrinopathies in patients. In this section, we will discuss the association of autoimmune endocrinopathies with drugs such as STZ, Vacor, amiodarone, IFNs, tacrolimus, and IL-2 in patients as well as the role of STZ, cyclosporine, the IFNs, and IL-2 in animal models of T1DM and autoimmune thyroiditis.

Streptozotocin

For several years, STZ, a glucosamine nitrosourea compound, was utilized in patients as a broad-spectrum antibiotic and more recently as a chemotherapeutic agent for neuroendocrine tumors; however, in several patients, hyperglycemia and glucose intolerance have been documented with this drug *(89,98)*. Later studies demonstrated that STZ administration can induce insulin-dependent diabetes in mice utilizing two STZ immunization regimens: ~2–3 days after single high-dose (90 mg/kg) intraperitoneal injection or ~5–6 days after five daily low-dose (40 mg/kg) intraperitoneal injections of this compound. Experiments utilizing the STZ-diabetes models have used either regimen. However, prior investigations suggest that multiple low doses of STZ may be less toxic to the mice undergoing this experimental regimen *(99)*. Nevertheless, investigators agree that this animal model of insulin-dependent diabetes provides a golden opportunity to study mechanisms that may be responsible for T1DM in patients as well as a vehicle to investigate the role of this autoimmune endocrinopathy in the development of diabetic nephropathy, obstetrical complications, and rejection or tolerance of pancreatic islet cells.

Several strains of mice have been found to be susceptible to STZ-induced insulin-dependent diabetes. These mice include male CD-1 mice, C57Bl/Ks mice *(100)*, male mice given multiple low doses of STZ (MSZ) *(99)*, and diabetic prone NOD mice before the onset of spontaneous insulinitis *(101)*. Interestingly, one study documented sex differences in susceptibility to STZ-induced diabetes using the multiple dose STZ regimen *(102)*. This study showed that susceptible male mice developed a higher hyperglycemic response than female mice, and this response was associated with testosterone. Hence, the STZ model of diabetes in mice could also be used to study the role of gender and genetics in the development of diabetes in this experimental model.

No single mechanism has been able to completely explain the development of insulin-dependent diabetes following STZ-administration in mice, although most studies agree that the final pathway responsible for diabetes following STZ administration involves direct toxicity to pancreatic beta cells. What is not clear, however, is which mechanism is primarily responsible for the destruction of pancreatic beta cells; hence, studies have suggested that several non-immune and immune mechanisms may have a vital role in this process. The most common non-immune mechanism is based on the finding that glucose transporter Glut-2 in pancreatic beta cells takes up STZ *(103)*. This study demonstrated that uptake of STZ by Glu-2 resulted in direct DNA damage by alkylation *(104)* or indirect DNA damage following the generation of nitric oxide (NO) *(105,106)*. The prevailing immune mechanism of STZ-induced insulin-dependent diabetes suggests that pancreatic beta cell injury occurs as a result of STZ-induced increases in CD8+ T cell and macrophage numbers as well as cytokine injury from IFN-γ producing T-helper and cytotoxic T cells *(107)*. Studies further characterizing these infiltrating T cells show that T cells infiltrating the islets of STZ-induced diabetic mice are relatively oligoclonal, expressing the Vβ8.2 T-cell receptor *(108)* and also show that diabetes can be adoptively transferred to naïve mice using T cells from STZ-treated mice *(109)*. Last, studies investigating the role of T-cell signaling in STZ-induced experimental diabetes have found that this disease requires T-cell recognition of self in inflamed pancreatic islets as well as CD28 costimulation *(110)*.

As might be expected, immune mechanisms believed to have a role in STZ-induced experimental diabetes often overlap with non-immune mechanisms, resulting in damage to pancreatic beta cells. In this fashion, Th1 cytokines such as tumor necrosis factor (TNF)-α, IFN-γ, and IL-1β produced by macrophages have been associated with diabetes following STZ administration *(111)*. Additionally, these same macrophages can damage pancreatic beta cells by generating oxygen-free radicals *(112)*. An additional mechanism that may be responsible for the production of oxygen-free radicals is through increased expression of inducible NO synthase *(113)* and the resultant production of NO and peroxynitrite. These studies show that the production of oxygen-free radicals is a final common pathway in the pathogenesis of STZ-induced experimental diabetes.

In the last few years, the importance of a non-immune mechanism involving direct DNA damage and subsequent repair has been extensively investigated. These studies may have been generated from the observation that NO can functionally inhibit beta cells, resulting in reduced insulin secretion *(114)* and ATP levels *(115)*, in addition to increased DNA damage *(116)* and cell death *(117)*. Studies clearly document the importance of DNA repair by poly (ADP-ribose) synthase also referred to as poly (ADP-ribose) polymerase in the mechanism of STZ-induced injury *(118,119)* and suggest that these studies may reveal future therapeutic targets for T1DM in patients.

Cyclosporin A

Cyclosporin A (CSA), a fungal metabolite, is an established and potent immunosuppressive agent primarily used in patients after undergoing organ transplantation *(120,121)*. Immunosuppression by CSA occurs through initial binding to intracellular cyclophilin and subsequently to calcium-dependent calcineurin. This binding to calcineurin inhibits activation of the *IL-2* gene and thus prevents expansion of T-cell clones through interference with the production of IL-2 from proliferating T cells *(122,123)*. Despite its role in immunosuppression, CSA has long been associated with organ-specific autoimmune disease in experimental mice *(124,125)* as well as glucose intolerance *(126)*, T1DM *(127)*, and more recently subacute thyroiditis in patients post-transplantation *(128)*.

Exact mechanisms responsible for CSA-associated autoimmune endocrinopathies in patients have not been completely clarified. Nevertheless, mechanisms for CSA-induced, organ-specific autoimmunity in mice have been investigated. Researchers have found that daily administration of CSA to newborn BALB/c mice induces gastritis, oophoritis, orchitis, adrenalitis, insulinitis, and thyroiditis with their associated serum autoantibodies 1 or 2 weeks following the cessation of CSA treatments *(125)*. These authors have suggested that organ-specific autoimmunity developed from the selective deficiency of regulatory T cells. Later studies suggested alternative mechanisms that also may be responsible for CSA-induced autoimmunity and suggested that CSA can induce thymic involution, inhibit deletion of low-affinity thymic clones, or prevent the development of T-cell clonal anergy *(129)*. Additionally, these authors noted that withdrawal of CSA can also induce a graft-vs-host response that may aggravate or induce autoimmune diseases such as autoimmune thyroiditis. These prior articles infer that the mechanism of CSA-induced autoimmune endocrinopathy targets T cells and T-cell function.

Other authors investigating the mechanisms of the CSA-induced autoimmune endocrinopathy, T1DM, have focused primarily on the effects of CSA on pancreatic beta cell function. These authors have showed that CSA reduced glucose-induced insulin secretion using in vitro cell cultures of rat pancreatic beta cells *(130,131)* and suggested that reduced insulin secretion occurred through two possible mechanisms. The first mechanism was through CSA-induced inhibition of insulin DNA or mRNA *(132)*, whereas the second mechanism was by CSA-induced direct damage of pancreatic beta cells *(133)*. A more recent article to address the mechanism of CSA action in pancreatic beta cells suggested an alternative mechanism for CSA-induced decreases in insulin. These authors showed that CSA decreased insulin secretion by interfering with the mitochondrial permeability transition pore *(134)* and suggested that CSA immunosuppressive effects occurred through calcineurin, whereas the diabetogenic effects occurred through the mitochondrial permeability transition pore.

The mechanism of CSA-induced autoimmune thyroiditis has not been as extensively investigated as that of T1DM, because a direct association with autoimmune thyroiditis in patients may be less clear. The first article to report subacute thyroiditis associated with CSA was in a patient on CSA, prednisolone, and chronic lithium, an agent well known to impair thyroid function *(88,128)*. Whether CSA contributed to the development of lithium-induced thyroid dysfunction was unclear from this report. Possibly, the role of CSA in autoimmune thyroiditis could be clarified using experimental models. However, investigations centering on the influence of CSA on thyroxin levels in experimental autoimmune thyroiditis showed a paradoxical effect of CSA where a high dose (360 mg/kg) prevented a decrease in thyroxin levels and a small dose (25–60 mg/kg) potentiated a decrease in serum thyroxin. Fortunately, earlier studies investigating CSA and organ-specific autoimmunity have familiarized us with paradoxical effects of CSA *(125)*. Hence, these articles investigating mechanisms of CSA-induced autoimmunity in mice may imply that similar mechanisms are responsible for CSA-induced autoimmunity in patients, but to date, there is no one mechanism that could explain the development of this phenomenon in patients.

Tacrolimus

Cyclosporin A is not the only calcineurin-inhibiting therapeutic agent that has been associated with the development of T1DM. Tacrolimus, also referred to in the literature as FK506, has been associated with T1DM in post-transplant patients. Tacrolimus is a macrolide antibiotic *(135)* that inhibits calcineurin by binding to an alternative calcineurin-associated immunophilin, tacrolimus-binding protein 12 *(136)*. It was introduced as an alternative to CSA with less potential for arterial hypertension and hyperlipidemia and no association with hirsuitism and gingival hyperplasia, two well-known complications of CSA *(137)*. Unfortunately, several studies suggest that patients receiving tacrolimus are more likely to develop T1DM when compared with CSA-treated patients, and this tendency is increased with the concomitant use of steroids *(94)*.

The mechanisms responsible for tacrolimus-induced T1DM in patients have not been fully elucidated. Previous studies have suggested direct toxicity to pancreatic beta cells, decreased insulin sensitivity or decreased insulin release, or synthesis by pancreatic beta cells as possible mechanisms to explain this phenomenon *(94,138,139)*. However, a thorough investigation of these mechanisms in experimental animal models will be useful. To date, there are no reports of tacrolimus-induced autoimmune thyroiditis in patients.

Amiodarone

Amiodarone is a benzofuranic derivative used to treat tachyarrhythmias, such as paroxysmal supraventricular tachycardia *(140)* as well as congestive heart failure *(141)* in patients. It has several unique pharmacological features including a relatively long half-life of around 40 days and a wide distribution to several key tissues including liver, heart, and thyroid. In addition to these features, it has a high iodine content of reportedly anywhere from 27% *(76)* to 37%, which results in increased exposure to iodine in patients treated with amiodarone for prolonged periods *(142,143)*. Not surprisingly, then, treatment of patients with amiodarone has been associated with thyroid dysfunction; however, whether or not amiodarone can cause thyroid autoimmunity remains controversial.

Nevertheless, most clinicians will agree that 14–18% of persons treated with amiodarone will develop abnormalities in thyroid function *(144)*, which are generally categorized into three types. The first type of amiodarone-induced abnormality results in thyrotoxicosis, more commonly seen in male patients with thyroid abnormalities, and caused by deiodination of thyroxin resulting in elevated serum-free T4 *(145)*. Studies suggest that the mechanism of this type of amiodarone-induced thyrotoxicosis, also termed AIT-1, is from a direct effect of amiodarone on thyroid cells from iodine-induced excess thyroid hormone (TH) synthesis *(146)*. Because of underlying thyroid abnormalities in these patients, the role of thyroid autoimmunity in this disease has been investigated. From these studies, researchers have concluded that humoral thyroid autoimmunity did not have a role in AIT-1 in patients without underlying thyroid disorders *(147)*. The second type of AIT, termed AIT-2, results in destructive thyroiditis in patients with no previously known abnormalities of the thyroid that occurs from the discharge of pre-formed hormones *(143)*. In AIT-2, most clinicians agree that thyroid autoimmunity is not an issue.

The third and last form of amiodarone-induced thyroid injury causes hypothyroidism and occurs more frequently in women with pre-existing thyroid injury, especially autoimmune thyroiditis *(143,144)*. Studies investigating the pathogenesis of amiodarone-induced hypothyroidism (AIH) suggest that damage from amiodarone occurs in areas already injured by autoimmune thyroiditis, resulting in susceptibility to iodine inhibition of TH and an inability to escape from Wolff–Chaikoff effect *(143)*. Even so, the association of AIH with autoimmunity lies with a pre-existing diagnosis of autoimmunity and not the development of new-onset autoimmunity. Clearly, from these mechanisms, amiodarone can induce thyroid injury; however, the development of thyroid autoimmunity may require an already injured thyroid gland. In fact, only one study transiently detected anti-thyroid peroxidase antibodies in patients following amiodarone treatment *(148)*. This study found that ~55% of patients developed these autoantibodies after starting amiodarone therapy *(148)*; however, later investigators were unable to reproduce these findings in other groups of patients *(149,150)*.

Rat Poison (Vacor)

Vacor is a rodenticide that can induce diabetes in rodents and humans *(90,91)*. However, in recent years, Vacor has been discussed primarily for its historical perspective. Before 1993, following inadvertent or intentional exposure to Vacor, individuals developed signs and symptoms similar to T1DM. The pathogenesis of diabetes in patients or mice is thought to be from direct toxicity to pancreatic beta cells using similar mechanisms found following administration of STZ, in addition to possible direct inhibition of NADH. Nevertheless the issue of autoimmunity following Vacor exposure has not been resolved.

Interferons and IL-2

The IFNs can be grouped into two classes: Type 1, which includes IFN-α and IFN-β, and Type 2, which includes IFN-γ *(151)*. Investigators have discovered several type 1 alpha IFNs but only one type 1 beta IFN, which may suggest that IFN-α may be capable of responding to a wider variety of environmental stimuli *(152)*. In fact, previous studies have demonstrated that challenging experimental systems with bacteria or lipopolysaccharide *(153)*, polyanions in addition to double-stranded DNA and RNA *(154)*, IL-2 *(155)*, IFN-γ *(156)*, hypoxia *(157)*, or vasoactive intestinal polypeptide *(158)* can induce IFN-α. Even so, investigators agree that viruses are the most potent inducers of IFN-α *(152,159)*. Hence, the antiviral properties of IFN-α have been utilized to treat persistent hepatitis B and C infections, and because of its diverse therapeutic effects, IFN-α is also used to treat leukemias, lymphoma, carcinoid tumors, and breast cancer *(160,161)*.

As a corollary to responding to various stimuli, IFN-α has various effects on the immune system. IFN-α can activate dendritic cells, stimulate T-helper cell and cytotoxic T-cell proliferation *(152)*, as well as promote immunoglobulin class switching *(162,163)*. Moreover, generation of these immune responses can occur through several avenues using specialized cell types, such as natural killer cells *(164)* and monocytes *(165)* and a number of cytokines including IL-1, IL-2, IL-4, IL-6, IL-8, IL-10, and IL-15 *(152)*. It is not surprising then that the ability of IFN-α to respond to a diverse array of stimuli and induce various effects on the immune system may predispose some patients receiving recombinant formulations of this drug or patients with elevated IFN-α to the development of autoimmune diseases.

Previous studies have associated the induction of natural IFN-α and the administration of recombinant IFN-α with the development of several autoimmune diseases in humans including systemic lupus erythematosus (SLE), T1DM, and thyroiditis. Our review of reports associating the induction of natural IFN-α with the development of autoimmune diseases demonstrated that SLE is the best documented of these diseases. Cross-sectional human studies clearly showed that SLE patients had elevated serum levels of IFN-α *(166, 167)*. Interestingly, these studies did not demonstrate recurring increases in IFN-β in these patients. Elevated levels of natural IFN-α were also documented in pancreatic biopsies from patients newly diagnosed with T1DM, and similar to SLE, IFN-β was not reliably elevated *(168,169)*. In contrast to these diseases, elevated expression of natural IFN-α has not been reported in autoimmune thyroiditis, although also documented in psoriasis *(170)*, Crohn's disease *(171)*, and celiac disease *(172)*.

The development of the autoimmune diseases T1DM and thyroiditis have been well documented following the administration of recombinant IFN-α. Yet, it cannot be ignored that several of these studies reporting an increase in the frequency of autoimmune diseases following IFN-α administration were performed in patients infected with chronic viral hepatitis *(173,174)*. Hence, the role of the concurrent infection in the development of T1DM and thyroiditis could not be separated. Even so, the first study correlating IFN-α with T1DM demonstrated increased autoantibody titers in a patient with hepatitis C who had T1DM-associated autoantibodies GAD and IAA before treatment with IFN-α *(175)*. Subsequent studies performed in Japan reported diabetes in 0.08–0.7% patients following IFN-α; however, these studies did not document autoantibody measurements in these patients *(173,174)*. A later study in hepatitis C patients then showed that the numbers of T1DM autoantibody-positive patients rose by 4%, from 3 to 7%, following treatment with IFN-α, further suggesting that recombinant IFN-α may have a role in the development of autoimmunity and T1DM in susceptible patients *(176)*.

Autoimmune thyroiditis following recombinant IFN-α is also well documented. Previous studies have recognized the types of autoimmune thyroiditis, the incidence, the potential risk factors, and the natural history of this disease in patients. These studies assist clinicians in potentially identifying high-risk patients before the onset of autoimmune thyroiditis. In this way, two types of autoimmune thyroid diseases have been associated with this therapy in patients: autoimmune hypothyroidism and thyrotoxicosis *(177)*. Although somewhat less investigated than SLE and T1DM following IFN-α, the incidence of IFN-α-associated autoimmune thyroiditis is surprisingly 6%. Not surprisingly, although, risk factors for developing autoimmune thyroid diseases resemble those associated with the development of T1DM following IFN-α and include female sex, malignancy or hepatitis C, pre-existing thyroid autoantibodies, prolonged IFN-α therapy, or therapy in combination with IL-2. Earlier studies investigating this phenomenon in hepatitis C patients suggested that, following recombinant

IFN-α, autoimmune thyroiditis in the majority of patients spontaneously resolves *(177)*; however, a recent study investigating the natural history of this type of thyroiditis suggests that thyroiditis may not resolve in some patients with hyperthyroidism who require therapy >5 years *(178)*.

Animal models of IFN-α-induced autoimmunity have assisted in the identification of mechanisms that may be responsible for IFN-α-associated autoimmunity in patients. The animal model of IFN-α-induced T1DM clearly demonstrates elevated IFN-α production by pancreatic islets cells before the onset of diabetes in STZ-treated mice *(179)*. Moreover, administration of anti-IFN-α antibodies could prevent the development of diabetes in these mice. Immunization with polyinosine/cytosine, an inducer of IFN-α accelerated the onset of T1DM in STZ-treated mice *(180)*. Additionally, further mechanistic investigations found that the induction of autoreactive T cells by IFN-α required the induction of intercellular adhesion molecule (ICAM)-1 and B7.2 *(181)*. To our knowledge, there are no animal models of IFN-α-induced autoimmune thyroiditis.

Low-dose IL-2 has been used as a systemic adjuvant with experimental cancer vaccines *(182)*. IL-2 is also used to promote the proliferation of antigen-specific T cells. However, administration of IL-2 has been associated with autoimmune diseases such as vitiligo, T1DM, and thyroiditis. One study evaluating the development of autoimmune diseases in patients treated with anti-tumor vaccines and low-dose IL-2 found that the most common autoimmune disease associated with this therapy was autoimmune thyroiditis (15.4%), whereas the frequency of T1DM (2%) was a distant third following vitiligo and visual and ocular inflammation *(97)*. Surprisingly, the majority of patients developing these diseases were male, suggesting that other mechanisms and not just autoimmunity could account for the development of thyroid dysfunction and hyperglycemia. To highlight this issue, in the case of thyroiditis, autoantibodies were not consistently measured before the onset of treatment and following the development of thyroiditis. However, in three patients, anti-thyroglobulin (Tg) and anti-microsomal antibodies were detected. In patients who developed hyperglycemia and diabetic ketoacidosis, autoantibodies were not documented. Nevertheless, these studies highlight the need for determining not only thyroid function and fasting hyperglycemia but also autoantibody status before the onset of treatment with IL-2. Additionally, the contribution of the anti-tumor vaccine to the development of autoimmunity has not been discussed.

AUTOIMMUNE ENDOCRINOPATHIES AND DIETARY FACTORS

Diet plays an important role in the development of an autoimmune endocrinopathy. Dietary factors such as fatty acids and sugars are often associated with autoimmune diabetes, and iodine, a micronutrient largely affects autoimmune thyroid diseases. Excessive consumption of foods with high nutritional values or "nutritional toxicity" has been referred to be a main cause of dysregulated glucose metabolism and obesity. Thus, nutritional habits in combination with behavioral factors determine the outcome of several autoimmune endocrinopathies.

T1DM and Dietary Factors

The prevalence of obesity has increased remarkably in the United States in the past decade, leading to increased risk of diabetes. The combination of eating large meals containing high amounts of fatty acids, fiber, cholesterol, and excess sugars with sedentary life style accounts for obesity. Obesity is often an adjunct to impaired glucose tolerance, dyslipidemia, hypertension, and type 2 diabetes. The dietary habits also vary with age, sex, and geographical distribution of the population. Although diet plays a major role in the development of endocrinopathies, only few studies have been performed that show a direct association between diet and T1DM. Interestingly, a study on 38 children aged 6–18 years showed a decreased sensitivity to insulin after intervention of 24-weeks exercise and controlled nutrition *(183)*. A large study comparing the effects of dietary changes among the non-migrated and migrated Indians to the United Kingdom showed a strong correlation between adapted high-fat diet and its effects on modulated insulin-like growth factor (IGF) and IGF-binding protein *(184)*. The study sets strong evidence for the role of environmental factors in disease etiology among genetically matched population. Both increased fatty acids and high glucose levels are shown to cause an excess stimulation of beta pancreatic cells, resulting in their functional impairment.

Very little is known about the immune-mediated effects that are caused because of excess glucose consumption; however, a direct effect of "hypersensitivity" has been observed. More studies are available that describe the effects of fatty acids on autoimmune diabetes. A study on transgenic mice with defective muscle insulin receptor signaling showed a correlation between impaired glucose tolerance and obesity *(185)*. The only fatty acids shown to be protective for glucose intolerance so far are the ones from the Omega 3 family *(186)*. The mechanisms suggested for fatty acid-induced beta-cell death involve the NF-κB signaling pathway mediated by cytokines such IL-1β and IFN-γ *(187)*. The initiation of NF-κB signaling leads to NO production, Fas expression, and beta-cell death *(188)*. However, another study has suggested that the mechanisms by which fatty acids and cytokines cause beta-cell death may be different and independent of NF-κB signaling *(189)*. Contrary to the above studies, the protective role of NF-κB activation in cytokine-mediated beta-cell death has also been described *(190)*. In summary, the effects of excess fatty acid exposure clearly involve an immune-mediated phenomenon of pancreatic beta-cell destruction; there may be more than one underlying mechanism.

Thyroid Disease and Dietary Factors

IODINE

Iodine has been known to be a major dietary factor involved in the manifestation of both hyperthyroidism (Graves' disease) and hypothyroidism (Hashimoto's thyroiditis). The interaction among genetic, hormonal, and environmental factors initiates disease. Results of epidemiological studies showing a strong association between iodine deficiency and thyroid dysfunction led to the implication of national policies on countrywide iodine supplementation in diets. Iodination of salt was introduced as a public health measure in the 1920s. The program was very successful and virtually eliminated endemic goiter in the United States *(191)*. However, the incidence of autoimmune thyroiditis increased concomitantly with the progressively increasing iodine content in the diet *(192–195)*. For example, a threefold increase in the prevalence of autoimmune thyroiditis among schoolchildren was noted once iodine deficiency was eliminated in an area of endemic goiter in northwestern Greece *(196)*. This increased iodine consumption is strongly implicated as a trigger for thyroiditis in genetically susceptible individuals *(197)*. Sources of dietary iodine include food and food additives (kelp and seaweed, iodinated salt, iodine additives to bread/flour, preservatives, and red coloring), therapeutics (amiodarone, vitamins, Lugol's solution, etc.), topical antiseptics, and contrast dyes *(198–200)*.

Besides the epidemiologic association mentioned previously, clinical studies have also associated elevated iodine intake with autoimmune thyroid diseases *(201–203)*. In one study, restriction of dietary iodine reversed the hypothyroidism in 12 of 22 patients. Seven patients with reversed hypothyroidism were re-fed iodine, and all of the seven patients became hypothyroid again *(197)*. Further clinical studies indicated that iodine restriction of many patients with primary hypothyroidism restored normal thyroid function *(204,205)*. Thus, high iodine intake facilitates the induction of autoimmune thyroid disease, but only in genetically predisposed individuals.

THYROGLOBULIN

The Tg molecule is an essential and abundant protein of the thyroid follicular cells on which the iodides are stored. Each chain of human Tg consists of 2748 amino acids, 67 (2.4%) of which are tyrosines *(206)*. Normally, no more than 25% of tyrosines are iodinated. Moreover, only four of the tyrosines per chain (positions 5, 2553, 2567, and 2746) are reputed to play a role in hormonogenesis *(207)*. These four tyrosines have high affinity for iodine. Early iodination takes place at these specific sites and in a particular sequence *(208,209)*. However, many other tyrosyl sites are available for the storage of iodine besides the four hormonogenic ones. The affinity of the other tyrosyl residues varies considerably according to their accessibility, neighboring groups, and ionization constant. With increasing degrees of iodination, structural modifications in Tg molecule may occur, leading to new molecular forms (27S or 37S) and to some extent change in its properties *(210)*. Increased binding of iodine into tyrosyl residues increases the stability of Tg and also increases its resistance to proteolysis *(211)*. The effect is presumably dependent on a greater hydrophobicity of the iodotyrosyl and iodothyronyl residues compared with tyrosyls alone *(212)*. Thus, increased iodination can have significant stereochemical effects on the Tg molecule, which can lead to the development of novel autoimmunogenic epitopes.

Variations in iodine content have also been shown to affect the immunogenic properties of Tg. Highly iodinated Tg is more immunogenic than poorly iodinated Tg. Studies in humans show that both antibody and in vitro T-cell responses decreased to background levels when Tg lacked iodine. Thyroglobulin re-iodination restored these responses *(213–215)*. Differing iodine content of human Tg can both create new epitopes and render others inaccessible, as recognized by monoclonal antibodies *(215)*. As in-depth research is difficult in human subjects, most of the mechanistic work has been performed using animal models.

Iodine-containing epitopes are more important in the induction of thyroid autoimmunity, because non-iodinated Tg fails to induce severe thyroiditis *(216,217)*. These important findings suggest that the critical effect of iodine may begin at the level of

T-cell recognition. Investigations on animal models such as (OS) chickens, (BB/W) rats, and NOD.H2^{h4} mice have provided firm support for the pathogenic role of iodine in autoimmune thyroid disease. Certain observations from animal studies remain consistent: (1) increased dietary iodine leads to earlier and more severe disease; (2) disease occurs only in a subset of genetically predisposed animals; (3) high-iodine diet increases the immune responses to Tg; and (4) iodine restriction retards lymphocytic infiltration.

THE NOD.H2^{H4} MOUSE

Among the animal models of thyroid diseases NOD.H2^{h4} has been the most relevant model of spontaneous autoimmune thyroiditis. NOD.H2^{h4} was developed at Merck Laboratories by Dr. Linda Wicker and colleagues. The mouse line was generated by crossing the NOD with the B10.A(4R) strains and extensively backcrossing to the NOD. The strain expresses the MHC-II (I-A^k) background permissive for thyroiditis *(218)*. None of the mice develop diabetes; however, a high proportion of older animals show an evidence of thyroiditis (50% in NOD.H2^{h4} vs 5% in the NOD strain). Furthermore, the incidence of thyroiditis in NOD.H2^{h4} rise to 90% if excess iodine is added to their drinking water *(219)*. The disease pathology is similar to that of autoimmune thyroiditis of humans, characterized by chronic infiltration of mononuclear cells, including CD4, CD8, B cells, macrophages, and dendritic cells *(220–222)*. Furthermore, severity of disease correlates with autoantibody to Tg. The previously described findings show a close analogy between mouse and human thyroiditis and that the NOD.H2^{h4} is a relevant model of human autoimmune thyroid disease.

INITIATION OF DISEASE PATHOLOGY

Both CD4 and CD8 T cells are required for the initiation of thyroiditis in the iodine-enhanced NOD.H2^{h4} model; however, only CD4 cells are required to maintain chronicity of the disease, because depletion of CD4 cells, but not of CD8, reduced disease severity, suggesting that CD8 cells are not necessary for maintaining progression to severe thyroiditis *(221)*. It is further demonstrated that B cells, especially early in life, were required for the initiation of disease in NOD.H2^{h4} mice *(223)*. These investigators depleted B cells with an anti-IgM treatment and found that thyroiditis was severely compromised *(223)*. Passive transfer of antibody or reconstitution of adults with B cells did not induce thyroiditis, suggesting further that there was early requirement for B cells and that B cells are important in antigen presentation. There is a little evidence for the effects of differentially iodinated Tg on the role of antigen-presenting cells (APCs), although THs and other iodinated compounds are known to play a role in the transition of monocytes to dendritic cells mediated by components such as granulocyte-monocyte colony-stimulating factor (GM-CSF), TNF-α, and IL-6 and are shown to considerably affect the immune responses *(224,225)*. Thus, it is possible that iodine acts by altering APCs directly to initiate the events that lead to thyroiditis. It is also likely that critical events in determining pathogenicity are downstream of these events. These results also suggest that the critical events for the initiation of diseases differ from the chronic stage of disease. Once the disease is established, no reduction in disease is found even after excess iodine is discontinued, suggesting that the initial stimuli are especially important in determining the future course of this disease.

IODINE AND ADHESION MOLECULES

Our recent studies showed that iodine provides an initial stimulus for ICAM-1 upregulation and leads to progression of thyroid disease. NOD.H2^{h4} mouse thyrocytes express ICAM-1 constitutively, which is considerably enhanced on a few weeks of iodine feeding (8,226). Further evidence came from our in vitro experiments where thyroid cells were isolated by magnetic beads and were cultured without any interference of mononuclear cells. An upregulated expression of ICAM-1 was noticed within 24 h after stimulation with iodine (8). Therefore, iodine by itself could foster increased expression of ICAM-1, which accounts for initial stimulus in disease.

ICAM-1 is shown to play a major role in early stages of inflammatory immune responses that help to determine the localization of inflammatory mononuclear cells. Several similar studies in humans have also reported an enhanced ICAM-1 expression in the thyroid glands of both Graves' disease and Hashimoto's thyroiditis patients (227,228). Using the NOD.H2^{h4} mouse model, we have expanded these findings to understand the mechanisms of ICAM-1 regulation.

The ICAM-1 gene promoter has multiple transcription binding sites with at least three different transcriptional initiation sites. Many stimuli can promote ICAM-1 expression that includes certain cytokines, viruses, radiation, retinoic acid, and oxidants. Iodine is taken up by the thyrocyte, organified, and stored on the Tg molecule through the enzymatic reaction of thyroperoxidase. During this process, reactive oxygen species (ROS) such as superoxide anion and hydrogen peroxide are generated. Both of these ROS are known to stimulate the *ICAM-1* gene promoter. In genetically susceptible individuals, this process is triggered through diverse small stimuli, so that ICAM-1 is overexpressed in the thyroid gland. In NOD.H2^{h4} mice ROS blocking with specific pharmacological inhibitors suppressed ICAM-1 expression on iodine treated thyrocytes in vitro (our unpublished data). The upregulated ICAM-1 was due solely to iodine, as no immune cells were present in the cultures. Thus, iodine can affect the thyrocyte *directly* as well as *indirectly* through the cytokine production by infiltrating lymphocytes.

ENDOCRINOPATHIES AND BEHAVIORAL FACTORS

T1DM and Cigarette Smoking

Cigarette smoking is a major public health concern in many countries and is considered a risk factor for T1DM. Only a few studies are available to provide direct evidence for the autoimmune nature of disease, and no study has revealed the immunogenic effects of tobacco on disease development. A retrospective study assessed the effects of smoking on circulating ICAM (cICAM)-1 in young adults. The levels of cICAM-1 were found to be significantly enhanced in a dose-dependent manner (229). Similarly, another study found increased levels of vascular ICAM (VCAM)-1 and endothelium ICAM (ECAM)-1 in T1DM patients with smoking habits. Most studies conducted are based on the information after the disease has established.

The exact mechanism responsible for smoking-induced T1DM is not clear; however, considering increased levels of plasma cICAM-1 and cVCAM-1, it may be speculated that enhanced inflammation, cell–cell interaction, and inflammatory cytokine secretion could be one mechanism of beta-cell destruction. In the absence of any antibody data, it is difficult to conclude whether the disease is truly of an autoimmune nature.

Thyroid Disease and Cigarette Smoking

A meta-analysis reviewed 25 studies pertaining to smoking history and Graves' disease with opthalmopathy and various forms of hyperthyroidism and hypothyroidism *(230)*. A dose response relationship was described between increasing risk of disease among current smokers. Stronger association (odds ratio 4.4) for ever-smoking subjects were seen with Graves' disease with ophthalmopathy. Strong association (odds ratio 3.3) among current smokers was found with Graves' disease compared with former smokers. Sex-specific analysis showed a stronger association of Graves' disease in women smokers. Fewer studies are available pertaining to smoking and hypothyroidism, Hashimoto's thyroiditis, or subclinical hypothyroidism *(230,231)*. In a study on 759 women in the Netherlands, a decreased prevalence of thyroid peroxidase antibodies was reported *(232)*. Yet, another study on 115,109 women reported smoking as a risk factor in Graves' hyperthyroidism (95% confidence interval), but the study does not present any antibody data *(233)*. The Denmark study on 132 same-sex, twin pairs showed a significant increase in clinically overt autoimmune thyroid disease in smokers as compared with their twin non-smokers *(234)*. Contradicting results were reported by National Health and Nutrition Examination Survey III (NHANES III) *(235)*. The study evaluated the levels of serum cotinine levels to distinguish smokers from non-smokers. A negative correlation among smokers and thyroid autoimmunity was found.

Very little is known about the mechanisms of cigarette smoking-induced thyroid diseases. Few studies show that thiocyanate a chemical substance generated by smoking may affect the thyroid gland functioning. Thiocyanate and perchlorate ions are known as inhibitors of iodine-trapping mechanism (*see* Endocrine Disease and Occupational Exposure). A relationship between cigarette smoking and Hashimoto's thyroiditis is well described *(234,236)*. High levels of serum thiocyanate were detected in smokers who had hypothyroidism but not hyperthyroidism *(236)*.

T1DM and Breastfeeding

Literature analysis showed a small protective effect of breastfeeding in infants and a few harmful effects of formula foods with respect to T1DM. Similarly, early introduction of cow's milk and dairy products to infants did not show any significant harmful effects on islet cell autoimmunity in children. A study on 10 children who progressed to T1DM showed no association between islet cell autoimmunity and duration of cow's milk or breastfeeding *(237)*. Similar findings were reported by the German baby diabetes study conducted on 1610 children *(238)*. However, children with increased genetic susceptibly (HLA-DQB1 alleles) were found to be at a higher risk for developing beta-cell autoimmunity after early introduction of cow's milk or short-term breastfeeding *(239)*. A recent pilot study has shown the interference of diet in the manipulation of spontaneous beta-cell autoimmunity in infants with HLA-DQB1 genotype. Therefore, most human studies have their limitations in providing a strong association between infant dietary factors and autoimmune diabetes.

Autoimmune Thyroiditis and Breastfeeding

Reduced breastfeeding practices because of changing life styles and demanding work needs of women have significant effects on infants' thyroid health. Breastfeeding is often replaced with several formula feeds with various combinations, which have put infants at a higher risk of thyroid autoimmune disease. More research studies have investigated the effects of infant formula foods and cows' milk feeding on children's health. Perchlorate, a goitrogenic anion, is well known as a competitive inhibitor of the sodium iodide transporter and has been widely detected in cow's milk throughout the United States. A study has indicated that almost 80% of perchlorate is metabolized in the lumen and could be a possible risk factor to cattle itself *(240)*. The remaining proportion that is fed from cows' milk could equally be goitrogenic in infants and can impair thyroid and neurodevelopment *(241)*. The effect of perchlorate on adults on the contrary had no significant effects on overall health of occupational workers that were exposed for an average of 1.7 years. No significant changes in the serum TSH and Tg concentrations were reported, but serum T4, free T4, and free T3 although slightly increased were significant as compared with controls *(242)*. Long-lasting protective effects of breastfeeding are well documented *(243,244)*. The effect of infant formula food is still controversial because of variations in iodine content in each preparation. A food survey study on eight infant formulas and 18 brands of cows' milk from 2001 to 2002 reported extremely high variations in iodine levels. The iodine content in infant food was found $23.5 \pm 13.8\,\mu g/5\,oz$ and in the cows' milk $116.0 \pm 22.1\,\mu g/250\,ml$. Thyroid gland volumes were found to be greatly reduced in infants who were partially or exclusively fed iodine-supplemented or iodine-free formula *(245)*. Interestingly, infants with mothers who had Hashimoto's thyroiditis or Graves' disease had normal thyroid functioning and T3, T4 levels on breastfeeding as compared with formula-fed infants *(246)*. More importantly, even with low maternal iodine status, breastfeeding compensated for iodine in infants *(247)*. Therefore, it is certain that breastfeeding protects from thyroid dysfunctions during early childhood.

ENDOCRINE DISEASE AND OCCUPATIONAL EXPOSURE

Exposure to industrial byproducts such as polychlorinated biphenyls, hexachlorobenzene, and organochlorine pesticides, thiocyanate and perchlorates, has been implicated in the development of autoimmune thyroid disease *(248,249)*. Increased levels of TSH, decreased T4, and anti-thyroid antibodies were detected in workers exposed to polychlorinated biphenyls in a manufacturing plant in East Slovakia *(250)*. Evidence of increased thyroid size and other thyroid-related defects because of exposure to dithiocarbomates and ethylenebisdithiocarbomates has been documented *(251,252)*. A longitudinal study on occupational workers in a factory of ammonia production plant studied the effects of perchlorate and thiocyanate on thyroid function. Both chemicals are associated with iodine uptake directly in the thyroid at the sodium–iodide symporter level. The study reported a small but significant increase in the levels of serum T4, free T4 and total T3 levels among the workers with 3-day (12 h/day) exposure compared with 3-day off workers *(242)*. It is important to consider the intensity and duration of exposure, combined with age, sex, and genetics that alter diseases pathology.

A large body of data are available from many examples of both animals and humans showing that chemicals directly initiate and exacerbate the pathological immune process, mutate genes, alter regulatory and immune effector pathways, and modify immune tolerance. Systemic allergenic reactions sometimes resemble an autoimmune-like phenomenon and progress to an autoimmune disease. In systemic allergenic reactions, an immune response may be directed to the chemical compound, whereas in autoimmune process, the immune reaction is directed toward the autoantigens. The basic mechanisms are summarized later in this chapter.

Chemicals or xenobiotics alter thyroid gland functioning either directly by disrupting the thyroid structure or indirectly by disrupting the action of regulatory enzymes involved at various levels of TH synthesis. THs T3 and T4 are produced in the thyroid gland from where they are released into the circulation and transported to different tissues. Chemicals such as thiocyanate and perchlorate inhibit the uptake of iodine at the symporter level or during thyrotropin stimulation, affecting TH synthesis *(253)*. Chemicals such as methimazole, aminotriazole, and thionamides inhibit TH synthesis by blocking organic binding of iodine to Tg molecules and thyroperoxidase activity *(253–255)*. Dithiocarbamates and ethylenebisdithiocarbamates on the one hand disrupt thyroid function similarly affecting the catalytic activity of thyroperoxidase *(252)*. Polyhalogenated aromatic hydrocarbons on the other hand affect TH synthesis at the tissue level by inducing enzymes such as uridine diphosphoglucuronosyl transferases that eliminate THs and affecting hepatic metabolism *(256–259)*.

Therefore, the mechanism of action of each compound may vary with its nature and so its effects on immune regulation.

Endocrine Diseases and Irradiation

Exposure of environmental radiation and its correlation with thyroidal dysfunction has generated considerable attention since the Chernobyl accident in 1986. The steam explosion from the Chernobyl nuclear reactor resulted in release of about 5% of the total radioactive core into the atmosphere and downwind. Over the last three decades, several studies on thyroid disease have been conducted on cohorts exposed to radiation in Chernobyl, Ukraine, Russia, and Belarus *(260)*. Studies on exposure to other ionizing radiations after the atomic bomb explosion in Hiroshima and Nagasaki have also been published. In the United States, the National Cancer Institute has provided a report in 1997 for the thyroid doses in the US population, resulting from fallouts from nuclear weapon testing at the Nevada Test Site *(261)*.

Thyroid Disease and Ionizing Radiation

Over the past two decades, several studies have suggested an association between environmental radiation exposure and risk of autoimmune thyroid disease. Most studies have assessed their diagnosis based on antithyroid antibodies, the size of thyroid gland, and ultrasonography of thyroid gland *(262)*. Significant increase in the incidence of hypothyroidism after radioactive iodine therapy was reported *(263)*. These studies establish a correlation between environmental radiation exposures with thyroid function.

Therapeutic use of radioactive isotope of iodine is over 50 years old, a dose of 15 mCi or 550 MBq is known to be safe. The thyroid being one of the most radiosensitive tissues is rapidly affected in terms of its function as well as pathophysiology because of radiation exposure. The genetic susceptibility of an individual together with dietary variations contributes to the initiation of the disease.

A study of 888 school children in the age group of 10–15 years from Chechelsk in Belarus assessed the effects of radiation exposure in a heavily contaminated area during the Chernobyl disaster *(264)*. Age-matched 521 children from Bobruisk, Belarus, were studied to represent a less-contaminated area. Thyroid examination was carried out in all the children; blood tests and ultrasonography were done in those who were found with enlarged thyroid glands/goiters. The study showed no statistical significant difference in thyroid function tests between the two groups of children. The incidence of diffused goiter was significantly higher ($p < 0.01$) in the less-contaminated region *(264)*.

Another study on occupational exposure to ionizing radiation in 4299 subjects described a high risk of autoimmune thyroid disease. TPO antibody was assessed, and ultrasound of the thyroid gland was performed in patients with higher antibody levels. Long-term exposure up to 5 years was evaluated. The results showed that subjects with long-term exposure to ionizing radiations were at a higher risk of developing autoimmune thyroid disease *(265)*.

In the animal studies, the pathophysiological effects of ionizing radiations leading to thyroid disease have been observed in a closed colony of beagle dogs. Thyroid neoplasia in addition to thyroid dysfunction has also been observed *(266)*.

Two different mechanisms by which radiation may cause an autoimmune phenomenon have been proposed. Radiation exposure may directly injure the thyroid cell or may affect the DNA methylation process of T cells, thereby indirectly modulating the immune responses.

SUMMARY OF MECHANISMS

Autoimmunity may be initiated by various mechanisms involving changes in autologous antigens or alterations in immune regulation (Fig. 1). The pathological consequence of an autoimmune response depends initially on the stimulation of helper/inducer T cells reactive with self-antigens. The activated CD4+ T cells secrete a combination of cytokines and other mediators that direct the quantity and quality of the subsequent immune response. Cytotoxic CD8+ T cells penetrate tissue spaces and attack cells bearing requisite surface antigens complexed with the appropriate MHC product. Their inflammogenic products indirectly damage tissues through delayed hypersensitivity-like reactions. Autoantibodies react with accessible cell antigens and mediate injury directly or indirectly. Mast cells, macrophages, and NK cells, activated by cytokines, have the potential to augment tissue damage. These several mechanisms do not operate in isolation; rather, multiple processes act in unison in most autoimmune diseases *(267,268)*.

The interference of an environmental factor with the ongoing immune process could alter the immune responses in various ways. The outcome of these interactions is essentially regulated by the quality, quantity, and duration of the exposure of one or more environmental factors. As we discuss here, the interaction may have an impact at the level of antigen processing, T- or B-cell responses, gene mutations or at thymic regulation.

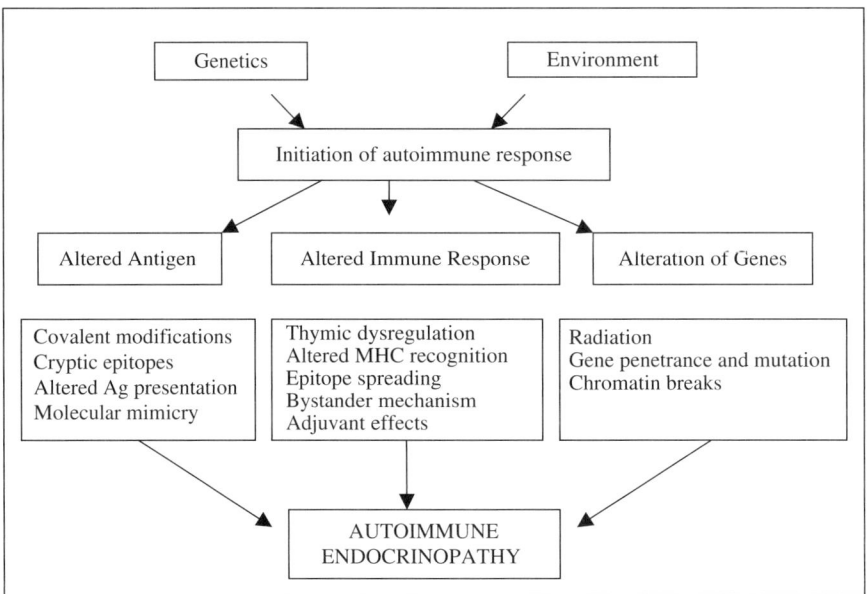

Fig. 1. Summary of mechanisms.

Altered Antigen

As a result of metabolic process, certain drugs and chemicals get converted into reactive electrophils, such as haptens or low-molecular weight compounds (LMWC). These LMWC are too small to be recognized by the T cells, but on conjugation with a larger self-protein, they may form new self-antigenic structure or a hapten–carrier complex, which can then induce an autoimmune-like response leading to an autoimmune disease. Termed as antigenic covalent modifications, these reactions form the basis of "hapten-hypothesis" *(269)*. These complexes are processed by MHC molecules of APCs and presented as neoantigens or altered self-antigens *(269)*. Initially, the immune responses are directed exclusively to the hapten or the altered self-antigen, but after a certain time period, autoimmune responses to native self-antigens may arise. For example, trifluoroacetyle (TFA) combines with the liver protein S100 to form hapten–carrier complex TFA-S100 and has been shown to induce autoimmune hepatitis in mice *(270)*. Another study on mice exposed to mercury ($HgCl_2$) revealed that T cells of treated mice first responded to mercury-modified fibrillarin, but after 8 weeks, a T-cell response to native fibrillarin epitope was also found *(271)*. This process, referred to as determinant or epitope spreading *(272,273)*, may explain why patients after exposure to certain drugs or other chemicals sometimes develop autoantibodies to unchanged self-antigens.

In certain cases of drugs such as procainamide and hydralazine, which are shown to induce a lupus-like autoimmune disorder, discontinuation of the drug causes the autoimmune reaction to cease. In such cases, it is believed that the initiation of an autoimmune response is directly dependent on the availability of the metabolic product (hapten) that contributes in the formation of altered self-antigen. Furthermore, these drugs are known to be activated by the acetylation pathway of drug metabolism. Slow acetylation of these drugs in genetically predisposed patients lead to accumulation of amines causing lupus-like disease. Removal of free amines from the systems recovered the patients (274). Similarly penicillamine has been associated with pemphigus and myasthenia gravis and other autoimmune diseases. Discontinuation of D-penicillamine favored the recovery of the patient (275). It is also suggested that the drug can unmask the antigens to have immunomodulatory effects (275). In these examples, ceasing of the administered drugs usually results in remission of disease. Such examples show that the response to altered antigen often does not extend to unaltered, native self-antigen.

Changed Antigen Processing—Structural Alteration of the Antigen

An autoimmune response may be caused by a chemical, drug, or metal ions by changes in antigen processing. It has been shown that interaction of certain metals such as gold and iron may interfere with antigen processing such that the cryptic epitopes end up in the MHC groove in a very high concentration, so that they can be presented to the T cells (276–278). Gold salts [Au (III)] rapidly oxidize proteins during their processing and causes changes in the mononuclear phagocytes. Once the antigen has been processed, T-cell recognition does not require the presence of gold. The APCs then deliver receptor-specific signals to T lymphocytes accompanied by costimulatory signals to elicit an autoimmune response (276). Chemicals such as para-substituted benzene derivatives have similarly been shown to cause changes in the structure of antigens that are recognized by the T cells (279). Therefore, interference of chemicals and metal salts may cause changes in antigen processing, resulting in its structural alteration and presentation of cryptic epitopes.

Altered Self/Altered MHC

Sometimes drugs containing metallic ions or their metabolic byproducts may directly alter MHC molecules when a hapten–carrier complex is being processed. This hypothesis is an extension of the hapten-hypothesis proposing that T cells recognize altered MHC primarily on the B cells of a healthy individual such that they provide "help" signals to autoreactive B cells carrying these molecules to produce autoantibodies (280,281). This hypothesis is supported mainly by studies with chemicals such as certain metals such as nickel and gold that can alter MHC molecule to induce an autoimmune disease (282). The T cells in this case recognize antigen that is presented by MHC molecules of a B cell, the help provided by T cells is therefore a non-cognate help because both cells recognize different antigens. Thus, B- and T-cell cooperation because of altered self may induce an autoimmune response initially triggered by a reactive chemical.

Cross-Reactivity/Molecular Mimicry

Epitopes of an infectious agent may closely resemble epitopes found in the host cells. The phenomenon is commonly described as molecular mimicry. Infectious agents or chemicals may stimulate autoimmune responses by inducing generation of cross-reactive T cells (283,284). Once the cross-reactive T cells are generated, the autoimmune responses lead to autoimmune disease. Cross-reactivity between the host antigen and a pathogen resulting in autoimmunity may occur at the T-cell level or at the antibody level. A study performed on human T cells isolated from rheumatoid heart disease patient revealed the molecular mimicry between streptococcal M protein and cardiac myosin *(283)*. The potential sites on T-cell clones for molecular mimicry were also identified *(283)*. In another example, CD4+ T-cell clones isolated from human Chagas disease cardiomyopathy patients were shown to cross-react with the immunodominant B13 protein of protozoan parasite *Trypanosoma cruzi*, describing a molecular mimicry with human cardiac myosin *(285)*. Furthermore, the definition of cross-reactivity implies that T cells may recognize not only the best-fitting MHC–peptide complex but also different peptides in the groove of a related MHC molecule *(286,287)*. It appears that T-cell clones are not stringent with respect to the structure of the peptide they recognize. For example, in the absence of the initiating agent, some T cells respond to syngeneic MHC complex of an autologous peptide. The implications of such reactions are that specificity of drug-reactive T cells may be highly MHC restricted yet not drug specific. Cross-reactivity of T cells thus caused by certain chemicals and drugs may play an important role in the recruitment and expansion of autoreactive T cell, resulting in an autoimmune disease.

Altered Gene Expression and Gene Penetrance

Normal T-cell functioning requires appropriate levels of DNA methylation. Defective methylation may lead to hyperactive or hypoactive genes. Ultraviolet radiation, drugs, and diet are common environmental factors that can alter the DNA methylation patterns. Richardson in 2003 *(288)* hypothesized that altered gene expression because of changes in DNA methylation may contribute to the pathogenesis of autoimmunity. Antiarrhythmic agents such as procainamide and hydrolyzine, which are known to induce lupus-like diseases, have been reported to inhibit DNA methylation in some cases *(289)*. This results in increased expression of the adhesion molecule leukocyte function-associated antigen-1 (LFA-1) and induction of autoreactivity in human and murine T cells *(290)*. In addition to the environmental factors, age-dependent changes in the T cell and DNA methylation may contribute to the development of some forms of autoimmunity in the elderly *(291)*.

Thymic Regulation

Neonatal thymectomy of 2- to 4-day-old mice can lead to organ-specific autoimmune disease *(292)*. These effects are probably because of the preferential removal of a population of CD4+ CD25+ regulatory T cells that have been characterized for their role in anti-tumor immunity as well as in the induction of autoimmunity *(293)*. Cyclophosphamide treatment exerts similar effects and can enhance autoimmunity *(294)*. Neonatal treatment with methylcholanthrene induces thymocyte apoptosis and is thought to disrupt the development of suppressor or regulatory T cells *(295)*. These examples of studies in mice suggest that non-specific suppressor cells are formed during the first three days of development and have an active role in self-tolerance *(292)*. Replenishing these cells through adoptive transfer reduces autoimmunity *(296)*.

CONCLUSIONS

Multiple genes and environmental factors interacting in various ways account for the etiology of autoimmune diseases. It is, however, difficult to search out individual factors initiating or modifying a particular disease. Incomplete gene penetrance may delay or obviate induction, so that not all susceptible individuals develop an autoimmune disease. Several disease susceptibility loci may interact differently, or different alleles may cause disease in different populations. In other words, it becomes difficult to identify disease susceptibility genes, ascertain the number and relationship of disease-associated loci and quantitate their effects in inheritance. To further understand the complex origin of an autoimmune disease, a full account of the numerous non-hereditary agents must be sorted out from genetic factors. Although, a great deal of circumstantial evidence strongly implicates infectious, chemical and physical agents act as adjuncts in the etiology of autoimmune disease, there are but few specific examples of environmental triggers in human autoimmune endocrinopathies and even less understanding of how they act.

REFERENCES

1. Hall R, Stanbury JB. Familial studies of autoimmune thyroiditis. *Clin Exp Immunol* 1967;2(Suppl):719–25.
2. Warram JH, Krolewski AS, Gottlieb MS, Kahn CR. Differences in risk of insulin-dependent diabetes in offspring of diabetic mothers and diabetic fathers. *N Engl J Med* 1984;311(3):149–52.
3. Roitt IM, Doniach D. A reassessment of studies on the aggregation of thyroid autoimmunity in families of thyroiditis patients. *Clin Exp Immunol* 1967;2(Suppl):727–36.
4. Barbesino G, Tomer Y, Concepcion E, Davies TF, Greenberg DA. Linkage analysis of candidate genes in autoimmune thyroid disease: 1. Selected immunoregulatory genes. International Consortium for the Genetics of Autoimmune Thyroid Disease. *J Clin Endocrinol Metab* 1998;83(5):1580–4.
5. Smyth D, Cooper JD, Collins JE, et al. Replication of an association between the lymphoid tyrosine phosphatase locus (LYP/PTPN22) with type 1 diabetes, and evidence for its role as a general autoimmunity locus. *Diabetes* 2004;53(11):3020–3.
6. Dittmar M, Kahaly GJ. Immunoregulatory and susceptibility genes in thyroid and polyglandular autoimmunity. *Thyroid* 2005;15(3):239–50.
7. Dallos T, Kovacs L. CTLA-4 and the genetic predisposition to autoimmunity. *Bratisl Lek Listy* 2005;106(2):55–62.
8. Sharma RB, Alegria JD, Talor MV, Rose NR, Caturegli P, Burek CL. Iodine and IFN-gamma synergistically enhance intercellular adhesion molecule 1 expression on NOD.H2h4 mouse thyrocytes. *J Immunol* 2005;174(12):7740–5.
9. Rose NR, Bacon LD, Sundick RS. Genetic determinants of thyroiditis in the OS chicken. *Transplant Rev* 1976;31:264–85.
10. Kaprio J, Tuomilehto J, Koskenvuo M, et al. Concordance for type 1 (insulin-dependent) and type 2 (non-insulin-dependent) diabetes mellitus in a population-based cohort of twins in Finland. *Diabetologia* 1992;35(11):1060–7.
11. Hyttinen V, Kaprio J, Kinnunen L, Koskenvuo M, Tuomilehto J. Genetic liability of type 1 diabetes and the onset age among 22,650 young Finnish twin pairs: a nationwide follow-up study. *Diabetes* 2003;52(4):1052–5.
12. Ringold DA, Nicoloff JT, Kesler M, Davis H, Hamilton A, Mack T. Further evidence for a strong genetic influence on the development of autoimmune thyroid disease: the California twin study. *Thyroid* 2002;12(8):647–53.
13. Whitacre CC. Sex differences in autoimmune disease. *Nat Immunol* 2001;2(9):777–80.
14. Chiovato L, Lapi P, Fiore E, Tonacchera M, Pinchera A. Thyroid autoimmunity and female gender. *J Endocrinol Invest* 1993;16(5):384–91.
15. Lu R, Burman KD, Jonklaas J. Transient Graves' hyperthyroidism during pregnancy in a patient with Hashimoto's hypothyroidism. *Thyroid* 2005;15(7):725–9.

16. Leclere J, Weryha G. Stress and auto-immune endocrine diseases. *Horm Res* 1989;31(1–2):90–3.

17. Karvonen M, Tuomilehto J, Libman I, LaPorte R. A review of the recent epidemiological data on the worldwide incidence of type 1 (insulin-dependent) diabetes mellitus. World Health Organization DIAMOND Project Group. *Diabetologia* 1993;36(10):883–92.

18. Rose Noel R. AM. From infection to autoimmunity: the adjuvant effect. *ASM News/Features* 2003;69(3):132–7.

19. Weets I, Kaufman L, Van der Auwera B, et al. Seasonality in clinical onset of type 1 diabetes in belgian patients above the age of 10 is restricted to HLA-DQ2/DQ8-negative males, which explains the male to female excess in incidence. *Diabetologia* 2004;47(4):614–21.

20. Onkamo P, Vaananen S, Karvonen M, Tuomilehto J. Worldwide increase in incidence of Type I diabetes–the analysis of the data on published incidence trends. *Diabetologia* 1999;42(12): 1395–403.

21. Viskari HR, Koskela P, Lonnrot M, et al. Can enterovirus infections explain the increasing incidence of type 1 diabetes? *Diabetes Care* 2000;23(3):414–6.

22. Forrest JM, Menser MA, Burgess JA. High frequency of diabetes mellitus in young adults with congenital rubella. *Lancet* 1971;2(7720):332–4.

23. Forrest JM, Menser MA, Harley JD. Diabetes mellitus and congenital rubella. *Pediatrics* 1969;44(3):445–7.

24. Forrest JM, Turnbull FM, Sholler GF, et al. Gregg's congenital rubella patients 60 years later. *Med J Aust* 2002;177(11–12):664–7.

25. Ou D, Mitchell LA, Metzger DL, Gillam S, Tingle AJ. Cross-reactive rubella virus and glutamic acid decarboxylase (65 and 67) protein determinants recognised by T cells of patients with type I diabetes mellitus. *Diabetologia* 2000;43(6):750–62.

26. McEvoy RC, Fedun B, Cooper LZ, et al. Children at high risk of diabetes mellitus: New York studies of families with diabetes and of children with congenital rubella syndrome. *Adv Exp Med Biol* 1988;246:221–7.

27. Ginsberg-Fellner F, Witt ME, Fedun B, et al. Diabetes mellitus and autoimmunity in patients with the congenital rubella syndrome. *Rev Infect Dis* 1985;7(Suppl 1):S170–6.

28. Kawasaki E, Eisenbarth GS. High-throughput radioassays for autoantibodies to recombinant autoantigens. *Front Biosci* 2000;5:E181–90.

29. Peterson C, Campbell IL, Harrison LC. Lack of specificity of islet cell surface antibodies (ICSA) in IDDM. *Diabetes Res Clin Pract* 1992;17(1):33–42.

30. Viskari H, Paronen J, Keskinen P, et al. Humoral beta-cell autoimmunity is rare in patients with the congenital rubella syndrome. *Clin Exp Immunol* 2003;133(3):378–83.

31. Gundersen E. Is diabetes of infectious origin? *J Infect Dis* 1927;41:197–202.

32. Helmke K, Otten A, Willems WR, et al. Islet cell antibodies and the development of diabetes mellitus in relation to mumps infection and mumps vaccination. *Diabetologia* 1986;29(1):30–3.

33. Parkkonen P, Hyoty H, Koskinen L, Leinikki P. Mumps virus infects beta cells in human fetal islet cell cultures upregulating the expression of HLA class I molecules. *Diabetologia* 1992;35(1):63–9.

34. Cavallo MG, Baroni MG, Toto A, et al. Viral infection induces cytokine release by beta islet cells. *Immunology* 1992;75(4):664–8.

35. Prince GA, Jenson AB, Billups LC, Notkins AL. Infection of human pancreatic beta cell cultures with mumps virus. *Nature* 1978;271(5641):158–61.

36. Hyoty H, Hiltunen M, Reunanen A, et al. Decline of mumps antibodies in type 1 (insulin-dependent) diabetic children and a plateau in the rising incidence of type 1 diabetes after introduction of the mumps-measles-rubella vaccine in Finland. Childhood Diabetes in Finland Study Group. *Diabetologia* 1993;36(12):1303–8.

37. Otonkoski T, Roivainen M, Vaarala O, et al. Neonatal type I diabetes associated with maternal echovirus 6 infection: a case report. *Diabetologia* 2000;43(10):1235–8.

38. Yoon JW, Austin M, Onodera T, Notkins AL. Isolation of a virus from the pancreas of a child with diabetic ketoacidosis. *N Engl J Med* 1979;300(21):1173–9.

39. Yoon JW, Onodera T, Jenson AB, Notkins AL. Virus-induced diabetes mellitus. XI. Replication of coxsackie B3 virus in human pancreatic beta cell cultures. *Diabetes* 1978;27(7):778–81.

40. Lau G. Acute fulminant, fatal coxsackie B virus infection: a report of two cases. *Ann Acad Med Singapore* 1994;23(6):917–20.

41. Helfand RF, Gary HE, Jr, Freeman CY, Anderson LJ, Pallansch MA. Serologic evidence of an association between enteroviruses and the onset of type 1 diabetes mellitus. Pittsburgh Diabetes Research Group. *J Infect Dis* 1995;172(5):1206–11.

42. Schernthaner G, Banatvala JE, Scherbaum W, et al. Coxsackie-B-virus-specific IgM responses, complement-fixing islet-cell antibodies, HLA DR antigens, and C-peptide secretion in insulin-dependent diabetes mellitus. *Lancet* 1985;2(8456):630–2.

43. Dahlquist GG, Forsberg J, Hagenfeldt L, Boman J, Juto P. Increased prevalence of enteroviral RNA in blood spots from newborn children who later developed type 1 diabetes: a population-based case-control study. *Diabetes Care* 2004;27(1):285–6.

44. Juhela S, Hyoty H, Hinkkanen A, et al. T cell responses to enterovirus antigens and to beta-cell autoantigens in unaffected children positive for IDDM-associated autoantibodies. *J Autoimmun* 1999;12(4):269–78.

45. Juhela S, Hyoty H, Roivainen M, et al. T-cell responses to enterovirus antigens in children with type 1 diabetes. *Diabetes* 2000;49(8):1308–13.

46. Kawashima H, Ihara T, Ioi H, et al. Enterovirus-related type 1 diabetes mellitus and antibodies to glutamic acid decarboxylase in Japan. *J Infect* 2004;49(2):147–51.

47. Nairn C, Galbraith DN, Taylor KW, Clements GB. Enterovirus variants in the serum of children at the onset of type 1 diabetes mellitus. *Diabet Med* 1999;16(6):509–13.

48. Yin H, Berg AK, Tuvemo T, Frisk G. Enterovirus RNA is found in peripheral blood mononuclear cells in a majority of type 1 diabetic children at onset. *Diabetes* 2002;51(6):1964–71.

49. Banatvala JE, Bryant J, Schernthaner G, et al. Coxsackie B, mumps, rubella, and cytomegalovirus specific IgM responses in patients with juvenile-onset insulin-dependent diabetes mellitus in Britain, Austria, and Australia. *Lancet* 1985;1(8443):1409–12.

50. Jones DB, Crosby I. Proliferative lymphocyte responses to virus antigens homologous to GAD65 in IDDM. *Diabetologia* 1996;39(11):1318–24.

51. D'Alessio DJ. A case-control study of group B Coxsackievirus immunoglobulin M antibody prevalence and HLA-DR antigens in newly diagnosed cases of insulin-dependent diabetes mellitus. *Am J Epidemiol* 1992;135(12):1331–8.

52. Salminen K, Sadeharju K, Lonnrot M, et al. Enterovirus infections are associated with the induction of beta-cell autoimmunity in a prospective birth cohort study. *J Med Virol* 2003;69(1):91–8.

53. Serreze DV, Wasserfall C, Ottendorfer EW, et al. Diabetes acceleration or prevention by a coxsackievirus B4 infection: critical requirements for both interleukin-4 and gamma interferon. *J Virol* 2005;79(2):1045–52.

54. Volta C, Carano N, Street ME, Bernasconi S. Atypical subacute thyroiditis caused by Epstein-Barr virus infection in a three-year-old girl. *Thyroid* 2005;15(10):1189–91.

55. Volpe R, Row VV, Ezrin C. Circulating viral and thyroid antibodies in subacute thyroiditis. *J Clin Endocrinol Metab* 1967;27(9):1275–84.

56. Mori K, Yoshida K, Funato T, et al. Failure in detection of Epstein-Barr virus and cytomegalovirus in specimen obtained by fine needle aspiration biopsy of thyroid in patients with subacute thyroiditis. *Tohoku J Exp Med* 1998;186(1):13–7.

57. Tran A, Quaranta JF, Benzaken S, et al. High prevalence of thyroid autoantibodies in a prospective series of patients with chronic hepatitis C before interferon therapy. *Hepatology* 1993;18(2):253–7.

58. Ganne-Carrie N, Medini A, Coderc E, et al. Latent autoimmune thyroiditis in untreated patients with HCV chronic hepatitis: a case-control study. *J Autoimmun* 2000;14(2):189–93.

59. Fernandez-Soto L, Gonzalez A, Escobar-Jimenez F, et al. Increased risk of autoimmune thyroid disease in hepatitis C vs hepatitis B before, during, and after discontinuing interferon therapy. *Arch Intern Med* 1998;158(13):1445–8.

60. Preziati D, La Rosa L, Covini G, et al. Autoimmunity and thyroid function in patients with chronic active hepatitis treated with recombinant interferon alpha-2a. *Eur J Endocrinol* 1995;132(5):587–93.

61. Antonelli A, Ferri C, Pampana A, et al. Thyroid disorders in chronic hepatitis C. *Am J Med* 2004;117(1):10–3.

62. Metcalfe RA, Ball G, Kudesia G, Weetman AP. Failure to find an association between hepatitis C virus and thyroid autoimmunity. *Thyroid* 1997;7(3):421–4.

63. Marazuela M, Garcia-Buey L, Gonzalez-Fernandez B, et al. Thyroid autoimmune disorders in patients with chronic hepatitis C before and during interferon-alpha therapy. *Clin Endocrinol (Oxf)* 1996;44(6):635–42.

64. Kawai H, Saito M, Takagi M, et al. Hashimoto's thyroiditis in HTLV-I carriers. *Intern Med* 1992;31(10):1213–6.

65. Mine H, Kawai H, Yokoi K, Akaike M, Saito S. High frequencies of human T-lymphotropic virus type I (HTLV-I) infection and presence of HTLV-II proviral DNA in blood donors with anti-thyroid antibodies. *J Mol Med* 1996;74(8):471–7.

66. Akamine H, Takasu N, Komiya I, et al. Association of HTLV-I with autoimmune thyroiditis in patients with adult T-cell leukaemia (ATL) and in HTLV-I carriers. *Clin Endocrinol (Oxf)* 1996;45(4):461–6.

67. Kawai H, Mitsui T, Yokoi K, et al. Evidence of HTLV-I in thyroid tissue in an HTLV-I carrier with Hashimoto's thyroiditis. *J Mol Med* 1996;74(5):275–78.

68. Kubonishi I, Kubota T, Sawada T, et al. An HTLV-I carrier with Graves' disease followed by uveitis: isolation of HTLV-I from thyroid tissue. *Int J Hematol* 1997;66(2):233–7.

69. Shenkman L, Bottone EJ. Antibodies to Yersinia enterocolitica in thyroid disease. *Ann Intern Med* 1976;85(6):735–9.

70. Bech K. Yersinia enterocolitica and thyroid autoimmunity. *Autoimmunity* 1990;7(4):291–4.

71. Bech K, Clemmensen O, Larsen JH, Thyme S, Bendixen G. Cell-mediated immunity of Yersinia enterocolitica serotype 3 in patients with thyroid diseases. *Allergy* 1978;33(2):82–8.

72. Weiss M, Ingbar SH, Winblad S, Kasper DL. Demonstration of a saturable binding site for thyrotropin in Yersinia enterocolitica. *Science* 1983;219(4590):1331–3.

73. Heyma P, Harrison LC, Robins-Browne R. Thyrotrophin (TSH) binding sites on Yersinia enterocolitica recognized by immunoglobulins from humans with Graves' disease. *Clin Exp Immunol* 1986;64(2):249–54.

74. Luo G, Seetharamaiah GS, Niesel DW, et al. Purification and characterization of Yersinia enterocolitica envelope proteins which induce antibodies that react with human thyrotropin receptor. *J Immunol* 1994;152(5):2555–61.

75. Gangi E, Kapatral V, El-Azami El-Idrissi M, Martinez O, Prabhakar BS. Characterization of a recombinant Yersinia enterocolitica lipoprotein; implications for its role in autoimmune response against thyrotropin receptor. *Autoimmunity* 2004;37(6–7):515–20.

76. Luo G, Fan JL, Seetharamaiah GS, et al. Immunization of mice with Yersinia enterocolitica leads to the induction of antithyrotropin receptor antibodies. *J Immunol* 1993;151(2):922–8.

77. Zhang H, Kaur I, Niesel DW, et al. Lipoprotein from Yersinia enterocolitica contains epitopes that cross-react with the human thyrotropin receptor. *J Immunol* 1997;158(4):1976–83.

78. Figura N, Di Cairano G, Lore F, et al. The infection by Helicobacter pylori strains expressing CagA is highly prevalent in women with autoimmune thyroid disorders. *J Physiol Pharmacol* 1999;50(5):817–26.

79. Larizza D, Calcaterra V, Martinetti M, et al. H. Helicobacter pylori infection and autoimmune thyroid disease in young patients: the disadvantage of carrying the human leukocyte antigen-DRB1*0301 allele. *J Clin Endocrinol Metab* 2006;91(1):176–9.

80. Fahmy MH, Said M, Amara F, Ghanem MH. Thyroid function in hepatic schistosomiasis. *Ann Trop Med Parasitol* 1978;72(4):353–6.

81. Nagayama Y, McLachlan SM, Rapoport B, Oishi K. Graves' hyperthyroidism and the hygiene hypothesis in a mouse model. *Endocrinology* 2004;145(11):5075–9.

82. Nagayama Y, Watanabe K, Niwa M, McLachlan SM, Rapoport B. Schistosoma mansoni and alpha-galactosylceramide: prophylactic effect of Th1 Immune suppression in a mouse model of Graves' hyperthyroidism. *J Immunol* 2004;173(3):2167–73.

83. Lindberg B, Ahlfors K, Carlsson A, et al. Previous exposure to measles, mumps, and rubella–but not vaccination during adolescence–correlates to the prevalence of pancreatic and thyroid autoantibodies. *Pediatrics* 1999;104(1):e12.

84. Toft J, Larsen S, Toft H. Subacute thyroiditis after hepatitis B vaccination. *Endocr J* 1998;45(1):135.

85. Tonooka N, Leslie GA, Greer MA, Olson JC. Lymphoid thyroiditis following immunization with group A streptococcal vaccine. *Am J Pathol* 1978;92(3):681–90.

86. Mancia G, Grassi G, Zanchetti A. New-onset diabetes and antihypertensive drugs. *J Hypertens* 2006;24(1):3–10.

87. Mason JM, Dickinson HO, Nicolson DJ, Campbell F, Ford GA, Williams B. The diabetogenic potential of thiazide-type diuretic and beta-blocker combinations in patients with hypertension. *J Hypertens* 2005;23(10):1777–81.

88. Roberts CG, Ladenson PW. Hypothyroidism. *Lancet* 2004;363(9411):793–803.

89. Herr RR, Eble TE, Bergy ME, Jahnke HK. Isolation and characterization of streptozotocin. *Antibiot Annu* 1959;7:236–40.

90. Prosser PR, Karam JH. Diabetes mellitus following rodenticide ingestion in man. *JAMA* 1978;239(12):1148–50.

91. Pont A, Rubino JM, Bishop D, Peal R. Diabetes mellitus and neuropathy following Vacor ingestion in man. *Arch Intern Med* 1979;139(2):185–7.

92. Sumrani N, Delaney V, Ding Z, et al. Posttransplant diabetes mellitus in cyclosporine-treated renal transplant recipients. *Transplant Proc* 1991;23(1 Pt 2):1249–50.

93. Keshavarz R, Mousavi MA, Hassani C. Diabetic ketoacidosis in a child on FK506 immunosuppression after a liver transplant. *Pediatr Emerg Care* 2002;18(1):22–4.

94. Ersoy A, Ersoy C, Tekce H, Yavascaoglu I, Dilek K. Diabetic ketoacidosis following development of de novo diabetes in renal transplant recipient associated with tacrolimus. *Transplant Proc* 2004;36(5):1407–10.

95. Wiersinga WM. Towards an animal model of amiodarone-induced thyroid dysfunction. *Eur J Endocrinol* 1997;137(1):15–7.

96. Trip MD, Wiersinga W, Plomp TA. Incidence, predictability, and pathogenesis of amiodarone-induced thyrotoxicosis and hypothyroidism. *Am J Med* 1991;91(5):507–11.

97. Chianese-Bullock KA, Woodson EM, Tao H, et al. Autoimmune toxicities associated with the administration of antitumor vaccines and low-dose interleukin-2. *J Immunother* 2005;28(4):412–9.

98. Evans JS, Gerritsen GC, Mann KM, Owen SP. Antitumor and hyperglycemic activity of streptozotocin (NSC-37917) and its cofactor, U-15,774. *Cancer Chemother Rep* 1965;48:1–6.

99. Wilson GL, Leiter EH. Streptozotocin interactions with pancreatic beta cells and the induction of insulin-dependent diabetes. *Curr Top Microbiol Immunol* 1990;156:27–54.

100. Rossini AA, Like AA, Dulin WE, Cahill GF, Jr. Pancreatic beta cell toxicity by streptozotocin anomers. *Diabetes* 1977;26(12):1120–4.

101. Reddy S, Sandler S. Age-dependent sensitivity to streptozotocin of pancreatic islets isolated from female NOD mice. *Autoimmunity* 1995;22(2):121–6.

102. Rossini AA, Williams RM, Appel MC, Like AA. Sex differences in the multiple-dose streptozotocin model of diabetes. *Endocrinology* 1978;103(4):1518–20.

103. Schnedl WJ, Ferber S, Johnson JH, Newgard CB. STZ transport and cytotoxicity. Specific enhancement in GLUT2-expressing cells. *Diabetes* 1994;43(11):1326–33.

104. Delaney CA, Dunger A, Di Matteo M, Cunningham JM, Green MH, Green IC. Comparison of inhibition of glucose-stimulated insulin secretion in rat islets of Langerhans by streptozotocin and methyl and ethyl nitrosoureas and methanesulphonates. Lack of correlation with nitric oxide-releasing or O6-alkylating ability. *Biochem Pharmacol* 1995;50(12):2015–20.

105. Turk J, Corbett JA, Ramanadham S, Bohrer A, McDaniel ML. Biochemical evidence for nitric oxide formation from streptozotocin in isolated pancreatic islets. *Biochem Biophys Res Commun* 1993;197(3):1458–64.

106. Kroncke KD, Fehsel K, Sommer A, Rodriguez ML, Kolb-Bachofen V. Nitric oxide generation during cellular metabolization of the diabetogenic N-methyl-N-nitroso-urea streptozotozin contributes to islet cell DNA damage. *Biol Chem Hoppe Seyler* 1995;376(3):179–85.

107. Albers R, de Heer C, Bol M, Bleumink R, Seinen W, Pieters R. Selective immunomodulation by the autoimmunity-inducing xenobiotics streptozotocin and HgCl2. *Eur J Immunol* 1998;28(4): 1233–42.

108. Herold KC, Bloch TN, Vezys V, Sun Q. Diabetes induced with low doses of streptozotocin is mediated by V beta 8.2+ T-cells. *Diabetes* 1995;44(3):354–9.

109. Arata M, Fabiano de Bruno L, Goncalvez Volpini WM, et al. Beta-cell function in mice injected with mononuclear splenocytes from multiple-dose streptozotocin diabetic mice. *Proc Soc Exp Biol Med* 1994;206(1):76–82.

110. Pechhold K, Patterson NB, Blum C, Fleischacker CL, Boehm BO, Harlan DM. Low dose streptozotocin-induced diabetes in rat insulin promoter-mCD80-transgenic mice is T cell autoantigen-specific and CD28 dependent. *J Immunol* 2001;166(4):2531–9.

111. Rabinovitch A, Suarez-Pinzon WL. Role of cytokines in the pathogenesis of autoimmune diabetes mellitus. *Rev Endocr Metab Disord* 2003;4(3):291–9.

112. Andrade J, Conde M, Sobrino F, Bedoya FJ. Activation of peritoneal macrophages during the prediabetic phase in low-dose streptozotocin-treated mice. *Adv Exp Med Biol* 1997;426:341–3.

113. Green IC, Cunningham JM, Delaney CA, Elphick MR, Mabley JG, Green MH. Effects of cytokines and nitric oxide donors on insulin secretion, cyclic GMP and DNA damage: relation to nitric oxide production. *Biochem Soc Trans* 1994;22(1):30–7.

114. Southern C, Schulster D, Green IC. Inhibition of insulin secretion by interleukin-1 beta and tumour necrosis factor-alpha via an L-arginine-dependent nitric oxide generating mechanism. *FEBS Lett* 1990;276(1–2):42–4.

115. Sandler S, Bendtzen K, Eizirik DL, Strandell E, Welsh M, Welsh N. Metabolism and beta-cell function of rat pancreatic islets exposed to human interleukin-1 beta in the presence of a high glucose concentration. *Immunol Lett* 1990;26(3):245–51.

116. Delaney CA, Green MH, Lowe JE, Green IC. Endogenous nitric oxide induced by interleukin-1 beta in rat islets of Langerhans and HIT-T15 cells causes significant DNA damage as measured by the 'comet' assay. *FEBS Lett* 1993;333(3):291–5.

117. Di Matteo MA, Loweth AC, Thomas S, et al. Superoxide, nitric oxide, peroxynitrite and cytokine combinations all cause functional impairment and morphological changes in rat islets of Langerhans and insulin secreting cell lines, but dictate cell death by different mechanisms. *Apoptosis* 1997;2(2):164–77.

118. Mabley JG, Suarez-Pinzon WL, Hasko G, et al. Inhibition of poly (ADP-ribose) synthetase by gene disruption or inhibition with 5-iodo-6-amino-1,2-benzopyrone protects mice from multiple-low-dose-streptozotocin-induced diabetes. *Br J Pharmacol* 2001;133(6):909–19.

119. Suarez-Pinzon WL, Mabley JG, Power R, Szabo C, Rabinovitch A. Poly (ADP-ribose) polymerase inhibition prevents spontaneous and recurrent autoimmune diabetes in NOD mice by inducing apoptosis of islet-infiltrating leukocytes. *Diabetes* 2003;52(7):1683–8.

120. Calne RY, Rolles K, White DJ, et al. Cyclosporin-A in clinical organ grafting. *Transplant Proc* 1981;13(1 Pt 1):349–58.

121. Powles RL, Clink HM, Spence D, et al. Cyclosporin A to prevent graft-versus-host disease in man after allogeneic bone-marrow transplantation. *Lancet* 1980;1(8164):327–9.

122. Sigal NH, Dumont FJ. Cyclosporin A, FK-506, and rapamycin: pharmacologic probes of lymphocyte signal transduction. *Annu Rev Immunol* 1992;10:519–60.

123. Brazelton TR, Morris RE. Molecular mechanisms of action of new xenobiotic immunosuppressive drugs: tacrolimus (FK506), sirolimus (rapamycin), mycophenolate mofetil and leflunomide. *Curr Opin Immunol* 1996;8(5):710–20.

124. Sakaguchi S, Sakaguchi N. Thymus and autoimmunity. Transplantation of the thymus from cyclosporin A-treated mice causes organ-specific autoimmune disease in athymic nude mice. *J Exp Med* 1988;167(4):1479–85.

125. Sakaguchi S, Sakaguchi N. Organ-specific autoimmune disease induced in mice by elimination of T cell subsets. V. Neonatal administration of cyclosporin A causes autoimmune disease. *J Immunol* 1989;142(2):471–80.

126. Krentz AJ, Dousset B, Mayer D, et al. Metabolic effects of cyclosporin A and FK 506 in liver transplant recipients. *Diabetes* 1993;42(12):1753–9.

127. Yamamoto H, Akazawa S, Yamaguchi Y, et al. Effects of cyclosporin A and low dosages of steroid on posttransplantation diabetes in kidney transplant recipients. *Diabetes Care* 1991;14(10):867–70.

128. Obuobie K, Al-Sabah A, Lazarus JH. Subacute thyroiditis in an immunosuppressed patient. *J Endocrinol Invest* 2002;25(2):169–71.

129. Prud'homme GJ, Parfrey NA, Vanier LE. Cyclosporine-induced autoimmunity and immune hyper-reactivity. *Autoimmunity* 1991;9(4):345–56.

130. Robertson RP. Cyclosporin-induced inhibition of insulin secretion in isolated rat islets and HIT cells. *Diabetes* 1986;35(9):1016–9.

131. Draznin B, Metz SA, Sussman KE, Leitner JW. Cyclosporin-induced inhibition of insulin release. Possible role of voltage-dependent calcium transport channels. *Biochem Pharmacol* 1988;37(20):3941–5.

132. Andersson A, Borg H, Hallberg A, Hellerstrom C, Sandler S, Schnell A. Long-term effects of cyclosporin A on cultured mouse pancreatic islets. *Diabetologia* 1984;27(Suppl):66–9.

133. Lucke S, Radloff E, Laube R, Hahn HJ. Morphology of the endocrine pancreas in cyclosporine-treated glucose-intolerant Wistar rats. *Anat Anz* 1991;172(5):351–8.

134. Dufer M, Krippeit-Drews P, Lembert N, Idahl LA, Drews G. Diabetogenic effect of cyclosporin A is mediated by interference with mitochondrial function of pancreatic B-cells. *Mol Pharmacol* 2001;60(4):873–9.

135. Goto T, Kino T, Hatanaka H, et al. Discovery of FK-506, a novel immunosuppressant isolated from Streptomyces tsukubaensis. *Transplant Proc* 1987;19(5 Suppl 6):4–8.

136. Goto T, Kino T, Hatanaka H, et al. FK 506: historical perspectives. *Transplant Proc* 1991;23(6):2713–7.

137. Crespo-Leiro MG. Calcineurin inhibitors in heart transplantation. *Transplant Proc* 2005;37(9):4018–20.

138. Tabasco-Minguillan J, Mieles L, Carroll P, Gavaler J, Van Thiel DH, Starzl TE. Insulin requirements after liver transplantation and FK-506 immunosuppression. *Transplantation* 1993;56(4):862–7.

139. Weir MR, Fink JC. Risk for posttransplant Diabetes mellitus with current immunosuppressive medications. *Am J Kidney Dis* 1999;34(1):1–13.

140. Reiffel JA, Estes NA, 3rd, Waldo AL, Prystowsky EN, DiBianco R. A consensus report on antiarrhythmic drug use. *Clin Cardiol* 1994;17(3):103–16.

141. Doval HC, Nul DR, Grancelli HO, Perrone SV, Bortman GR, Curiel R. Randomised trial of low-dose amiodarone in severe congestive heart failure. Grupo de Estudio de la Sobrevida en la Insuficiencia Cardiaca en Argentina (GESICA). *Lancet* 1994;344(8921):493–8.

142. Rao RH, McCready VR, Spathis GS. Iodine kinetic studies during amiodarone treatment. *J Clin Endocrinol Metab* 1986;62(3):563–8.

143. Bogazzi F, Bartalena L, Gasperi M, Braverman LE, Martino E. The various effects of amiodarone on thyroid function. *Thyroid* 2001;11(5):511–9.

144. Martino E, Bartalena L, Bogazzi F, Braverman LE. The effects of amiodarone on the thyroid. *Endocr Rev* 2001;22(2):240–54.

145. Martino E, Aghini-Lombardi F, Bartalena L, et al. Enhanced susceptibility to amiodarone-induced hypothyroidism in patients with thyroid autoimmune disease. *Arch Intern Med* 1994;154 (23):2722–6.

146. Chiovato L, Martino E, Tonacchera M, et al. Studies on the in vitro cytotoxic effect of amiodarone. *Endocrinology* 1994;134(5):2277–82.

147. Martino E, Macchia E, Aghini-Lombardi F, et al. Is humoral thyroid autoimmunity relevant in amiodarone iodine-induced thyrotoxicosis (AIIT)? *Clin Endocrinol (Oxf)* 1986;24(6):627–33.

148. Monteiro E, Galvao-teles A, Santos ML, et al. Antithyroid antibodies as an early marker for thyroid disease induced by amiodarone. *Br Med J (Clin Res Ed)* 1986;292(6515):227–8.

149. Safran M, Martino E, Aghini-Lombardi F, et al. Effect of amiodarone on circulating antithyroid antibodies. *BMJ* 1988;297(6646):456–7.

150. Weetman AP, Bhandal SK, Burrin JM, Robinson K, McKenna W. Amiodarone and thyroid autoimmunity in the United Kingdom. *BMJ* 1988;297(6640):33.

151. Diaz MO, Bohlander S, Allen G. Nomenclature of the human interferon genes. *J Interferon Cytokine Res* 1996;16(2):179–80.

152. Stewart TA. Neutralizing interferon alpha as a therapeutic approach to autoimmune diseases. *Cytokine Growth Factor Rev* 2003;14(2):139–54.

153. Vilcek J, Ng MH. Potentiation of the action of interferon by extracts of Escherichia coli. *Virology* 1967;31(3):552–5.

154. Merigan TC. Induction of circulating interferon by synthetic anionic polymers of known composition. *Nature* 1967;214(86):416–7.

155. Reyes VE, Ballas ZK, Singh H, Klimpel GR. Interleukin 2 induces interferon alpha/beta production in mouse bone marrow cells. *Cell Immunol* 1986;102(2):374–85.

156. Zhou A, Chen Z, Rummage JA, et al. Exogenous interferon-gamma induces endogenous synthesis of interferon-alpha and -beta by murine macrophages for induction of nitric oxide synthase. *J Interferon Cytokine Res* 1995;15(10):897–904.

157. Chakrabarti D, Huang X, Beck J, et al. Control of islet intercellular adhesion molecule-1 expression by interferon-alpha and hypoxia. *Diabetes* 1996;45(10):1336–43.

158. Chelbi-Alix MK, Brouard A, Boissard C, Pelaprat D, Rostene W, Thang MN. Induction by vasoactive intestinal peptide of interferon alpha/beta synthesis in glial cells but not in neurons. *J Cell Physiol* 1994;158(1):47–54.

159. Devendra D, Eisenbarth GS. Interferon alpha–a potential link in the pathogenesis of viral-induced type 1 diabetes and autoimmunity. *Clin Immunol* 2004;111(3):225–33.

160. Sumi M, Tauchi T, Takaku T, Ohyashiki JH, Ohyashiki K. [Successful treatment with interferon-alpha in a case of acute myeloid leukemia with del (20q) following polycythemia vera]. *Rinsho Ketsueki* 2005;46(11):1208–12.

161. Makita M, Nakamura K, Kono A. [Successful rituximab treatment in a patient with refractory hairy cell leukemia-Japanese variant and suffering from acute respiratory distress]. *Rinsho Ketsueki* 2005;46(11):1196–201.

162. Rodriguez MA, Prinz WA, Sibbitt WL, Bankhurst AD, Williams RC, Jr. alpha-Interferon increases immunoglobulin production in cultured human mononuclear leukocytes. *J Immunol* 1983;130(3):1215–9.

163. Finkelman FD, Svetic A, Gresser I, et al. Regulation by interferon alpha of immunoglobulin isotype selection and lymphokine production in mice. *J Exp Med* 1991;174(5):1179–88.

164. Rawlinson L, Dalton BJ, Rogers K, Rees RC. The influence of interferon alpha and gamma, singly or in combination on human natural cell mediated cytotoxicity. *Biosci Rep* 1989;9(5):549–57.

165. Webb DS, Zur Nedden D, Miller DM, Zoon KC, Gerrard TL. Enhancement of monocyte-mediated tumoricidal activity by multiple interferon-alpha species. *Cell Immunol* 1989;124(1):158–67.

166. Hooks JJ, Moutsopoulos HM, Geis SA, Stahl NI, Decker JL, Notkins AL. Immune interferon in the circulation of patients with autoimmune disease. *N Engl J Med* 1979;301(1):5–8.

167. Preble OT, Black RJ, Friedman RM, Klippel JH, Vilcek J. Systemic lupus erythematosus: presence in human serum of an unusual acid-labile leukocyte interferon. *Science* 1982;216(4544):429–31.

168. Foulis AK, Farquharson MA, Meager A. Immunoreactive alpha-interferon in insulin-secreting beta cells in type 1 diabetes mellitus. *Lancet* 1987;2(8573):1423–7.

169. Huang X, Yuang J, Goddard A, et al. Interferon expression in the pancreases of patients with type I diabetes. *Diabetes* 1995;44(6):658–64.

170. Schmid P, Itin P, Cox D, McMaster GK, Horisberger MA. The type I interferon system is locally activated in psoriatic lesions. *J Interferon Res* 1994;14(5):229–34.

171. Fais S, Capobianchi MR, Silvestri M, Mercuri F, Pallone F, Dianzani F. Interferon expression in Crohn's disease patients: increased interferon-gamma and -alpha mRNA in the intestinal lamina propria mononuclear cells. *J Interferon Res* 1994;14(5):235–8.

172. Monteleone G, Pender SL, Wathen NC, MacDonald TT. Interferon-alpha drives T cell-mediated immunopathology in the intestine. *Eur J Immunol* 2001;31(8):2247–55.

173. Fattovich G, Giustina G, Favarato S, Ruol A. A survey of adverse events in 11,241 patients with chronic viral hepatitis treated with alfa interferon. *J Hepatol* 1996;24(1):38–47.

174. Okanoue T, Sakamoto S, Itoh Y, et al. Side effects of high-dose interferon therapy for chronic hepatitis C. *J Hepatol* 1996;25(3):283–91.

175. Fabris P, Betterle C, Floreani A, et al. Development of type 1 diabetes mellitus during interferon alfa therapy for chronic HCV hepatitis. *Lancet* 1992;340(8818):548.

176. Fabris P, Floreani A, Tositti G, Vergani D, De Lalla F, Betterle C. Type 1 diabetes mellitus in patients with chronic hepatitis C before and after interferon therapy. *Aliment Pharmacol Ther* 2003;18(6):549–58.

177. Koh LK, Greenspan FS, Yeo PP. Interferon-alpha induced thyroid dysfunction: three clinical presentations and a review of the literature. *Thyroid* 1997;7(6):891–6.

178. Doi F, Kakizaki S, Takagi H, et al. Long-term outcome of interferon-alpha-induced autoimmune thyroid disorders in chronic hepatitis C. *Liver Int* 2005;25(2):242–6.

179. Huang SW, Taylor GE. Immune insulitis and antibodies to nucleic acids induced with streptozotocin in mice. *Clin Exp Immunol* 1981;43(2):425–9.

180. Moriyama H, Wen L, Abiru N, et al. Induction and acceleration of insulitis/diabetes in mice with a viral mimic (polyinosinic-polycytidylic acid) and an insulin self-peptide. *Proc Natl Acad Sci USA* 2002;99(8):5539–44.

181. Chakrabarti D, Hultgren B, Stewart TA. IFN-alpha induces autoimmune T cells through the induction of intracellular adhesion molecule-1 and B7.2. *J Immunol* 1996;157(2):522–8.

182. Smith KA. Lowest dose interleukin-2 immunotherapy. *Blood* 1993;81(6):1414–23.

183. Carrel A, Meinen A, Garry C, Storandt R. Effects of nutrition education and exercise in obese children: the Ho-Chunk Youth Fitness Program. *WMJ* 2005;104(5):44–7.

184. Heald AH, Sharma R, Anderson SG, et al. Dietary intake and the insulin-like growth factor system: effects of migration in two related populations in India and Britain with markedly different dietary intake. *Public Health Nutr* 2005;8(6):620–7.

185. Moller DE, Chang PY, Yaspelkis BB, 3rd, Flier JS, Wallberg-Henriksson H, Ivy JL. Transgenic mice with muscle-specific insulin resistance develop increased adiposity, impaired glucose tolerance, and dyslipidemia. *Endocrinology* 1996;137(6):2397–405.

186. Ebbesson SO, Risica PM, Ebbesson LO, Kennish JM, Tejero ME. Omega-3 fatty acids improve glucose tolerance and components of the metabolic syndrome in Alaskan Eskimos: the Alaska Siberia project. *Int J Circumpolar Health* 2005;64(4):396–408.

187. Rakatzi I, Mueller H, Ritzeler O, Tennagels N, Eckel J. Adiponectin counteracts cytokine- and fatty acid-induced apoptosis in the pancreatic beta-cell line INS-1. *Diabetologia* 2004;47(2):249–58.

188. Liu D, Cardozo AK, Darville MI, Eizirik DL. Double-stranded RNA cooperates with interferon-gamma and IL-1 beta to induce both chemokine expression and nuclear factor-kappa B-dependent apoptosis in pancreatic beta-cells: potential mechanisms for viral-induced insulitis and beta-cell death in type 1 diabetes mellitus. *Endocrinology* 2002;143(4):1225–34.

189. Kharroubi I, Ladriere L, Cardozo AK, Dogusan Z, Cnop M, Eizirik DL. Free fatty acids and cytokines induce pancreatic beta-cell apoptosis by different mechanisms: role of nuclear factor-kappaB and endoplasmic reticulum stress. *Endocrinology* 2004;145(11):5087–96.

190. Chang I, Kim S, Kim JY, et al. Nuclear factor kappaB protects pancreatic beta-cells from tumor necrosis factor-alpha-mediated apoptosis. *Diabetes* 2003;52(5):1169–75.

191. Oddie TH, Fisher DA, McConahey WM, Thompson CS. Iodine intake in the United States: a reassessment. *J Clin Endocrinol Metab* 1970;30(5):659–65.

192. Braverman LE. Iodine induced thyroid disease. *Acta Med Austriaca* 1990;17(Suppl 1):29–33.

193. Weaver DK, Batsakis JG, Nishiyama RH. Relationship of iodine to "lymphocytic goiters". *Arch Surg* 1969;98(2):183–6.

194. Phillips DI, Nelson M, Barker DJ, Morris JA, Wood TJ. Iodine in milk and the incidence of thyrotoxicosis in England. *Clin Endocrinol (Oxf)* 1988;28(1):61–6.

195. Pennington JA. A review of iodine toxicity reports. *J Am Diet Assoc* 1990;90(11):1571–81.

196. Zois C, Stavrou I, Kalogera C, et al. High prevalence of autoimmune thyroiditis in schoolchildren after elimination of iodine deficiency in northwestern Greece. *Thyroid* 2003;13(5):485–9.

197. Tajiri J, Higashi K, Morita M, Umeda T, Sato T. Studies of hypothyroidism in patients with high iodine intake. *J Clin Endocrinol Metab* 1986;63(2):412–7.

198. Basaria S, Cooper DS. Amiodarone and the thyroid. *Am J Med* 2005;118(7):706–14.

199. Rao RR, Chatt A. Determination of nanogram amounts of iodine in foods by radiochemical neutron activation analysis. *Analyst* 1993;118(10):1247–51.

200. Allegrini M, Pennington JA, Tanner JT. Total diet study: determination of iodine intake by neutron activation analysis. *J Am Diet Assoc* 1983;83(1):18–24.

201. Braverman LE, Ingbar SH, Vagenakis AG, Adams L, Maloof F. Enhanced susceptibility to iodide myxedema in patients with Hashimoto's disease. *J Clin Endocrinol Metab* 1971;32(4):515–21.

202. Konno N, Makita H, Yuri K, Iizuka N, Kawasaki K. Association between dietary iodine intake and prevalence of subclinical hypothyroidism in the coastal regions of Japan. *J Clin Endocrinol Metab* 1994;78(2):393–7.

203. Roti E, Uberti ED. Iodine excess and hyperthyroidism. *Thyroid* 2001;11(5):493–500.

204. Yoon SJ, Choi SR, Kim DM, et al. The effect of iodine restriction on thyroid function in patients with hypothyroidism due to Hashimoto's thyroiditis. *Yonsei Med J* 2003;44(2):227–35.

205. Kasagi K, Iwata M, Misaki T, Konishi J. Effect of iodine restriction on thyroid function in patients with primary hypothyroidism. *Thyroid* 2003;13(6):561–7.

206. Malthiery Y, Lissitzky S. Primary structure of human thyroglobulin deduced from the sequence of its 8448-base complementary DNA. *Eur J Biochem* 1987;165(3):491–8.

207. Rawitch AB, Chernoff SB, Litwer MR, Rouse JB, Hamilton JW. Thyroglobulin structure-function. The amino acid sequence surrounding thyroxine. *J Biol Chem* 1983;258(4):2079–82.

208. Gavaret JM, Deme D, Nunez J, Salvatore G. Sequential reactivity of tyrosyl residues of thyroglobulin upon iodination catalyzed by thyroid peroxidase. *J Biol Chem* 1977;252(10):3281–5.

209. Palumbo G, Gentile F, Condorelli GL, Salvatore G. The earliest site of iodination in thyroglobulin is residue number 5. *J Biol Chem* 1990;265(15):8887–92.

210. Van der Walt B, Van Jaarsveld P. Bovine 37S iodoprotein: isolation and characterization. *Arch Biochem Biophys* 1972;150(2):786–91.

211. Lamas L, Ingbar SH. The effect of varying iodine content on the susceptibility of thyroglobulin to hydrolysis by thyroid acid protease. *Endocrinology* 1978;102(1):188–97.

212. Schneider AB, Edelhoch H. The properties of thyroglobulin. XIX. The equilibrium between guinea pig thyroglobulin and its subunits. *J Biol Chem* 1970;245(4):885–90.

213. Rasooly L, Rose NR, Saboori AM, Ladenson PW, Burek CL. Iodine is essential for human T cell recognition of human thyroglobulin. *Autoimmunity* 1998;27(4):213–9.

214. Saboori AM, Rose NR, Burek CL. Iodination of human thyroglobulin (Tg) alters its immunoreactivity. II. Fine specificity of a monoclonal antibody that recognizes iodinated Tg. *Clin Exp Immunol* 1998;113(2):303–8.

215. Saboori AM, Rose NR, Bresler HS, Vladut-Talor M, Burek CL. Iodination of human thyroglobulin (Tg) alters its immunoreactivity. I. Iodination alters multiple epitopes of human Tg. *Clin Exp Immunol* 1998;113(2):297–302.

216. Dai YD, Rao VP, Carayanniotis G. Enhanced iodination of thyroglobulin facilitates processing and presentation of a cryptic pathogenic peptide. *J Immunol* 2002;168(11):5907–11.

217. Champion BR, Page K, Rayner DC, Quartey-Papafio R, Byfield PG, Henderson G. Recognition of thyroglobulin autoantigenic epitopes by murine T and B cells. *Immunology* 1987;62(2):255–63.

218. Vladutiu AO, Rose NR. Autoimmune murine thyroiditis relation to histocompatibility (H-2) type. *Science* 1971;174(14):1137–9.

219. Weatherall D, Sarvetnick N, Shizuru JA. Genetic control of diabetes mellitus. *Diabetologia* 1992;35(Suppl 2):S1–7.

220. Bonita RE, Rose NR, Rasooly L, Caturegli P, Burek CL. Kinetics of mononuclear cell infiltration and cytokine expression in iodine-induced thyroiditis in the NOD-H2h4 mouse. *Exp Mol Pathol* 2003;74(1):1–12.

221. Braley-Mullen H, Sharp GC, Medling B, Tang H. Spontaneous autoimmune thyroiditis in NOD. H-2h4 mice. *J Autoimmun* 1999;12(3):157–65.

222. Yu S, Medling B, Yagita H, Braley-Mullen H. Characteristics of inflammatory cells in spontaneous autoimmune thyroiditis of NOD.H-2h4 mice. *J Autoimmun* 2001;16(1):37–46.

223. Braley-Mullen H, Yu S. Early requirement for B cells for development of spontaneous autoimmune thyroiditis in NOD.H-2h4 mice. *J Immunol* 2000;165(12):7262–9.

224. Mooij P, Simons PJ, de Haan-Meulman M, de Wit HJ, Drexhage HA. Effect of thyroid hormones and other iodinated compounds on the transition of monocytes into veiled/dendritic cells: role of granulocyte-macrophage colony-stimulating factor, tumour-necrosis factor-alpha and interleukin-6. *J Endocrinol* 1994;140(3):503–12.

225. Mooij P, de Haan-Meulman M, de Wit HJ, Drexhage HA. Thyroid hormones and their iodinated breakdown products enhance the capability of monocytes to mature into veiled cells. Blocking effects of alpha-GM-CSF. *Adv Exp Med Biol* 1993;329:633–6.

226. Bonita RE, Rose NR, Rasooly L, Caturegli P, Burek CL. Adhesion molecules as susceptibility factors in spontaneous autoimmune thyroiditis in the NOD-H2h4 mouse. *Exp Mol Pathol* 2002;73(3):155–63.

227. Bagnasco M, Caretto A, Olive D, Pedini B, Canonica GW, Betterle C. Expression of intercellular adhesion molecule-1 (ICAM-1) on thyroid epithelial cells in Hashimoto's thyroiditis but not in Graves' disease or papillary thyroid cancer. *Clin Exp Immunol* 1991;83(2):309–13.

228. Bagnasco M, Pesce GP, Caretto A, et al. Follicular thyroid cells of autoimmune thyroiditis may coexpress ICAM-1 (CD54) and its natural ligand LFA-1 (CD11a/CD18). *J Allergy Clin Immunol* 1995;95(5 Pt 1):1036–43.

229. Zoppini G, Targher G, Cacciatori V, Guerriero A, Muggeo M. Chronic cigarette smoking is associated with increased plasma circulating intercellular adhesion molecule 1 levels in young type 1 diabetic patients. *Diabetes Care* 1999;22(11):1871–4.

230. Vestergaard P. Smoking and thyroid disorders–a meta-analysis. *Eur J Endocrinol* 2002;146(2): 153–61.

231. Vestergaard P, Rejnmark L, Weeke J, et al. Smoking as a risk factor for Graves' disease, toxic nodular goiter, and autoimmune hypothyroidism. *Thyroid* 2002;12(1):69–75.

232. Strieder TG, Prummel MF, Tijssen JG, Endert E, Wiersinga WM. Risk factors for and prevalence of thyroid disorders in a cross-sectional study among healthy female relatives of patients with autoimmune thyroid disease. *Clin Endocrinol (Oxf)* 2003;59(3):396–401.

233. Holm IA, Manson JE, Michels KB, Alexander EK, Willett WC, Utiger RD. Smoking and other lifestyle factors and the risk of Graves' hyperthyroidism. *Arch Intern Med* 2005;165(14):1606–11.

234. Brix TH, Hansen PS, Kyvik KO, Hegedus L. Cigarette smoking and risk of clinically overt thyroid disease: a population-based twin case-control study. *Arch Intern Med* 2000;160(5):661–6.

235. Belin RM, Astor BC, Powe NR, Ladenson PW. Smoke exposure is associated with a lower prevalence of serum thyroid autoantibodies and thyrotropin concentration elevation and a higher prevalence of mild thyrotropin concentration suppression in the third National Health and Nutrition Examination Survey (NHANES III). *J Clin Endocrinol Metab* 2004;89(12):6077–86.

236. Fukata S, Kuma K, Sugawara M. Relationship between cigarette smoking and hypothyroidism in patients with Hashimoto's thyroiditis. *J Endocrinol Invest* 1996;19(9):607–12.

237. Couper JJ, Steele C, Beresford S, et al. Lack of association between duration of breast-feeding or introduction of cow's milk and development of islet autoimmunity. *Diabetes* 1999;48(11):2145–9.

238. Ziegler AG, Schmid S, Huber D, Hummel M, Bonifacio E. Early infant feeding and risk of developing type 1 diabetes-associated autoantibodies. *JAMA* 2003;290(13):1721–8.

239. Kimpimaki T, Erkkola M, Korhonen S, et al. Short-term exclusive breastfeeding predisposes young children with increased genetic risk of Type I diabetes to progressive beta-cell autoimmunity. *Diabetologia* 2001;44(1):63–9.

240. Capuco AV, Rice CP, Baldwin RLt, et al. Fate of dietary perchlorate in lactating dairy cows: Relevance to animal health and levels in the milk supply. *Proc Natl Acad Sci USA* 2005;102(45):16152–7.

241. Kirk AB, Martinelango PK, Tian K, Dutta A, Smith EE, Dasgupta PK. Perchlorate and iodide in dairy and breast milk. *Environ Sci Technol* 2005;39(7):2011–7.

242. Braverman LE, He X, Pino S, et al. The effect of perchlorate, thiocyanate, and nitrate on thyroid function in workers exposed to perchlorate long-term. *J Clin Endocrinol Metab* 2005;90(2):700–6.

243. Strbak V, Skultetyova M, Michalickova J, et al. Effect of breast-feeding on infant thyroid activity: 3 year follow up–longitudinal study. *Endocrinol Exp* 1986;20(2–3):257–66.

244. Strbak V, Skultetyova M, Hromadova M, Randuskova A, Macho L. Late effects of breast-feeding and early weaning: seven-year prospective study in children. *Endocr Regul* 1991;25(1–2):53–7.

245. Bohles H, Aschenbrenner M, Roth M, von Loewenich V, Ball F, Usadel KH. Development of thyroid gland volume during the first 3 months of life in breast-fed versus iodine-supplemented and iodine-free formula-fed infants. *Clin Investig* 1993;71(1):13–20.

246. Mizuta H, Amino N, Ichihara K, et al. Thyroid hormones in human milk and their influence on thyroid function of breast-fed babies. *Pediatr Res* 1983;17(6):468–71.

247. Smyth PP, Hetherton AM, Smith DF, Radcliff M, O'Herlihy C. Maternal iodine status and thyroid volume during pregnancy: correlation with neonatal iodine intake. *J Clin Endocrinol Metab* 1997;82(9):2840–3.

248. Brouwer A, Longnecker MP, Birnbaum LS, et al. Characterization of potential endocrine-related health effects at low-dose levels of exposure to PCBs. *Environ Health Perspect* 1999;107 (Suppl 4):639–49.

249. Sala M, Sunyer J, Otero R, et al. Health effects of chronic high exposure to hexachlorobenzene in a general population sample. *Arch Environ Health* 1999;54(2):102–9.

250. Langer P, Tajtakova M, Fodor G, et al. Increased thyroid volume and prevalence of thyroid disorders in an area heavily polluted by polychlorinated biphenyls. *Eur J Endocrinol* 1998;139(4):402–9.

251. Steenland K, Cedillo L, Tucker J, et al. Thyroid hormones and cytogenetic outcomes in backpack sprayers using ethylenebis(dithiocarbamate) (EBDC) fungicides in Mexico. *Environ Health Perspect* 1997;105(10):1126–30.

252. Marinovich M, Guizzetti M, Ghilardi F, Viviani B, Corsini E, Galli CL. Thyroid peroxidase as toxicity target for dithiocarbamates. *Arch Toxicol* 1997;71(8):508–12.

253. McNabb FM, Larsen CT, Pooler PS. Ammonium perchlorate effects on thyroid function and growth in bobwhite quail chicks. *Environ Toxicol Chem* 2004;23(4):997–1003.

254. Capen CC. Mechanistic data and risk assessment of selected toxic end points of the thyroid gland. *Toxicol Pathol* 1997;25(1):39–48.

255. Capen CC, Martin SL. The effects of xenobiotics on the structure and function of thyroid follicular and C-cells. *Toxicol Pathol* 1989;17(2):266–93.

256. Hill RN, Crisp TM, Hurley PM, Rosenthal SL, Singh DV. Risk assessment of thyroid follicular cell tumors. *Environ Health Perspect* 1998;106(8):447–57.

257. Hurley PM. Mode of carcinogenic action of pesticides inducing thyroid follicular cell tumors in rodents. *Environ Health Perspect* 1998;106(8):437–45.

258. Hill RN, Erdreich LS, Paynter OE, Roberts PA, Rosenthal SL, Wilkinson CF. Thyroid follicular cell carcinogenesis. *Fundam Appl Toxicol* 1989;12(4):629–97.

259. Capen CC. Mechanisms of chemical injury of thyroid gland. *Prog Clin Biol Res* 1994;387:173–91.

260. Jacob P, Kenigsberg Y, Zvonova I, et al. Childhood exposure due to the Chernobyl accident and thyroid cancer risk in contaminated areas of Belarus and Russia. *Br J Cancer* 1999;80(9):1461–9.

261. Institute NC. Estimated exposure and thyroid doses received by the American people from Iodine-131 in fallout following Nevada Atmospheric Nuclear Bomb Test. US Department of Health and Human Resources, Washington, DC NIH Pub No 97-4264 1997.

262. Eheman CR, Garbe P, Tuttle RM. Autoimmune thyroid disease associated with environmental thyroidal irradiation. *Thyroid* 2003;13(5):453–64.

263. DeGroot LJ. Effects of irradiation on the thyroid gland. *Endocrinol Metab Clin North Am* 1993;22(3):607–15.

264. Sugenoya A, Asanuma K, Hama Y, et al. Thyroid abnormalities among children in the contaminated area related to the Chernobyl accident. *Thyroid* 1995;5(1):29–33.

265. Volzke H, Werner A, Wallaschofski H, et al. Occupational exposure to ionizing radiation is associated with autoimmune thyroid disease. *J Clin Endocrinol Metab* 2005;90(8):4587–92.

266. Lu ST, Michaelson SM, Quinlan WJ. Sequential pathophysiologic effects of ionizing radiation on the beagle thyroid gland. *J Natl Cancer Inst* 1973;51(2):419–41.

267. Rose NR. Mechanisms of autoimmunity. *Semin Liver Dis* 2002;22(4):387–94.

268. Rose NR. Pathogenic mechanisms in autoimmune diseases. *Clin Immunol Immunopathol* 1989;53 (2 Pt 2):S7–16.

269. Griem P, Wulferink M, Sachs B, Gonzalez JB, Gleichmann E. Allergic and autoimmune reactions to xenobiotics: how do they arise? *Immunol Today* 1998;19(3):133–41.

270. Njoku DB, Talor MV, Fairweather D, Frisancho-Kiss S, Odumade OA, Rose NR. A novel model of drug hapten-induced hepatitis with increased mast cells in the BALB/c mouse. *Exp Mol Pathol* 2005;78(2):87–100.

271. Kubicka-Muranyi M, Kremer J, Rottmann N, et al. Murine systemic autoimmune disease induced by mercuric chloride: T helper cells reacting to self proteins. *Int Arch Allergy Immunol* 1996;109 (1):11–20.

272. Lehmann PV, Sercarz EE, Forsthuber T, Dayan CM, Gammon G. Determinant spreading and the dynamics of the autoimmune T-cell repertoire. *Immunol Today* 1993;14(5):203–8.

273. Sercarz EE, Lehmann PV, Ametani A, Benichou G, Miller A, Moudgil K. Dominance and crypticity of T cell antigenic determinants. *Annu Rev Immunol* 1993;11:729–66.

274. Reidenberg MM. Aromatic amines and the pathogenesis of lupus erythematosus. *Am J Med* 1983;75(6):1037–42.

275. Jan V, Callens A, Machet L, Machet MC, Lorette G, Vaillant L. [D-penicillamine-induced pemphigus, polymyositis and myasthenia]. *Ann Dermatol Venereol* 1999;126(2):153–6.

276. Griem P, Panthel K, Kalbacher H, Gleichmann E. Alteration of a model antigen by Au(III) leads to T cell sensitization to cryptic peptides. *Eur J Immunol* 1996;26(2):279–87.

277. Griem P, Gleichmann E. [Gold antirheumatic drug: desired and adverse effects of Au(I) and Au(III) [corrected] on the immune system. *Z Rheumatol* 1996;55(5):348–58.

278. Bowlus CL. The role of iron in T cell development and autoimmunity. *Autoimmun Rev* 2003;2(2):73–8.

279. Wulferink M, Dierkes S, Gleichmann E. Cross-sensitization to haptens: formation of common haptenic metabolites, T cell recognition of cryptic peptides, and true T cell cross-reactivity. *Eur J Immunol* 2002;32(5):1338–48.

280. Gleichmann H. Studies on the mechanism of drug sensitization: T-cell-dependent popliteal lymph node reaction to diphenylhydantoin. *Clin Immunol Immunopathol* 1981;18(2):203–11.

281. van Elven EH, van der Veen FM, Rolink AG, Issa P, Duin TM, Gleichmann E. Diseases caused by reactions of T lymphocytes to incompatible structures of the major histocompatibility complex. V. High titers of IgG autoantibodies to double-stranded DNA. *J Immunol* 1981;127(6):2435–8.

282. Romagnoli P, Spinas GA, Sinigaglia F. Gold-specific T cells in rheumatoid arthritis patients treated with gold. *J Clin Invest* 1992;89(1):254–8.

283. Ellis NM, Li Y, Hildebrand W, Fischetti VA, Cunningham MW. T cell mimicry and epitope specificity of cross-reactive T cell clones from rheumatic heart disease. *J Immunol* 2005;175(8):5448–56.

284. Guilherme L, Cunha-Neto E, Coelho V, et al. Human heart-infiltrating T-cell clones from rheumatic heart disease patients recognize both streptococcal and cardiac proteins. *Circulation* 1995;92(3):415–20.

285. Iwai LK, Juliano MA, Juliano L, Kalil J, Cunha-Neto E. T-cell molecular mimicry in Chagas disease: identification and partial structural analysis of multiple cross-reactive epitopes between Trypanosoma cruzi B13 and cardiac myosin heavy chain. *J Autoimmun* 2005;24(2):111–7.

286. Pichler WJ. Modes of presentation of chemical neoantigens to the immune system. *Toxicology* 2002;181–182:49–54.

287. Depta JP, Pichler WJ. Cross-reactivity with drugs at the T cell level. *Curr Opin Allergy Clin Immunol* 2003;3(4):261–7.

288. Richardson B. DNA methylation and autoimmune disease. *Clin Immunol* 2003;109(1):72–9.

289. Uetrecht J. Current trends in drug-induced autoimmunity. *Autoimmun Rev* 2005;4(5):309–14.

290. Richardson B, Powers D, Hooper F, Yung RL, O'Rourke K. Lymphocyte function-associated antigen 1 overexpression and T cell autoreactivity. *Arthritis Rheum* 1994;37(9):1363–72.

291. Richardson BC. Role of DNA methylation in the regulation of cell function: autoimmunity, aging and cancer. *J Nutr* 2002;132(8 Suppl):2401S–5S.

292. Kojima A, Tanaka-Kojima Y, Sakakura T, Nishizuka Y. Spontaneous development of autoimmune thyroiditis in neonatally thymectomized mice. *Lab Invest* 1976;34(6):550–7.

293. Wei WZ, Jacob JB, Zielinski JF, et al. Concurrent induction of antitumor immunity and autoimmune thyroiditis in CD4+ CD25+ regulatory T cell-depleted mice. *Cancer Res* 2005;65(18):8471–8.

294. Vladutiu AO. Autoimmune thyroiditis: conversion of low-responder mice to high-responders by cyclophosphamide. *Clin Exp Immunol* 1982;47(3):683–8.

295. Silverman DA, Rose NR. Spontaneous and methylcholanthrene-enhanced thyroiditis in BUF rats. I. The incidence and severity of the disease, and the genetics of susceptibility. *J Immunol* 1975;114 (1 Pt 1):145–7.

296. Taguchi O, Nishizuka Y. Self tolerance and localized autoimmunity. Mouse models of autoimmune disease that suggest tissue-specific suppressor T cells are involved in self tolerance. *J Exp Med* 1987;165(1):146–56.

II AUTOIMMUNE THYROID DISEASE

4 Animal Models of Autoimmune Thyroid Disease

Marian Ludgate, *BSc, PhD*

CONTENTS

Summary

Autoimmune thyroid diseases (AITD) cover the spectrum from hypothyroid Hashimoto's thyroiditis (HT) to hyperthyroid Graves' disease (GD). The main autoimmune targets are thyroglobulin (TG), thyroid peroxidase (TPO), and the thyrotropin receptor (TSHR). Autoantibodies and specific T cells directed against all three autoantigens can be detected in the circulation of HT and GD patients and also in a significant proportion of the healthy population. In AITD, as in other autoimmune conditions, the central question remains how is immune tolerance overcome? In vivo models, mostly induced in rodents, have contributed to our understanding of the mechanisms operating and many hundreds of papers, spanning from 1956 to the present day, have been published describing the results obtained. Most of the information has been derived from experimental autoimmune thyroiditis models induced with TG, an antigen that, based on current knowledge, seems to be of lesser importance in human AITD. Nevertheless, many of the basic precepts underlying autoimmunity, for example the importance of the major histocompatability complex II and the existence of immunoregulatory T cells, have been identified using TG-based models, and these are described. Reports based on induction of disease with TPO, the driving antigen in HT, are not very numerous but include a seminal paper that clearly demonstrates the redundancy of autoantibodies and the central role of T cells in pathogenesis. In contrast, autoantibodies to the TSHR cause GD and much of the chapter is devoted to models attempting to mimic GD, and these have been the subject of considerable effort since its cloning in 1989. This has culminated with the recent publication of monoclonal antibodies with thyroid stimulating activity either measured in vitro or in vivo.

Key Words: Hashimoto's thyroiditis, Graves' disease, animal models, thyroiditis, hyperthyroidism, hypothyroidism, autoantibodies, thyrotropin receptor, thyroglobulin, thyroid peroxidase.

From: *Contemporary Endocrinology: Autoimmune Diseases in Endocrinology*
Edited by: A. P. Weetman © Humana Press, Totowa, NJ

INTRODUCTION

The concept of autoimmunity was proposed following two observations by two separate groups of investigators working on opposite sides of the Atlantic; (1) the binding of a serum component, from patients with thyroiditis, to sections of thyroid tissue *(1)* and (2) the induction of thyroiditis in rabbits immunized with thyroid extract *(2)*. Both of these occurred in 1956, and in the intervening years, considerable progress has been made in understanding the mechanisms in operation. In the case of thyroid autoimmunity, this has extended to the recognition that at least three proteins central to thyrocyte function are targets of the response *(3)*. Beyond the thyroid, many diseases previously described as idiopathic were found to have an autoimmune pathogenesis *(4)*.

Much of the information has been derived from the study of animal models of autoimmunity, both spontaneous and induced. Spontaneous models of thyroid autoimmunity are rather scarce, and the underlying autoimmune response is restricted chiefly to thyroglobulin (TG). Examples include the obese strain chicken and the BB rat. These are reviewed in refs. 5 and 6 and will not be explored further in this chapter.

The success of any induced animal model is based on how closely it resembles its human counterpart. Hashimoto's thyroiditis (HT) and Graves' disease (GD) cover the spectrum from hypothyroidism to hyperthyroidism, accompanied by destruction or hypertrophy of the gland. Despite these differences, they also share many features including a higher proportion of women affected than men, a strong genetic predisposition (polymorphisms in human leukocyte antigen [HLA]-DR, cytotoxic T-lymphocyte-associated antigen [CTLA])-4 and so on and susceptibility to environmental variables such as iodine intake *(7)*.

For convenience, the models of experimental autoimmune thyroiditis (EAT) will be described according to the inducing thyroid antigen, namely TG, thyroid peroxidase (TPO) or the thyrotropin receptor (TSHR).

TG-INDUCED MODELS OF EAT

The mature 660-kD TG protein is a glycosylated homodimer of two identical 300-kD subunits and functions as the substrate and storage protein for thyroid hormones in the follicular lumen *(8)*. It is the most abundant thyroid protein, and thus, it is not surprising that the first demonstrated autoimmune response, both in animals and in humans, was to TG. Following the initial report, the model, essentially comprising injection of TG plus adjuvant, was adapted for use in mice, and disease susceptibility was shown to be strain specific and in particular dependent on the H-2 haplotype *(9)*. Subsequent studies led to (1) the identification of pathogenic peptide fragments of TG, (2) the role of iodide in modulating TG antigenicity, (3) the passive transfer of disease through T cells, and (4) the establishment of disease-inducing T-cell clones (reviewed in ref. *10*).

An alternative protocol involved eliminating the T-cell population in rats. This was achieved by thymectomy in early life or in later life accompanied by sub-lethal irradiation of the bone marrow *(11)*. The T-cell depleted rats developed thyroiditis consequent to an autoimmune response to TG. In common with the model induced using TG plus adjuvant, the response was found to be strain specific, again pointing to

the importance of major histocompatibility complex (MHC) class II-encoded susceptibility. Furthermore, it was demonstrated to be more prevalent in female animals, which
could be protected by administration of testosterone; this diminished the thyroiditis,
although TG antibody titers remained high *(12)*.

There are two human scenarios that resemble this model, although the resulting
immune response is to the TSHR and not TG.

1. In patients with multiple sclerosis (MS) treated in vivo with Campath1, a humanized
   monoclonal to the pan-lymphocyte antigen CD52, >95% of their circulating T lymphocytes were eliminated, and there was considerable amelioration of their disease. Eighteen
   months after this treatment, T-cell numbers had returned to 35% (mostly CD8+, and
   in the CD4+ population, the CD45RO:RA ratio was low) and B cells to 180% of
   pre-treatment values. Furthermore, less interferon (IFN)-γ was produced upon in vitro
   activation of the T cells post-treatment. Cytokines play a pivotal role in the pathogenesis of all autoimmune diseases, with IFN-γ and interleukin (IL)-4 indicating Th1
   (cell-mediated) and Th2 (humoral) responses, respectively *(13)*. Most organ-specific
   autoimmune conditions display a Th1 pattern. Of 47 MS patients treated (30 female),
   14 (11 female) developed GD with TSAB. The deviation from Th1 to Th2, although
   beneficial for MS, was permissive for GD and stresses the importance of balance
   in maintaining appropriate immune responsiveness *(14)* (Alasdair Coles). Of interest,
   the same treatment has been applied to more than 600 patients with other Th1-type
   autoimmune diseases but without this complication.
2. A multi-center study of patients positive for human immunodeficiency virus, and who
   received highly active antiretroviral therapy, identified 17 with autoimmune thyroid
   disease (AITD), 15 of whom had GD. The estimated combined prevalence was 7/234
   for women and 2/1289 for men. The authors attributed this late complication of immune
   reconstitution to immune dysregulation *(15)*.

Adequate immunoregulation depends on a range of mechanisms that maintain
discrimination between self and non-self. These include elimination of autoreactive
T cells in the thymus, peripheral tolerance and anergy—the need for a second signal in
the immune synapse. Mature CD4+ thymocytes contain a high frequency of cells with
the potential to differentiate into regulatory T cells in the periphery *(16)* in sufficient
numbers to prevent disease. The radiation- and thymectomy-induced thyroiditis model
provides clear evidence for the existence of such a process, because disease is prevented
by reconstituting animals with peripheral CD4+ cells from syngeneic donors *(17)*.
These cells have a "memory" phenotype (CD45RC-), suggesting that recognition of
specific antigen in the periphery is an essential development step. Peripheral regulatory
T cells that prevent thyroiditis are not found in rats whose thyroids were ablated by
radio-iodine treatment *in utero*, although the thymus maintains the capacity to generate
them *(18)*. These experiments suggest an involvement of antigen-specific immunosuppression in the pathogenesis of AITD *(19)*. However, very different results were
obtained when the TSHR was the immunogen, comparing the induced response in
wild-type (WT) and TSHR knock-out animals (*see* TSHR-Induced Models).

In HT, disruption of thyroid follicular structure with progressive destruction of the
gland leads to hypothyroidism *(7,20)*. CD8+ T lymphocytes play an important role
in mediating the cytotoxic processes *(21,22)* that culminate in the destruction of the
cells by either necrosis or apoptosis *(20,23)*. In the necrotic process perforin plays
a central role *(24)*, as demonstrated by the correlation between perforin expression

in infiltrating lymphocytes and T-cell-mediated cytotoxicity (21,25). The Fas–FasL system is the most studied apoptotic pathway (26), and thyrocytes can express the death receptor Fas, but little is known about its regulation. Giordano et al. demonstrated that Fas was not expressed on thyrocytes unless IL-1β was present (27), whereas others reported the constitutive expression of this protein on thyroid cells (28). In EAT, it has been demonstrated that the expression of FasL on thyroid cells strongly inhibited lymphocytic infiltration, with simultaneous reduction of the anti-TG proliferative and cytotoxic T-cell responses, as well as autoantibody production (29). The effects were dependent on FasL levels, because only elevated expression was protective, whereas low-level expression exacerbated the disease by attracting inflammatory cells. In the same model, the Fas/FasL pathway may contribute to resolution of thyroiditis by the activity of CD8+ lymphocytes (30), perhaps by upregulating FasL on thyrocytes which in turn kill Fas+ inflammatory CD4+ cells and thus limit thyrocyte destruction.

TPO-INDUCED MODELS OF EAT

TPO is a glycosylated hemoprotein that catalyzes the iodination and coupling of tyrosyl residues in TG to produce thyroid hormones, T3 and T4 (31). Despite its location, on the apical surface of the thyrocyte, it is the target of both humoral and cell-mediated autoimmune responses, which underlie the pathogenesis of HT (32). Thus, animal models induced by TPO should resemble more closely human disease. The first report, from Kotani and colleagues (33), used biochemically purified TPO from pig thyroids to induce thyroiditis and TPO antibodies in C57BL/6 mice. Other mouse strains were resistant to disease induction. The authors also generated a T-cell line, which was capable of transferring disease to naïve syngeneic recipients. In subsequent studies, a thyroiditogenic epitope of TPO was identified in a peptide corresponding to TPO residues 774–788 (34). This precise model has not been reproduced by others but use of the cDNA (see TSHR-induced models) for human TPO, in combination with IL-12 or GM–CSF, induced TPO antibodies but minimal thyroiditis in the C57BL/6 strain. When the protocol was applied to HLA-DR3 transgenic non-obese diabetic (NOD) mice, thyroiditis was present in nearly one quarter of the animals and the TPO antibodies produced recognized the immunodominant regions of TPO, as defined using human autoantibodies (35). The C57BL/6 (but not CBA) strain is also susceptible to HT-like disease induced with bacterially generated mouse TPO fusion protein (36). In none of these protocols, does the thyroiditis comprise follicular destruction leading to hypothyroidism.

Although much emphasis has been placed on the fact that the induced TPO antibodies resemble the human equivalent, a recent report questions the relevance of the humoral response to the pathogenesis of HT. The authors made use of T-cell clones derived from the thyroid infiltrate of a patient with HT. The clone selected recognizes a cryptic epitope of TPO (residues 536–547), and the extracellular domains (ECDs) of its TCRA and TCRB were ligated to the intracellular domains of the mouse TCRA and TCRB. The resulting construct was used to generate transgenic mice, both on a rag$^{+/+}$ and rag$^{-/-}$ background, the latter to exclude the possibility of endogenous TCRα chains. The transgenic mice expressed the humanized TCR in the thymus and in CD4$^+$ and CD8$^+$ T cells. By 20 weeks of age, the transgenic animals were significantly heavier than their littermates and had significantly lower circulating T4 accompanied by elevated TSH. Their thyroids had extensive lymphocytic infiltration, small follicles and evidence of thyrocyte destruction, correlating with massive epithelial apoptosis. The inter-follicular spaces were filled with clusters of CD4$^+$ and CD8$^+$ T cells. Because the mice are recombinase deficient, they did not have TPO autoantibodies. The model confirms a pathogenic role for T cells specific for cryptic epitopes in AITD *(37)*. In subsequent studies, the mice were shown to have a significant reduction in CD4$^+$ CD25(hi) regulatory T cells *(38)*.

TSHR-INDUCED MODELS

Graves' disease is a common autoimmune condition caused by thyroid-stimulating antibodies (TSAb), which mimic the action of TSH *(39)*. As both the growth and the function of the thyroid are controlled by TSH *(40)*, TSAb lead to hyperthyroidism and diffuse goiter. The target of the autoimmune response in GD is the TSHR *(41)*. There are several lines of evidence suggesting that it may also provide a link between the thyroid and the orbit resulting in thyroid eye disease (TED), including the demonstration of functional TSHR in the adipose compartment, and that patients with TED tend to have the highest titers of TSAb *(42–45)*.

The TSHR is a G-protein-coupled receptor, composed of two subunits. There is a 398 residue ECD of ~55 kD that provides the high-affinity TSH-binding domain *(46)*. The ECD is attached by disulfide bonds to the 346 residue membrane-spanning region (MSR) of ~40 kD, which has the characteristic serpentine portion responsible for signal transduction. The process of generating the two subunits *(47)* may release a highly immunogenic portion of the TSHR into the circulation, which has the capacity to stimulate affinity maturation of receptor antibodies, some of which will be TSAB or thyroid-blocking antibodies (TBAb). The structure also permits the ECD to act as a tethered inverse agonist, which switches to a true agonist in the presence of TSH *(48)*. Other post-translational modifications of the TSHR required for TSH activation include tyrosine sulfation *(49)* and glycosylation on four of the six potential N-linked sites *(47)*. Recent studies have employed the ECD tethered to the cell surface by a glycophophatidyl inositol (GPI) link. The affinity of TSH for ECD–GPI is much higher than that for the holoreceptor on intact cells *(50)*, and TSAb (but not TBAb) preferentially recognize ECD–GPI compared with the holoreceptor *(51)*, a feature which has been exploited in a TSHR-induced model (*see* TSHR-Induced Models).

Despite recognizing that TSAb cause GD and that GD and TED share a common autoantigen, very little progress has been made in understanding the mechanisms responsible for breaking immune tolerance. The low expression of TSHR in the thyroid has impeded the development of animal models and made it necessary to resort to recombinant methods to produce the quantities of receptor protein required for autoimmunization protocols. Consequently, although TG-induced models have been in existence for 50 years, TSHR-induced models are a far more recent development.

Most in vitro protein production methods, from synthetic peptides through prokaryotic expression in bacteria and eukaryotic expression in insect or mammalian cells, have been tried with varying degrees of success (reviewed in ref. *52*). I will review the models that come closest to reproducing the main features of GD and TED, that is (1) elevated circulating thyroxine and/or suppressed TSH; (2) antibodies to the

TSHR, at least thyrotropin-binding-inhibiting immunoglobulins (TBII) and preferably TSAb; (3) changes in thyroid architecture and size; (4) lymphocytic non-destructive thyroiditis; (5) clinical signs of hyperthyroidism such as weight loss; (6) female animals more susceptible than male; and (7) orbital changes similar to those seen in TED, including disordered structure of extraocular muscles, edema, infiltration by immune cells, and fat accumulation.

The first clear induction of TSAb was achieved by immunizing AKR/N mice with fibroblasts transfected, so that they have stable expression of a MHC class II molecule, H-2k (homologous with the mice) and the full-length human TSHR *(53)*. When female mice were injected six times, at two weekly intervals, with 10^7 fibroblasts by the intraperitoneal route, about 20% of them developed increased thyroxine levels and TSAb. In addition, the thyroids of the animals were enlarged and displayed microscopic hypertrophy and hypercellularity but no lymphocytic infiltration. The same authors then repeated the protocol but used fibroblasts expressing chimeras of the TSHR and luteinizing hormone receptor (LHR), along with H-2k *(54)*. The aim was to define regions of the TSHR that are required and/or sufficient to induce disease. TBII (but not TSAb) were induced in mice treated with cells expressing a chimera lacking the carboxyl part of the ECD of the TSHR but not when the fibroblasts expressed a receptor construct lacking the amino end of the ECD. The absence of TSAb and elevated thyroxine, in all except animals receiving cells expressing the full-length human TSHR, confirm the requirement for numerous discontinuous residues in the ECD for complete autoreactivity to the TSHR.

The model has been confirmed *(55)* by modifying the protocol to include adjuvants most likely to stimulate T-lymphocyte helper 1 (Th1) or Th2 immune cells. These subsets of T lymphocytes, although both of a helper phenotype, are associated with either predominantly cell-mediated immunity, in the case of Th1, or humoral antibody production (including the immunoglobulin [Ig]E isotype) for Th2. The adjuvants, complete Freund's for Th1 and alum for Th2, were administered at the same time as the fibroblasts expressing H-2k and the human TSHR. Nine of 19 mice receiving alum had increased thyroxine levels and goiters and with an earlier onset than in mice not receiving the alum (9 vs 11 weeks). In contrast, induction of hyperthyroidism was slower in the mice treated with complete Freund's adjuvant (14 weeks). No difference in susceptibility was noted between male and female animals.

The most recent variation to this approach used cells expressing H-2d and the full-length murine TSHR to induce TSAb and hyperthyroxinemia in the majority of treated BALBc mice examined at 26 weeks *(56)*. The animals also exhibited weight loss, and, late in the disease process, their thyroids displayed focal necrosis and lymphocytic infiltration. The success of the model (which can also induce a response when TPO is the expressed thyroid antigen) may well reside in the expression of the B7.1 costimulatory molecule by the fibroblasts, rendering them capable of antigen presentation *(57)*.

Modelling GD and TED has been attempted by transferring TSHR-primed T cells to naive syngeneic recipients. Our experiments used unfractionated T cells and a CD4+-enriched population with the in vivo TSHR priming step performed using the ECD of the receptor produced as a maltose-binding protein fusion (ECD–MBP) in bacteria or genetic immunization (*see* TSHR-induced models). In both cases, in vivo priming was followed by an in vitro priming period using ECD–MBP. In the first study *(58)*, BALBc and NOD recipients were examined 16 days after the transfer of syngeneic receptor-primed T cells, and both strains of mice displayed thyroiditis but of very different phenotype. In the BALBc mice, B cells and immunoreactivity for IL-4 and IL-10 were found, but in the NOD mice, there was a minimal B-cell infiltrate and immunoreactivity for IFN-γ, indicating the respective Th2 and Th1 nature of the induced disease. In neither strain had antibodies developed to the receptor in the recipient animals at this early stage, although these antibodies were present in the donor mice.

Although these studies were in progress, we and others were able to demonstrate TSHR transcripts and protein in the human orbit, particularly in the adipose compartment *(43–45)*. Consequently, in more recent experiments *(59)*, to determine the kinetics of disease induced using unfractionated T cells and a CD4+-enriched population, the mouse orbits were also examined. In both BALBc and NOD recipients, the Th2 and Th1 nature of induced thyroiditis respectively was confirmed and found to persist for the 12-week duration of the experiment. At 4 weeks, TSHR antibodies, including TBII, had been induced in both strains, and these too persisted throughout the experiment. Changes in thyroid hormone levels were more difficult to evaluate, especially in the BALBc strain. In NOD recipients of TSHR-primed T cells, thyroxine levels were reduced, as might be expected from the destructive thyroiditis induced in this strain. Four weeks after transfer, BALBc recipients of TSHR-primed and control-non-primed T cells had reduced thyroxine levels, which slowly recovered in the latter. At 8 and 12 weeks, some BALBc recipients of receptor-primed T cells had increased thyroxine, relative to the control-non-primed recipients.

When examining the orbits, all of the NOD recipients of primed and non-primed cells displayed normal histology with intact, well-organized muscle fiber architecture. BALBc orbits of primed (but not non-primed) T cells appeared strikingly different. The muscle fibers were disorganized and separated by periodic acid Schiff-positive edema. There were accumulation of adipose tissue and infiltration by immune cells, especially mast cells. These changes were observed in 17 of 25 BALBc recipients of receptor-primed cells and did not correlate with TBII or T4 levels. However, orbital changes were observed only in mice having the most severe thyroiditis with 25–30% of the gland occupied by interstitium, which also correlated with the most skewed Th2 response, B:T cell ratio 1.6–1.9 and IL-4:INF-γ ratio >2.5.

One of the most ingenious protocols involves immunization with the cDNA for the full-length human TSHR cloned into a eukaryotic expression vector, a protocol that has also been applied for TPO *(60)*. One assumes that the cDNA is taken up into the myocytes at the site of injection (usually the anterior tibialis) and subsequently expressed at the surface of these cells. Myocytes do not express MHC class II or the costimulatory molecules necessary to activate T cells. Consequently, there must be a phase, perhaps triggered by inflammation of the muscle, in which professional antigen-presenting cells become involved, maybe by phagocytosing fragmented receptor/TPO released from myocytes.

Fourteen of 15 female BALBc mice treated with receptor cDNA developed antibodies to the TSHR measured by flow cytometry, and the majority contained TBII activity. One serum contained TSAb, resulting in 800% increase in cAMP production and which persisted for 18 weeks. Thyroid hormone levels remained normal throughout the experiment. All mice displayed severe thyroiditis with many infiltrating B cells, but instead of thyroid destruction, there were signs of epithelial thickening and budding.

The method was then applied to the NMRI outbred strain of mice with exciting results *(61)*. Thirty male and 30 female mice underwent the genetic immunization protocol, and virtually all developed receptor antibodies detectable by flow cytometry. Nine of the 30 males displayed signs of hypothyroidism with reduced T4. Five of 29 females developed stable hyperthyroidism with circulating TSAb accompanied by increased thyroxine but undetectable TSH levels. In addition, Th2-dependent thyroiditis and orbital changes, including infiltration by mast cells and macrophages, were induced. Analysis of the MHC haplotype of the mice revealed that they were predominantly H-2q, irrespective of whether disease had been induced or not. This highlights the importance of non-MHC genes in the development of GD and also TED, which in the words of the authors "provides the most convincing murine model of GD available to date."

All of these experiments had been performed in the animal unit in Brussels. More recently, we attempted to establish the models in the United Kingdom and found that the characteristics of the induced pathology are completely different, even when using identical Balb/cbyJico mice from the same supplier *(62)*. Although >95% of mice in both locations had antibodies recognizing the native conformation of the TSHR, as detected by flow cytometry, only a small proportion of the Balb/cbyJico mice immunized in Brussels had TSAB (and consequently raised T4) contrasting with up to 50% in Cardiff, even when using a fusion protein. However, thyroiditis was not induced in any of the TSHR-treated mice in Cardiff. We immunized 15 Balb/cbyJico mice using TSHR cDNA and the same using a TSHR fusion protein of which 15 and 12, respectively survived for analysis. From our earlier work, we would have expected at least nine mice to have thyroiditis and three of these to display orbital changes akin to TED. None of the animals developed thyroiditis or TED.

Part of the reason for this discrepancy is the possible overestimation of thyroiditis in the previous studies, caused by the high level of ectopic thymus we have found in the substrain from this supplier. Previously published thyroid histology demonstrates "inflammatory clusters at the periphery of the thyroid", which bear all the hallmarks of ectopic thymus tissue being encapsulated with and adjacent to the parathyroid gland. It should be stressed that the references also state that "cell infiltrates were also found between the follicles", and these are clearly visible in the relevant figures. However, recent flow cytometry studies of normal whole thyroid digests demonstrate significant amounts of resident immune cells *(63)*. Such a quantifiable technique would differentiate more convincingly between populations of resident and infiltrating immune cells. Any experimental animal with peripheral focal thyroiditis should have its relationship to the parathyroid described to prevent misinterpretation of ectopic thymus for a pathological lymphocytic infiltration, particularly given the high incidence of thymic ectopy reported in BALB/c (and CBA/J) mice *(63,64)*. Similarly, ocular muscle anatomy is complex and easily disturbed if muscle contraction occurs before fixation *(65)*. We obtained contraction artefacts, which could be misinterpreted as edema, in both immunized and control mice.

Given the identical genetic makeup of the animals studied, the results indicate an important influence of environment in shaping the TSHR-induced response. One potential difference between the two locations is in the iodine intake. The local feed has 1 mg/kg iodine, whereas the feed used in Brussels has 4.5 mg/kg iodine. Apart from the many reports of iodine influencing autoimmunity in rodents and humans (reviewed in Chap. 3), an enriched iodine diet (water containing 6.5 mg/L) can transiently increase the amount of thyroid-associated ectopic thymic tissue in Wistar rats *(66)*.

Neither the Brussels nor the Cardiff animal units are specific pathogen free (SPF), and in both, genetic immunization produces antibodies recognizing the native receptor, in contrast to other investigators *(67,68)*. Some differences in cytokine profile are apparent, for example in Cardiff, levels of IL-4 were low but measurable, unlike secretion of IFN-γ, which largely remained below the limit of detection in all mice. This differs from the findings of Pichurin et al. *(67)* in which genetic immunization of BALB/c mice, in an SPF facility, did not induce antibodies to the TSHR, and splenocytes stimulated with a receptor preparation produced significant IFN-γ but no IL-4.

With some rare examples of thyroiditis induced late in disease *(56)* and even allowing for overestimation, it is only in the Brussels animal unit that BALB/cbyJico mice develop TSHR-induced lymphocytic infiltration. A similar frustration is encountered in models of type 1 diabetes in which protocols based on injection of antigen (GAD or insulin) plus adjuvant or β-cell-specific expression of a viral antigen in combination with T cells with the relevant receptor fail to induce autoimmune diabetes. In the latter case, diabetes ensued following infection with live virus, which was postulated to overcome the state of ignorance (reviewed in ref. *69*). The mechanism in operation has been elegantly demonstrated to be activation of Toll-like receptors (TLRs). In this case, agonists of TLR3 or TLR7 were able to mimic the action of the live virus, and the effects are mediated through IFN-α *(70)*. The TLRs receive signals from bacteria and viruses *(71)*, and these experiments highlight the importance of infection, and the innate immune system, in the development of antigen-specific autoimmunity. TLR stimulation may be one of the contributions of an adjuvant, and, to my knowledge, only Freund's adjuvant (favors Th1) and alum (favors Th2) have been applied to TSHR-induced AITD *(55)*. A recent poster presentation reports that TSHR-immunized mice in a conventional unit (as in Brussels or Cardiff) have higher and more persistent TSAB levels than those in SPF conditions *(72)*. It could be enlightening to compare the serology of mice (preferably from the same supplier) from various units conducting such experiments.

The last study employed a protocol in which mice are immunized with adenovirus expressing the human TSHR. First described by Nagayama and colleagues *(73)*, $3 \times$ IM injections of 10^{11} viral particles, induced GD-like hyperthyroidism (elevated T4, TSAB but no thyroiditis) in 55% female/33% male BALB/c and 25% of female C57BL/6 mice. Female mice of other strains, including CBA/J, DBA/1J, and SJL/J, did not develop disease. The model has then been applied in a series of investigations reported by Rapoport and McLachlan and their co-workers. The first *(74)* used three forms of human TSHR: (1) full-length WT, (2) a mutant from which is incapable of cleavage, and (3) the free A subunit (ECD). Thyrotoxicosis and thyroid enlargement were induced in >80% ECD treated compared with 30–50% in the WT and 10–20% in the non-cleaving receptor immunized animals. Titers of TSHR antibodies, measured by enzyme linked immunosorbent assay (ELISA) or as thyrotropin-binding-inhibiting immunoglobulins

(TBII), were similar in all three groups of animals. This contrasted with TSAB and TBAB activities of which the ECD group had the highest TSAB but lowest TBAB, with the opposite in the non-cleaving receptor treated mice; once again the WT animals were at an intermediate level. The authors conclude that shed A subunits induce or amplify the immune response leading to hyperthyroidism. We have employed the ECD-GPI, in a flow cytometry protocol, to demonstrate the presence of IgG, IgA, and IgE class antibodies to the TSHR not only in GD but also in 8–12% of normal healthy individuals (75). These non-functional antibodies would not cause thyroid dysfunction, but such individuals may be at higher risk of developing GD, just as healthy TPO-positive people are more likely to progress to HT. The amplification of the immune response, leading to the evolution of TSAb, could be through increased cleavage, for instance by an estrogen-regulated metalloprotease, or by TLR stimulation following infection or treatment with IFN-α (76). TSHR expression is increased in GD compared with other thyroid pathologies or with normal glands (77,78). It is possible that TSHR gene polymorphisms (79) have a role in controlling the expression level thereby conferring predisposition to GD in individuals harboring them.

Several other conclusions can be drawn from the adenovirus model in BALB/c mice: lower doses of virus induce autoantibodies more closely resembling GD (80) and factors other than TSHR T-cell epitopes contribute to the induction of hyperthyroidism (81). When applied to other strains, it was found that even though TSAB were present in C57BL/6 mice, the accompanying high titer of TBAb prevented overt hyperthyroidism, in contrast to the situation in BALB/c mice. In the NOD mouse, the presence of thyroiditis (which occurs spontaneously in this strain) did not correlate with the magnitude of the TSHR-induced response, suggesting that the receptor may not be the autoantigen responsible for the lymphocytic infiltration found in some GD patients (82). The adenoviral and other models of GD have recently been the subject of an insightful review from these authors (83).

In related studies, TSHR null mice were generated on the C57BL/6 background. The magnitude and/or type of immune response induced to other self-proteins have been reported to differ in WT animals compared with the null equivalent (84,85). The TSHR null mice and their WT counterparts received cDNA for the full-length human TSHR. The results obtained were surprising, because TSHR antibodies, whether measured by ELISA as TBII or by flow cytometry, were similarly induced in both groups of animals. Furthermore, splenocyte responses to TSHR protein were not significantly different, and T cells from the two strains recognized the same TSHR peptides (86). If we think back to the experiments using thyroidectomized rats, these animals had no regulatory T cells that would prevent induction of thyroiditis in the thymectomy/irradiation model. We would expect the TSHR null mice to be the same and thus, devoid of regulatory T cells, to be highly susceptible to TSHR-induced immunity. This has certainly been the experience with other experimental models of autoimmune disease (84,85). Does this imply that tolerance mechanisms for the receptor differ from other self-proteins? Or is it a consequence of the strain of mouse studied (C57BL/6) being only partially susceptible to the immunization protocol employed?

Finally, it is probably true to say that many of the TSHR-induced models are the byproducts of attempts to generate monoclonal TSAb. The considerable efforts that have been expended by many investigators have been rewarded with the publication, in

December 2002, of the production and characterization of three different monoclonal antibodies with TSAb activity. Three differing approaches were used: (1) adenoviral injections into hamsters *(87)*, (2) cDNA immunization of NMRI mice *(88)*, and (3) cDNA immunization of BALB/cbyJico mice *(89)*. In each case, the full-length human TSHR was employed as immunogen, and even though the sera contained strong TSAb, many hundreds of hybridomas had to be screened to identify the monoclonal equivalent. The monoclonals had EC_{50} values in the nanomolar range, displaced TSH, TSAb, and TBAb from the TSHR in binding experiments and functioned as Fabs, a feature shared by their human counterparts *(87–89)*. Furthermore, when two such monoclonal TSAb were injected into mice, biological and histological signs of hyperthyroidism were induced, accompanied by an inflammatory reaction in the thyroid gland *(90)*.

CONCLUSIONS

The science of autoimmunity began (in part) with an animal model, and in vivo studies have been central in defining many of the fundamental principles including the role of the MHC II gene cluster, the mechanisms of central tolerance induction, and the existence of antigen-specific immunoregulatory cells. Although there are many theories as to how immune tolerance is broken, there is little convincing data to support some of them such as molecular mimicry. We know that individuals expressing certain MHC haplotypes and polymorphisms in CTLA-4 will have circulating self-reactive T cells and are predisposed to develop autoimmune disease. The antigen that becomes the target of the response may depend on polymorphic variation in an organ-specific protein, for example, the TSHR *(79)*. The environment must provide the trigger to tip the balance toward chronic autoreactivity, and activation of TLRs, by viral or bacterial products, may well contribute as has been shown for experimental autoimmune disease *(70,91)*. The next challenge will be to identify which TLRs are implicated in AITD, initially in various induced models and ultimately in patients with HT and GD.

REFERENCES

1. Roitt IM, Doniach D, Campbell RN, Vaughan Hudson R. Autoantibodies in Hashimoto's disease (lymphadenoid goiter). *Lancet* 1956;2:820–821.
2. Rose NR, Witebsky E. Studies on organ specificity. V. Changes in thyroid glands of rabbits following active immunization with rabbit thyroid extracts. *J Immunol* 1956;76:417–427.
3. Ludgate M, Vassart G. The molecular-genetics of 3 thyroid autoantigens – thyroglobulin, thyroid peroxidase and the thyrotropin receptor. *Autoimmunity* 1990;7:201–211.
4. Lorenz HM, Herrmann M, Kalden JR. The pathogenesis of autoimmune diseases. *Scand J Clin Lab Invest* 2001;61:16–26(Suppl. 235).
5. Sundick RS, Bagchi N, Brown TR. The obese strain chicken as a model for human Hashimoto's thyroiditis. *Exp Clin Endocrinol Diabetes* 1996;104:4–6(Suppl. 3).
6. Delemarre FGA, Simons PJ, Drexhage HA. The BB rat as a model for autoimmune thyroiditis: Relevance for the pathogenesis of human disease. *Exp Clin Endocrinol Diabetes* 1996;104:10–12(Suppl. 3).
7. Weetman AP. Autoimmune thyroid disease: propagation and progression. *Eur J Endocrinol* 2003;148:1–9.
8. Van de Graaf SAR, Ris-Stalpers C, Pauws E, Mendive FM, Targovnik HM, de Vijlder JJM. Structure update - up to date with human thyroglobulin. *J Endocrinol* 2001;170:307–321.

9. Vladitui A, Rose N. Autoimmune murine thyroiditis. Relation to histocompatabiltiy (H-2) type. *Science* 1971;174:1137–1140.

10. Kong, Y-CM, Giraldo, AA. Experimental autoimmune thyroiditis in the mouse and rat. In *Autoimmune Disease Models* (Irun Cohen, Ariel Miller, eds). Elsevier. *Academic Press, San Diego*; 1994;123–145.

11. Penhale WJA, Farmer A, McKenna RP, Irvine WJ. Spontaneous thyroiditis in thymectomised and irradiated Wistar rats. *Clin Exp Immunol* 1973;15:122.

12. Ahmed SA, Young PR, Penhale WJ. Beneficial effect of testosterone in the treatment of chronic autoimmune thyroiditis in rats. *J Immunol* 1986;136:143–147.

13. Singh VK, Mehrotra S, Agarwal SS. The paradigm of Th1 and Th2 cytokines: its relevance to autoimmunity and allergy. *Immunol Res* 1999;20:147–161.

14. Coles AJ, Wing N, Smith S et al. Pulsed monoclonal antibody treatment and autoimmune thyroid disease in multiple sclerosis. *Lancet* 1999;354:1691–1695.

15. Chen F, Day SL, Metcalfe RA et al. Characteristics of autoimmune thyroid disease occurring as a late complication of immune reconstitution in patients with advanced human immunodeficiency virus (HIV) disease. *Medicine* 2005;84:98–106.

16. Saoudi A, Seddon B, Fowell D, Mason D. The thymus contains a high frequency of cells that prevent autoimmune diabetes on transfer into prediabetic recipients. *J Exp Med* 1996;184:2393–2398.

17. Seddon B, Mason D. Regulatory T cells in the control of autoimmunity: the essential role of transforming growth factor beta and interleukin 4 in the prevention of autoimmune thyroiditis in rats by peripheral CD4(+)CD45RC- cells and CD4(+)CD8(-) thymocytes. *J Exp Med* 1999;189:279–288.

18. Seddon B, Mason D. Peripheral autoantigen induces regulatory T cells that prevent autoimmunity. *J Exp Med* 1999;189:877–882.

19. Volpe R. Suppressor T lymphocyte dysfunction is important in the pathogenesis of autoimmune thyroid disease: a perspective. *Thyroid* 1993;3:345–352.

20. Dayan CM, Daniels GH. Chronic autoimmune thyroiditis. *N Engl J Med* 1996;335:99–107.

21. Hammond LJ, Palazzo FF, Shattock M, Goode AW, Mirakian R. Thyrocyte targets and effectors of autoimmunity: a role for death receptors? *Thyroid* 2001;11:919–927.

22. Wu Z, Podack ER, McKenzie JM, Olsen KJ, Zakarija M. Perforin expression by thyroid-infiltrating T cells in autoimmune thyroid disease. *Clin Exp Immunol* 1994;98:470–477.

23. Barry M, Bleackley RC. Cytotoxic T lymphocytes: all roads lead to death. *Nat Rev Immunol* 2002;2:401–409.

24. Stassi G, De Maria R. Autoimmune thyroid disease: new models of cell death in autoimmunity. *Nat Rev Immunol* 2002;2:195–204.

25. Stepp SE, Mathew PA, Bennett M, de Saint Basile G, Kumar V. Perforin: more than just an effector molecule. *Immunol Today* 2000;21:254–256.

26. De Maria R, Testi R. Fas-FasL interactions: a common pathogenetic mechanism in organ-specific autoimmunity. *Immunol Today* 1998;19:121–125.

27. Giordano C, Stassi G, De Maria R, Todaro M, Richiusa P, Papoff G, Ruberti G, Bagnasco M, Testi R, Galluzzo A. Potential involvement of Fas and its ligand in the pathogenesis of Hashimoto's thyroiditis. *Science* 1997;275:960–963.

28. Phelps E, Wu P, Bretz J, Baker JR Jr. Thyroid cell apoptosis. A new understanding of thyroid autoimmunity. *Endocrinol Metab Clin North Am* 2000;29:375–388.

29. Batteux F, Lores P, Bucchini D, Chiocchia G. Transgenic expression of Fas ligand on thyroid follicular cells prevents autoimmune thyroiditis. *J Immunol* 2000;164:1681–1688.

30. Wei Y, Chen K, Sharp GC, Yagita H, Braley-Mullen H. Expression and regulation of Fas and Fas ligand on thyrocytes and infiltrating cells during induction and resolution of granulomatous experimental autoimmune thyroiditis. *J Immunol* 2001;167:6678–6686.

31. Libert F, Ruel J, Ludgate M, Swillens S, Alexander N, Vassart G, Dinsart C. Thyroperoxidase, an auto-antigen with a mosaic structure made of nuclear and mitochondrial gene modules. *EMBO J* 1987;6:4193–4196.

32. McLachlan SM, Rapoport B. The molecular biology of thyroid peroxidase: cloning, expression and role as autoantigen in autoimmune thyroid disease. *Endocr Revs* 1992;13:192–206.

33. Kotani T, Umeki K, Hirai K, Ohtaki S. Experimental murine thyroiditis induced by porcine thyroid peroxidase and its transfer by the antigen-specific T cell line. *Clin Exp Immunol* 1990;80:11–18.

34. Kotani T, Umeki K, Yagihashi S, Hirai K, Ohtaki S. Identification of thyroiditogenic epitope on porcine thyroid peroxidase for C57bl/6 mice. *J Immunol* 1992;148:2084–2089.

35. Flynn JC, Gardas A, Wan Q, Gora M, Alsharabi G, Wei WZ, Giraldo AA, David CS, Kong YM, Banga JP. Superiority of thyroid peroxidase DNA over protein immunization in replicating human thyroid autoimmunity in HLA-DRB1*0301. *Clin Exp Immunol* 2004;137:503–512.

36. Ng HP, Banga JP, Kung AWC. Development of a murine model of autoimmune thyroiditis induced with homologous mouse thyroid peroxidase. *Endocrinology* 2004;145:809–816.

37. Quaratino S, Badami E, Pang YY, Bartok I, Dyson J, Kioussis D, Londei M, Maiuri L. Degenerate self-reactive human T-cell receptor causes spontaneous autoimmune disease in mice. *Nat Med* 2004;10:920–926.

38. Badami E, Maiuri L, Quaratino S. High incidence of spontaneous autoimmune thyroiditis in immunocompetent self-reactive human T cell receptor transgenic mice. *J Autoimmun* 2005;24:85–91.

39. Rees Smith B, Mclachlan S, Furmaniak J. Autoantibodies to the thyrotropin receptor. *Endocr Rev* 1998;9:106–120.

40. Vassart G, Dumont JE. The thyrotropin receptor and the regulation of thyrocyte function and growth. *Endocr Rev* 1992;13:596–611.

41. Paschke R, Ludgate M. The thyrotropin receptor and thyroid disease. *N Engl J Med* 1997;337: 1675–1681.

42. Khoo DHC, Ho SC, Seah LL et al. The combination of absent thyroid peroxidase antibodies and high thyroid stimulating immunoglobulins identifies a group at markedly increased risk of ophthalmopathy. *Thyroid* 1999;9:1175–1180.

43. Crisp M, Lane C, Halliwell M et al. Thyrotropin receptor transcripts in human adipose tissue. *J Clin Endocrinol Metab* 1997;82:2003–2005.

44. Bahn R, Dutton C, Natt N et al. Thyrotropin receptor expression in Graves' orbital adipose/connective tissues; potential autoantigen in Graves' Ophthalmopathy. *J Clin Endocrinol Metab* 1998;83:998–1002.

45. Crisp M, Starkey K, Ham J et al. Adipogenesis in thyroid eye disease. *Invest Ophthalmol Vis Sci* 2000;41:3249–3255.

46. Misrahi M, Loosfelt H, Gross B, Atger M, Jolivet A, Savouret JF, Milgrom E. Characterization of the thyroid stimulating hormone receptor. *Curr Opin Endocrinol Diabetes* 1994;175:175–183.

47. Rapoport B, Chazenbalk GD, Juame JC, McLachlan SM. The thyrotropin (TSH) receptor: interaction with TSH and autoantibodies. *Endocr Rev* 1998;19:673–716.

48. Vlaeminck-Guillem V, Ho SC, Rodien P, Vassart G, Costagliola S. Activation of the cAMP pathway by the TSH receptor involves switching of the ectodomain from a tethered inverse agonist to an agonist. *Mol Endocrinol* 2002;16:736–746.

49. Costagliola S, Paneels V, Bonomi M, Koch J, Many MC, Smits G, Vassart G. Tyrosine sulfation is required for agonist recognition by glycoprotein hormone receptors. *EMBO J* 2002;21:504–513.

50. Costagliola S, Khoo D, Vassart G. Production of bioactive amino-terminal domain of the thyrotropin receptor via insertion in the plasma membrane by a glycosylphosphatidylinositol anchor. *FEBS Lett* 1998;436:427–433.

51. Chazenbalk GD, Pichurin P, Chen CR, Latrofa F, Johnstone AP, McLachlan SM, Rapoport B. Thyroid stimulating autoantibodies in Graves' disease preferentially recognise the free A subunit, not the thyrotropin holoreceptor. *J Clin Invest* 2002;110:209–217.

52. Ludgate M. Animal models of Graves' disease. *Eur J Endo* 2000;142:1–8.

53. Shimojo N, Kohno Y, Yamaguchi KI et al. Induction of Graves'-like disease in mice by immunization with fibroblasts transfected with the thyrotropin receptor and a class II molecule. *Proc Natl Acad Sci USA* 1996;93:11074–11079.

54. Kikuoka S, Shimojo N, Yamaguchi KI et al. The formation of thyrotropin receptor (TSHR) antibodies in a Graves' animal model requires the N-terminal segment of the TSHR extracellular domain. *Endocrinology* 1998;139:1891–1898.

55. Kita M, Ahmad L, Marians RC et al. Regulation and transfer of a murine model of thyrotropin receptor antibody mediated Graves' Disease. *Endocrinology* 1999;140:1392–1398.

56. Kaithamana S, Fan JL, Osuga Y et al. Induction of experimental autoimmune Graves' disease in BALB/c mice. *J Immunol* 1999;163:5157–5167.

57. Yan XM, Guo J, Pichurin P, Tanaka K, Jaume JC, Rapoport B, McLachlan SM. Cytokines, IgG subclasses and costimulation in a mouse model of thyroid autoimmunity induced by injection of fibroblasts co-expressing MHC class II and thyroid autoantigens. *Clin Exp Immunol* 2000;122:170–179.

58. Costagliola S, Many MC, StalmansFalys M et al. Transfer of thyroiditis, with syngeneic spleen-cells sensitized with the human thyrotropin receptor, to naive BALB/c and nod mice. *Endocrinology* 1996;137:4637–4643.

59. Many MC, Costagliola S, Detrait M et al. Development of an animal model of autoimmune thyroid eye disease. *J Immunol* 1999;162:4966–4974.

60. Costagliola S, Rodien P, Many MC et al. Genetic immunization against the human thyrotropin receptor causes thyroiditis and allows production of monoclonal antibodies recognizing the native receptor. *J Immunol* 1998;160:1458–1465.

61. Costagliola S, Many MC, Denef JF et al. Genetic immunisation of outbred mice with thyrotropin receptor cDNA provides a model of Graves' disease. *J Clin Invest* 2000;105:803–811.

62. Baker G, Mazziotti G, von Ruhland C, Ludgate M. Re-evaluating thyrotropin receptor induced mouse models of Graves' disease & ophthalmopathy. *Endocrinology* 2005;146:835–844.

63. Caturegli P, Rose N, Kimura M, Kimura H, Tzou S. Studies on murine thyroiditis: new insights from organ flow cytometry. *Thyroid* 2003;13:419–426.

64. Vladutiu A, Rose N. Aberrant thymus tissue in rat and mouse thyroid. *Experientia* 1972;28:79–81.

65. Muhlendyck H, Syed A. Fixation artefacts in the external eye muscles in biopsy examinations. (A light microscopy and electron microscopy study). *Buch Augenarzt* 1978;73:181–191.

66. Mooij P, de Wit H, Drexhage H. A high iodine intake in Wistar rats results in the development of a thyroid-associated ectopic thymic tissue and is accompanied by a low thyroid autoimmune reactivity. *Immunology* 1994;81:309–316.

67. Pichurin P, Yan XM, Farilla L, Guo J, Chazenbalk GD, Rapoport B, McLachlan SM. Naked TSH receptor DNA vaccination: A TH1 T cell response in which interferon-gamma production, rather than antibody, dominates the immune response in mice. *Endocrinology* 2001;142:3530–3536.

68. Rao PV, Watson PF, Weetman AP, Carayanniotis G, Banga JP. Contrasting activities of thyrotropin receptor antibodies in experimental models of Graves' disease induced by injection of transfected fibroblasts or deoxyribonucleic acid vaccination. *Endocrinology* 2003;144:260–266.

69. Bach JF. A Toll-like trigger for autoimmune disease. *Nat Med* 2005;11:120–121.

70. Lang et al. Toll-like receptor engagement converts T-cell autoreactivity into overt autoimmune disease. *Nat Med* 2005;11:138–145.

71. Hemmi H et al. A toll-like receptor recognizes bacterial DNA. *Nature* 2000;408:740–745.

72. Bhattacharyya KK, Coenen MJ, Bahn RS. Effect of environmental pathogens on the TSHR-directed immune response in an animal model of Graves' disease. *Thyroid* 2005;15:422–426.

73. Nagayama Y et al. A novel murine model of Graves' hyperthyroidism with intramuscular injection of adenovirus expressing the thyrotropin receptor. *J Immunol* 2002;168:2789–2794.

74. Chen CR et al. The thyrotropin receptor autoantigen in Graves' disease is the culprit as well as the victim. *J Clin Invest* 2003;111:1897–1904.

75. Metcalfe R, Jordan N, Watson P, Gullu S, Wiltshire M, Crisp M, Evans C, Weetman A, Ludgate M. Demonstration of IgG, IgA and IgE autoantibodies to the human thyrotropin receptor using flow cytometry. *J Clin Endocrinol Metab* 2002;87:1754–1761.

76. Fentiman IS, Thomas BS, Balkwill FR, Rubens RD, Hayward JL. Primary hypothyroidism associated with interferon therapy of breast cancer. *Lancet* 1985;1:1166.

77. Sequeira M, Jasani B, Fuhrer D, Wheeler M, Ludgate M. Demonstration of reduced in vivo surface expression of activating mutant thyrotropin receptors in thyroid sections. *Eur J Endocrinol* 2002;146:163–171.

78. Starkey KJ, Janezic A, Jones G, Jordan N, Baker G, Ludgate M. Adipose thyrotropin receptor expression is elevated in Graves' and thyroid eye diseases ex vivo and indicates adipogenesis in progress in vivo. *J Mol Endocrinol* 2003;30:369–380.

79. Dechairo BM et al. Association of the TSHR gene with Graves' disease: the first disease specific locus. *Eur J Hum Genetics* 2005;13:1223–1230.

80. Chen CR et al. Low dose immunization with adenovirus expressing the thyroid stimulating hormone receptor A-subunit deviates the antibody response toward that of autoantibodies in human Graves' disease. *Endocrinology* 2004;145:228–233.

81. Pichurin PN, Chen CR, Nagayama Y, Pichurina O, Rapoport B, McLachlan SM. Evidence that factors other than particular thyrotropin receptor T cell epitopes contribute to the development of hyperthyroidism in murine Graves' disease. *Clin Exp Immunol* 2004;135:391–397.

82. Chen CR, Aliesky H, Pichurin PN, Nagayama Y, McLachlan SM, Rapoport B. Susceptibility rather than resistance to hyperthyroidism is a dominant in a thyrotropin receptor adenovirus-induced animal model of Graves' disease as revealed by BALB/c-C57BL/6 hybrid mice. *Endocrinology* 2004;145:4927–4933.

83. McLachlan SM, Nagayama Y, Rapoport B. Insight into Graves' hyperthyroidism from animal models. *Endocr Rev* 2005;26:800–832.

84. Amagai M, Tsunoda K, Suzuki H, Nishifuji K, Koyasu S, Nishikawa T. Use of autoantigen-knockout mice in developing an active autoimmune disease model for pemphigus. *J Clin Invest* 2000;105:625–631

85. Harrington CJ, Paez A, Hunkapiller T, Mannikko V, Brabb T, Ahearn M, Beeson C, Goverman J. Differential tolerance is induced in T cells recognizing distinct epitopes of myelin basic protein. *Immunity* 1998;8:571–580

86. Pichurin PN et al. Thyrotropin receptor knockout mice: studies on immunological tolerance to a major thyroid autoantigen. *Endocrinology* 2004;145:1294–1301.

87. Ando T, Latif R, Protsker A, Moran T, Nagayama Y, Davies TF. A monoclonal thyroid stimulating antibody. *J Clin Invest* 2002;110:1667–1674.

88. Sanders J et al. Thyroid-stimulating monoclonal antibodies. *Thyroid* 2002;12:1043–1050.

89. Costagliola S et al. Generation of a mouse monoclonal TSH receptor antibody with stimulating activity. *Biochem Biophys Res Commun* 2002;299:891–896.

90. Costagliola S et al. Delineation of the discontinuous-conformational epitope of a monoclonal antibody displaying full in vitro and in vivo thyrotropin activity. *Mol Endocrinol* 2004;18:3020–3034.

91. Rifkin IR, Leadbetter EA, Busconi L, Viglianti G, Marshak-Rothstein A. Toll-like receptors, endogenous ligands, and systemic autoimmune disease. *Immunol Rev* 2005;204:27–42.

5 Thyroid Autoantigens

Philip F. Watson, PhD, and Nagat Saeed, PhD

Contents

Summary

Identification and characterization of key antigenic targets is an important step in understanding the development and pathogenic mechanisms of autoimmune disease. Fifty years after the initial description of thyroid autoimmunity and identification of the major autoantigens, the disease remains the best understood form of human organ-specific autoimmunity. The structure and function of the major thyroid antigens, together with recent advances in our understanding of the corresponding autoimmune responses to these targets, will be discussed in this chapter.

Key Words: Thyroglobulin, thyroid peroxidase, thyrotropin receptor, thyroid-stimulating antibodies, epitopes.

INTRODUCTION

Autoimmune thyroid disease (AITD), the archetypal example of organ-specific autoimmunity, comprises several disorders that together constitute the most common form of autoimmune disease affecting approximately 1% of the population *(1)*. Autoimmune hypothyroidism (AH) is generally divided into goitrous (Hashimoto's thyroiditis [HT]) and non-goitrous primary myxedema. HT features extensive lymphocytic infiltration of the thyroid gland, often with the formation of germinal centers, whereas in myxedema progressive fibrosis and atrophy of the gland proceed with little inflammatory infiltrate.

Autoimmune hyperthyroidism or Graves' disease (GD) affects approximately 2% of women and 0.2% of men *(1)*. The disease is characterized by the presence of thyroid-stimulating antibodies (TSAbs) that target the thyrotropin receptor (TSHR) and act as agonists, resulting in chronic overstimulation and thyrotoxicosis *(2)*. Lymphocytic

From: *Contemporary Endocrinology: Autoimmune Diseases in Endocrinology*
Edited by: A. P. Weetman © Humana Press, Totowa, NJ

infiltration is also a feature of GD, though this tends to be less abundant and more focal in nature than that observed in HT *(2)*.

Thyroid-associated ophthalmopathy (TAO) and pretibial myxedema (PTM) are two extrathyroidal manifestations of GD, the etiology of which remains unclear. TAO, the more common and clinically more significant of the two, features edema and lymphocytic infiltration of the retro-orbital soft fatty tissues and the retro-orbital muscles. Given the association with GD, investigations into the pathogenesis of TAO have focused on the concept of an autoimmune process directed at a component common to both tissues, though to date there is no conclusive evidence to support a particular candidate antigen *(3)*.

Evidence for a genetic predisposition to AITD is well established from both family and twin studies with sibling-risk estimated to be between 5 and 10 for individual diseases *(4,5)*. Cumulative data from a range of genetic studies support the hypothesis that the occurrence of AITD is the result of a complex interaction between environmental factors an array of susceptibility genes *(6)*. The most clearly established genetic associations with AITD are that of the major histocompatibility complex (MHC), in particular human leukocyte antigen (HLA)-DR3 *(2)*, and more recently the immunomodulatory gene *CTLA-4 (6)*. The contributions of these genes to the overall risk of AITD are relatively minor and suggest a role for additional, as yet undetermined, genetic factors. Candidate genes include the major thyroid autoantigenic targets, and the current evidence regarding the potential role of these genes as susceptibility factors will be reviewed next.

AITD represents a most useful model of organ-specific autoimmunity, not least as the major autoantigens involved: thyroglobulin (TG), thyroid peroxidase (TPO), and TSHR were identified some five decades ago and have been the subject of intense investigation over this period. It could be said that each thyroid antigen provides insights into different facets of the autoimmune process, from the role of post-translational modification in the immunobiology of TG, to the cytotoxic cellular destructive processes associated with the immune response to TPO, and finally the critical role of TSHR autoantibodies in the pathology of GD. Understanding the nature of thyroid autoantigens, from their biological function in the thyroid gland to their role as targets for the immune system, and as potential genetic determinants in disease susceptibility, offers insights into the etiology and the pathogenesis of AITD and, by extension, other organ-specific autoimmune conditions. This account will provide a summary of current knowledge and recent advances in this field.

THYROGLOBULIN

Structure and Function

TG is a large 660-kDa homodimeric glycoprotein and the major protein product of the thyroid gland. TG is synthesized in the endoplasmic reticulum of thyroid follicular cells (thyrocytes) and, following post-translational modification, mainly glycosylation, is secreted into the thyroid lumen where it accumulates. TPO catalyzes the iodination of TG tyrosine residues to form monoiodotyrosines and di-iodotyrosines, and subsequent oxidative coupling of these iodotyrosines produces TG molecules bearing tetra-iodothyronine (T_4) or tri-iodothyronine (T_3) at specific hormonogenic sites *(7)*. Release of thyroid hormones into the circulation takes place following limited extracellular proteolysis of stored $TG–T_4/T_3$ complexes and lysosomal-mediated liberation of T_3 and T_4 *(7)*. Human TG (hTG) monomer is a 2748-residue polypeptide with a predicted molecular weight of approximately 303 kDa *(8)*. The amino-terminal 70% of the primary sequence features a number of regions of internal homology that can be subdivided into three groups based on sequence conservation: 10 type 1 domains containing 60 amino acids and featuring proline, cysteine, and glycine residues in conserved positions suggesting a conserved three-dimensional (3D) structure; three relatively short type 2 domains containing 14–17 residues; and five type 3 domains that feature repeated cysteine residues *(9)*. The carboxy terminal region of TG has homology to acetylcholinesterase, with similarity ranging from 20% overall but increasing to 60% in specific regions *(9)*. This feature has been the subject of discussion and investigation, but the significance of this similarity remains unclear. The identification of autoantibodies directed against the carboxy-terminal portion of TG and cross-reactive with acetycholinesterase suggested a possible connection between TG immunoreactivity and targets expressed in eye muscle, but low frequency of such antibodies in GD patient sera mitigated against there being a causal role for this phenomenon in TAO *(10)*. Immunologically TG possesses a number of interesting features. Unlike other thyroid antigens, it is not sequestered but released into the circulation together with T_3 and T_4 *(11)*. The release of TG into the circulation and the anatomical connection between the lymphatic system of the thyroid gland and the eyes led to the suggestion that deposition of TG in the orbit could initiate an immune process that either precipitated or contributed to TAO *(12)*. More recent evidence however indicates that the interaction of circulating TG with orbital tissues is so weak as to make this an unlikely pathogenic mechanism *(13)*. There is evidence that the degree of iodination influences the immune response to TG, suggesting the possibility that dominant epitopes may either contain iodine or are modified by iodination *(11)*. The concept of "cryptic self" extends this hypothesis to include the additional post-translational modifications that are a feature of TG biosynthesis and function and suggests a pathogenic mechanism based on the unmasking of hidden epitopes and subsequent breakdown of tolerance *(11)*.

Genetics

The TG structural gene is located on chromosome 8q24.2–q24.3 and extends over some 300 kbp *(9)*. A number of polymorphisms of TG gene have been described, and TG has been investigated as a candidate risk factor for AITD with mixed results. A genome-wide sib-pair linkage analysis identified region 8q23–q24 as a potential AITD susceptibility locus in the Japanese population *(14)*, and a subsequent case–control study demonstrated a weak association between a TG microsatellite (Tgms2) and AITD, though it could not be determined if this association was due to the TG gene or an adjacent locus in linkage disequilibrium *(15)*. A large case–control study based on UK patients demonstrated an increased frequency of Tgms2 in the patient group, but the rarity of the associated allele prevented a familial analysis and conclusive demonstration of a causal connection rather than chance *(16)*. A case–control analysis of three more common (non-conservative) single base polymorphisms in exons 10, 12, and 33 indicated an association with AITD in the Caucasian population *(17)*, though another larger case–control study failed to confirm this association in the UK population *(18)*. Thus, while the linkage of chromosomal region 8q23–q24 has been confirmed independently as a risk locus for AITD, whether this is due to the TG gene or another adjacent gene remains unclear.

T-Cell Epitopes

Mice immunized with TG or TG peptides develop experimental autoimmune thyroiditis (EAT), a T-cell mediated disease with similarities to HT *(2)*. The induction of EAT with TG has been shown to be MHC dependent *(2)*, and work from several groups has identified 13 thyroiditogenic T-cell epitopes (Fig. 1) *(19)*. Eight of these were identified in murine TG (mTG) and three in hTG, and two (1–12, 2549–2560) were conserved sites of hormonogenesis and identical in both species. Peptide 2549–2560 contains T_4 at position 2553 and has been shown to be a potent stimulus for both proliferative and cytotoxic T-cell responses *(11)*. By contrast, two other T_4-containing peptides (2559–2570 and 2737–2748) lack immunogenicity, indicating that the T_4 hapten is not in itself sufficient to elicit a T-cell response *(11)*. Studies with an analogue peptide (2549–2560) containing thyronine but lacking the four iodine atoms of T_4 showed that iodination per se does not render a peptide immunogenic but iodine atoms can contribute to peptide–MHC complexes and generate a specific T-cell response *(11)*. It is not known whether iodination of other non-hormonogenic TG peptides can generate T-cell epitopes by this mechanism, but this phenomenon provides a possible explanation for observations such as the reduced immunogenicity of TG with low iodine content in mice and rats and conversely the increased immuno-genicity of highly iodinated TG *(11)*. Finally, it has been shown that a number of peptides, synthetically or biochemically derived, that contain T-cell epitopes are also targets of B-cell responses (Fig. 1), and this has highlighted the possibility that TGAb binding can modulate the processing and presentation of immunogenic peptides and thus potentially contribute to the autoimmune process perhaps by promoting the spread of the immune response to cryptic T-cell epitopes *(11)*.

B-Cell Epitopes

TG autoantibodies (TGAbs) are a common marker of AITD and can be present at a high level in patient sera *(20)*. Natural autoantibodies to TG are also present in normal individuals *(21)* and anti-TG antibodies feature in monogammaglobulinopathies *(22)*, suggesting that TG is a common target for both normal and pathogenic B-cell responses. However, TGAbs from AITD patients recognize a narrower range of epitopes with high affinity, reach higher titres, and, in contrast to natural antibodies, exhibit somatic hyper-mutation *(23)*. The role of TGAb in disease is unclear as they do not fix complement and do not appear to contribute to complement-mediated tissue destruction *(24)*. However, cytotoxic TGAb have been described in HT *(25)*, and it has been suggested that the formation of opsonized immune complexes can promote B-cell and T-cell proliferation in response to self-antigens in AITD *(11)*.

Early attempts to determine epitopes used fragments of TG produced mixed results with AITD patient sera. Screening of λgt11 fragment libraries using rabbit TG-antisera identified linear epitopes, but none of these were recognized by AITD patient sera *(26)*. Consistent data were only achieved with the use of intact native antigen, suggesting that, in common with other thyroid autoantigens, the majority of patient epitopes are conformational *(27)*. Analysis of IgG and IgM TGAb has been reported from peripheral

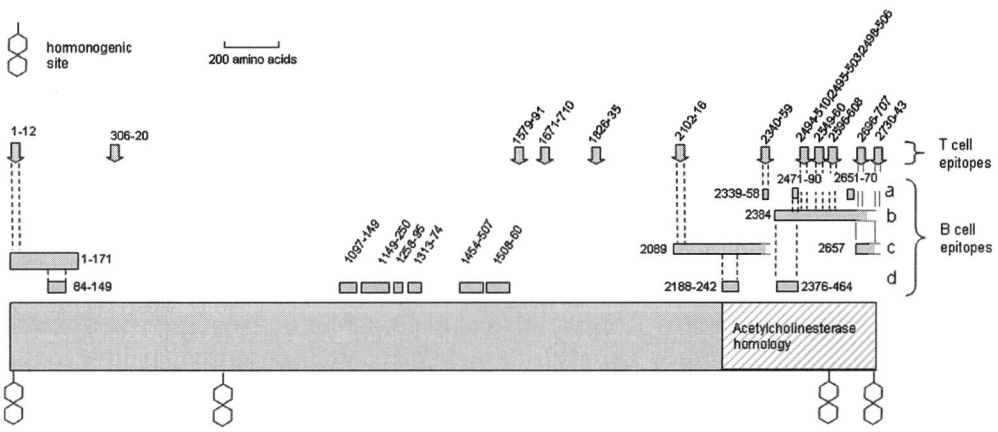

Fig. 1. Diagrammatic representation of the polypeptide chain of hTG showing the location of epitopes recognized by human TGAb and immunopathic peptides causing EAT in mice. T and B cell epitopes are indicated by boxes and identified by numbering of N- and C-terminal amino acids. Peptides in which the C-terminus is only predicted are identified by the N-terminal residue number alone and dotted lines at the C-terminal end. (a) Chemically synthesized peptides; (b) fragments produced by oxidative cleavage; (c) peptides produced by chemical or enzymatic cleavage; (d) recombinantly expressed peptides. Overlapping regions of different epitopes are connected by vertical dashed lines (dotted lines for presumptive C-termini). Figure reproduced with permission *(19)*.

blood, intrathyroidal lymphocytes, and lymph node tissue from several patients with HT using both conventional hybridoma and phage display approaches *(28)*. Although the limited number of patient studies carried out to date suggests that the available monoclonals probably represent only a fraction of the TGAb patient repertoire, some useful insights have been provided by analysis of these reagents. In one study of TGAbs isolated from a patient combinatorial library (κ and λ), the heavy chains used were all from the relatively common (frequently rearranged) VH-3-23 family *(23)*. Interestingly, these TG Fabs shared both heavy gene usage and epitope specificity with a previously isolated conventional hTG mAb 3C42 *(29)*. A second combinatorial approach utilized an alternative screening method to increase the diversity of recovered mAbs, and the resultant pool of 64 monoclonals were used in competition studies to define two major patient epitopes and several minor TG epitopes *(28)*. One major epitope was recognized by mAb 3C42, though this antibody was also able to inhibit TG binding by normal euthyroid sera suggesting that this epitope may also be common to the natural autoantibody repertoire *(28)* and raising the intriguing possibility that some of the AITD patient TGAb repertoire may arise from affinity maturation of natural autoantibodies.

THYROID PEROXIDASE

Structure

TPO is a membrane-bound glycoprotein expressed on the apical surface of thyroid follicular cells. TPO contains a prosthetic heme group and, in a reaction dependent upon iodide and H_2O_2, catalyzes the iodination of tyrosine residues on TG and the condensation of these iodinated groups to generate diiodothyronines T_3 and T_4 *(30)*.

Structurally, TPO is most related to human myeloperoxidase (MPO) with approximately 42% amino acid similarity. TPO has an additional 197-amino acid extension comprising two domains, the first similar to a complement control protein repeat motif (CCP) and the second similar to the epidermal growth factor (EGF) low-density lipoprotein receptor families *(31)*. This region is followed by a single transmembrane domain and intracellular carboxy terminus (Fig. 2A).

Genetics

The cDNA for human TPO was simultaneously isolated by a number of groups in 1987 *(32–34)*. The full-length gene encodes a polypeptide of 933 amino acids, though a number of splice variants exist *(30)*. The human TPO gene is located on chromosome 2 and spans approximately 150 kbp *(33,35)*. A number of genetic variants of TPO have been identified in studies of congenital defects in iodine fixation and hypothyroidism *(30)*; however, no known polymorphisms of TPO are associated with risk of AITD, and the most powerful study to date revealed no linkage to the corresponding chromosomal region *(36)*.

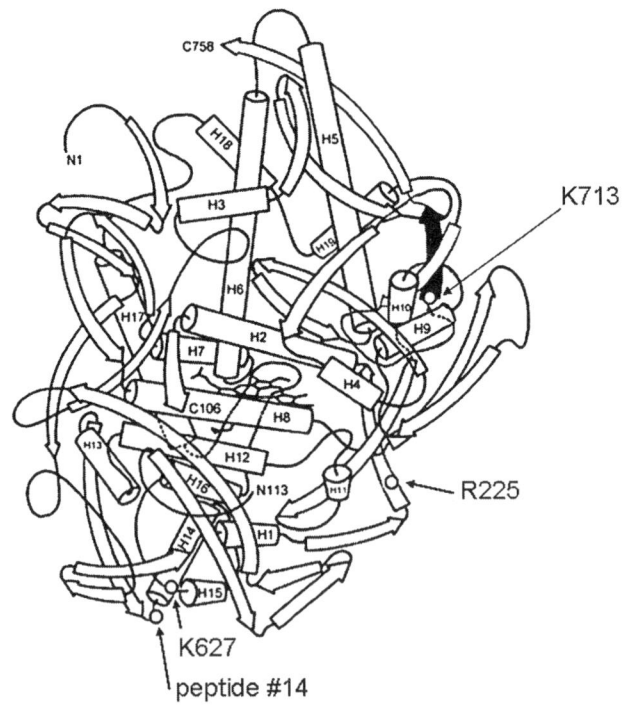

Fig. 2. Representation of the three-dimensional structure of TPO, based on the known structure of MPO (reproduced with permission from Zeng and Fenna 1992 *(61)*). Only one TPO monomer is depicted, and TPO amino acid residues 1-121 (corresponding residues cleaved from mature MPO) have been omitted. The mAb47 epitope is shown shaded in black. The relative positions of R225, K627, and peptide #14, and the predicted TPO structural features are estimates based on the homology between the TPO and MPO primary sequences.

T-Cell Epitopes

Compared with the body of work surrounding TPO autoantibodies relatively little has been reported regarding T-cell responses to TPO. In contrast to human disease, a clear role for TPO has not been demonstrated in the various known spontaneous animal models of AITD *(37–39)*. Historically, TG has been the antigen of choice for animal models of AITD, and the majority of T-cell studies have been carried out on patient intrathyroidal and circulating T cells using synthetic peptides and recombinant TPO fragments. Investigation of expanded T-cell clones recovered from thyroid infiltrate indicated that the response to TPO was diverse in terms of HLA dependency and identified at least two separate T-cell epitopes *(40)*. Subsequent studies from different groups have demonstrated reactivity to a range of TPO peptide epitopes (summarized in Table 1) *(41–46)*. Interestingly, a potentially cross-reactive epitope present in TPO and TG was identified *(47)*, and a corresponding synthetic peptide was able to stimulate splenocytes from mice immunized with TG or TPO *(48)*. In recent years, the central role of regulatory T cells in the etiology of human autoimmunity has become increasingly clear, and studies of T-cell responses in animal models of thyroiditis have assumed a greater importance. Importantly, a novel animal model of EAT was recently developed in which mice transgenic for a human TPO peptide-specific (536–548) T-cell receptor molecule developed spontaneous destructive thyroiditis and hypothyroidism *(49)*. Vaccination of BALB/c mice with TPO-DNA in a plasmid led to the generation of TPO antibodies and T-cell responses to a diverse response to a range of peptides encompassing the TPO ectodomain and the identification of two dominant T-cell epitopes, one of which was also recognized by AITD patients *(50)*. In summary, current data suggest that the response to TPO not restricted but directed to a range of epitopes spread throughout the TPO ectodomain.

Table 1
Summary of Synthetic Thyroid Peroxidase (TPO) Peptides
Recognized by T Cells in Autoimmune Thyroid Disease

Amino acids	TPO sequence
100–119	AMKRKVNLKTQQSQHPTD *(41,42)*
110–129	QQSQHPTDALSEDLLSIIA *(43)*
211–230	HVIQVSNEVVTDDDRYSDLL *(43)*
415–432	NRLAAALKALNAHWSADA *(44,45)*
420–434	ALKALNAHWSADAVY *(41)*
439–457	KVVGALHQIITLRDYIPRI *(44)*
463–481	AFQQYVGPYEGYDSTANPTV *(44)*
535–551	LDPLIRGLLARPAKLQ *(40)*
536–547	DPLIRGLLARPAK *(46)*
625–645	LYKHPDNIDVWLGGGLAENFLP *(41)*
632–645	IDVWLGGLAENFLP *(40)*

B-Cell Epitopes

It was long recognized that approximately 90% of AITD patients have antibodies to the "microsomal antigen;" with the isolation of the TPO cDNA sequence, it became clear that TPO and the "microsomal antigen" *(51)* were identical. TPO autoantibodies are diagnostic for AITD and found in approximately 90% of HT patient and 75% of GD patient sera *(52)*. Antibody responses to TPO are pathologically significant as in contrast to TG and TSHR, anti-TPO antibodies are able to fix complement *(24)* and mediate cell destruction via the complement cascade *(53)*. It has also been shown that TPOAb can mediate NK cytotoxic responses *(25,54)*.

The advent of the molecular revolution offered the hope of rapid advances in the analysis of antigen recognition and epitope mapping, and indeed a number of studies followed the initial TPO cDNA cloning. Using high-titre patient sera, two linear epitopes were described *(55)*, and one of these, C21, overlaps completely with the epitope of a murine monoclonal mAb47 *(56)*, both recognizing residues 713–717 *(57)*. However, while it was reported that some patient sera could recognize various linear determinants of denatured forms of TPO, including tryptic peptides and recombinant protein fragments, with subsequent access to patient mAb, it soon became clear that the majority of AITD patient sera recognize a limited number of highly conformational TPO epitopes and that the bulk of patient TPOAb binding mapped to an immunodominant region (IDR) comprising two adjacent and partially overlapping sub-domains termed A and B *(58)*. It also became apparent that relatively simplistic epitope-mapping methods, including recombinant expression of deletion and substitution mutants, and synthetic peptide arrays, would not be applicable in the case of complex conformational epitopes. Competition studies using a series of murine mAbs defined an IDR, and this was subsequently refined to include two overlapping but distinct sub-regions termed A and B *(58)*. Competition studies showed that the murine mAbs specific for these regions could block approximately 90% of patient serum binding. Although defining the bulk properties of patient sera is a useful step in estimating the antibody diversity, mapping of patient B-cell epitopes depends ultimately on the availability of human monoclonal reagents. The development of recombinant antibody technology led to significant advances with a number of groups isolating a range of patient monoclonal Fabs that could compete with patient sera and the original murine mAbs for binding to the IDRs *(59,60)*. It was unfortunate that the human IDR nomenclature became then reversed with respect to the original studies and here the original murine nomenclature will be used. Mapping of conformational epitopes presents several challenges. Synthetic peptides do not provide the correct conformation, and molecular approaches such as deletion or substitution mutagenesis are essentially precluded as both can have unpredictable affects on the 3D structure of the target antigen. One approach to this task was based on the use of chimeric molecules in which regions of the immunologically distinct but closely related protein MPO, for which the crystal structure is available *(61)*, were exchanged with corresponding regions of TPO, exploiting structural conservation to preserve native conformation in the recombinant molecule. Evidence for the exquisitely specific nature of patient antibody recognition was provided by an initial substitution study based simply on primary sequence homology. Despite the high degree of conservation between TPO and MPO, exchange of selected regions led to loss of antibody recognition in seven of eight chimeric molecules *(62)*. A subsequent study used crystallographic data to guide the exchanges, and here, by contrast, the chimeric molecules were recognized by patient sera and monoclonal Fab *(63)*, showing that the native structure had been preserved in the chimera and emphasizing the importance of a guided approach based on knowledge of 3D structure. Recently, in an innovative and elegant approach, a series of rabbit antisera were raised against amino acid sequences loops that, based on structural modelling, were predicted to be exposed on the TPO surface. Exploiting steric hindrance, it was possible using these reagents to identify residues 599–617 as critical for recognition of IDR-B by mAbs and patient sera *(64)*. The complexity of these studies is highlighted by the somewhat conflicting data regarding IDR-A. It was reported that mAb47 could compete with some region A region patient Fabs *(65,66)*, suggesting that residues in the region 713–717 contributed to IDR-A. This contradicted earlier studies in which IDR-A-specific Fabs could not compete with mAb47 for TPO binding *(60)*. However, when used at a higher concentration one these Fabs (TR1.9) did weakly compete with mAb47, and a subsequent footprinting study identified a lysine residue at position 713 as critical for TR1.9 binding *(67)*. This observation was also supported by a targeted mutagenesis study *(68)*. It now appears that the overlapping subdomains A and B map to residues on opposite poles of one face of the TPO molecule (Fig. 2). The IDR-B-specific residues identified by the rabbit anti-peptide sera (599–617) lie between putative helices 13 and 14 apparently remote from IDR-A-specific residues 713–717 (Fig. 2). Possible explanations for these data could include the fact that B-cell epitopes are generally larger than 5 amino acids, so it is possible that region 713–717 contributes to a larger epitope that depends on additional residues, which may be shared with IDR-B, and that the affinity of the A and B mAbs depends on different amino acid residues spread out across the IDR region. Further mutagenesis studies confirmed this model and highlighted residues R225 and K627 as critical components of IDR-A and IDR-B, respectively *(69)*, and N642 was identified as marking the boundary of IDR-B for A and B *(64)*.

THYROTROPIN RECEPTOR

Structure and Function

In humans, TSH activates both the cAMP and, at higher concentrations, the phospholipase C-diacylglycerol pathways. The cAMP cascade upregulates a range of thyroid hormone synthesis and stimulates thyrocyte growth *(70)*. In common with other glycoprotein hormone receptors, TSHR is a member of the leucine-rich-repeat-containing (LGR) subfamily of G-protein-coupled receptors (GPCRs) characterized by a large extracellular domain containing multiple leucine-rich repeats (LRRs) and a rhodopsin-like domain of seven-transmembrane (7TM) helices *(71)*. In contrast to other GPCRs, the LGRs have large ectodomains and bind protein ligands including glycoprotein hormones. The TSHR has yet to be crystallized, but recently the structure of the related follicle-stimulating hormone receptor (FSHR) was determined and the resulting information offers insights into the structure and function of the LGR subfamily of receptors *(72)*. The LRRs form a curved tube arrangement in which the leucine residues form part of a buried framework supporting a concave inner surface composed of parallel relatively flat β-sheets (Fig. 3). Parallel β-sheets are a rare feature more commonly found in the interior of proteins where helices or other β-sheets pack against them *(73)*. The complementarity of LRR protein receptor-binding sites is relatively poor, and it appears that high-affinity ligand binding is mediated by multiple contact points across the β-sheet surface and intrinsic plasticity of the structure *(74)*. It is

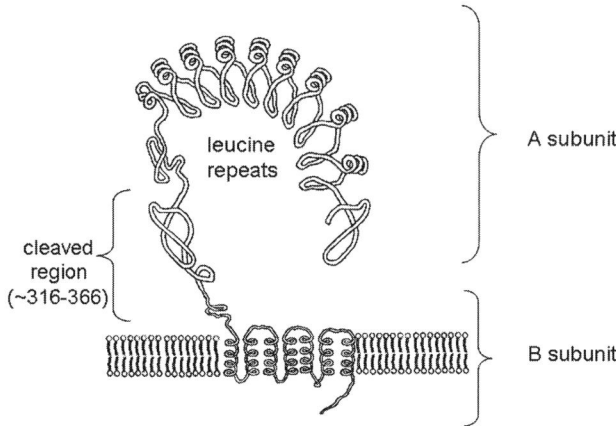

Fig. 3. The subunit structure of TSHIR. Following intramolecular cleavage a region of approximately 50 amino acids is lost, forming a two subunit structure. The large extracellular A subunit is the site of patient antibody recognition and contains the nine leucine-rich repeat (LRR) domain responsible for hormone biniding. Subunit A and the transmembrane and intracellular subunit B are linked by disulfide bonds *(75)*.

thought that the LRR structure is oriented normal to the cell surface and binds the central cysteine belt region *(72)* of FSH in a cupped hand configuration with the ligand perpendicular to the cell membrane, allowing loops of the FSH α-chain to interact with the 7TM domain. Given the structural conservation of glycoprotein hormones, it is likely that the other glycoprotein receptors of the family, including TSHR, will function in a similar fashion. It is thought that the signal is transduced by a conformational change in the receptor due to hormone binding, but the mechanism remains unclear. There is evidence that these receptors can dimerize on the cell surface and this has been observed with TSHR *(75)*.

A unique feature of TSHR is that, compared with similar related LGRs such the gonadotropin receptor, it features an additional 50 amino acid insert in the ectodomain, and a proportion of mature receptor undergoes intramolecular cleavage leading degradation of this peptide and the generation of two distinct subunits (A and B) covalently linked by disulfide bonds *(75)*. Subunit A comprises the extracellular TSH-binding domain, and subunit B includes the 7TM and intracellular domains. Evidence suggests that a proportion of subunit A is shed from the cell surface and subunit B predominates *(75)*. The physiological significance of this distinctive feature of the TSHR is currently unclear. A second unique feature of the TSHR is the presence of constitutive activity in the absence of ligand. This intrinsic activation is suppressed in part by the TSHR A subunit, and the ectodomain has been described as a tethered inverse agonist for this reason *(76)*. This seems to be unique to the TSHR though whether this is associated with the subunit structure is unknown. Another interesting feature of TSHR is the high degree of glycosylation; up to 45% by weight of the extracellular domain is in the form of carbohydrate *(75)*.

As the major immune target in GD TSHR has been proposed by a number of groups as the putative cross-reactive antigen in TAO *(3)*. A number of studies have correlated the levels of TSAb and TBAb with TAO clinical activity score, but the significance of this association is not clear (reviewed in ref. *3*). Several laboratories have reported the expression of TSHR cDNA and protein in a range of orbital preparations *(3)*. However, TSHR transcripts have also been reported in a number of other extrathyroidal tissues, and further studies will be required to confirm a specific association with TAO. Recent successes in the development of animal models of GD by immunization with TSHR protein or cDNA have led to accounts of orbital changes associated with the immune response to the receptor, but a convincing and reproducible model of TAO has yet to be established *(77)*.

Genetics

TSHR cDNA was cloned independently by a number of groups *(78–80)* and shown to encode a primary polypeptide of 764 amino acids. The TSHR gene covers more than 60 kbp on chromosome 14q31 and is split into 10 exons *(81,82)*. As a major thyroid autoantigen TSHR has been analyzed as a candidate gene for susceptibility to AITD in a number of studies with mixed results. A single base polymorphism leading to a Pro52Thr substitution was identified in a group of GD patients with TAO, and subsequent studies suggested that this polymorphism was associated with the occurrence of GO *(83)* and AITD in the female population *(84)*. However, neither of these reports could be confirmed *(85,86)*, and another study failed to observe any association between a TSHR microsatellite marker and GD *(87)*. More recently, a genome-wide screen based on 56 multiplex AITD families found evidence of linkage between GD and a chromosome 14q region near to but distinct from the *TSHR* gene *(88)*. By contrast, Hiratani et al. *(89)* carried out a large association study and showed that several single-nucleotide polymorphisms (SNPs) in intron 7 of TSHR were associated with GD in the Japanese population. These data are supported by a separate UK multi-family study involving two separate association studies in which a TSHR SNP was found to be associated with the occurrence of GD, the first disease-specific locus to be identified *(90)*.

T-Cell Epitopes

The majority of studies of T-cell responses to TSHR have been carried out using patient peripheral blood mononuclear cells (PBMCs), though in some cases T-cell lines expanded from thyroid infiltrate have been employed. Use of synthetic peptides overcomes the requirement for antigen processing and enables mapping of epitopes. T-cell reactivity to a range of TSHR peptides has been described *(91)* (summarized in Fig. 4), and these cover the entire extracellular domain, in some cases extending into the transmembrane region. Considering that in general these proliferative responses are relatively minor, and in some cases comparable with those obtained from controls *(75)*, it is difficult to draw firm conclusions regarding patient T-cell reactivity to TSHR. By grading the T-cell responses, a number of major epitopes have been identified including residues 52–71, 142–161, 202–221, and 247–266 *(91)* but no single dominant epitope.

Autoimmunity represents a breakdown in tolerance to self-proteins. Central tolerance is the process by which immature T cells undergo a process of education in the thymus and develop tolerance to peptides derived from self-proteins expressed in thymic epithelium. Low levels of TSHR mRNA and protein have been detected in rodent and human thymic tissue, and it is assumed that central tolerance plays a significant

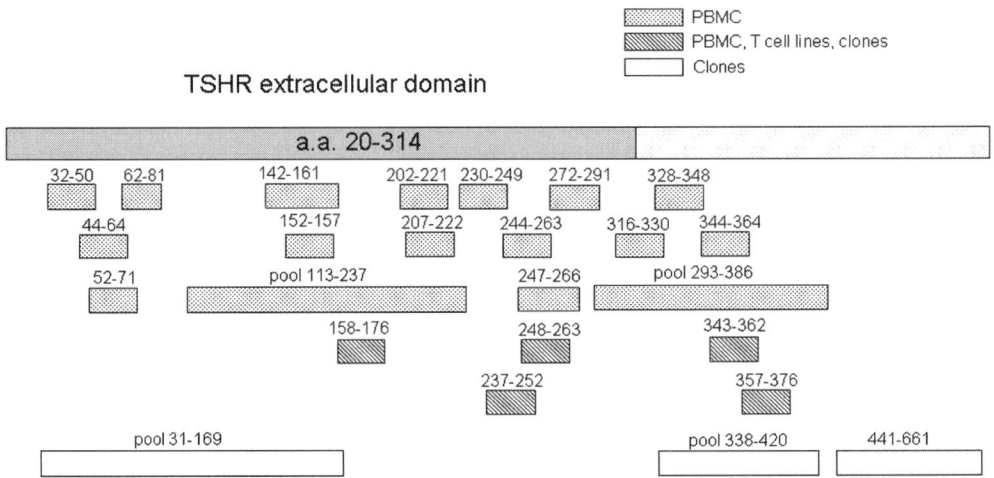

Fig. 4. Synthetic TSHIR peptides and mixed peptide pools that stimulate proliferation in Graves' PBMC, T cell lines, or clones *(75)*. Peptide pools are indicated, together with the first and last amino acid residues of the spanned range.

role in preventing thyroid autoimmunity. It has now become clear that the situation may be more complex than originally thought. Recently, a TSHR-knockout mouse was developed in which expression of TSHR mRNA and protein was abolished *(92)*. Although these mice clearly fail to develop central tolerance to TSHR and so recognize it as a foreign protein, immunization with TSHR DNA generated an immune response in an equivalent percentage of animals to that observed with wild-type control mice and led to similar humoral and cellular TSHR responses in both groups *(93)*. These observations suggest that TSHR may not fit in with general models of central tolerance and suggest a role for alternative regulatory pathways such as peripheral tolerance and regulatory T cells in the control of immune responses to the TSHR and thyroid autoimmunity in general. Recently, it was reported that therapeutic trials of a T-cell depleting mAb led to the appearance of GD in a large proportion of treated patients *(94)*, and similar results have been reported in patients featuring immune dysregulation while undergoing HIV treatment *(95)*. These data, together with emerging clarity in the often controversial field of regulatory T cells, suggest that the function of specific T-cell subsets *(26)*, and more specifically, T-cell suppression, may be an important factor in the aetiology of GD and AITD *(96)*.

B-Cell Epitopes

Given the pathological role of TSHR autoantibodies in GD, the identification of the corresponding B-cell epitopes has been a major research objective since the original description of TSAb. Knowledge of the autoantibody binding sites would not only contribute to our understanding of pathology but would also open up new opportunities for targeted therapeutic approaches. Attempts to classify TSHRAb have been based on the different assays used for detection and quantification. Bioassays in which stimulation of TSHR expressed on thyrocytes or transgenic cell lines is measured by direct or indirect determination of cAMP levels are the most direct method of

TSAb detection and quantification. Assays based on the ability of TSHRAb to block binding of TSH to the receptor define the classification of TSH binding inhibiting immunoglobulins (TBII). Early insights into the nature of the TSHRAb-binding sites were derived from determination of TBII activity, and it was shown that a large proportion of patient TSHRAb could block TSH binding, and this largely correlated with TSAb activity. TBII measurements also defined a second class of THSRAb that were able to block TSH binding but not stimulate the receptor, and these thyroid-blocking antibodies (TBAb) are thought to be the basis of hypothyroidism in a subset of AITD patients *(97)*. The nature of these antibodies and in particular what features determine whether an antibody exhibits TSAb or TBAb activity are still subjects of some debate *(75)*. Most recent data suggest that the residues associated with TSH binding and the epitopes for blocking and stimulating antibodies are probably all in close proximity *(98)*, and it has been suggested that TBAbs are actually functionally equivalent to weak TSHR agonists *(99)*. Initial studies of serum TSAbs did show that they were restricted to the λ-immunoglobulin subclass *(100)*, but more detailed studies of TSAbs, and in particular the corresponding TSHR epitopes, were often conflicting—not least as it was often overlooked that in the absence of monoclonal reagents the properties described were a property of the patient sera and not necessarily characteristics of individual TSAbs, an unknown fraction of the circulating TSHRAb.

Attempts to dissect the TSHR autoantibody response in detail have presented a number of particular difficulties. First, the levels of circulating patient TSHRAb are much lower than those of other thyroid antigens such as TPO *(75)*. Second, TSHRAbs recognize highly conformational epitopes, and even the degree of glycosylation appears to be an important factor, though whether this is directly associated with antibody recognition or secondary to receptor misfolding is currently unknown *(75)*. TSHR is highly glycosylated with up to 45% by weight of the extracellular domain in the form of carbohydrate *(75)*. Finally, until recently, the absence of a suitable animal model of GD was a significant obstacle. No spontaneous animal model of GD is known, and for more than a decade, attempts to generate TSAbs by immunization with various forms of recombinant receptor invariably failed, though a range of non-functional TSHRAbs were readily produced *(75)*.

A significant breakthrough came with the development of the first successful animal model of GD by Shimojo et al. *(101)* based on the multiple injection of mice with syngeneic fibroblasts stably transfected with MHC class II and TSHR. The majority of mice developed TSHRAb, as determined by TBII assay, and approximately 20% developed TSAbs and elevated serum thyroxine.

This approach was reproduced in modified form by a number of other groups. Davies et al. *(102)* immunized hamsters with stably transfected chinese hamster ovary cells expressing the TSH receptor, together with conventional adjuvants, and hyper-thyroidism was observed in approximately 30% of animals. An alternative approach, based on DNA vaccination in the form of intramuscular injections of eucaryotic expression vectors encoding the TSH receptor, produced hyperthyroidism in outbred mice *(103)* though at a lower rate than the fibroblast approach, and there has been some difficulty in reproducing this model *(104)*. The most effective animal model of GD exploits adenoviral vectors encoding the TSH receptor to generate in vivo receptor expression following intramuscular injection *(105)*. This approach has been reproduced by different groups in both mice and hamsters and is highly efficient with approximately 100% TSHRAb induction and in the case of BALB/c mice approximately 50–60% induction of TSAb activity *(104)*. These models have provided a number of insights into the pathogenesis of GD. All but one of the mouse models relied upon in vivo expression of receptor *(105)*, whereas previous attempts to induce TSAb by immunization with various forms of TSH receptor and adjuvant were uniformly unsuccessful *(106)*. A possible explanation is provided by the recent observation that GD patient TSAbs preferentially recognize free TSHR ectodomain rather than the two-subunit form or corresponding single full-length polypeptide *(105)*, suggesting that the A may be the most effective immunogenic form. One possibility is that in vivo expression and subunit A shedding may bias the immune response towards receptor-stimulating epitopes, and this is supported by evidence from adenovirus-mediated immunization using truncated receptor constructs *(107)*.

Following on from the successful development of animal models, the year 2002 saw three independent accounts of the successful isolation of animal TSAb monoclonal antibodies *(108–110)*. These were followed shortly afterwards by the report of a single human TSAb monoclonal *(98)*, this the result of a prodigious screening effort involving TBI assay of 16,500 wells. These monoclonals fulfilled a number of the criteria that have been defined for TSAb *(111)*; they stimulated the receptor at ng/ml concentrations, they had high affinity for the receptor, and they recognized conformational epitopes and not synthetic peptides *(105)*. Interestingly, the human TSAb was much more active in bioasssay than the best of the animal monoclonals with maximal receptor obtained at an IgG concentration of 10 ng/ml compared with approximately 20,000 ng/ml for the mouse/hamster mAbs *(105)*. Patient sera with stimulating or blocking activity were able to compete with monoclonals for receptor binding, indicating the corresponding epitopes for agonist and antagonist activity are in proximity or similar *(105)*.

Finally, the availability of monoclonals also eliminated much of the uncertainty surrounding the question of valency and TSAb. Fab fragment was also stimulatory and there was no requirement for bivalency or crosslinking of antibody for function. The isolation of monoclonal stimulating antibodies will allow the first detailed analysis of the functional basis of different TSHR epitopes and the development of novel assays free from the complications associated with the use of mixed sera.

OTHER THYROID ANTIGENS

Sodium Iodide Symporter Antibodies

Sodium iodide symporter (NIS) is a membrane glycoprotein that mediates active transport of I^- into thyroid follicular cells and thus plays a key role in thyroid hormone biosynthesis *(112)*. Following the isolation of NIS cDNA, it was shown that sera from GD and HT patients could recognize recombinant NIS protein in Western blots and inhibit iodide uptake *(113)*. Using a NIS bioassay, it was reported that approximately 30% of tested GD sera were able to inhibit NIS-mediated iodide transport *(114)*. In another study, 22% of GD and 24% of HT patient sera were positive in an in vitro translation immunoprecipitation assay, and a large proportion of the positive samples from this assay were also shown to inhibit iodide uptake *(115)*. By contrast, a study based on an alternative bioassay found only a small proportion of samples had I^- uptake inhibiting activity, and this was lost upon IgG purification or dialysis *(116)*.

The evidence for NIS as a thyroid autoantigen is to some extent contradictory, though it seems unlikely that the symporter represents a major antigen.

Megalin (gp330)

Megalin is a member of the low-density lipoprotein (LDL) receptor family that binds a range of varied ligands and mediates its endocytosis via coated pits. Megalin is expressed on a limited range of absorptive epithelial cells including thyroid follicular cells, where it has been shown to be a high-affinity receptor for TG and critical for TG endocytosis *(117,118)*. Megalin was identified as an autoantigen in rat model of membranous glomerulonephritis and based on this association investigated as a potential antigen in AITD. Using a flow cytometric assay, antibodies to megalin were demonstrated in 13 of 26 autoimmune thyroiditis patient and 2 of 19 GD patient sera *(119)*. The significance of these findings remains to be clarified, but it is of interest that though none of the patients in the previously described study had evidence of renal disease, a recent case report described a pediatric case of autoimmune thyroiditis and membraneous nephropathy *(120)*, suggesting the possibility that megalin may, in some cases, play a role as a common antigen in the two disorders.

REFERENCES

1. Tunbridge WMG, Evered DC, Hall R, Appleton D, Brewis M, Clark F, Evans JG, Young E, Bird T, Smith PA. Spectrum of thyroid disease in a community – Whickham survey. *Clinical Endocrinology* 1977;7:481–493.
2. Weetman AP, McGregor AM. Autoimmune thyroiditis: further developments in our understanding. *Endocrine Reviews* 1994;15:788–830.
3. Prabhakar BS, Bahn RS, Smith TJ. Current perspective on the pathogenesis of Graves' disease and ophthalmopathy. *Endocrine Reviews* 2003;24:802–835.
4. Brix TH, Kyvik KO, Christensen K, Hegedus L. Evidence for a major role of heredity in Graves' disease: a population-based study of two Danish twin cohorts. *The Journal of Clinical Endocrinology and Metabolism* 2001;86:930–934.
5. Brix TH, Kyvik KO, Hegedus L. A population-based study of chronic autoimmune hypothyroidism in Danish twins. *The Journal of Clinical Endocrinology and Metabolism* 2000;85:536–539.
6. Tomer Y, Davies TF. Searching for the autoimmune thyroid disease susceptibility genes: from gene mapping to gene function. *Endocrine Reviews* 2003;24:694–717.
7. van de Graaf SAR, Ris-Stalpers C, Pauws E, Mendive FM, Targovnik HM, de Vijlder JJM. Structure update – up to date with human thyroglobulin. *The Journal of Endocrinology* 2001;170:307–321.
8. Malthiery Y, Lissitzky S. Primary structure of human thyroglobulin deduced from the sequence of its 8448-base complementary-DNA. *European Journal of Biochemistry* 1987;165:491–498.
9. Malthiery Y, Marriq C, Bérge-Lefranc JL, Franc JL, Henry M, Lejeune PJ, Ruf J, Lissitzky S. Thyroglobulin structure and function – recent advances. *Biochimie* 1989;71:195–210.
10. Geen J, Howells RC, Ludgate M, Hullin DA, Hogg SI. The prevalence of anti-acetylcholinesterase antibodies in autoimmune disease. *Autoimmunity* 2004;37:579–585.
11. Carayanniotis G. The cryptic self in thyroid autoimmunity: The paradigm of thyroglobulin. *Autoimmunity* 2003;36:423–428.
12. Kriss JP, Pleshako V, Rosenblu A, Holderne M, Sharp G, Utiger R. Studies on pathogenesis of ophthalmopathy of Graves' disease. *The Journal of Clinical Endocrinology and Metabolism* 1967;27:582–593.

13. Lisi S, Botta R, Agretti P, Sellari-Franceschini S, Marcocci C, Pinchera A, Marino M. Poorly specific binding of thyroglobulin to orbital fibroblasts from patients with Graves' ophthalmopathy. *Journal of Endocrinological Investigation* 2005;28:420–424.

14. Sakai K, Shirasawa S, Ishikawa N, Ito K, Tamai H, Kuma K, Akamizu T, Tanimura M, Furugaki K, Yamamoto K, Sasazuki T. Identification of susceptibility loci for autoimmune thyroid disease to 5q31-q133 and Hashimoto's thyroiditis to 8q23-q24 by multipoint affected sib-pair linkage analysis in Japanese. *Human Molecular Genetics* 2001;10:1379–1386.

15. Tomer Y, Greenberg DA, Concepcion E, Ban Y, Davies TF. Thyroglobulin is a thyroid specific gene for the familial autoimmune thyroid diseases. *The Journal of Clinical Endocrinology and Metabolism* 2002;87:404–407.

16. Collins JE, Heward JM, Carr-Smith J, Daykin J, Franklyn JA, Gough SCL. Association of a rare thyroglobulin gene microsatellite variant with autoimmune thyroid disease. *The Journal of Clinical Endocrinology and Metabolism* 2003;88:5039–5042.

17. Ban Y, Greenberg DA, Concepcion E, Skrabanek L, Villanueva R, Tomer Y. Amino acid substitutions in the thyroglobulin gene are associated with susceptibility to human and murine autoimmune thyroid disease. *Proceedings of the National Academy of Sciences of the United States of America* 2003;100:15119–15124.

18. Collins JE, Heward JM, Howson JMM, Foxall H, Carr-Smith J, Franklyn JA, Gough SCL. Common allelic variants of exons 10, 12, and 33 of the thyroglobulin gene are not associated with autoimmune thyroid disease in the United Kingdom. *The Journal of Clinical Endocrinology and Metabolism* 2004;89:6336–6339.

19. Gentile F, Conte M, Formisano S. Thyroglobulin as an autoantigen: what can we learn about immunopathogenicity from the correlation of antigenic properties with protein structure? *Immunology* 2004;112:13–25.

20. Tomer Y. Anti-thyroglobin autoantibodies in autoimmune thyroid disease: cross reactive or pathogenic? *Clinical Immunology and Immunopathology* 1997;82:3–11.

21. Coutinho A, Kazatchkine MD, Avrameas S. Natural autoantibodies. *Current Opinion in Immunology* 1995;7:812–818.

22. Yativ N, Buskila D, Blank M, Burek CL, Rose NR, Shoenfeld Y. The detection of antithyroglobulin activity in human serum monoclonal immunoglobulins (monoclonal gammopathies). *Immunological Research* 1993;12:330–337.

23. McIntosh R, Watson P, Weetman A. Somatic hypermutation in autoimmune thyroid disease. *Immunological Reviews* 1998;162:219–231.

24. Belyavin G, Trotter WR. Immunological reactions in thyroid disease. *Lancet* 1959;1:784–784.

25. Bogner U, Schleusener H, Wall JR. Antibody-dependent cell-mediated cytotoxicity against human thyroid cells in Hashimoto's thyroiditis but not Graves' disease. *The Journal of Clinical Endocrinology and Metabolism* 1984;59:734–738.

26. Dong Q, Ludgate M, Vassart G. Towards an antigenic map of human thyroglobulin – identification of 10 epitope-bearing sequences within the primary structure of thyroglobulin. *The Journal of Endocrinology* 1989;122:169–176.

27. Shimojo N, Saito K, Kohno Y, Sasaki N, Tarutani O, Nakajima H. Antigenic determinants on thyroglobulin – comparison of the reactivities of different thyroglobulin preparations with serum antibodies and T-cells of patients with chronic thyroiditis. *The Journal of Clinical Endocrinology and Metabolism* 1988;66:689–695.

28. Latrofa F, Phillips M, Rapoport B, McLachlan SM. Human monoclonal thyroglobulin autoantibodies: Epitopes and immunoglobulin genes. *The Journal of Clinical Endocrinology and Metabolism* 2004;89:5116–5123.

29. Prentice L, Kiso Y, Fukuma N, Horimoto M, Petersen V, Grennan F, Pegg C, Furmaniak J, Smith BR. Monoclonal thyroglobulin autoantibodies – variable region analysis and epitope recognition. *The Journal of Clinical Endocrinology and Metabolism* 1995;80:977–986.

30. Ruf J, Carayon P. Structural and functional aspects of thyroid peroxidase. *Archives of Biochemistry and Biophysics* 2006;445:269–277.

31. Libert F, Ruel J, Ludgate M, Swillens S, Alexander N, Vassart G, Dinsart C. Thyroperoxidase, an auto-antigen with a mosaic structure made of nuclear and mitochondrial gene modules. *The EMBO Journal* 1987;6:4193–4196.

32. Magnusson RP, Chazenbalk GD, Gestautas J, Seto P, Filetti S, Degroot LJ, Rapoport B. Molecular-cloning of the complementary deoxyribonucleic-acid for human thyroid peroxidase. *Molecular Endocrinology* 1987;1:856–861.

33. Kimura S, Kotani T, McBride OW, Umeki K, Hirai K, Nakayama T, Ohtaki S. Human thyroid peroxidase – complete cDNA and protein-sequence, chromosome mapping, and identification of 2 alternately spliced messenger-RNAs. *Proceedings of the National Academy of Sciences of the United States of America* 1987;84:5555–5559.

34. Libert F, Ruel J, Ludgate M, Swillens S, Alexander N, Vassart G, Dinsart C. Complete nucleotide-sequence of the human thyroperoxidase-microsomal antigen cDNA. *Nucleic Acids Research* 1987;15:6735–6735.

35. Devijlder JJM, Dinsart C, Libert F, Vankessel AG, Bikker H, Bolhuis PA, Vassart G. Regional localization of the gene for thyroid peroxidase to human-chromosome 2pter-P12. *Cytogenetics and Cell Genetics* 1988;47:170–172.

36. Taylor JC, Gough SC, Hunt PJ, Brix TH, Chatterjee K, Connell JM, Franklyn JA, Hegedus L, Robinson BG, Wiersinga WM, Wass JAH, Zabaneh D, Mackay I, Weetman AP. A genome-wide screen in 1119 relative pairs with autoimmune thyroid disease. *The Journal of Clinical Endocrinology and Metabolism* 2006;91:646–653.

37. Wick G, Most J, Schauenstein K, Kromer G, Dietrich H, Ziemiecki A, Fassler R, Schwarz S, Neu N, Hala K. Spontaneous autoimmune-thyroiditis – a birds eye-view. *Immunology Today* 1985;6:359–364.

38. Allen EM, Appel MC, Braverman LE. The effect of iodide ingestion on the development of spontaneous lymphocytic thyroiditis in the diabetes-prone BB/W rat. *Endocrinology* 1986;118:1977–1981.

39. Rasooly L, Burek CL, Rose NR. Iodine-induced autoimmune thyroiditis in NOD-H-2(h4) mice. *Clinical Immunology and Immunopathology* 1996;81:287–292.

40. Dayan CM, Londei M, Corcoran AE, Grubeck-Loebenstein B, James RFL, Rapoport B, Feldmann M. Autoantigen recognition by thyroid-infiltrating T-cells in Graves-disease. *Proceedings of the National Academy of Sciences of the United States of America* 1991;88:7415–7419.

41. Fisfalen ME, Palmer EM, van Seventer GA, Soltani K, Sawai Y, Kaplan E, Hidaka Y, Ober C, DeGroot LJ. Thyrotropin-receptor and thyroid peroxidase-specific T cell clones and their cytokine profile in autoimmune thyroid disease. *Clinical and Experimental Immunology* 1997;82:3655–3663.

42. Fisfalen ME, Soliman M, Okamoto Y, Soltani K, DeGroot LJ. Proliferative responses of T-cells to thyroid antigens and synthetic thyroid peroxidase peptides in autoimmune thyroid-disease. *The Journal of Clinical Endocrinology and Metabolism* 1995;80:1597–1604.

43. Kawakami Y, Fisfalen ME, DeGroot LJ. Proliferative responses of peripheral blood mononuclear cells from patients with autoimmune thyroid disease to synthetic peptide epitopes of human thyroid peroxidase. *Autoimmunity* 1992;13:17–26.

44. Tandon N, Freeman M, Weetman AP. T cell responses to synthetic thyroid peroxidase peptides in autoimmune thyroid disease. *Clinical and Experimental Immunology* 1991;86:56–60.

45. Fukuma N, McLachlan SM, Rapoport B, Goodacre J, Middleton SL, Philips DIW, Pegg CAS, Rees Smith B. Thyroid autoantigens and human T cell responses. *Clinical and Experimental Immunology* 1990;82:275–283.

46. Quaratino S, Thorpe CJ, Travers PJ, Londei M. Similar antigenic surfaces, rather than sequence homology, dictate T-cell epitope molecular mimicry. *Proceedings of the National Academy of Science United States of America* 1995;92:10398–10402.

47. McLachlan SM, Rapoport B. Evidence for a potential common T-cell epitope between human thyroid peroxidase and human thyroglobulin with implications for the pathogenesis of autoimmune thyroid-disease. *Autoimmunity* 1989;5:101–106.

48. Hoshioka A, Kohno Y, Katsuki T, Shimojo N, Maruyama N, Inagaki Y, Yokochi T, Tarutani O, Hosoya T, Niimi H. A common T-cell epitope between human thyroglobulin and human thyroid peroxidase is related to murine experimental autoimmune-thyroiditis. *Immunology Letters* 1993;37:235–239.

49. Quaratino S, Badami E, Pang YY, Bartok I, Dyson J, Kioussis D, Londei M, Maiuri L. Degenerate self-reactive human T-cell receptor causes spontaneous autoimmune disease in mice. *Nature Medicine* 2004;10:920–926.

50. Guo J, Pichurin PN, Morris JC, Rapoport B, McLachlan SM. "Naked" deoxyribonucleic acid vaccination induces recognition of diverse thyroid peroxidase T cell epitopes. *Endocrinology* 2004;145:3671–3678.

51. Czarnocka B, Ruf J, Ferrand M, Carayon P, Lissitzky S. Purification of the human thyroid peroxidase and its identification as the microsomal antigen involved in autoimmune thyroid-diseases. *FEBS Letters* 1985;190:147–152.

52. Mariotti S, Caturegli P, Piccolo P, Barbesino G, Pinchera A. Antithyroid peroxidase autoantibodies in thyroid-diseases. *The Journal of Clinical Endocrinology and Metabolism* 1990;71:661–669.

53. Chiovato L, Bassi P, Santini F, Mammoli C, Lapi P, Carayon P, Pinchera A. Antibodies producing complement-mediated thyroid cytotoxicity in patients with atrophic or goitrous autoimmune-thyroiditis. *The Journal of Clinical Endocrinology and Metabolism* 1993;77:1700–1705.

54. McLachlan SM, Atherton MC, Pegg CAS, Young ET, Clark F, Smith BR. Mechanisms of thyroid destruction in autoimmune thyroid-disease. *The Journal of Endocrinology* 1987;112:285–285.

55. Libert F, Ludgate M, Dinsart C, Vassart G. Thyroperoxidase, but not the thyrotropin receptor, contains sequential epitopes recognized by autoantibodies in recombinant peptides expressed in the pUEX vector. *The Journal of Clinical Endocrinology and Metabolism* 1991;73:857–860.

56. Finke R, Seto P, Ruf J, Carayon P, Rapoport B. Determination at the molecular-level of a B-cell epitope on thyroid peroxidase likely to be associated with autoimmune thyroid-disease. *The Journal of Clinical Endocrinology and Metabolism* 1991;73:919–921.

57. Bresson D, Cerutti M, Devauchelle G, Pugniere M, Roquet F, Bes C, Bossard C, Chardes T, Peraldi-Roux S. Localization of the discontinuous immunodominant region recognized by human anti-thyroperoxidase autoantibodies in autoimmune thyroid diseases. *The Journal of Biological Chemistry* 2003;278:9560–9569.

58. Ruf J, Toubert ME, Czarnocka B, Durandgorde JM, Ferrand M, Carayon P. Relationship between immunological structure and biochemical-properties of human thyroid peroxidase. *Endocrinology* 1989;125:1211–1218.

59. McLachlan SM, Rapoport B. Genetic and epitopic analysis of thyroid peroxidase (TPO) autoantibodies – markers of the human thyroid autoimmune-response. *Clinical and Experimental Immunology* 1995;101:200–206.

60. Chazenbalk GD, Costante G, Portolano S, McLachlan SM, Rapoport B. The immunodominant region on human thyroid peroxidase recognized by autoantibodies does not contain the monoclonal-antibody 47/C21 linear epitope. *The Journal of Clinical Endocrinology and Metabolism* 1993;77:1715–1718.

61. Zeng J, Fenna RE. X-ray crystal structure of canine myeloperoxidase at 3 Å resolution. *Journal of Molecular Biology* 1992;226:185–207.

62. Nishikawa T, Nagayama Y, Seto P, Rapoport B. Human thyroid peroxidase-myeloperoxidase chimeric molecules – tools for the study of antigen recognition by thyroid peroxidase autoantibodies. *Endocrinology* 1993;133:2496–2501.

63. Nishikawa T, Rapoport B, McLachlan SM. The quest for the autoantibody immunodominant region on thyroid peroxidase: Guided mutagenesis based on a hypothetical three-dimensional model. *Endocrinology* 1996;137:1000–1006.

64. Hobby P, Gardas A, Radomski R, McGregor AM, Banga JP, Sutton BJ. Identification of an immunodominant region recognized by human autoantibodies in a three-dimensional model of thyroid peroxidase. *Endocrinology* 2000;141:2018–2026.

65. Guo J, McIntosh RS, Czarnocka B, Weetman AP, Rapoport B, McLachlan SM. Relationship between autoantibody epitopic recognition and immunoglobulin gene usage. *Clinical and Experimental Immunology* 1998;111:408–414.

66. Jones FG, Ziemnicka K, Sanders J, Wolstenholme A, Fiera R, Furmaniak J, Smith BR. Analysis of autoantibody epitopes on human thyroid peroxidase. *Autoimmunity* 1999;30:157–169.

67. Guo J, Yan XM, McLachlan SM, Rapoport B. Search for the autoantibody immunodominant region on thyroid peroxidase: epitopic footprinting with a human monoclonal autoantibody locates a facet on the native antigen containing a highly conformational epitope. *Journal of Immunology* 2001;166:1327–1333.

68. Bresson D, Pugniere M, Roquet F, Rebuffat SA, N-Guyen B, Cerutti M, Guo J, McLachlan SM, Rapoport B, Estienne V, Ruf J, Chardes T, Peraldi-Roux S. Directed mutagenesis in region 713–720 of human thyroperoxidase assigns 713KFPED717 residues as being involved in the B domain of the discontinuous immunodominant region recognized by human autoantibodies. *The Journal of Biological Chemistry* 2004;279:39058–39067.

69. Gora M, Gardas A, Watson PF, Hobby P, Weetman AP, Sutton BJ, Banga JP. Key residues contributing to dominant conformational autoantigenic epitopes on thyroid peroxidase identified by mutagenesis. *Biochemical and Biophysical Research Communications* 2004;320:795–801.

70. Tonacchera M, Van Sande J, Parma J, Duprez L, Cetani F, Costagliola S, Dumont JE, Vassart G. TSH receptor and disease. *Clinical Endocrinology* 1996;44:621–633.

71. Szkudlinski MW, Fremont V, Ronin C, Weintraub BD. Thyroid-stimulating hormone and thyroid-stimulating hormone receptor structure-function relationships. *Physiological Reviews* 2002;82:473–502.

72. Fan QR, Hendrickson WA. Structure of human follicle-stimulating hormone in complex with its receptor. *Nature* 2005;433:269–277.

73. Kobe B, Deisenhofer J. The leucine-rich repeat – a versatile binding motif. *Trends in Biochemical Sciences* 1994;19:415–421.

74. Kobe B, Deisenhofer J. Mechanism of ribonuclease inhibition by ribonuclease inhibitor protein based on the crystal structure of its complex with ribonuclease A. *Journal of Molecular Biology* 1996;264:1028–1043.

75. Rapoport B, Chazenbalk GD, Jaume JC, McLachlan SM. The thyrotropin (TSH) receptor: interaction with TSH and autoantibodies. *Endocrine Reviews* 1998;19:673–716.

76. Vlaeminck-Guillem V, Ho SC, Rodien P, Vassart G, Costagliola S. Activation of the cAMP pathway by the TSH receptor involves switching of the ectodomain from a tethered inverse agonist to an agonist. *Molecular Endocrinology* 2002;16:736–746.

77. Baker G, Mazziotti G, von Ruhland C, Ludgate M. Reevaluating thyrotropin receptor-induced mouse models of Graves' disease and ophthalmopathy. *Endocrinology* 2005;146:835–844.

78. Parmentier M, Libert F, Maenhaut C, Lefort A, Gerard C, Perret J, Vansande J, Dumont JE, Vassart G. Molecular-cloning of the thyrotropin receptor. *Science* 1989;246:1620–1622.

79. Nagayama Y, Kaufman KD, Seto P, Rapoport B. Molecular-cloning, sequence and functional expression of the cDNA for the human thyrotropin receptor. *Biochemical and Biophysical Research Communications* 1989;165:1184–1190.

80. Misrahi M, Loosfelt H, Atger M, Sar S, Guiochonmantel A, Milgrom E. Cloning, sequencing and expression of human TSH receptor. *Biochemical and Biophysical Research Communications* 1990;166:394–403.

81. Rousseaumerck MF, Misrahi M, Loosfelt H, Atger M, Milgrom E, Berger R. Assignment of the human thyroid stimulating hormone receptor (TSHR) gene to chromosome-14q31. *Genomics* 1990;8:233–236.

82. Gross B, Misrahi M, Sar S, Milgrom E. Composite structure of the human thyrotropin receptor gene. *Biochemical and Biophysical Research Communications* 1991;177:679–687.

83. Bahn RS, Dutton CM, Heufelder AE, Sarkar G. A genomic point mutation in the extracellular domain of the thyrotropin receptor in patients with Graves ophthalmopathy. *The Journal of Clinical Endocrinology and Metabolism* 1994;78:256–260.

84. Cuddihy RM, Dutton CM, Bahn RS. A polymorphism in the extracellular domain of the thyrotropin receptor Is highly associated with autoimmune thyroid-disease in females. *Thyroid* 1995;5:89–95.

85. Watson PF, French A, Pickerill AP, McIntosh RS, Weetman AP. Lack of association between a polymorphism in the coding region of the thyrotropin receptor gene and Graves-disease. *The Journal of Clinical Endocrinology and Metabolism* 1995;80:1032–1035.

86. Kotsa KD, Watson PF, Weetman AP. No association between a thyrotropin receptor gene polymorphism and Graves' disease in the female population. *Thyroid* 1997;7:31–33.

87. deRoux N, Shields DC, Misrahi M, Ratanachaiyavong S, McGregor AM, Milgrom E. Analysis of the thyrotropin receptor as a candidate gene in familial Graves' disease. *The Journal of Clinical Endocrinology and Metabolism* 1996;81:3483–3486.

88. Tomer Y, Barbesino G, Greenberg DA, Concepcion E, Davies TF. Mapping the major susceptibility loci for familial Graves' and Hashimoto's diseases: Evidence for genetic heterogeneity and gene interactions. *The Journal of Clinical Endocrinology and Metabolism* 1999;84:4656–4664.

89. Hiratani H, Bowden DW, Ikegami S, Shirasawa S, Shimizu A, Iwatani Y, Akamizu T. Multiple SNPs in intron 7 of thyrotropin receptor are associated with Graves' disease. *The Journal of Clinical Endocrinology and Metabolism* 2005;90:2898–2903.

90. Dechairo BM, Zabaneh D, Collins J, Brand O, Dawson GJ, Green AP, Mackay I, Franklyn JA, Connell JM, Wass JA, Wiersinga WM, Hegedus L, Brix T, Robinson BG, Hunt PJ, Weetman AP, Carey AH, Gough SC. Association of the TSHR gene with Graves' disease: the first disease specific locus. *European Journal of Human Genetics* 2005;13:1223–1230.

91. Martin A, Nakashima M, Zhou A, Aronson D, Werner AJ, Davies TF. Detection of major T cell epitopes on human thyroid stimulating hormone receptor by overriding immune heterogeneity in patients with Graves' disease. *The Journal of Clinical Endocrinology and Metabolism* 1997;82:3361–3366.

92. Marians RC, Ng L, Blair HC, Unger P, Graves PN, Davies TF. Defining thyrotropin-dependent and -independent steps of thyroid hormone synthesis by using thyrotropin receptor-null mice. *Proceedings of the National Academy of Sciences of the United States of America* 2002;99:15776–15781.

93. Pichurin PN, Pichurina O, Marians RC, Chen CR, Davies TF, Rapoport B, McLachlan SM. Thyrotropin receptor knockout mice: Studies on immunological tolerance to a major thyroid autoantigen. *Endocrinology* 2004;145:1294–1301.

94. Coles AJ, Wing N, Smith S, Coraddu F, Greer S, Taylor C, Weetman A, Hale G, Chatterjee VK, Waldmann H, Compston A. Pulsed monoclonal antibody treatment and autoimmune thyroid disease in multiple sclerosis. *Lancet* 1999;354:1691–1695.

95. Chen F, Day SL, Metcalfe RA, Sethi G, Kapembwa MS, Brook MG, Churchill D, de Ruiter A, Robinson S, Lacey CJ, Weetman AP. Characteristics of autoimmune thyroid disease occurring as a late complication of immune reconstitution in patients with advanced human immunodeficiency virus (HIV) disease. *Medicine* 2005;84:98–106.

96. Volpe R. Suppressor T-lymphocyte dysfunction is important in the pathogenesis of autoimmune thyroid-disease – a perspective. *Thyroid* 1993;3:345–352.

97. Chiovato L, Vitti P, Bendinelli G, Santini F, Fiore E, Capaccioli A, Tonacchera M, Mammoli C, Ludgate M, Pinchera A. Detection of antibodies blocking thyrotropin effect using chinese-hamster ovary cells transfected with the cloned human TSH receptor. *Journal of Endocrinological Investigation* 1994;17:809–816.

98. Sanders J, Evans M, Premawardhana L, Depraetere H, Jeffreys J, Richards T, Furmaniak J, Smith BR. Human monoclonal thyroid stimulating autoantibody. *Lancet* 2003;362:126–128.

99. Morgenthaler NG. New assay systems for thyrotropin receptor antibodies. *Current Opinion in Endocrinology and Diabetes* 1999;6:251–260.

100. Weetman AP, Yateman ME, Ealey PA, Black CM, Reimer CB, Williams RC, Shine B, Marshall NJ. Thyroid-stimulating antibody-activity between different immunoglobulin-G subclasses. *The Journal of Clinical Investigation* 1990;86:723–727.

101. Shimojo N, Kohno Y, Yamaguchi K, Kikuoka S, Hoshioka A, Niimi H, Hirai A, Tamura Y, Saito Y, Kohn LD, Tahara K. Induction of Graves-like disease in mice by immunization with fibroblasts transfected with the thyrotropin receptor and a class II molecule. *Proceedings of the National Academy of Sciences of the United States of America* 1996;93:11074–11079.

102. Ando T, Imaizumi M, Graves P, Unger P, Davies TF. Induction of thyroid-stimulating hormone receptor autoimmunity in hamsters. *Endocrinology* 2003;144:671–680.

103. Costagliola S, Many MC, Denef JF, Pohlenz J, Refetoff S, Vassart G. Genetic immunization of outbred mice with thyrotropin receptor cDNA provides a model of Graves' disease. *The Journal of Clinical Investigation* 2000;105:803–811.

104. Nagayama Y. Animal models of Graves' hyperthyroidism. *Endocrine Journal* 2005;52:385–394.

105. McLachlan SM, Rapoport B. Thyroid stimulating monoclonal antibodies: overcoming the road blocks and the way forward. *Clinical Endocrinology* 2004;61:10–18.

106. McLachlan SM, Nagayama Y, Rapoport B. Insight into Graves' hyperthyroidism from animal models. *Endocrine Reviews* 2005;26:800–832.

107. Chen CR, Pichurin P, Nagayama Y, Latrofa F, Rapoport B, McLachlan SM. The thyrotropin receptor autoantigen in Graves' disease is the culprit as well as the victim. *The Journal of Clinical Investigation* 2003;111:1897–1904.

108. Ando T, Latif R, Pritsker A, Moran T, Nagayama Y, Davies TF. A monoclonal thyroid-stimulating antibody. *The Journal of Clinical Investigation* 2002;110:1667–1674.

109. Costagliola S, Franssen JDF, Bonomi M, Urizar E, Willnich M, Bergmann A, Vassart G. Generation of a mouse monoclonal TSH receptor antibody with stimulating activity. *Biochemical and Biophysical Research Communications* 2002;299:891–896.

110. Sanders J, Jeffreys J, Depraetere H, Richards T, Evans M, Kiddie A, Brereton K, Groenen M, Oda Y, Furmaniak JG, Smith BR. Thyroid-stimulating monoclonal antibodies. *Thyroid* 2002;12:1043–1050.

111. McLachlan SM, Rapoport B. Monoclonal, human autoantibodies to the TSH receptor – The holy grail and why are we looking for it? *The Journal of Clinical Endocrinology and Metabolism* 1996;81:3152–3154.

112. Dohan O, De la Vieja A, Paroder V, Riedel C, Artani M, Reed M, Ginter CS, Carrasco N. The sodium/iodide symporter (NIS): characterization, regulation, and medical significance. *Endocrine Reviews* 2003;24:48–77.

113. Endo T, Kogai T, Nakazato M, Saito T, Kaneshige M, Onaya T. Autoantibody against Na$^+$/I$^-$ symporter in the sera of patients with autoimmune thyroid disease. *Biochemical and Biophysical Research Communications* 1996;224:92–95.

114. Ajjan RA, Findlay C, Metcalfe RA, Watson PF, Crisp M, Ludgate M, Weetman AP. The modulation of the human sodium iodide symporter activity by Graves' disease sera. *The Journal of Clinical Endocrinology and Metabolism* 1998;83:1217–1221.

115. Ajjan RA, Kemp EH, Waterman EA, Watson PF, Endo T, Onaya T, Weetman AP. Detection of binding and blocking autoantibodies to the human sodium-iodide symporter in patients with autoimmune thyroid disease. *The Journal of Clinical Endocrinology and Metabolism* 2000;85:2020–2027.

116. Chin HS, Chin DKH, Morgenthaler NG, Vassart G, Costagliola S. Rarity of anti-Na$^+$/I-symporter (NIS) antibody with iodide uptake inhibiting activity in autoimmune thyroid diseases (AITD). *The Journal of Clinical Endocrinology and Metabolism* 2000;85:3937–3940.

117. Marinò M, Zheng G, McCluskey RT. Megalin (gp330) is an endocytic receptor for thyroglobulin on cultured Fisher rat thyroid cells. *The Journal of Biological Chemistry* 1999;274:12898–12904.

118. Lisi S, Segnani C, Mattii L, Botta R, Marcocci C, Dolfi A, McCluskey RT, Pinchera A, Bernardini N, Marino M. Thyroid dysfunction in megalin deficient mice. *Molecular and Cellular Endocrinology* 2005;236:43–47.

119. Marinò M, Chiovato L, Friedlander JA, Latrofa F, Pinchera A, McCluskey RT. Serum antibodies against megalin (gp330) in patients with autoimmune thyroiditis. *The Journal of Clinical Endocrinology and Metabolism* 1999;84:2468–2474.

120. Illies F, Wingert AM, Bald M, Hoyer PF. Autoimmune thyroiditis in association with membranous nephropathy. *Journal of Pediatric Endocrinology & Metabolism* 2004;17:99–104.

6 Graves' Disease

Simon H. S. Pearce, MD, FRCP

CONTENTS

INTRODUCTION
EPIDEMIOLOGY
GENETIC AND ENVIRONMENTAL FACTORS
IMMUNOPATHOGENESIS
DIAGNOSIS
TREATMENT
FUTURE DEVELOPMENTS
REFERENCES

Summary

Hyperthyroid Graves' disease is one of the most common autoimmune disorders, affecting about 1% of women. It is most frequent in the 4th decade of life. There is a genetic predisposition to Graves' disease, determined by alleles at the major histocompatibility complex, cytotoxic T-lymphocyte-associated antigen, protein tyrosine phosphatase non-receptor 22, and other less well-defined chromosomal loci. Additional, non-genetic, factors that have an influence are cigarette use, pregnancy, estrogen use, and stressful life events. The hyperthyroidism is caused by thyroid-stimulating hormone (TSH) receptor stimulating autoantibodies that lead to excess thyroid hormone production and thyroid growth. Thyroid peroxidase autoantibodies are also frequently found and may be important in thyrocyte destruction and perpetuation of autoimmunity. Graves' disease may be treated with thionamide antithyroid drugs, radioiodine, or thyroid surgery. No treatment is perfect and each has its pros and cons. The recent isolation of monoclonal human TSH receptor antibodies may lead to more sensitive tests for thyroid-stimulating autoantibodies. A key challenge is to define novel therapies that lead to more certain and safe remission of hyperthyroidism without ablation of thyroid function.

Key Words: Autoimmune hyperthyroidism, thionamide, radioiodine, TSH receptor, thyroid peroxidase, autoantibody, goiter.

INTRODUCTION

Graves' disease is unique among autoimmune conditions in that the target tissue is stimulated by the immune response, rather than being progressively destroyed by it. This, coupled with the early identification of circulating thyroid-stimulating autoantibodies as the immunological hallmark of the condition, has led to Graves' disease acting as a paradigm for research into autoimmune endocrinopathies. The curious

From: *Contemporary Endocrinology: Autoimmune Diseases in Endocrinology*
Edited by: A. P. Weetman © Humana Press, Totowa, NJ

combination of thyroid disease and ophthalmopathy has also sparked interest in the condition over more than a century, and there are several aspects of this association that remain unexplained. Detailed discussion of Graves' ophthalmopathy can be found in Chap. 9, and basic mechanisms and animal models of autoimmune thyroid disease (AITD) are reviewed in Chaps. 1–4. This chapter reviews the pathophysiology, immunology, and clinical features of human hyperthyroid Graves' disease.

EPIDEMIOLOGY

Graves' disease is one of the most common autoimmune disorders and affects women about seven times more frequently than men. Its prevalence varies, with 0.5–1% of women having had hyperthyroidism in different westernized populations (1,2). More accurately, the 12-year follow-up of the Nurses Health II study in North America found an incidence of 0.04% per year for Graves' disease (3) and this is corroborated by a 20-year follow-up study from the North East of England, which showed an incidence of hyperthyroidism of 0.08% per year in women (4). Graves' disease is more prevalent in countries that are iodine replete (5). Graves' disease may occur at any time from early childhood to old age, and there is a peak in incidence in the fourth decade with the mean age at diagnosis being between 35 and 40 years in most large series (3). It is often found in women around the time of pregnancy, during which time hyperthyroidism is often mild and easy to control, with a tendency to remission by the third trimester. However, there is typically relapse of GD 4–8 months post-partum. Thyroid eye disease (Graves' ophthalmopathy; GO) is a frequent accompaniment to hyperthyroid Graves' disease, with eyelid manifestations or surface symptoms being found in about 40% of hyperthyroid subjects. In contrast, functionally significant thyroid eye disease (most commonly manifest as proptosis and extraocular muscle involvement) has a relative predilection for older subjects and occurs equally frequently in both sexes (6).

GENETIC AND ENVIRONMENTAL FACTORS

Genetics

Graves' disease is a complex genetic condition, meaning that alleles at several different chromosomal loci, along with non-genetic factors, are thought to contribute to disease pathogenesis in varying degrees in each affected individual. Between one-quarter and one-third of GD patients have a first-degree relative with either Graves' or another AITD, suggesting a significant contribution of genetic factors (7). Detailed twin studies have also suggested that inherited factors make the dominant contribution to disease susceptibility, perhaps contributing up to 79% of the risk (8). An index of the heritability of a disorder can be gained by assessing the risk to a sibling of an affected individual compared with that of the unrelated background population. For GD, this relative risk estimate, termed λ_s, has been estimated to between 10 and 15 (7), which is comparable to that found for other common autoimmune disorders.

Among genes known to contribute to GD susceptibility, alleles at three loci have been identified to have moderate or large effects: the major histocompatibility complex (*MHC*, including *HLA* alleles), the cytotoxic T-lymphocyte antigen-4 locus (*CTLA4*), and the protein tyrosine phosphatase-22 (*PTPN22*) gene, which encodes the lymphoid tyrosine phosphatase protein (Fig. 1). Alleles at each of these loci underlie

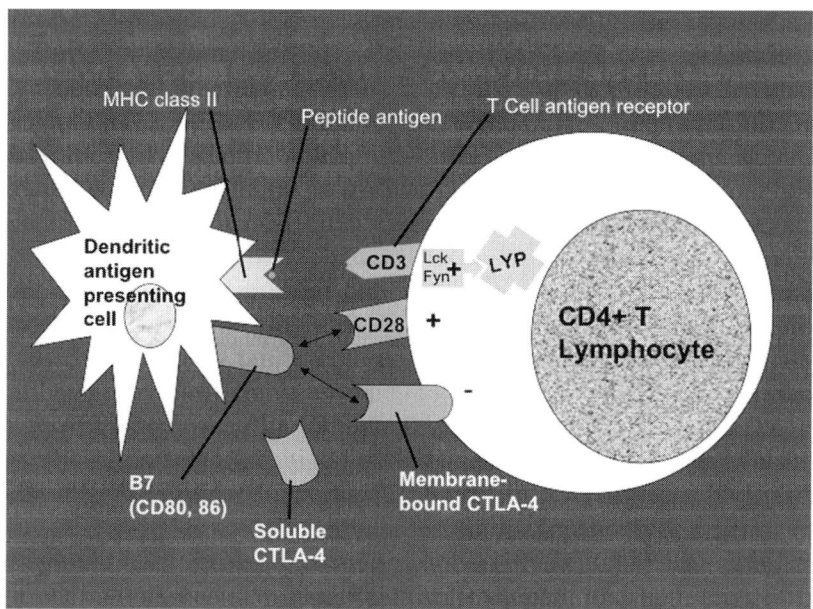

Fig. 1. An antigen-presenting cell (APC) interacting with a T lymphocyte. The dendritic APC presents a cleaved peptide antigen bound to the groove of the tetrameric class II major histocompatibility complex (MHC) molecule. This is recognized by a T lymphocyte with an antigen receptor (CD3 complex) of appropriate affinity for the peptide/MHC combination. For the lymphocyte to become activated a second signal must be delivered by the interaction of a costimulatory molecule with B7 molecules expressed on the APC. CD28 is a positive costimulator allowing lymphocyte proliferation and activation, but cytotoxic T-lymphocyte-associated antigen (CTLA4) is an inhibitory costimulator, causing the lymphocyte to become quiescent or to apoptose. Soluble CTLA4 (sCTLA4) may have a role as a natural inhibitor of CD28 engagement, by binding to APC B7 molecules with a higher affinity than CD28 and thereby stopping the costimulatory activation of the lymphocyte via CD28-B7 interaction. Subjects with the susceptibility allele for AITD at *CTLA4* have relatively less sCTLA4 mRNA *(21)* and if reflected at the protein level, this could allow a greater activation signal to T lymphocytes, by stronger costimulatory activity. Lymphoid tyrosine phosphatase (LYP) is encoded by the *PTPN22* gene, and the autoimmunity-associated SNP codes for an arginine (wild-type) to tryptophan change. The LYP molecule inhibits Lck signalling following TCR (CD3) engagement, however the tryptophan variant of LYP is more highly active than the arginine variant, paradoxically causing more potent downregulation of signaling *(23)*.

the susceptibility to many common autoimmune disorders including autoimmune hypothyroidism, type 1 diabetes, rheumatoid arthritis, celiac disease, autoimmune Addison's disease, and systemic lupus erythematosis, as well as Graves' disease. These immune-response genes determine the "general" predisposition to autoimmunity that accounts for much of the co-occurrence of other autoimmune conditions with AITD *(9)*. In addition to these general autoimmune disease alleles, there are likely to be "target-organ" specific genes that determine whether the thyroid is affected by the autoimmune disease and the course of the autoimmune disease (e.g., hyperthyroidism or hypothyroidism; transient or permanent). The genetic factors established for GD will be briefly reviewed next; more detailed analysis is given in Chap. 2.

The association of GD with alleles of the *MHC* on chromosome 6p21 has long been established *(10,11)*. The dominant association in white populations of European descent is with *HLA-DR3* carrying haplotypes (*DRB1*0301-DQB1*0201-DQA1*0501*) (*12,13*). This haplotype is carried by 25–30% of unaffected individuals but is consistently over-represented among those with GD, of whom about 50% carry the haplotype. Recent studies have resequenced the *DRB1* gene in many GD subjects and suggest that a critical amino acid for disease susceptibility is arginine at position 74 (*14,15*). Even so, the odds ratio for the *DR3* haplotype in GD is about 2, and *MHC* does not have the dominant genetic effect in GD that is found in other autoimmune disorders (e.g., type 1 diabetes or rheumatoid arthritis). This is manifest by the lack of strong evidence for genetic linkage to 6p21 in many studies (*16–18*) and suggests that loci other than *MHC* also have major effects. The fact that 50% of GD subjects carry "non-*DR3*" HLA alleles may also indicate that there is not one unique immunogenic or pathogenic peptide that is always involved in triggering the T-cell response in GD.

Alleles in the 3′ region of the *CTLA4* gene on chromosome 2q33 have been extensively associated with GD. CTLA4 is involved in the regulation of the costimulatory ("second") signal in T-lymphocyte activation and so was a good candidate gene. Initial investigations by Yanagawa and colleagues (*19*) were confirmed with a gamut of replication studies in many different GD populations (reviewed in ref. *20*). The true disease susceptibility allele at *CTLA4* remains to be defined but probably lies within a 6-kb region including the 3′ untranslated region (UTR) of the gene (*21*). The susceptibility haplotype at *CTLA4* is carried by about 50% of the healthy white population, and its prevalence increases to 60% in subjects with GD, with an odds ratio for the most associated allele of about 1.5 (*21*). The mechanism by which these non-coding polymorphisms might modulate the immune response is far from clear. One recent study has suggested a role for *CTLA4* polymorphisms in T-cell differentiation and lineage commitment, with genotypes being correlated to the number of circulating $CD4^+$, $CD25^+$ T regulatory lymphocytes (*22*).

An additional locus that has come to light in the last year is *PTPN22*, which encodes the lymphoid tyrosine phosphatase (LYP). A coding polymorphism, arginine to tryptophan at codon 620, activates the LYP molecule, paradoxically causing more potent inhibition of the T-cell antigen receptor (CD3)-signaling kinases, following engagement with MHC antigen (*23*). The tryptophan allele is carried by about 7% of healthy subjects in white populations but is over-represented in GD subjects with a prevalence of about 13% (*24,25*). The odds ratio for the effect of this allele is about 1.8, but because of its comparative rarity (*24,25*), it contributes slightly less to overall population Graves' disease susceptibility than *CTLA4*. It remains to be seen how the effect of this variant on TCR signaling predisposes to autoimmunity.

Disease-specific loci for GD have started to be identified in recent years. After a period of negative investigations into the thyroid-stimulating hormone (TSH) receptor gene, alleles of SNP markers have now been shown to have unequivocal association with GD in two distinct patient cohorts (*26,27*). The associated polymorphism lies within the regulatory regions of the extracellular domain of the receptor, and fine mapping studies are in progress to more fully define the disease-associated allele and hence the mechanism for the disease effect (*26,27*). In contrast, several studies have shown weak evidence for association of GD with SNP and microsatellite markers in the thyroglobulin (*Tg*) gene (*28,29*). On aggregate, these studies of the *Tg* gene have not shown convincing evidence for association with GD (although the effect may be different in autoimmune hypothyroidism) *(30)*. *Tg* is a huge, 48 exon, gene and further work, to define and test the enormous diversity of haplotypes, is currently awaited.

Environment

Of environmental influences, cigarette smoking and stress are the best defined risk factors for GD *(31)*. Although many studies have demonstrated a clear association of smoking with Graves' ophthalmopathy, a meta-analysis of eight studies shows an odds ratio of 3.3 (95% confidence intervals 2.1–5.2) for the effect of current smoking on Graves' disease *(32)*. However, the mechanism of this effect is unclear. Two recent studies have looked in detail at thyroid autoantibody production in smokers and both show a protective effect of current smoking for thyroid peroxidase (TPO) antibody positivity *(33,34)*. There is also an association of current smoking with a trend toward a lower TSH value in large populations *(34)*, but this may be a chemical effect of smoke thiocyanates or other substances on thyroid hormone production or metabolism, rather than an immunomodulatory effect.

Since the first descriptions of Graves' disease, stress has been suggested to have a role in pathogenesis. Several studies of the prevalence of Graves' disease during times of national conflict have shown significantly increased rates *(35,36)*, (reviewed in ref. *37*), however, there have also been simultaneous major dietary changes within these wartime populations. Graves' patients from many cultural backgrounds have also been shown to have experienced more "negative life events" (e.g., death of family member) in the year before the onset of their disease *(38,39)*. This appears to be true, even after carefully controlling for the hyperthyroid state using non-autoimmune hyperthyroid subjects *(40)*. There are many mechanisms by which stress could be acting through altered immune function to precipitate Graves' disease in a predisposed individual *(37)*, although no correlation has been shown between stressful life events and TPO antibody status *(41)*.

Pregnancy and estrogen use also have significant influences on the occurrence of Graves' disease. As mentioned, previous pregnancy is a common risk factor for Graves' disease with an odds ratio of more than six in one study *(33)*. In contrast, estrogen use (most commonly in the form of the combined oral contraceptive pill) is protective against Graves' disease *(33)*. This protective effect holds true even when corrected for the lack of pregnancy in estrogen users. The mechanism for the effects of pregnancy on Graves' disease may relate to a relative suppression of immune function during pregnancy and a rebound of immune activity in the postpartum period, which may have some analogy to the immune reconstitution Graves' disease seen in other circumstances (*see* paragraph below).

Modulation of normal immune function, by infection, allergy, or iatrogenic manipulation, is associated with Graves' disease in various circumstances. During recovery from a severe immunosuppressive insult, a reconstituted and relatively antigen-naïve immune system, presumably recently re-exposed to thyroid antigens, can lead to Graves' disease. This immune reconstitution GD occurs in up to 30% of multiple sclerosis patients, following the T-cell-depleting (anti-CD52) Campath-H1 treatment *(42)*, and in a small number of patients (2–5%) recovering T-cell function following successful highly active antiretroviral therapy for HIV infection *(43)*.

Probably by a different mechanism, a minority of Graves' cases appear to have a clear temporal link to an attack of allergic illness (typically allergic rhinitis) with high serum IgE levels preceding the onset of, or relapse, of symptoms *(44,45)*. It has been speculated that the Th2 (humoral) arm of the immune system is active in these circumstances and provides a permissive environment for thyroid antibody generation. Although there are many reports of different infectious agents, or serum antibodies toward such organisms, being associated with Graves' disease *(46,47)*, (reviewed in ref. *48*), many of these studies are small and have not been convincingly reproduced *(49)*. Importantly, Graves' patients represent a population with a distinct immunogenetic profile (e.g., 50% of whites with GD are HLA-DR3 positive), and studies looking at infectious factors need to be designed with an HLA-matched healthy control group before such reports can be considered credible.

IMMUNOPATHOGENESIS

Antibodies that stimulate the TSH receptor (TSHR) are the essential driver for the hyperthyroidism and thyrocyte hyperplasia that characterize Graves' disease *(50)*. These stimulating antibodies, termed TSAbs, are demonstrable by sensitive immunoassays in >95% of Graves' subjects *(51)*. TSAbs are predominantly of the IgG1 subclass and target a conformational and discontinuous epitope in the amino-terminal region of the leucine-rich repeat motif in the extracellular domain of the TSHR *(52)* (Fig. 2). The TSHR has the unique feature for a glycoprotein hormone receptor of being cleaved and re-formed from two disulfide-linked subunits (termed A & B) during its processing for cell surface expression. Curiously, it appears that TSAbs have a higher affinity for the cleaved off, "shed," extracellular A domain of the receptor than for the intact "holoreceptor," and indeed, immunization with the A domain also generates higher TSHR-stimulating activity in murine models than with intact receptor *(53,54)*. Binding of these TSAbs activates the intracellular G proteins coupled to the TSHR, and this induces transcription of the genes encoding Tg, the thyroid hormone-generating enzymes (including TPO), and the sodium iodide transporter through the cyclic-AMP and phospholipase-C pathways. Thyroid hormone production, secretion, and thyrocyte growth results. As well as TSAbs, subjects with Graves' disease and other AITD may have circulating antibodies that block the effects of TSH (or of TSHR-stimulating antibodies) on TSHR activation. The presence of these blocking antibodies, co-existing with circulating TSAbs, is partly responsible for the fluctuating nature of the hyperthyroidism that is sometimes seen in Graves' disease. In addition, high titer blocking antibodies are responsible for the occasional individual with hyperthyroid Graves' disease who presents after a prolonged period of hypothyroidism.

Whether the immune response directed against the TSHR is the initiating immunological event for Graves' disease may never be fully clarified; however, there are circulating antibodies to several other thyroid antigens in the majority of subjects with Graves' disease. These include antibodies directed against TPO, thyroglobulin, the sodium iodide symporter, and some other less well-defined thyrocyte components. Of these, anti-TPO (formerly known as microsomal) antibodies are pathogenically the most important and also the most frequent, being found in up to 90% of Graves' subjects using sensitive assays *(55)*. These anti-TPO antibodies may be of various subclasses

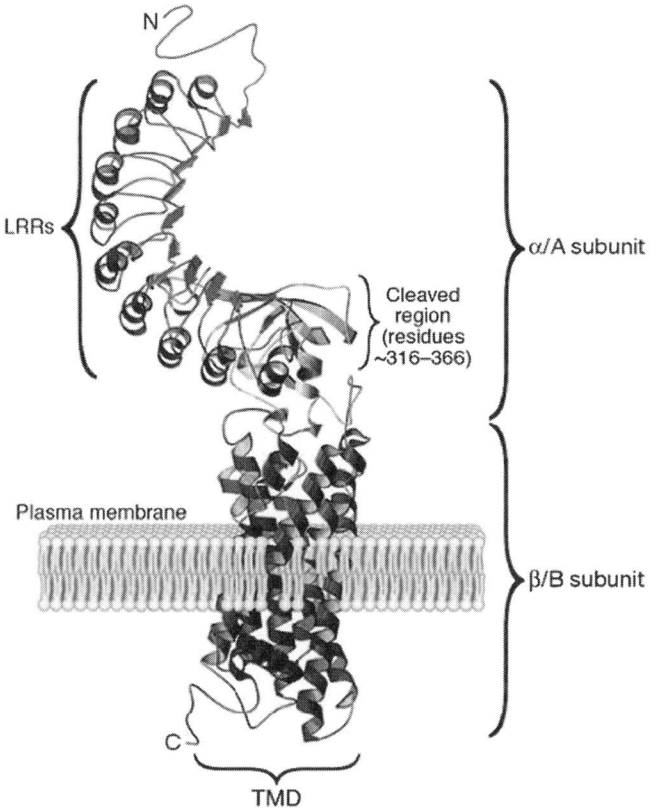

Fig. 2. Ribbon diagram of the putative structure of the TSH receptor. The large extra-cellular "A" domain contains 9 leucine-rich repeat (LRR) regions, which is attached to the transmembrane and intracellular tail of the receptor ("B" domain) by disulfide bonds. The sites of TSHR-stimulating antibody binding have been mapped to discontinuous and conformational epitopes involving the amino-terminal portion of the LRR domain.

(immunoglobulin [Ig]G-1, -2 or -4) and uniquely among thyroid autoantibodies have the capacity to fix complement and to mediate thyrocyte damage through antibody-dependent cell-mediated cytotoxicity *(56,57)*. In contrast to the low concentration THSR-stimulating antibodies, which circulate in nanogram per milliliter quantities in Graves' disease, TPO antibodies are commonly found at 1000-fold or higher concentrations. Naturally occurring TPO antibodies tend to be directed against certain specific and highly conformational "immunodominant" epitopes of TPO *(58,59)* (Fig. 3). Interestingly, these patterns of TPO antibody response (epitopic fingerprints) are stable, persisting for many years; they are also inherited in a dominant fashion *(60)*. In contrast to anti-TSHR antibodies, anti-TPO antibodies do not seem to affect the enzymatic function of TPO in vivo.

In the untreated state, the thyroid gland in Graves' disease, as well as being enlarged by thyrocyte hyperplasia, also contains an extensive B- and T-cell lymphocytic infiltrate. The thyroid autoantibodies are produced predominantly from these intrathyroidal B cells/plasma cells *(61)*, which cluster into lymphoid follicles. Antibodies are also produced to a lesser degree from activated B cells in adjacent lymph nodes, spleen,

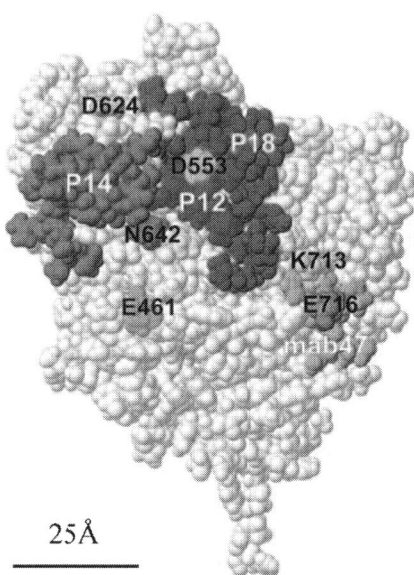

25Å

Fig. 3. Space-filling diagram of the putative structure of the myeloperoxidase-like domain of thyroid peroxidase. Thyroid peroxidase (TPO) acts as a cell surface homodimer, and has a large myeloper-oxidase (MPO)-like domain, with two smaller, complement control protein (CCP)-like and EGF-like domains (not shown). There are specific TPO epitopes that are predominantly recognized by autoantibodies in human autoimmune thyroid diseases. The TPO peptides that block autoantibody binding to these immunodominant regions are shown mapped out on the surface of the MPO-like domain, but in reality these epitopes involve additional residues on the CCP-like domain in a three-dimensional conformation *(96)*.

or thymus. These B cells, in turn, are regulated by activated intrathyroidal T cells, which are of restricted T-cell antigen receptor diversity *(62)*, suggesting derivation from a limited number of precursor T cells. Once established, it is likely that the immune response in the thyroid is maintained by a number of factors, including the ability of thyrocytes themselves, as well as the intrathyroidal B cells, to present antigen to T cells and the overexpression of TPO and Tg that is driven by TSHR stimulation. It can certainly be envisaged that a circle of perpetuation might occur, whereby antibody-mediated TSHR stimulation triggers increased TPO and Tg expression, leading to formation of anti-TPO and Tg antibodies and progressive thyrocyte antigen release, which re-primes the immune response.

DIAGNOSIS

Clinical Presentation

The symptoms of thyrotoxicosis are often non-specific, so patients with Graves' disease may present in numerous ways. The start of symptoms is gradual and often poorly defined with most subjects having felt unwell for 3–6 months before seeking medical attention. If the onset of thyrotoxic symptoms can be pinned down to a single day or few days, then the diagnosis is most frequently that of a destructive thyroiditis rather than Graves' disease. Weight loss despite an increase in appetite is found in 80% of subjects, although in a minority the increase in appetite, coupled with the free availability of calorie-dense food, leads to weight gain. Pervasive exhaustion may alternate with periods of restlessness and hyperactivity. Heat intolerance is also common, with the need to wear fewer clothes and sweating at night being characteristic. Palpitations at rest or on minimal exertion, or shortness of breath during light exercise are common at all ages. Tremor of the hands may be noted, along with inappropriate feelings of anxiety, apprehension, or jumpiness. Poor sleep with mental overactivity and physical hyperkinesis at night may be a problem. Intestinal transit-time is shortened, leading to more frequent defecation. Menstrual bleeding may be light, decreased in frequency, or absent.

Thyroid tenderness or pain is not a feature. Less commonly reported symptoms are thirst, nausea, generalized itch, and diffuse scalp hair loss. In 5–10% of people, the first symptoms are because of Graves' ophthalmopathy (*see* Chap. 9), with itchy, gritty, or watering eyes, or an abnormal appearance. Individuals with asymmetrical ophthalmopathy tend to present earlier with change in appearance. In the elderly, there may be little to suggest thyrotoxicosis. Feelings of lethargy, along with reduced appetite may lead to a diagnosis of depression. Alternatively, the onset of atrial fibrillation may precipitate a cardiac presentation with dyspnea and/or congestion. In childhood, hyperactivity, short attention span, behavioral problems, and increased linear growth are found.

The subject may have difficulty sitting still, with constant fidgeting of the hands. The face, neck, and upper chest wall are often flushed. The palms may be warm and sweaty, with a symmetrical fine tremor when hands are outstretched. A diffuse goiter can be visible or palpable, with a systolic phase bruit found over it. There is often tachycardia unless beta-blockers are being taken, and rapid atrial fibrillation may be present, particularly in the elderly. Systolic blood pressure may be elevated. There may be hepatomegaly or splenomegaly. The ankles may be swollen with pitting edema or rarely because of infiltrative thyroid dermopathy (pretibial myxedema). However, the latter is more commonly manifest as discrete violaceous plaques on the shin or dorsum of the foot. Hyperreflexia is common and proximal musculature can be weak. Frank spasticity and pseudobulbar paresis are late features. Rapid onset of severe and generalized muscle weakness suggests hypokalemic periodic paralysis: a syndrome most common in men of Asian descent that is precipitated by thyrotoxicosis. Signs of Graves' ophthalmopathy, including lid retraction, lid or conjunctival redness and edema, proptosis and restricted ocular motility may be present. Rare signs of Graves' disease include chorea, onycholysis, or acropachy of the nails.

Investigation

Elevation of one or both serum-free thyroid hormones together with an undetectable TSH (on a third generation assay) confirms the diagnosis of thyrotoxicosis. About 5% of subjects, most commonly elderly, present with elevation of free T3 alone, with normal free T4 and undetectable TSH. This "T3 thyrotoxicosis" is often a manifestation of relatively mild hyperthyroidism and may respond better to medical treatment. Elevation of free T4 alone, with normal free T3 and undetectable TSH may be found in someone with co-existing major illness (a combination of thyrotoxicosis and sick-euthyroid syndrome) but is also typical of iodine-induced thyrotoxicosis or exogenous levothyroxine use. If there is doubt about the chronicity or severity of symptoms, then it is good practice to repeat the abnormal thyroid function tests after a short period, as a rapid fluctuation may be the clue to the diagnosis of destructive (silent) thyroiditis. If the TSH is low but detectable, then the diagnosis is almost certainly not Graves' disease and further investigations are needed. Individuals with a persistently undetectable TSH but normal free thyroid hormones (in the absence of pituitary disease and drug effects) are said to have subclinical hyperthyroidism and need further investigation (i.e., serum thyroid antibodies, Holter monitor, DEXA bone scan). There is little clear evidence to guide treatment in this situation (63,64), but in the presence of atrial fibrillation or established osteoporosis, such subjects warrant treatment for their mild hyperthyroidism (65).

In the presence of clear extrathyroidal signs of Graves' disease (e.g., proptosis, dermopathy), no further testing beyond free thyroid hormone(s) and TSH is necessary. In the absence of these features, an attempt to secure an etiological diagnosis should be made. The gold-standard test is a highly sensitive TSHR-stimulating antibody assay, which will be positive in >95% of subjects with Graves' disease (51). But other serum antibody tests, including indirect assay of TSH-stimulating antibodies by TSH-binding inhibitory immunoglobulin (TBI or TBII) or TPO antibody assay are commonly employed and have >90% sensitivity for Graves' disease. In the absence of a positive antibody test, or in the presence of a nodular thyroid on palpation, the thyroid gland should be imaged. Although an ultrasound examination may give a diagnosis of multinodular goiter, a radionuclide image with either ^{99m}Tc or ^{123}I gives functional data as to the presence and distribution of functioning thyroid tissue. Where both tests are available, radionuclide imaging with measurement of isotope uptake may be the preferable investigation for a positive diagnosis of Graves' disease. Other investigations may be worthwhile depending on the clinical situation and likely treatment plan. If there is significant tachycardia, it is good practice to document the rhythm by ECG, and subjects with atrial fibrillation should proceed to a more detailed cardiac evaluation. If antithyroid drug treatment is planned, then a blood count and white cell differential at baseline may be helpful for the future. A negative pregnancy test is mandatory if radioiodine treatment is to be undertaken. Microcytosis, elevation of serum alkaline phosphatase, and mildly deranged liver enzymes are often found; mild hypercalcemia is rare.

TREATMENT

The treatment options for hyperthyroid Graves' disease include thionamide antithyroid drug treatment, radioiodine therapy, or thyroid surgery. All thyrotoxic patients may gain symptomatic benefit from beta blockade, but this is contraindicated in those with asthma. Higher doses (e.g., 80 mg tds of propranolol or more) may be needed to gain heart-rate control in severe thyrotoxicosis, as there is accelerated drug metabolism in this situation. Individuals with atrial fibrillation should also be considered for anticoagulation. Currently, there is no perfect treatment for Graves' hyperthyroidism (66). Each modality has its own pros and cons, and patient preference is frequently a deciding factor.

Thionamide Treatment

The thionamide antithyroid drugs, propylthiouracil, carbimazole, and its active metabolite methimazole, have been in use to treat Graves' disease for >50 years.

After prolonged administration, they induce remission of hyperthyroidism in about 50% of those treated *(67,68)*. Thionamides act as preferential substrates for iodination by TPO *(69)*, competing with thyroglobulin to prevent iodotyrosine formation, and as the iodinated drug derivative is metabolized peripherally, there is gradual depletion of the thyroidal iodine stores *(70)*. Initial treatment with methimazole or carbimazole is preferable to propylthiouracil as the drugs can be taken once or twice daily, rather than 8 hourly, and the longer half-life leads to more rapid control *(71)*.

The majority of subjects with hyperthyroid Graves' disease are rendered euthyroid (as judged by normal free thyroid hormones) by 4- to 8-weeks treatment with methimazole (30 mg daily) or carbimazole (40 mg daily). Only those with large goiter, recent iodide exposure, or with poor treatment compliance may need to be treated for longer or with larger thionamide doses. After euthyroidism is achieved, two different regimens can be employed. In the first regimen, termed "block-replace," the dose of thionamide is kept constant (e.g., carbimazole 40 mg daily), blocking thyroid hormone production, and levothyroxine is added in a suitable dose to maintain euthyroidism (e.g., 100 μg daily for a woman, 125 μg daily for a man). In the second regimen, termed "titrated," the thionamide dose is progressively lowered at regular intervals to allow endogenous synthesis of thyroid hormone to continue in a regulated fashion, with only a partial blockade to hormone production.

In both regimens, there is approximately a 50% remission rate if treatment is continued for between 6 and 18 months and then stopped (Table 1) *(72,73)*. The relative merits and drawbacks of the two treatment regimens are summarized in Table 1. The disadvantage to antithyroid drug treatment with either regimen relates to the uncertainty that the individual may not achieve remission after treatment is stopped and the potential adverse effects of the antithyroid drugs *(70,74)*. A pruritic rash, which is often transient, is seen in about 5% of subjects taking antithyroid drugs. The much rarer but occasionally lethal problem of thionamide-induced agranulocytosis occurs in 1 in 300–500 subjects *(74)*, and patients embarking on antithyroid drug treatment for any length of time should have clear (and ideally written) instructions to discontinue treatment and seek a blood count should fever and sore throat develop. Agranulocytosis occurs most frequently in the first 3 months of treatment (with a median time of about 30 days) and is rare after 6 months *(75)*.

A recent Cochrane evidence-based medicine review has performed meta-analysis of all randomized controlled trials of thionamides and suggests that titrated regimens are

Table 1
Methods of Administering Antithyroid Drugs

Block–replace regimen	*Titrated dose regimen*
Stable euthyroidism	Prone to periods of hypo- and hyperthyroidism
Less clinic visits, less monitoring	More clinic visits, more monitoring
Higher rate of adverse reaction	Lower risk of adverse reaction
Optimal remission rate after 6–12 months	Optimal remission rate after 12–18 months
No prediction of remission by dose changes	Prediction of early remission by successful dose reduction
No significant difference in early or late remission rates between either regimen	

preferable, as they have a lower incidence of adverse reactions *(73)*. However, this recommendation is not relevant to current practice as the block-replace treatment arms in the three of the four trials that provided evidence of adverse effects used what would now be considered as high-dose treatment (i.e., carbimazole 60 mg daily or higher dosages). Nevertheless, the adverse effects of thionamides, including agranulocytosis, are clearly dose-dependent, and subjects should be carefully observed when higher dosages are necessary to gain control of hyperthyroidism. Occasional subjects feel persistently unwell despite euthyroidism on antithyroid drugs. It is worth investigating these for evidence of Addison's disease, pernicious anemia, or celiac disease. The ideal Graves' patient to treat with antithyroid drugs is someone with a high chance of remission after treatment. Thus, individuals of older age, female sex, small thyroid size, no extrathyroidal manifestations, mild hyperthyroxinemia at presentation, and low-titer TSHR antibodies are most likely to have a successful outcome from drug treatment *(76,77)*.

Radioiodine

[131]I (radioiodine, RAI) is a beta and gamma radiation emitter, which is rapidly concentrated by the thyroid after oral ingestion. The active beta particles have a short 2-mm radius of activity and induce DNA damage in the thyrocytes and surrounding non-epithelial thyroid cells, leading to necrosis, followed by fibrosis and atrophy. Over 6 weeks to 6 months following RAI treatment, most individuals with Graves' disease are rendered sequentially euthyroid and then hypothyroid *(78)*. Although there have been many attempts to use careful dosimetry to estimate the optimal dose of RAI for each individual *(79)*, many centers administer a pragmatic dose that results in eu- or hypothyroidism in 70–90% of subjects treated. The exact dose and its efficacy depends on the iodide nutritional status of the local population, the restriction to iodide intake imposed on the subject before administration, and whether antithyroid drugs are used and how long they are stopped before administration *(80)*. In the United Kingdom, doses of 370 to 550 MBq (10–15 mCi) are routinely used to treat Graves' disease in different centers. There is a small risk of exacerbating hyperthyroidism (or even precipitating thyroid storm) in the month following RAI treatment because of release of pre-formed hormone. For subjects with large goiters, moderate to severe thyrotoxicosis, known ischemic heart disease, or arrhythmic tendency, it is recommended to pre-treat with thionamide until the subject is euthyroid, to reduce this risk *(81)*. Propylthiouracil in particular *(80)*, but also other thionamides, should be stopped several days *(3–14)* before RAI is administered. These can be restarted 2 weeks after the dose, with or without thyroxine, if ongoing control of thyrotoxicosis is critical.

RAI is absolutely contraindicated in pregnancy and lactation, and subjects are advised to avoid new pregnancy for 6 months after the treatment. RAI is best avoided in childhood and adolescence while subjects are still growing (<18 years), as the thyroid at this age is probably more vulnerable to the deleterious effects of ionizing radiation. Several studies have looked in detail at cancer risk following therapeutic RAI use in adults, and the data are strongly reassuring that cancers at all major sites are no different or less frequent in RAI-treated individuals than in the background population *(82,83)*. The limited long-term follow-up data for RAI use in childhood and adolescence are also reassuring *(84)*. Some patients believe that taking RAI will render them infertile or lead to alopecia. These fairly common but unfounded preconceptions should be directly addressed. Radioiodine is relatively contraindicated in individuals with active inflammatory Graves' ophthalmopathy, as thyroid antigen release and subsequent hypothyroidism may be associated with deterioration of eye disease *(85)*. However, this is rarely observed in subjects who do not smoke or with inactive ophthalmopathy, as long as prompt levothyroxine replacement is undertaken *(86)*. RAI is a good treatment for subjects who want a predictable cure from their Graves' disease and for whom the high probability of lifelong levothyroxine treatment afterward is an acceptable consequence. RAI is the treatment of choice for individuals with severe Graves' disease, males, and those with large goiter but without active (inflammatory) ophthalmopathy *(87)*.

Thyroid Surgery

Total (or near total) thyroidectomy is a highly effective and predictable treatment for Graves' disease. Individuals with Graves' disease who have relapsed following adequate medical therapy, those with active Graves' ophthalmopathy or with a cosmetically undesirable goiter are all well suited to surgical intervention. Patients who have had severe hyperthyroidism with circulatory disturbance treated by iodine load, having been unable to tolerate thionamides, may also be best treated with early surgery *(88)*. Long-term complications of thyroid surgery should occur in <2% of operations. These include hypocalcemia as a result of hypoparathyroidism, which is most frequently transient and vocal cord paresis because of operative compromise of the recurrent laryngeal nerve.

Historically, subtotal thyroidectomy has often been performed for Graves' disease, on the basis that the small amount of residual tissue was enough to avoid hypothyroidism and levothyroxine prescription. In the modern era, where the majority of patients who are treated by thyroidectomy have aggressive or difficult to control Graves' disease, the risk of recurrent hyperthyroidism from the TSAb-stimulated thyroid remnant outweighs this small benefit *(89,90)*. Techniques for less invasive thyroid surgery are currently being developed *(91)*, and could be suitable for subjects with Graves' disease. Patients need to be rendered euthyroid before surgery, and where thionamides cannot be used, iodine loading with potassium iodide, Lugol's iodine, or oral cholecystographic contrast media (iopanoic acid 1 g daily) for 5–10 days is sufficient to achieve euthyroidism in almost all cases *(92)*.

Special Situations

Antithyroid drug treatment with titrated dose propylthiouracil is the treatment of choice for Graves' disease during pregnancy *(93)*. In this situation, block–replace regimens risk fetal hypothyroidism and goiter. There is also a possible risk of aplasia cutis and embryopathy with carbimazole or methimazole *(94,95)*. The dose of propylthiouracil may be progressively dropped throughout the pregnancy, and often, the drug can be discontinued in the third trimester. The onset of intractable vomiting in a newly diagnosed thyrotoxic is likely to herald pregnancy. There is a risk of TSAb-mediated fetal or neonatal hyperthyroidism in pregnant women whose Graves' disease has been treated with RAI or surgery; assay of maternal TSAb during pregnancy will allow anticipation of this rare but treatable complication. Breastfeeding is safe with all three antithyroid drugs.

As previously described, RAI should be avoided in active inflammatory Graves' ophthalmopathy. Antithyroid drug treatment in a block and replace regimen is probably the optimal treatment, until the ophthalmopathy becomes inactive *(86)*. If this cannot be tolerated, then total thyroidectomy is a good option. In childhood and adolescence, the chances of remission following thionamide treatment are lower. If compliance with medication is good, such subjects may be best treated with longer-term thionamide. This can be withdrawn at an age when RAI treatment has become a more acceptable option.

FUTURE DEVELOPMENTS

With the recent isolation of monoclonal human TSHR-stimulating antibodies, more sensitive antibody assays to confirm Graves' disease are set to become widely available *(51)*. Genomic investigation into the association with the TSHR locus are likely to shed light on why some people develop Graves' disease, whereas others in the same family develop autoimmune hypothyroidism. There are also likely to be results of genome scans for association in Graves' disease cohorts in the next 5 years, and these will lead to a leap in novel biological insights into AITD. It is disappointing that the therapeutic armamentarium for the management of Graves' disease remains unchanged since the introduction of RAI and thionamides in the 1940s. However, it is possible that novel and specific treatments will stem from knowledge gained from genomics and from the detailed molecular studies of thyroid antigens that are also currently moving at a fast pace *(52–54,96)*.

REFERENCES

1. Tunbridge WM, Evered DC, Hall R, et al. The spectrum of thyroid disease in a community: the Whickham survey. *Clin Endocrinol* 1977; 7: 481–493.
2. Hollowell JG, Staehling NW, Flanders WD, et al. Serum TSH, T(4), and thyroid antibodies in the United States population (1988 to 1994): National Health and Nutrition Examination Survey (NHANES III). *J Clin Endocrinol Metab* 2002; 87: 489–499.
3. Holm IA, Manson JE, Michels KB, Alexander EK, Willett WC, Utiger RD. Smoking and other lifestyle factors and the risk of Graves' hyperthyroidism. *Arch Int Med* 2005; 165: 1606–1611.
4. Vanderpump MP, Tunbridge WM, French JM, et al. The incidence of thyroid disorders in the community; a twenty year follow up. *Clin Endocrinol* 1995; 43: 55–68.
5. Laurberg P, Pedersen KM, Vestergaard H, Sigurdsson G. High incidence of multinodular toxic goitre in the elderly population in a low iodine intake area vs. high incidence of Graves' disease in the young in a high iodine intake area: comparative surveys of thyrotoxicosis epidemiology in East-Jutland Denmark and Iceland. *J Intern Med* 1991; 229: 415–420.
6. Perros P, Crombie AL, Matthews JN, Kendall-Taylor P. Age and gender influence the severity of thyroid-associated ophthalmopathy: a study of 101 patients attending a combined thyroid-eye clinic. *Clin Endocrinol* 1993; 38: 367–372.
7. Vaidya B, Kendall-Taylor P, Pearce SHS. The genetics of autoimmune thyroid disease. *J Clin Endocrinol Metab* 2002; 87: 5385–5397.
8. Brix TH, Kyvik KO, Christensen K, Hegedus L. Evidence for a major role of heredity in Graves' disease: a population-based study of two Danish twin cohorts. *J Clin Endocrinol Metab* 2001; 86: 930–934.
9. Criswell LA, Pfeiffer KA, Lum RF, et al. Analysis of families in the multiple autoimmune disease genetics consortium (MADGC) collection: the PTPN22 620W allele associates with multiple autoimmune phenotypes. *Am J Hum Genet* 2005; 76: 561–571.

10. Grumet FC, Payne RO, Konishi J, Kriss JP. HL-A antigens as markers for disease susceptibility and autoimmunity in Graves' disease. *J Clin Endocrinol Metab* 1974; 39: 1115–1119.

11. Farid NR, Sampson L, Noel EP, et al. A study of human leukocyte D locus related antigens in Graves' disease. *J Clin Invest* 1979; 63: 108–113.

12. Yanagawa T, Mangklabruks A, Chang YB, et al. Human histocompatability leukocyte antigen-DQA1*0501 allele associated with genetic susceptibility to Graves' disease in a Caucasian population. *J Clin Endocrinol Metab* 1993; 76: 1569–1574.

13. Heward JM, Allahabadia A, Daykin J, et al. Linkage disequilibrium between the human leukocyte antigen class II region of the major histocompatibility complex and Graves' disease: replication using a population case control and family-based study. *J Clin Endocrinol Metab* 1998; 83: 3394–3397.

14. Ban Y, Davies TF, Greenberg DA, et al. Arginine at position 74 of the HLA-DR beta 1 chain is associated with Graves' disease. *Genes Immun* 2004; 5: 203–208.

15. Simmonds MJ, Howson JM, Heward JM, et al. Regression mapping of association between the human leukocyte antigen region and Graves' disease. *Am J Hum Genet* 2005; 76: 157–163.

16. Tomer Y, Barbesino G, Greenberg DA, Concepcion ES, Davies TF. Mapping the major susceptibility loci for familial Graves' and Hashimoto's diseases: evidence for genetic heterogeneity and gene interactions. *J Clin Endocrinol Metab* 1999; 84: 4656–4664.

17. Sakai K, Shirasawa S, Ishikawa N, et al. Identification of susceptibility loci for autoimmune thyroid disease to 5q31-q33 and Hashimoto's thyroiditis to 8q23-q24 by multipoint affected sib-pair linkage analysis in Japanese. *Hum Mol Genet* 2001; 10: 1379–1386.

18. Vaidya B, Imrie H, Perros P, et al. The cytotoxic T lymphocyte antigen-4 is a major Graves' disease locus. *Hum Mol Genet* 1999; 8: 1195–1199.

19. Yanagawa T, Hidaka Y, Guimaraes V, Soliman M, DeGroot LJ. CTLA4 gene polymorphism associated with Graves' disease in a Caucasian population. *J Clin Endocrinol Metab* 1995; 80: 41–45.

20. Vaidya B, Pearce SHS. The emerging role of the CTLA4 gene in autoimmune endocrinopathies. *Eur J Endocrinol* 2004; 150: 619–626.

21. Ueda H, Howson JM, Heward JM, et al. Association of the T-cell regulatory gene CTLA4 with susceptibility to autoimmune disease. *Nature* 2003; 423: 506–511

22. Atabani SF, Thio CL, Divanovic S, et al. Association of CTLA4 polymorphism with regulatory T cell frequency. *Eur. J. Immunol* 2005; 35: 2157–2162.

23. Vang T, Congia M, Macis MD, et al. Autoimmune-associated lymphoid tyrosine phosphatase is a gain of function variant. *Nat Genet* 2005; 37: 1300–1302; doi:10.1038/ng1673.

24. Velaga MR, Wilson V, Jennings CE, et al. The codon 620 tryptophan allele of the lymphoid tyrosine phosphatase (LYP) gene is a major determinant of Graves' Disease. *J Clin Endocrinol Metab* 2004; 89, 5862–5865.

25. Smyth D, Cooper JD, Collins JE, et al. Replication of an association between the lymphoid tyrosine phosphatase locus (LYP/PTPN22) with type 1 diabetes, and evidence for its role as a general autoimmunity locus. *Diabetes* 2004; 53: 3020–3023.

26. Hiratani H, Bowden DW, Ikegami S, et al. Multiple SNPs in intron 7 of thyrotropin receptor are associated with Graves' disease. *J Clin Endocrinol Metab* 2005; 90: 2898–2903.

27. Dechairo BM, Zabaneh D, Collins J, et al. Association of the TSHR gene with Graves' disease: the first disease-specific locus. *Eur J Hum Genet* 2005; 13: 1223–1230.

28. Ban Y, Greenberg DA, Concepcion E, Skrabanek L, Villanueva R, Tomer Y. Amino acid substitutions in the thyroglobulin gene are associated with susceptibility to human and murine autoimmune thyroid disease. *Proc Natl Acad Sci USA* 2003; 100: 15119–15124.

29. Collins JE, Heward JM, Carr-Smith J, Daykin J, Franklyn JA, Gough SC. Association of rare thyroglobulin gene microsatellite variants with autoimmune thyroid disease. *J Clin Endocrinol Metab* 2003; 88: 5039–5042.

30. Collins JE, Heward JM, Howson JM, et al. Common allelic variants of exons 10, 12, and 33 of the thyroglobulin gene are not associated with autoimmune thyroid disease in the United Kingdom. *J Clin Endocrinol Metab* 2004; 89: 6336–6339.

31. Prummel MF, Strieder T, Wiersinga WM. The environment and autoimmune thyroid disease. *Eur J Endocrinol* 2004; 150: 605–618.

32. Vestergaard P. Smoking and thyroid disorders - a meta-analysis. *Eur J Endocrinol* 2002; 146: 153–161.

33. Strieder TG, Prummel MF, Tijssen JG, Endert E, Wiersinga WM. Risk factors for and prevalence of thyroid disorders in a cross-sectional study among healthy female relatives of patients with autoimmune thyroid disease. *Clin Endocrinol* 2003; 59: 396–401.

34. Belin RM, Astor BC, Powe NR, Ladenson PW. Smoke exposure is associated with a lower prevalence of serum thyroid autoantibodies and thyrotropin concentration elevation and a higher prevalence of mild thyrotropin concentration suppression in the third National Health and Nutrition Examination (NHANESIII). *J Clin Endocrinol Metab* 2004; 89: 6077–6086.

35. Grelland R. Thyrotoxicosis at Ullevål hospital in the years 1934-44 with a special view of frequency of the disease. *Acta Med Scand* 1946; 125: 108–138.

36. Paunkovic N, Paunkovic J, Pavlovic O, Paunovic Z. The significant increase in incidence of Graves' disease in eastern Serbia during the civil war in the former Yugoslavia. *Thyroid* 1998; 8: 37–41.

37. Mizokami T, Wu LA, El-Kaissi S, Wall JR. Stress and thyroid autoimmunity. *Thyroid* 2004; 14: 1047–1055.

38. Winsa B, Adami HO, Bergstrom R, et al. Stressful life events and Graves' disease. *Lancet* 1991; 338: 1475–1479.

39. Yoshiuchi K, Kumano H, Nomura S, et al. Stressful life events and smoking were associated with Graves' disease in women, but not in men. *Psychosomat Med* 1998; 60: 182–185.

40. Matos-Santos A, Nobre EL, Costa JG, et al. Relationship between the number and impact of stressful life events and the onset of Graves' disease and toxic nodular goitre. *Clin Endocrinol* 2001; 55: 15–19.

41. Strieder TG, Prummel MF, Tijssen JG, Brosschot JF, Wiersinga WM. Stress is not associated with thyroid peroxidase autoantibodies in euthyroid women. *Brain Behav Immun* 2005; 19: 203–206.

42. Coles AJ, Wing M, Smith S, et al. Pulsed monoclonal antibody treatment and autoimmune thyroid disease in multiple sclerosis. *Lancet* 1999; 354: 1691–1695.

43. Chen F, Day SL, Metcalfe RA, et al. Characteristics of autoimmune thyroid disease occurring as a late complication of immune reconstitution in patients with advanced human immunodeficiency virus (HIV) disease. *Medicine (Baltimore)* 2005; 84: 98–106.

44. Hidaka Y, Amino N, Iwatani Y, et al. Recurrence of thyrotoxicosis after attack of allergic rhinitis in patients with Graves' disease. *J Clin Endocrinol Metab* 1993; 77: 1667–1670.

45. Sato A, Takemura Y, Yamada T, et al. A possible role of immunoglobulin E in patients with hyperthyroid Graves' disease. *J Clin Endocrinol Metab* 1999; 84: 3602–3605.

46. Strieder TG, Wenzel BE, Prummel MF, Tijssen JG, Wiersinga WM. Increased prevalence of antibodies to enteropathogenic Yersinia enterocolitica virulence proteins in relatives of patients with autoimmune thyroid disease. *Clin Exp Immunol* 2003; 132: 278–282.

47. Munakata Y, Kodera T, Saito T, Sasaki T. Rheumatoid arthritis, type 1 diabetes and Graves' disease after acute parvovirus B19 infection. *Lancet* 2005; 366: 780.

48. Tomer Y, Davies TF. Infection, thyroid disease and autoimmunity. *Endocrin Rev* 1993; 14: 107–120.

49. Arscott PA, Rosen ED, Koenig RJ, et al. Immunoreactivity to Yersinia enterocolitica antigens in patients with autoimmune thyroid disease. *J Clin Endocrinol Metab* 1992; 75: 295–300.

50. Adams DD, Fastier FN, Howie JB, Kennedy TH, Kilpatrick JA, Stewart RD. Stimulation of the human thyroid by infusion of plasma containing LATS protector. *J Clin Endocrinol Metab* 1974; 39: 826–832.

51. Smith BR, Bolton J, Young S, et al. A new assay for thyrotropin receptor autoantibodies. *Thyroid* 2004; 14: 830–835.

52. Costagliola S, Bonomi M, Morgenthaler NG, et al. Delineation of the discontinuous-conformational epitope of a monoclonal antibody displaying full in vitro and in vivo thyrotropin activity. *Mol Endocrinol* 2004; 18: 3020–3034.

53. Chazenbalk GD, Pichurin P, Chen CR, et al. Thyroid-stimulating autoantibodies in Graves' disease preferentially recognize the free A subunit, not the thyrotropin holoreceptor. *J Clin Invest* 2002; 110: 209–217.

54. Chen CR, Pichurin P, Nagayama Y, Latrofa F, Rapoport B, McLachlan SM. The thyrotropin receptor autoantigen in Graves' disease is the culprit as well as the victim. *J Clin Invest* 2003; 111: 1897–1904.

55. Beever K, Bradbury J, Phillips D, et al. Highly sensitive assays of autoantibodies to thyroglobulin and thyroid peroxidase. *Clin Chem* 1989; 35: 1949–1954.

56. Weetman AP, Cohen S. The IgG subclass distribution of thyroid autoantibodies. *Immunol Lett* 1986; 13: 335–341.

57. Khoury EL, Hammond L, Bottazzo GF, Doniach D. Presence of organ-specific "microsomal" autoantigen on the surface of human thyroid cells in culture: its involvement in complement-mediated cytotoxicity. *Clin Exp Immunol* 1981; 45: 319–328.

58. Chazenbalk GD, Portolano S, Russo D, Hutchinson JS, Rapoport B, McLachlan S. Human organ-specific autoimmune disease. Molecular cloning and expression of an autoantibody gene repertoire for a major autoantigen reveals an antigenic immunodominant region and restricted immunoglobulin gene usage in the target organ. *J Clin Invest* 1993; 92: 62–74.

59. Arscott PL, Koenig RJ, Kaplan MM, Glick GD, Baker JR Jr. Unique autoantibody epitopes in an immunodominant region of thyroid peroxidase. *J Biol Chem* 1996: 271: 4966–4973.

60. Jaume JC, Guo J, Pauls DL, et al. Evidence for genetic transmission of thyroid peroxidase autoantibody epitopic "fingerprints". *J Clin Endocrinol Metab* 1999; 84: 1424–1431.

61. Weetman AP, McGregor AM, Lazarus JH, Hall R. Thyroid antibodies are produced by thyroid derived lymphocytes. *Clin Exp Immunol* 1982; 48: 196–200.

62. Nakashima M, Martin A, Davies TF. Intrathyroidal T cell accumulation in Graves' disease: delineation of mechanisms based on in situ T cell receptor analysis. *J Clin Endocrinol Metab* 1996; 81: 3346–51.

63. Surks M, Ortiz E, Daniels GH, et al. Subclinical thyroid disease; scientific review and guidelines for diagnosis and management. *JAMA* 2004; 291: 228–238.

64. Biondi B, Palmieri EA, Klain M, Schlumberger M, Filetti S, Lombardi G. Subclinical hyperthyroidism: clinical features and treatment options. *Eur J Endocrinol* 2005; 152: 1–9.

65. McDermott MT, Woodmansee WW, Haugen BR, Smart A, Ridgway EC. The management of subclinical hyperthyroidism by thyroid specialists. *Thyroid* 2003; 13: 1133–1139.

66. Torring O, Tallstedt L, Wallin G, et al. Graves' hyperthyroidism: treatment with antithyroid drugs, surgery, or radioiodine-a prospective, randomized study. *J Clin Endocrinol Metab* 1996; 81: 2986–2993.

67. Solomon DH, Beck JC, Vanderlaan WP. Prognosis of hyperthyroidism treated by antithyroid drugs. *J Am Med Assoc* 1953; 152: 201–205.

68. Reinwein D, Benker G, Lazarus JH, Alexander WD. A prospective randomised trial of antithyroid drug dose in Graves' disease therapy. *J Clin Endocrinol Metab* 1993; 76: 1516–1521.

69. Engler H, Taurog A, Luthy C, Dorris ML. Reversible and irreversible inhibition of thyroid peroxidase catalysed iodination by thioureylene antithyroid drugs. *Endocrinology* 1983; 112: 86–95.

70. Marchant B, Lees JF, Alexander WD. Antithyroid drugs. *Pharmacol Ther B* 1978; 3: 305–348.

71. Okamura K, Ikenoue H, Shiroozu A, Sato K, Yoshinari M, Fujishima M. Reevaluation of the effects of methylmercaptoimidazole and propylthiouracil in patients with Graves' hyperthyroidism. *J Clin Endocrinol Metab* 1987; 65: 719–723.

72. Cooper DS. Antithyroid drugs. *N Engl J Med* 2005; 352: 905–917.

73. Abraham P, Avenell A, Watson WA, Park CM, Bevan JS. Antithyroid drug regimen for treating Graves' hyperthyroidism. *Cochrane Database Syst Rev* 2004; (2): CD003420.pub2; doi: 10.1002/14651858.CD003420.pub2.

74. Bartalena L, Bogazzi F, Martino E. Adverse effects of thyroid hormone preparations and antithyroid drugs. *Drug Saf* 1996; 15: 53–63.

75. Pearce SHS. Spontaneous reporting of adverse reaction to carbimazole and propylthiouracil in the United Kingdom. *Clin Endocrinol* 2004: 61; 589–594.

76. Young ET, Steel NR, Taylor JJ, et al. Prediction of remission after antithyroid drug treatment of Graves' disease. *Quart J Med* 1988; 66: 175–189.

77. Allahabadia A, Daykin J, Holder RL, et al. Age and gender predict the outcome of treatment for Graves' hyperthyroidism. *J Clin Endocrinol Metab* 2000; 85: 1038–1042.

78. Wartofsky L. Radioiodine therapy for Graves' disease: case selection and restrictions recommended to patients in North America. *Thyroid* 1997; 7: 213–216.

79. Catargi B, Leprat F, Guyot M, Valli N, Ducassou D, Tabarin A. Optimized radioiodine therapy of Graves' disease: analysis of the delivered dose and of other possible factors affecting outcome. *Eur J Endocrinol* 1999; 141: 117–121.

80. Imseis RE, Vanmiddlesworth L, Massie JD, Bush AJ, Vanmiddlesworth NR. Pretreatment with propylthiouracil but not methimazole reduces the therapeutic efficacy of iodine-131 in hyperthyroidism. *J Clin Endocrinol Metab* 1998; 83: 685–687.

81. Lazarus JH. Guidelines for the use of radioiodine in the management of hyperthyroidism: a summary. *J R Coll Physicians Lond* 1995; 29: 464–469.

82. Ron E, Doody MM, Becker DV, et al. Cancer mortality following treatment for adult hyperthyroidism. *JAMA* 1998; 280: 347–355.

83. Franklyn JA, Maisonneuve P, Sheppard M, Betteridge J, Boyle P. Cancer incidence and mortality after radioidine treatment for hyperthyroidism: a population-based cohort study. *Lancet* 1999; 353: 2111–2115.

84. Read CH, Tansey MJ, Menda Y. A 36-year retrospective analysis of the efficacy and safety of radioactive iodine in treating young Graves' patients. *J Clin Endocrinol Metab* 2004; 89: 4229–4233.

85. Tallstedt L, Lundell G, Torring O et al. Occurrence of ophthalmopathy after treatment for Graves' hyperthyroidism. The Thyroid Study Group. *N Engl J Med* 1992; 326: 1733–1738.

86. Perros P, Kendall-Taylor P, Neoh C, Frewin S, Dickinson J. A prospective study of the effects of radioiodine therapy for hyperthyroidism in patients with minimally active Graves' ophthalmopathy. *J Clin Endocrinol Metab* 2005; 90: 5321–5323.

87. Allahabadia A, Daykin J, Sheppard MC, Gough SC, Franklyn JA. Radioiodine treatment of hyperthyroidism-prognostic factors for outcome. *J Clin Endocrinol Metab* 2001; 86: 3611–3617.

88. Scholz GH, Hagemann E, Arkenau C, et al. Is there a place for thyroidectomy in older patients with thyrotoxic storm and cardiorespiratory failure? *Thyroid* 2003; 13: 933–940.

89. Lal G, Ituarte P, Kebebew E, Siperstein A, Duh QY, Clark OH. Should total thyroidectomy become the preferred procedure for surgical management of Graves' disease? *Thyroid* 2005; 15: 569–574.

90. Ku CF, Lo CY, Chan WF, Kung AW, Lam KS. Total thyroidectomy replaces subtotal thyroidectomy as the preferred surgical treatment for Graves' disease. *ANZ J Surg* 2005; 75: 528–531.

91. Miccoli P, Berti P, Materazzi G, Minuto M, Barellini L. Minimally invasive video-assisted thyroidectomy: five years of experience. *J Am Coll Surg* 2004; 199: 243–248.

92. Panzer C, Beazley R, Braverman L. Rapid preoperative preparation for severe hyperthyroid Graves' disease. *J Clin Endocrinol Metab* 2004; 89: 2142–2144.

93. Glinoer D. Thyroid hyperfunction during pregnancy. *Thyroid* 1998; 8: 859–864.

94. Clementi M, Di Gianantonio E, Pelo E, Mammi I, Basile RT, Tenconi R. Methimazole embryopathy: delineation of the phenotype. *Am J Med Genet* 1999; 83: 43–46.

95. Barbero P, Ricagni C, Mercado G, Bronberg R, Torrado M. Choanal atresia associated with prenatal methimazole exposure: three new patients. *Am J Med Genet A* 2004; 129: 83–86.

96. Gora M, Gardas A, Wiktorowicz W, et al. Evaluation of conformational epitopes on thyroid peroxidase by antipeptide antibody binding and mutagenesis. *Clin Exp Immunol* 2004; 136: 137–144.

7 Autoimmune Hypothyroidism

Francesco Latrofa, MD,
and Aldo Pinchera, MD

Contents

Summary

Hypothyroidism is defined as the lack of action of thyroid hormones on target tissues. The term autoimmune hypothyroidism identifies situations with insufficient thyroid function caused by an autoimmune thyroid diseases autoimmune destruction of the thyroid gland. The most common form of autoimmune thyroid diseases is chronic or lymphocytic autoimmune thyroiditis (Hashimoto's thyroiditis). Prevalence of autoimmune hypothyroidism is high. In its initial stage, chronic autoimmune thyroiditis is characterized by the presence of hallmarks of thyroid autoimmunity and normal thyroid function. As a consequence of the autoimmune attack to the gland, hypothyroidism may develop, usually slowly and insidiously, through a subclinical phase (normal thyroid hormone and slightly elevated thyroid-stimulating hormone [TSH] levels) and an eventual phase of overt insufficiency (low thyroid hormones and frankly elevated TSH levels). Etiology and pathogenesis of chronic autoimmune thyroiditis and mechanisms leading to the hypothyroid phase remain elusive. However, some predisposing genetic factors and some triggering environmental factors have been identified. The role of antigen-presenting cells, of T- and B-cell response, and of effector mechanisms in the immunopathogenesis of chronic autoimmune hypothyroidism has been extensively investigated. Clinical presentation and consequences of autoimmune hypothyroidism vary according to patient's age and duration and severity of hypothyroidism. The picture is peculiar in the elderly, and the effects are particularly negative in fetuses and newborns. Circulating thyroid autoantibodies and a hypoecogenic pattern at thyroid ultrasound are the two hallmarks of AITD. Treatment of hypothyroidism is based on the administration of synthetic levo-thyroxine (L-T4), whereas the usefulness of combined treatment with liothyronine (L-T3) is uncertain and difficult to manage. Opinions about treatment of subclinical hypothyroidisms diverge largely, but it should be supported, or at least not discouraged. Because of the awareness about negative consequences of maternal hypothyroidism on the

From: *Contemporary Endocrinology: Autoimmune Diseases in Endocrinology*
Edited by: A. P. Weetman © Humana Press, Totowa, NJ

fetus development, screening or intensive case finding for chronic autoimmune hypothyroidism in women of childbearing aging is unanimously recommended.

Key Words: Thyroid, chronic autoimmune thyroiditis, Hashimoto's thyroiditis, hypothyroidism, thyroid autoantibodies, levo-thyroxine, liothyronine, screening, pregnancy.

INTRODUCTION

Hypothyroidism is defined as the lack of action of thyroid hormones on target tissues. It can be caused by transient or permanent thyroid failure (primary hypothyroidism), by lack of thyroid stimulation by thyroid-stimulating hormone (TSH) (secondary or central hypothyroidism) or by resistance to thyroid hormone (Table 1). The causes of primary hypothyroidism are autoimmune, iatrogenic ("definitive" treatment of thyroid disease with radioiodine or thyroidectomy, external neck radiotherapy or treatment with anti-thyroid or other drugs), subacute thyroiditis, severe iodine deficiency, natural goitrogens, infiltrative diseases of the thyroid (amyloidosis, sclerodermia), congenital abnormalities (congenital defects in thyroid hormone biosynthesis, inactivating mutations of the TSH receptor [TSHR], and thyroid dysgenesis).

The term autoimmune hypothyroidism identifies some situations with insufficient thyroid function caused by an autoimmune destruction of the thyroid gland. The most common forms of AITD are chronic or lymphocytic autoimmune thyroiditis (with its goitrous, subatrophic, or atrophic variants). Other AITD include postpartum thyroiditis (PPT), painless (or sporadic) thyroiditis, focal thyroiditis, and juvenile thyroiditis. Riedel's thyroiditis, which is characterized by a progressive fibrosis, has an uncertain pathogenesis. Although Hashimoto's thyroiditis, according to the author's definition in 1912, identified its goitrous variant only, this term is used frequently as synonymous of chronic autoimmune thyroiditis. The autoimmune process is similar in the goitrous and atrophic (idiopathic myxedema) variants of chronic autoimmune thyroiditis, and it is uncertain whether they are distinct entities or represent two ends of a spectrum of autoimmune thyroid destruction. No clear evidence for progression between the goitrous and the atrophic form of chronic autoimmune thyroiditis has been reported.

A large number of surveys, until recently, have established the high prevalence of autoimmune hypothyroidism. With the possible exception of areas with severe iodine deficiency, chronic autoimmune thyroiditis is the most common cause of spontaneous hypothyroidism. In its initial stage, chronic autoimmune thyroiditis is characterized by the presence of hallmarks of thyroid autoimmunity and normal thyroid function. As a consequence of the autoimmune attack to the gland, hypothyroidism develops, usually slowly and insidiously through a subclinical phase (normal thyroid hormone and slightly elevated TSH levels) and an eventual phase of overt insufficiency (low thyroid hormones and frankly elevated TSH levels) *(1)*. The etiology and pathogenesis of chronic autoimmune thyroiditis and the mechanism leading to the hypothyroid phase of autoimmune hypothyroidism remain not clear. The clinical presentation and the effects of autoimmune hypothyroidism vary according to the age of patients. Mild maternal hypothyroidism can affect fetal neurodevelopment. More rarely, maternal autoantibodies to the TSHR (TSHR autoantibodies) with blocking activity (TSHR-B autoantibodies) can induce transient neonatal hypothyroidism. Juvenile autoimmune

Table 1
Classification of Hypothyroidism

Primary (transient or permanent)	Autoimmune (thyroiditis)	Chronic (lymphocytic)
		Goitrous (Hashimoto's thyroiditis)
		Atrophic (idiopathic mixedema)
		Post-partum
		Painless (sporadic)
		Focal
		Juvenile
	Subacute thyroiditis	
	Riedel's thyroiditis	
	Iatrogenic	Post-radioiodine
		Post-thyroidectomy
		External radiotherapy
		Anti-thyroid and other drugs (thionamides, iodine, amiodarone, lithium, interferon-α, interleukin-2, granulocyte-macrophage colony-stimulating factor)
	Severe iodine deficiency	
	Natural goitrogens	
	Infiltrative diseases of the thyroid	Amyloidosis
		Sclerodermia
	Congenital abnormalities	Defects in thyroid hormone biosynthesis
		Inactivating mutations of the thyroid-stimulating hormone receptor (TSHR)
		Thyroid dysgenesis
	Transient neonatal hypothyroidism	Transplacental passage of maternal TSHR-B autoantibodies
		Iodine deficiency
		Iodine excess
		Administration of antithyroid agents to the mother
Secondary or central	Pituitary disease	
	Hypothalamic disease	
Thyroid hormone resistance		

hypothyroidism can affect physical and sexual development. Clinical presentation of hypothyroidism in the elderly is peculiar. Whereas the need for treatment of clinical hypothyroidism and its management are universally accepted, the necessity of treating subclinical hypothyroidism is discussed. The need of screening for autoimmune hypothyroidism is debated as well.

Juvenile thyroiditis is usually characterized by a moderate lymphocytic infiltration and may have a transient course. A mild degree of infiltration and no evidence of thyroid dysfunction are the distinctive features of focal or minimal thyroiditis. A period of transient thyrotoxicosis and a phase of transient or permanent hypothyroidism are typical of PPT and painless sporadic thyroiditis.

EPIDEMIOLOGY

The prevalence of chronic autoimmune thyroiditis and hypothyroidism is influenced by gender, age, and the environment.

Some degree of lymphocytic infiltration at autopsy is present in the thyroid in 32% of adult women and in 8% of adult men and is more common over 50 years (2). Thyroid autoantibodies correlate with the presence of focal thyroiditis in biopsy and at autopsy (3). Their frequency and distribution are greatly influenced by the technique of detection. In the Whickham survey, thyroglobulin (Tg) autoantibodies were reported in 2% of population, whereas thyroperoxidase (TPO) autoantibodies (microsomial antibodies) were positive in 7% of subjects (10% of women and 3% of men); the figures in females over 75 years of age were 7% for Tg autoantibodies and 9% for TPO autoantibodies (4). Similar results have been recently reported in populations living in iodine-sufficient areas (5,6). Taking as control a group of people aged <50 years, the prevalence of TPO autoantibodies and Tg autoantibodies was significantly greater in subjects aged 70–85 years but not in centenarians (7). In addition, the prevalence of TPO autoantibodies and Tg autoantibodies was higher in unselected or hospitalized elderly patients and lower in centenarians and in "younger" healthy elderly as compared with an apparently normal population (8). Therefore, the appearance of thyroid autoantibodies in elderly subjects might be related to age-associated disease, and healthy older subjects might represent a selected population with an unusually efficient immune system (9). The influence of age, sex, and iodine intake on the prevalence of hypothyroidism is similar to that on thyroid autoantibodies. In large epidemiological studies on populations living in iodine-sufficient areas, hypothyroidism occurs in 1–9.5% of the general population and in 3–20% over 75 years (4–6), whereas only 0.2% of people living in an iodine-deficient area were hypothyroid (10). In the Wickham survey, spontaneous overt hypothyroidism was 1% in women and <0.1% in men, the mean serum concentration of TSH was significantly higher in subjects with positive antibody tests, and 50% of subjects with circulating thyroid autoantibodies had serum TSH >6 mUI/L (4). In the same survey, subclinical hypothyroidism was present in 8% of women and in 3% of men and increased with aging. Similar results have been reported by recent surveys (5,6). The prevalence of subclinical hypothyroidism was lower in an iodine-deficient area (3.8% of adults) (10). Indeed, it has been shown that small differences in iodine intake influence greatly the incidences of overt hypothyroidism and hyperthyroidism (11). Thus, subclinical hypothyroidism is two- to fourfold more common than the corresponding overt condition and is more frequently in women, in elderly, and in iodine-sufficient areas.

Risk factors for hypothyroidism have been determined in the 20-year follow-up study of the Whickham survey (12). The mean incidence of spontaneous hypothyroidism in women was 3.5/1000/year, and the risk increased with age to 13.7/1000 in women between 75 and 80 years. In men the risk was 0.6/1000/year. The risk factors for having developed hypothyroidism at 20-year follow up in women were elevated TSH (odds ratio 14) and positive thyroid autoantibodies (odds ratio 13); when elevated TSH and positive thyroid autoantibodies were combined, the odds ratio was 38. The results were similar in men. Thyroiditis is the cause of euthyroid goiter in about half of children and adolescent living in iodine-sufficient areas. Its prevalence in these areas is 1.2% *(13)*. The disease is rare in children younger than 5 years.

GENETIC AND ENVIRONMENTAL FACTORS (TABLE 2)

Genetic Factors

A bulk of epidemiological studies have established that the prevalence of chronic autoimmune thyroiditis is higher within some families and that chronic autoimmune thyroiditis and Graves' disease (AITD) frequently occur in members of the same family. The prevalence of thyroid autoantibodies is higher in first-degree relatives of patients with chronic autoimmune thyroiditis, and a high correlation rate for thyroid

Table 2
Factors Involved in the Pathogenesis of Autoimmune Hypothyroidism

Genetic	Genes	HLA class I and class II
		Tumor necrosis factor
		T-cell receptor
		Immunoglobulin
		Cytokine regulatory
		Thyroid autoantigens
		Thyroperoxidase
		Thyroglobulin
		TSH-receptor
	Genetic syndromes	Turner's syndrome
		Down's syndrome
Endogenous	Sex hormones	
	Sex chromosomes	
	Glucocorticoids	
	Low birth weight	
	Stress	
Environmental	Infectious agents	Congenital rubella syndrome
		Hepatitis C virus infection
	Iodine	
	Drugs	Amiodarone
		Lithium
		Interferon-α
		Interleukin-2
		Granulocyte-macrophage colony-stimulating factor
	Radiation	Internal: 131-I (fallout, treatment)
		External: head and neck irradiation

autoantibodies is reported in twins *(14)*. Although the results differ, partially as a consequence of the different parameters evaluated in different studies, the relative risk reported for chronic autoimmune thyroiditis in siblings (between 10 and 45) clearly indicate that genetic predisposition is relevant in chronic autoimmune thyroiditis *(15)*.

Human leukocyte antigens (HLA) class I and *class II* genes, *tumor necrosis factor* genes *(TNF)*, *T-cell receptor (TCR)* genes, *immunoglobulin (Ig)* genes, and *cytokine regulatory genes* have been implicated in susceptibility to thyroid autoimmunity.

An increased frequency of HLA-DR3, DR4, and DR5 has been reported in white patients with chronic autoimmune thyroiditis and in PPT but not in other ethnic groups *(16)*. As the relative risk for people bearing this HLA alleles is low *(2–7)* and specific HLA loci often fail to segregate with the expression of the autoimmunity within families *(17–19)*, it has been accomplished that HLA genes cannot be the only factors contributing to the genetic predisposition of chronic autoimmune thyroiditis *(15,20)*.

The role of the three major thyroid-specific genes *(TPO, Tg, and TSHR)* in AITD has been investigated. The epitopic specificity of TPO autoantibodies is inherited dominantly *(21)*, but *TPO* gene is not linked nor associated with chronic autoimmune thyoiditis *(22)*. Neither *TSHR* gene shows any correlation with AITD *(23)*. Amino acid substitutions of *Tg* gene have been recently correlated with susceptibility for AITD both in humans and in experimental autoimmune thyroiditis (EAT) *(24)*.

A higher prevalence of chronic autoimmune thyroiditis has been reported in some chromosomal abnormalities. In Turner's syndrome, both thyroid antibody *(25)* and hypothyroidism *(26)* are more common. However, linkage studies on the correlation between chromosome X and AITD were not conclusive *(20)*. AITD are more common in patients with Down's syndrome *(27,28)*, but serum markers of thyroid autoimmunity are not more frequent in the parents of Down's patients with thyroid disease *(29)*.

As few genes conferring a low risk have been identified to date, it has been accomplished that genetic predisposition to chronic autoimmune thyroiditis is probably complex and induced by several genes with reduced penetrance *(20)*. In addition, different genetic backgrounds, probably with different types of inheritance, can determine an identical phenotype *(15)*.

There is a predisposition to develop other autoimmune diseases associated with chronic autoimmune thyroiditis. Patients with chronic autoimmune thyroiditis have autoantibodies to adrenal cortex (1–2%), pancreatic islet cells (1–3%), gastric parietal cells (10–30%), intrinsic factor (1%), DNA, phospholipids, or IgG *(30)*.

Endogenous Factors

The endogenous factors that have been proposed to play a role in chronic autoimmune thyroiditis include sex hormones, glucocorticoids, and low birth weight.

Sexual dimorphism is apparent in normal immune function and in autoimmune diseases in humans as well as in animals. Most organ- and non-organ-specific autoimmune diseases are more prevalent in women than in men. In addition, a sex-related susceptibility is apparent in models of both spontaneous and induced EAT and of other autoimmune diseases *(31)*. The sexual dimorphism of immune and autoimmune responses can be because of the influence exerted on the immune system by genes carried by sex chromosomes (X or Y) or by sex hormones. The levels of estrogens and androgens can influence the prevalence of autoimmune diseases in animals *(31,32)*.

Estrogens may modulate the function of the antigen-presenting cells (APCs), influencing their cytokine profile, differentiation, and migration *(33)*. However, estrogens were not able to increase TPO expression on human thyroid cells *(34)*. Stress does not seem to play a crucial role in the induction of chronic autoimmune thyroiditis, but it could affect susceptibility through cortisol secretion variations, as shown in animals *(35)*. The prevalence of high thyroid autoantibody concentrations in monozygotic twins has been related to their birth weight *(36)*.

Environmental Factors

Environmental factors involved in autoimmune thyroiditis include infectious agents, iodine, treatment with amiodarone, interferon (IFN)-α, interleukin (IL)-2, granulocyte-macrophage colony-stimulating factor (GM-CSF), ionizing radiation, and toxins.

Only few reports relating chronic autoimmune thyroiditis and viral infections (congenital rubella syndrome and hepatitis C virus infection) have been published so far *(37,38)*.

The role of iodine intake in the development of EAT is well known. In addition, epidemiological surveys have demonstrated the role of dietary iodine in human autoimmunity. After introduction of iodization programs into iodine-deficient regions, an increased prevalence of thyroid autoantibodies and lymphocytic infiltration was reported *(39)*. As already mentioned, iodine intake modifies the incidence of overt hypothyroidism as a consequence of direct effect on thyroid function and on thyroid autoimmunity. Patients with chronic autoimmune thyroiditis treated with iodine have an enhanced susceptibility to develop hypothyroidism *(40)*.

Amiodarone-induced hypothyroidism is more common than amiodarone-induced thyrotoxicosis in iodine-sufficient areas *(41)*. Female sex and positive TPO autoantibodies represented a relative risk of 7.9 and 7.3, respectively, for amiodarone-induced hypothyroidism, and when both were present, the risk was 13.5 *(42)*. Thus, pre-existing chronic autoimmune disease is a risk factor for the occurrence of hypothyroidism in amiodarone-treated patients *(43)*. The most likely pathogenetic mechanism is that the thyroid gland, damaged by chronic autoimmune thyroiditis, is unable to escape from the acute Wolff–Chaikoff effect after the iodine load and therefore to resume a normal hormone synthesis *(44)*. In addition, iodine-induced damage to the thyroid may add to that caused by the pre-existing chronic autoimmune thyroiditis, thus accelerating the trend toward hypothyroidism. Amiodarone-induced hypothyroidism is more frequently persistent in TPO autoantibody-positive patients and more commonly transient in TPO autoantibody-negative patients *(43)*. The majority of studies indicate that the occurrence of de novo TPO autoantibodies after amiodarone treatment, reported by some authors, is unlikely (reviewed in ref. *44*). In the presence of thyroid autoimmunity, treatment with lithium may increase thyroid antibody concentration and may induce subclinical or overt hypothyroidism *(45)*. The development of thyroid antibodies, transient thyrotoxicosis, hypothyroidism, or both has been reported after therapy with IFN-α *(46)*, IL-2 *(47,48)*, and granulocyte-macrophage colony-stimulating factor (GM-CSF) *(49)*. Patients with pre-existing circulating antibodies are at higher risk for thyroid dysfunction. However, in 15% of patients with no evidence of thyroid autoimmunity, treatment with IFN-α will induce high serum TPO autoantibody concentration or thyroid dysfunction *(50)*.

Thyroid can be exposed to external and internal radiation. Internal radiation can be the consequence of indirect exposure after environmental disasters (fallout) or after therapeutic irradiation with 131-I. External radiations are the consequence of direct exposure after environmental disasters or therapeutic irradiation for diseases of the head and the neck. The effects of environmental irradiation on thyroid autoimmunity are controversial *(51)*. Hypothyroidism was correlated with exposure to fallout from a hydrogen bomb explosion releasing short-lived radioiodine isotopes *(52)*. About 6–8 years after the Chernobyl accident, a significant increase in thyroid autoimmunity without evidence of thyroid dysfunction was found in children exposed to radioactive fallout *(53)*. Pubertal age in girls was a risk factor for increased prevalence of thyroid autoimmunity. In a subsequent analysis with a longer follow-up, no increase has been found by the same group (Pinchera and Elisei, unpublished data), suggesting that this phenomenon is transient. In persons exposed as children to 131-I released in the atmosphere from the Hanford nuclear site, the radiation did not correlate neither with chronic autoimmune thyroiditis nor with autoimmune hypothyroidism 40 years after exposure *(54)*. Although a significant relationship between thyroid radiation dose and autoimmune hypothyroidism was observed in atomic bomb survivors in Nagasaki 40 years after the atomic bomb explosion *(55)*, neither anti-thyroid antibodies nor autoimmune hypothyroidism correlated with thyroid radiation dose in Hiroshima and Nagasaki atomic bomb survivors 55–58 years after radiation exposure *(56)*. The role of occupational exposure to ionizing radiation in inducing AITD, which has been reported recently *(57)*, needs confirmation in larger studies. The occurrence of hypothyroidism after neck and head irradiation has been long recognized and histological lymphocytic thyroiditis after low-dose irradiation exposure during childhood has been demon- strated *(58)*. AITD were more frequent in patients exposed to multiple fluoroscopic examination, although the difference was not statistically significant *(59)*. Hypothy- roidism has been reported after irradiation for Hodgkin's disease *(60)*. 131-I treatment can induce a transient rise of titers in thyroid autoantibody-positive patients *(61)* and the appearance of thyroid autoantibodies in autoantibody-negative patients *(62,63)*.

Smoking may increase the risk of hypothyroidism in patients with chronic autoimmune thyroiditis *(64)*.

IMMUNOPATHOGENESIS

Autoimmune hypothyroidism results from an interaction of endogenous and environ- mental factors with thyroid and non-thyroid genes, leading to activation of thyroid- autoreactive T cells and ultimately hypothyroidism through immune-mediated inflam- mation and thyroid tissue destruction. A number of mechanisms are involved in this process.

Antigen Presentation

Antigen presentation from APCs expressing HLA class II stimulates T cells through TCRs, in the presence of costimulatory molecules. This process initiates and maintains immune response. In the absence of costimulatory molecules, the presentation of antigens on APCs induces T-cell inactivation or anergy.

As previously reported, some predisposing genes, including HLA and thyroid- specific genes, have been implicated in chronic autoimmune thyroiditis. In keeping with this view is the recent demonstration that amino acid substitutions in the Tg gene interact with HLA-DR3 in conferring susceptibility to human and murine AITD *(24)*. It is envisaged that Tg gene may predispose to AITD by many mechanisms: sequence changes in Tg may make the molecule more immunogenic or may change its interaction with HLA class II molecules *(24)*.

The observation that thyroid follicular cells from patients with chronic autoimmune thyroiditis express on their surface HLA class II molecules *(65,66)* and that TPO and HLA class II expression in thyroid follicular cells is a dynamic phenomenon under the influence of TSH, TSHR-S autoantibodies, and IFN-γ *(67)*, led to the suggestion that they may act as facultative APCs. More recently, costimulatory molecules have been demonstrated on thyroid cells from patients with AITD *(68–71)*. Taken together, these findings support the role of thyroid follicular cells as APCs, at least in the perpetuation of chronic autoimmune thyroiditis, whereas their importance in the initiation of the autoimmune process remains uncertain *(72)*.

The function of APCs in chronic autoimmune thyroiditis is complex and diverse among the different cell types involved. In particular, thyroid follicular cells may act as facultative APCs by unmasking a "cryptic" epitope of TPO, leading to thyroid immune response *(73)*, whereas competent APC dendritic cells, in addition to exert a stimulatory action on T cells, may also induce anergy of a T-cell clone specific for human TPO epitope *(74)*.

T-Cell Responses

The pivotal role of T cells in inducing chronic autoimmune thyroiditis has recently been demonstrated by the induction of hypothyroidism associated with histological changes of thyroiditis in a transgenic mouse model, which was unable to produce antibodies *(75)*.

The reported restriction of the *V*α gene usage of TCRs among T cells infiltrating the thyroid in AITD, which raised the possibility of a clonal restriction of T-cell response in thyroid autoimmune disease *(76)*, has not been confirmed *(77)*.

More recently, a role of cytotoxic T-lymphocyte antigen (CTLA)-4, the protein involved in the down regulation of activated T cells and thus in tolerance, has been proposed. In particular, a polymorphism of the *CTLA-4* gene, which reduces the mRNA expression of the soluble form of this protein, represents a risk for the development of AITD *(78)*.

B-Cell Responses

TPO, Tg, and TSHR are the most important thyroid autoantigens, giving rise to autoantibodies detectable in the serum of patients with chronic autoimmune thyroiditis. Autoantibodies to megalin and to thyroid hormones have been reported, whereas the presence of autoantibodies to Na/I symporter is uncertain (reviewed in ref. *79*).

TPO autoantibodies are present in >80% and Tg autoantibodies in up to 80% of patients with chronic autoimmune thyroiditis *(80–82)*. The variable heavy (H) and light (L)-chain composition of TPO autoantibodies and Tg autoantibodies and the usage of different H and L chain V region genes encoding Tg autoantibodies and TPO autoantibodies derived from the same patient *(83)* indicate that a polyclonal

B-cell response is involved in thyroid autoimmunity. Both TPO autoantibodies and Tg autoantibodies are predominantly of IgG class. In patients with chronic autoimmune thyroiditis, Tg autoantibodies are predominantly IgG2 *(84)*. IgA class Tg autoantibodies and TPO autoantibodies are also present *(85)*. TPO autoantibodies and Tg autoantibodies recognize the respective human autoantigens with high affinity and better than antigens from other species. Human TPO autoantibodies recognize conformational epitopes on two overlapping domains, each of which subdivided into two subdomains and, less commonly, linear epitopes *(86)*. TPO autoantibodies can fix complement. The observations that Tg autoantibodies do not fix the complement, that are present in otherwise healthy subjects *(80)*, and that their levels do not correlate with the severity of chronic autoimmune thyroiditis support the concept that these autoantibodies are not pathogenetic. As previously reported, chronic autoimmune thyroiditis is more common in iodine-sufficient areas. The degree of iodination of Tg changes its antigenicity with respect to mouse monoclonal antibody binding *(87)*. In EAT, enhanced iodination of Tg facilitates the selective presentation of a cryptic pathogenetic peptide to APCs *(88)*. Human Tg autoantibodies recognize conformational epitopes preferentially. The view that the binding of Tg autoantibodies from patients with AITD is restricted to two major (and several minor) epitopic regions on Tg has been recently confirmed *(89)*. In addition, the overlap of Tg epitope recognition by Tg autoantibodies from patients with Graves' disease and chronic autoimmune thyroiditis was demonstrated by inhibition studies using two human monoclonal Tg autoantibodies *(90)*. At variance, evaluating inhibition of binding of Tg autoantibody-positive sera to Tg by a panel of mouse monoclonal Tg autoantibodies, recognition was more restricted for patients with AITD than for patients with non-toxic goiter (and normal individuals) *(91)*.

The finding of autoantibodies cross-reacting with Tg and TPO (TgPO Ab) in patients with chronic autoimmune thyroiditis *(92,93)*, which suggested a role for cross-reactivity of B-cell response to Tg and TPO *(94)*, has not been confirmed *(83)*.

TSHR autoantibodies play a direct role in the pathogenesis of AITD. They are detectable in most patients with Graves' disease, in whom they act as TSH agonist, activating TSHR and inducing hyperthyroidism and goiter (TSHR-stimulating [TSHR-S autoantibodies]). Conversely, TSHR autoantibodies are present in a minority of patients with chronic autoimmune thyroiditis, in whom they exert a TSH antagonist action, thus inducing hypothyroidism and thyroid atrophy (TSHR-B autoantibodies). Currently, TSHR autoantibodies can be detected by radioreceptor assays or by bioassays *(95)*. Direct assays for TSHR autoantibody detection are also available. Radioreceptor assays are based on the ability of TSHR autoantibodies to compete for the binding of radiolabeled TSH to the TSHR (TSH-binding inhibitory assay, TBI) and thus cannot differentiate TSHR-S from TSHR-B autoantibodies. The differentiation is possible by bioassay, which measures in cultured cells expressing the TSHR the ability of TSHR autoantibodies to directly stimulate cyclic AMP production (TSHR-S autoantibodies) or vice versa to block cyclic AMP production induced by TSH simulation (TSHR-B autoantibodies). In a TBI assay, only 15% of patients with chronic autoimmune thyroiditis resulted positive as compared with nearly 100% of patients with Graves' disease *(96)*. By bioassay, TSHR-B autoantibodies are present in up to 20% of patients with the atrophic variant of chronic autoimmune thyroiditis and less frequently in those with the goitrous variant *(97,98)*. At variance with TSHR autoantibodies from patients with Graves' disease *(99,100)*, TSHR-B autoantibodies are not class-restricted, and therefore, their origin is probably polyclonal *(101)*. TSHR autoantibody epitopes comprise discontinuous sequences of the polypeptide chain that are contiguous in the folded protein under native conditions *(102)*. Whereas TSHR-S autoantibodies interact mainly with the N-terminal components of the ectodomain, TSHR-B autoantibodies interact to a greater extent with the C terminus and to a lower degree with the N terminus and the midregion of the TSHR *(102,103)*. Accordingly, immunization of mice with the N-terminal component of the TSHR or with the TSHR holoreceptor generated preferentially TSHR-S and TSHR-B autoantibodies, respectively *(104)*. Whereas the epitope(s) for TSHR-S autoantibodies are partially sterically hindered on the holoreceptor by the plasma membrane, those for TSHR-B autoantibodies are fully accessible *(105)*. Thyroid autoantibody production requires the presence of thyroid autoantigens as indicated by their disappearance after total thyroid ablation obtained by thyroidectomy plus 131-I treatment *(106)*.

Megalin (gp330) binds Tg with high affinity and participates in its transcytosis across thyroid cells *(107)*. Autoantibodies to megalin were detected in 50% of patients with chronic autoimmune thyroiditis and in some patients with Graves' disease and thyroid carcinoma but not in normal subjects *(108)*. Autoantibodies to T4 and T3 *(109)* have been reported. A role of Na/I symporter as autoantigen in thyroid autoimmunity has been proposed by some authors *(110,111)* but excluded by others *(112–114)*.

Effector Mechanisms

Both cell-mediated and humoral mechanisms are responsible for thyroid damage in chronic autoimmune thyroiditis.

CELL-MEDIATED MECHANISMS

T-cell-mediated cytotoxicity plays a role in EAT, by the release of soluble cytolytic mediators such as perforin and granzymes, resulting in death of thyroid cells. This mechanism is probably important in human chronic autoimmune thyroiditis as well. An additional mechanism resides in the release of cytokine following lymphocytic infiltration, which contributes to thyroid cell damage and death. Intrathyroidal cytokines can increase the expression of intercellular adhesion molecule (ICAM)-1 on thyroid cells, with the consequent binding to its cognate receptor (lymphocyte function-associated antigen [LFA]-1), present on lymphocytes. This sequence of events exert a cytotoxic effect on thyroid cells. In addition, a role for Fas (CD 95) has been proposed in chronic autoimmune thyroiditis. Fas, a death-signaling receptor, is known to induce peripheral deletion of chronically activated T cells when activated by its ligand (Fas L) on their surface. The finding that Fas expression could be induced by IL-1 on thyroid cells from patients with chronic autoimmune thyroiditis led to the suggestion that the interaction of Fas with Fas L is a mechanism of cell death in this disease *(115)*. Subsequent studies provided no support to this interpretation *(116,117)*.

HUMORAL MECHANISMS

TPO autoantibodies can fix complement and have been shown to induce cytotoxic of thyroid cells in vitro *(118)*. TPO autoantibodies have been detected within thyroid follicules of patients with chronic autoimmune thyroiditis *(119)*, raising the question of their in vivo cytotoxic role. As the prerequisite for their access to intrafollicular TPO is the disruption of tight junctions between thyroid cells, TPO autoantibodies probably exert a secondary destructive mechanism. Babies born to mothers with circulating TPO autoantibodies are euthyroid because TPO autoantibodies have no direct access to their target. Cytotoxic activity of TPO autoantibodies does not correlate with their concentration *(118)* and is restricted to IgG1 subclass, at least in vitro *(120)*. Tg autoantibodies are unable to fix the complement but may form Tg–Tg autoantibody immune complexes along the basal membrane of thyroid follicles, inducing complement attack and subsequent release of proinflammatory molecules. By binding natural killer (NK) cells through their Fc, both types of thyroid autoantibodies can cause antibody-dependent cell-mediated cytotoxicity. The importance of this mechanism in chronic autoimmune thyroiditis is unclear *(121,122)*. TPO autoantibodies and TSHR autoantibodies may also exert a direct effect on thyroid cells. TPO autoantibodies have been reported to inhibit the enzymatic activity of TPO in vitro by some *(123)* but not all authors *(124,125)*. TSHR-B autoantibodies contribute to the development of hypothyroidism in some patients with the atrophic form of chronic autoimmune thyroiditis and in few patients with goitrous chronic autoimmune thyroiditis *(97)*. The occasional reports of a temporal association between disappearance of TSHR-B autoantibodies and remission of hypothyroidism and that of a transient neonatal hypothyroidism induced by maternal TSHR-B autoantibodies crossing the placenta in neonates born to mothers with TSHR-B autoantibodies *(126,127)* are in keeping with this view. The hypothesis that maternal TSHR-B autoantibodies crossing the placenta might play a crucial role in athyreotic myxedematous cretinism *(128)* has been excluded by the demonstration that these autoantibodies are present only in a minority of mothers of athyreotic subjects *(129)*. The *de novo* appearance of TSHR-B autoantibodies after 131-I treatment of Graves' disease, which was proposed as a prevalent cause in inducing hypothyroidism following 131-I treatment *(130)*, has not been confirmed *(131)*.

Histological Findings

Histological findings of chronic autoimmune thyroiditis encompass a spectrum of pathological changes, from a large goiter to an atrophic gland, from scattered clusters of infiltrating lymphocytes to extensive chronic inflammation and scarring with almost complete loss of follicular epithelium (reviewed in ref. *132*). If the thyroiditis is slight and focal, then the thyroid is normal in size and contains scattered infiltrates of T and B cells and few plasma cells. Some infiltrates contain lymphoid follicular centers. The involved thyroid follicles are atrophic and devoid of colloid. Focal lymphocytic thyroiditis might represent the early form of autoimmune thyroiditis. When lymphocytic infiltration is more extensive, occasional follicular cells undergo metaplasia toward oxyphilic cells. In more advanced cases of autoimmune thyroiditis, little or no normal parenchyma is visible, many follicles are small and contain little amount of colloid, and infiltrates of lymphocytes, plasma cells, and macrophages become extensive. Lymphoid follicular cells are numerous, the amount of connective tissue is increased, and some thyroid follicular cells are atrophic or damaged, hyperplastic or metaplastic (oncocytic or Hürthle cells).

Chronic Autoimmune Thyroiditis and Pregnancy

Amelioration of the clinical course of chronic autoimmune thyroiditis during pregnancy is the consequence of the heightened state of immune tolerance in this period. The large amounts of estrogens and progesterone during pregnancy have been implicated in this immunomodulation and in particular in the shift from Th1 to Th2 response *(133)*. An additional mechanism is the production by trophoblastic cells of special substances such as a special major histocompatibility complex class I molecule (HLA-G). As a consequence of the rebound of the immune response following delivery, exacerbation of autoimmune thyroiditis or development of PPT may occur. An additional mechanism of post-partum thyroid autoimmunity is attributed to fetal microchimerism. This phenomenon consists of the migration of fetal cells into maternal tissues during pregnancy. Intrathyroidal fetal microchimerism has been reported in thyroid specimens of women with chronic autoimmune thyroiditis *(134,135)*, leading to the concept that a graft-vs-host reaction is important in post-partum thyroid autoimmunity.

DIAGNOSIS

Clinical Presentation

In the natural history of chronic autoimmune thyroiditis, the presence of hallmarks of thyroid autoimmunity with normal thyroid function usually precedes the development of hypothyroidism (Table 3). The progression from euthyroidism to hypothyroidism may take several years. The presence of a goiter may be the first clinical manifestation of chronic autoimmune thyroiditis. In some patients, the diagnosis is based on the finding of positive circulating thyroid autoantibodies and of the typical hypoecogenicity at thyroid ultrasound. In other cases, the first finding is a slightly elevated TSH concentration, which is detected accidentally, in the absence of symptoms and signs of hypothyroidism (subclinical hypothyroidism). When the thyroid damage is more severe, a mild-to-severe clinical hypothyroidism is present. Clinical expression of hypothyroidism is mainly influenced by its rate of development and patient's age. When progression of hypothyroidism is rapid, as after withdrawal of replacement therapy or total thyroidectomy, symptoms are well recognized, whereas when it is slow, as in chronic autoimmune thyroiditis, its appearance may be insidious and its severity variable. In most adult patients with the goitrous form of chronic autoimmune

Table 3
Clinical Presentation of Autoimmune Hypothyroidism

- Goiter
- Positive circulating thyroid autoantibodies
- Hypoecogenicity and/or thyroid atrophy at ultrasound
- Slightly elevated circulating thyroid-stimulating hormone (TSH) levels and normal thyroid hormones (subclinical hypothyroidism)
- Frankly elevated TSH levels and low thyroid hormones (clinical hypothyroidism)
- Symptoms and signs of hypothyroidism

thyroiditis, few and mild symptoms are present, and sometimes, they are recognized only retrospectively, after restoration of euthyroidism with thyroid hormone treatment. In the elderly, the atrophic form of chronic autoimmune thyroiditis may cause a particularly insidious and severe form of hypothyroidism, which may eventually lead to myxedema coma. Diagnostic indexes that score the presence or absence of symptoms and signs of hypothyroidsm have been proposed *(136,137)*.

As previously reported, mildly increased serum TSH levels and elevated thyroid autoantibody levels are predictive of subsequent thyroid failure *(12,138)*. In a 20-year follow-up study of goitrous juvenile thyroiditis, hypothyroidism developed in 33% of patients *(13)*.

SYMPTOMS OF OVERT HYPOTHYROIDISM IN ADULTHOOD

Overt hypothyroidism of adulthood induces changes in almost every organ system (Table 4) *(139)*. Cutaneous changes are frequent and include cold intolerance, nail abnormality, thickening and dryness of hair and skin, edema of hands, face, and eyelids, change in shape of face, malar flush, non-pitting edema, alopecia, and pallor. Unusual coldness of the arms and legs is common.

Multiple alterations of the cardiovascular system are present. Bradycardia parallels the decrease in body metabolic rate. Loss of the inotropic and chronotropic actions of the thyroid hormones reduces myocardial contractility, thus both stroke volume and hearth rate and consequently cardiac output at rest. Narrowing of pulse pressure, prolongation of circulation time, and decreased blood flow to the tissues are because of the increase of peripheral vascular resistance at rest and reduction of blood volume.

Table 4
Manifestations of Overt Hypothyroidism

Cutaneous	Cold intolerance
	Nail abnormality
	Thickening and dryness of hair and skin
	Edema of hands, face, and eyelids
	Change in shape of face
	Malar flush
	Non-pitting edema
	Alopecia
	Pallor
	Decreased sweat secretion
Cardiovascular	Dyspnea
	Decreased exercise tolerance
	Angina
	Low pulse rate
	Increased systemic vascular resistance
	Diastolic hypertension
	Cardiomegaly
	Pericardial effusion
	Peripheral non-pitting edema
	Low-voltage ECG, non-specific ST-T changes

Gastrointestinal	Anorexia
	Gaseous distension
	Constipation
	Prolonged gastric emptying
	Prolonged intestinal transit time
	Slowed intestinal absorption
	Ascites
	Elevated liver enzymes
	Gallbladder hypotonia
	Atrophy of the gastric and intestinal mucosa, immune gatritis
Neurologic	Somnolence, lethargy
	Slow speech
	Impaired cognitive functions
	Headache
	Paraesthesias
	Cerebellar ataxia
	Deafness
	Vertigo
	Delayed relaxation of deep tendon reflexes
	Low-voltage EEG, slow α-wave activity
Psychiatric	Depression
	Bipolar disorders
	Affective psychosis
Musculoskeletal	Generalized muscular hypertrophy
	Easy fatigue
	Slowness of movements
	Articular and muscular pain
	Stiffness of the extremity
Female and male reproductive system	Oligomenorrhea, amenorrhea, polymenorrhea, menorrhagia
	Diminished libido
	Fetal wastage and abortion in the first trimester
	Impotence
Metabolic changes	Reduced basal metabolic rate
	Reduced protein synthesis and degradation
	Reduced glucose absorption and assimilation
	Increased sensitivity to exogenous insulin
	Increased total cholesterol, LDL-cholesterol, and triglycerides
	Normochromic or macrocytic anemia

Because myocardial oxygen consumption is decreased more than blood supply to the myocardium, angina is uncommon. The hemodynamic alterations at rest resemble those of congestive heart failure, but, in response to exercise, cardiac output increases and peripheral vascular resistance decreases normally, unless the hypothyroid state is severe. As a consequence of the increase of peripheral resistance, blood pressure raises mildly. Diastolic hypertension is usually restored to normal after treatment. All these cardiovascular alterations induce few symptoms. The occurrence of angina before or after the beginning of substitutive treatment indicates the presence of coronary artery disease.

Respiratory troubles are rarely a serious complaint in hypothyroid patients. Fatigue and particularly dyspnea on exertion are reported commonly by hypothyroid patients but also by well-being people and patients with other diseases. The severity of hypothyroidism parallels the incidence of impaired ventilatory drive. Carbon dioxide narcosis may be a cause of myxedema coma. Sleep apnea syndrome and upper airway obstruction can be present.

Poor appetite can be a leading symptom in hypothyroid patients. Weight gain is reported by most patients but is of modest amount and due largely to retention of fluid. True obesity is uncommon. Constipation is frequent and is because of lowered food intake and decreased peristaltic activity; it may mimic mechanical ileus. Gaseous distension may be a troublesome symptom. As a result of decreased energy metabolism and heat production, the basal metabolic rate is low, the appetite decreases, and the patients suffer of cold intolerance and slightly low basal body temperature.

In adults, severe hypothyroidism induces neurologic symptoms such as somnolence, slow speech, impaired cognitive functions, loss of initiative, memory defects, headache, paraesthesia, deafness, and vertigo. An unusual complacency, fatigue, and pronounced somnolence or even lethargy should suggest the possibility of severe hypothyroidism. Cerebellar ataxia is present in rare cases of long-standing hypothyroidism. Sensory phenomena are common. Numbness and tingling of the extremities are frequent, as well as carpal tunnel syndrome and other mononeuropathies, which cause nocturnal paraesthesia and pain. Deafness is a characteristic symptom of hypothyroidism and is because of both conduction and nerve impairment. Serous otitis media is common. Vestibular abnormalities and night blindness can be present. These symptoms respond to treatment with thyroid hormone. Psychiatric symptoms are common and include depression, bipolar disorders, and affective psychosis. Reasoning power is preserved, except in the terminal stage. The emotional level seems low, and irritability is decreased. Hypothyroidism should be suspected in any patient presenting with depression.

Muscle symptoms such as myalgia, stiffness, cramps, slowness of movements, and easy fatigability are often the predominating features and sometimes the sole manifestations of hypothyroidism. Hoffman's syndrome identifies hypothyroid adult with increased muscle mass because of pseudohypertrophy, which mainly involves gastrocnemius, deltoid, and trapezius muscles.

Articular and muscular pain and stiffness of the extremity may mistakenly suggest the diagnosis of rheumatoid arthritis or polymyalgia rheumatica.

Bleeding symptoms are uncommon. Hypothyroid women of fertile age have changes in cycle length and amount of bleeding. Oligomenorrhea is the most common symptoms; amenorrhea, polymenorrhea, and menorrhagia are also reported *(140)*. Severe hypothyroidism in women is associated with diminished libido and failure of ovulation. Hypothyroidism is associated with more fetal wastage and abortion in the first trimester. In adult men, hypothyroidism may cause diminished libido and impotence.

Ocular manifestations typical of Graves' ophthalmopathy are uncommon in autoimmune hypothyroidism and may represent different stages of a common disorder or, more probably, distinct entities with common pathogenetic mechanisms.

PHYSICAL FINDINGS

The typical goiter of Hashimoto's thyroiditis of adult patients is firm, moderate in size, lobulated; well-defined nodules are unusual. Both lobes are enlarged, but usually asymmetrically. Goiter may develop gradually over many years and rarely enlarges rapidly. In the atrophic form of chronic autoimmune thyroiditis, thyroid volume is reduced.

The main physical findings of overt hypothyroidism include changes of skin, face, hands, voice, thyroid, and reflexes.

The epidermis is dry, rough, cool, and covered with fine superficial scales, as a consequence of decreased cutaneous metabolism, reduced secretion of sweat and sebaceous glands, vasoconstriction, and hyperkeratosis of the stratum corneum. Subcutaneous fat may be increased, particularly above the clavicles. The hands and feet show a broad appearance, because of thickening of subcutaneous tissue. The diffuse pallor and pale waxy surface color is because of vasoconstriction, excess fluid, and mucopolysaccharide accumulation in the dermis and coexistent anemia. Yellowish discoloration of the skin is caused by the elevation of carotene concentrations. The face is puffy, pale, and expressionless at rest; sometimes it appears round or moonlike (Fig. 1). The palpebral fissure may be narrowed. The tongue is usually large and appears smooth if pernicious anemia coexists. The voice is husky, low-pitched, and coarse. The speech is slow. The hair is sparse, dry, dull, and coarse, grows slowly, and falls out readily. Loss of scalp, genital, and beard hair may occur. Hair may be lost from the temporal aspects of the eyebrows; however, this sign may be present in other diseases. In men, the beard becomes sparse. The nails are thickened, brittle, and striated. The non-pitting swelling is because of an abnormal accumulation of salts, mucopolysaccharides, and protein in the interstitial spaces of the skin, with the consequent increase of water-binding capacity. Capillary permeability is augmented in hypothyroidism.

Tendon reflexes are slow, especially during the relaxation time, as a consequence of a decrease in the rate of muscle contraction. Patients with hypothyroid myopathy may present with firm, large, well-developed muscles, especially in the arms and legs. More commonly, physical examination of muscles is unimpressive.

Cardiovascular signs such as low pulse rate, diastolic hypertension with narrowing of pulse pressure, cardiomegaly, and peripheral non-pitting edema are present. The heart sounds may be diminished in intensity, because of pericardial effusion. Ascites is unusual in hypothyroidism and can occur in association with pleural and pericardial effusion.

LABORATORY TESTS

The serum levels of creatine phosphokinase, aspartate and alanine aminotransferases and lactate dehydrogenase may be increased. In most patients, isoenzyme distribution indicates its origin from the skeletal rather than the cardiac muscle.

Hypothyroidism reduces the basal metabolic rate. Synthesis and particularly degradation of proteins are decreased with the result that nitrogen balance is usually slightly

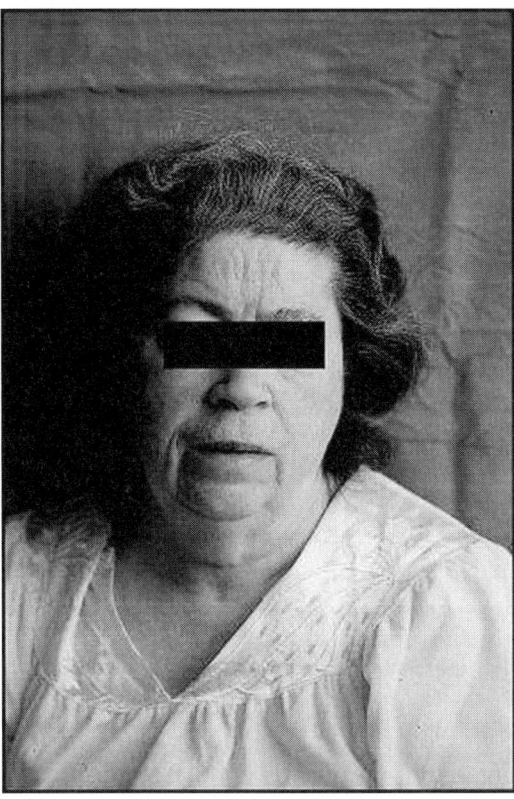

Fig. 1. A patient with autoimmune hypothyroidism (*see* Table 4).

positive. Absorption of glucose from the gastrointestinal tract is reduced, and peripheral glucose assimilation is retarded. Owing to reduced insulin degradation, sensitivity to exogenous insulin is increased, but hypoglycemia is rare. Various abnormalities in plasma lipid concentrations occur: triglycerides, phospholipids, and low-density lipoprotein (LDL) cholesterol are elevated. These changes bear in general a reciprocal relationship with the levels of thyroid hormones. The increased serum cholesterol is caused by a transient proportionally greater retardation in degradation than in synthesis, in particular of the LDL cholesterol.

About 5–25% of patients have been reported to have circulating autoantibodies directed against the gastric parietal cells or intrinsic factor, and a small minority have pernicious anemia because of impaired absorption of vitamin B12.

Anemia is a common finding of hypothyroidism. It is usually mild and may be normochromic and normocytic, as a consequence of decreased production of erythropoietin and depression of bone marrow, or macrocytic, as a consequence of deficiency of vitamin B12 and folate. An additional cause of anemia is iron deficiency, resulting from blood loss because of menorrhagia and poor iron absorption secondary to achlorhydria. Leukocytes and thrombocytes are usually normal. The most frequent defects in hemostasis are prolonged bleeding time, decreased platelet adhesiveness, and low plasma concentrations of factor VIII and of Von Willebrand factor. The clinical relevance of these abnormalities is usually limited.

As a consequence of a mild decrease of renal blood flow and glomerular filtration rate, a slight increase of serum creatinine and uric acid can be present. Occasionally, minimal proteinuria is reported. The total body sodium content is increased, but its serum concentrations tend to be low. Plasma potassium, calcium, and phosphorus levels are usually normal.

CHANGES OF OTHER ENDOCRINE GLANDS

The dramatic retardation of growth observed in hypothyroid children is caused by a deficient secretion of growth hormone (GH) and by an impairment of its action. In severe hypothyroidism, prolactin levels may rise as a consequence of an increased production of thyrotropin-releasing hormone. The total serum concentrations of both testosterone and estradiol are reduced because of a diminution of the concentration of the carrier sex hormone-binding globulin (SHBG). Thus, their absolute free concentrations remain normal. Hypothyroid patients have subtle abnormalities of pituitary adrenal function that may be correlated with the severity and duration of hypothyroidism.

INSTRUMENTAL CHANGES

Electrocardiogram changes include sinus bradycardia, prolongation of the PR interval, low amplitude of the P wave and of the QRS complex, alterations of the ST segment, and flattened or inverted T waves, which are all suggestive of myocardial ischemia. Complete heart block is uncommon. Ventricular premature beats and ventricular tachycardia may occur. These changes disappear with thyroid hormone treatment. Echocardiographic findings include a prolongation of the pre-ejection time and pericardial effusion, which is more common and severe in long-standing, severe hypothyroidism.

Atrophy of the gastric and intestinal mucosa and myxedematous infiltration of the bowel wall may be present at histological examination. Immune gastritis is often observed in autoimmune hypothyroid patients, and as many as 50% of patients have achlorhydria.

Electroencephalographic changes include slow α-wave activity and general loss of amplitude. Cognitive tests of patients with moderate-to-severe hypothyroidism indicate difficulties in performing calculations, recent memory loss, reduced attention span, and slow reaction time. Electromyography abnormalities are not specific. Patients with muscle hypertrophy lack the classic electromyography findings of myotonia.

Measurement of the resting energy expenditure is rarely performed nowadays. In patients with complete athyreosis, it falls between 35 and 45% below normal.

CLINICAL ASPECTS OF AUTOIMMUNE HYPOTHYROIDISM AT DIFFERENT AGES

Congenital Hypothyroidism. Autoimmunity is a rare cause of transient congenital hypothyroidism *(129,141,142)*. Infants born to mothers with chronic autoimmune thyroiditis and circulating TSHR-B autoantibodies may show a transient hypothyroidism because of the inhibition of their thyroid function by TSHR-B autoantibodies crossing the placenta, which gradually disappear within 3–4 months after delivery. Severe hypothyroidism is a rare occurrence and is associated with high-titer, high-affinity TSHR-B autoantibodies that inhibit fetal thyroid function throughout gestation *(126)*.

Acquired Hypothyroidism in Infancy, Childhood, and Adolescence. Chronic autoimmune thyroiditis is the most common cause of acquired hypothyroidism in children and adolescents living in iodine-sufficient areas. The atrophic variant seems more common in infants, whereas the goitrous variety is more frequent in adolescents. Clinical presentation is mainly influenced by the age of the onset of the disease and the rapidity of its progression. Hypothyroidism may affect the development of the central nervous system when it occurs in the first 3 years of life, whereas its detrimental effects on skeletal growth and maturation, pubertal development, and adult height occur until puberty is complete. Longitudinal bone growth is mainly sensitive to hypothyroidism.

Acquired autoimmune hypothyroidism in infants is rare. Symptoms and signs develop after 6 months of age and resemble those infants with congenital hypothyroidism not detected by screening *(143)*. Deceleration in linear growth and delay or arrest in the developmental milestones are also present. Because of the rapid development of hypothyroidism, skeletal maturation and eruption of primary teeth are not delayed. Early recognition and prompted treatment are essential to prevent neurologic damage and possible mental retardation *(143)*.

Hypothyroidism acquired after 3 years of age does not affect school performance and progression. Deceleration of linear growth with preservation of weight gain is the predominant clinical feature, associated with goiter, easy fatigability, and changes in school and athletic performance. True obesity is rare. Some children have muscle weakness and muscle pseudohypertrophy (Kocher-Debré-Sémélaigne syndrome). A profound delay in dental and skeletal maturation, often with radiographic evidence of epiphyseal dysgenesis, is present in younger children. The bone age is often younger than the height age.

Older children and adolescents with hypothyroidism may show symptoms and signs similar to those that occur in adults. Non-specific symptoms such as fatigue, excessive sleeping habits, anemia, and headache may occur. School performance may be normal. Harsh skeletal and growth retardation and delayed eruption of permanent teeth are the characteristic findings of severe hypothyroidism at this age. Pubertal development may occur at a normal age or may be delayed. Sexual precocity is rare and is characterized by breast development, galactorrhea, and vaginal bleeding, in absence of sexual hair. Isolated menarche has been reported. In boys, precocious testicular enlargement may occur. The testicles are histologically immature if hypothyroidism precedes puberty and show tubular involution if the onset is after puberty. Testosterone secretion is not increased. In some children, the effect of sex steroids on bone maturation seems to override that of hypothyroidism, leading to an adult height below genetic potential.

Autoimmune hypothyroidism occurs more frequently in children with Turner's and Down's syndromes and with type 1 diabetes.

Hypothyroidism in the Elderly. In the elderly chronic autoimmune thyroiditis is usually atrophic. The clinical features of autoimmune hypothyroidism described in younger patients are often absent, and several symptoms and signs including fatigue, weakness, cold intolerance, dry skin, hair loss, constipation, poor appetite, depression and/or mental deterioration, hearing loss, cardiomegaly and congestive heart failure may be confused with changes of "normal" aging (reviewed in ref. *144*). The most relevant clinical findings that are suspicious for hypothyroidism in the elderly are increased level of cholesterol, constipation, congestive heart failure, and macrocytic anemia. Neurological manifestations (syncope, seizure, impaired cerebellar function, and carpal tunnel syndrome) and arthritic complaints are common. Owing to the cardiovascular involvement, dyspnea and chest pain are common. As a consequence of reduced appetite, some elder hypothyroid patients lose weight. Neuropsychiatric symptoms are common, and depression may be the presenting symptom of hypothyroidism. Dementia is rarely a direct consequence of hypothyroidism and reverts after restoration of euthyroidism with thyroid hormone treatment.

MYXEDEMA COMA

Myxedema coma, a rare but dreadful event, is more common in older subjects and represents the extreme of hypothyroidism. It generally occurs in the winter months and can be precipitated by non-thyroidal illness, drugs, exposure to cold, and stress. In the absence of a known prior thyroid dysfunction, the diagnosis can be cumbersome. Cold intolerance, constipation to paralytic ileus, progressive deterioration of mental status to stupor, and coma are the typical symptoms. Localized neurological signs, marked hypotension, bradycardia, periorbital edema, and dry skin are the usual signs. Laboratory findings include hypercapnia, hypoglycemia, hypoxemia, hyponatremia, and elevated creatine phosphokinase. Cardiac enlargement is present at thoracic radiography, bradycardia, low voltage, and non-specific ST wave changes at ECG. Echocardiography shows decreased left ventricular contractility and cardiac workload. The mortality rate is very high, unless vigorous treatment with thyroid hormones and supportive measures are given immediately.

HYPOTHYROIDISM DURING PREGNANCY

Severe hypothyroidism is associated with stillbirth and prematurity. Gestational hypertension is two to three times more common in hypothyroid women and can cause premature delivery with low birth weight. Thyroid hormones are essential for brain development. Indeed, euthyroid neonates born to mothers who were hypothyroid during pregnancy achieve a lower intelligence quotient later in life (145,146), whereas fetal death and congenital abnormalities are not increased in properly treated hypothyroid pregnant women (147).

SUBCLINICAL HYPOTHYROIDISM

Subclinical hypothyroidism, particularly in the presence of TSH levels >10 mIU/L, has been associated with neuromuscular symptoms (148), increased cholesterol levels, and other lipid abnormalities (5,149,150), cardiac alterations (151,152) and vascular impairment (153,154). Subclinical hypothyroidism has recently been reported to be an independent risk factor for atherosclerosis and myocardial infarction in postmenopausal women (155) and in men (156). However, other authors have reported that subclinical hypothyroidism does not alter mortality rate (157). Many studies on this issue have recently been criticized because they do not meet the "evidence-based medicine" criteria (158).

Recent stimulating data have to be taken into account in the discussion of subclinical hypothyroidism. First, variations of FT4 in the individuals are narrower than variations within the reference range of a population, and therefore, an FT4 value that is normal for the population when associated with an increased TSH level probably reflects an abnormal low FT4 for the individual patient *(159)*. Second, a recent large epidemiological study has shown that the upper limit of serum TSH in a population living in an iodine-sufficient area and with no evidence of thyroid autoimmunity does not exceed 2.5 mIU/L *(6)*. Thus, the suggestion has been made by some *(160)* but not all authors *(161)* to consider 2.5 mU/L as the upper limit of the normal range of TSH. Finally, as mildly elevated TSH may normalize over time *(162)*, it is generally recommended to confirm this finding by a second determination.

ASSOCIATION WITH OTHER DISEASES

Thyroid autoimmunity, independently from the thyroid status, might interfere with the female reproductive function and the outcome of the pregnancy. Positive thyroid autoantibodies have been associated with an increased rate of abortion *(163,164)*. In female patients of infertile couples, the relative risk for AITD is slightly increased (1.95) (reviewed in ref. *165*), and a lower rate of success of assisted reproduction, because of a higher risk of miscarriage, has been reported in women with circulating thyroid autoantibodies by some but not all studies *(166)*. The link between these two conditions is unknown.

Chronic autoimmune thyroiditis is a component of the type II autoimmune polyglandular syndrome, which is characterized by the coexistence of at least two of the following disorders: Addison's disease, chronic autoimmune thyroiditis, type 1 diabetes mellitus, atrophic gastritis (with or without pernicious anemia), vitiligo, alopecia, myasthenia gravis, and hypophysitis *(30)*. Association of primary autoimmune hypothyroidism and primary adrenal insufficiency is known as Schmidt's syndrome. A latency of months or years is observed from the clinical manifestation of the first to the last disease, but the clinical manifestations are preceded by the appearance of circulating specific antibody *(167)*. Premature ovarian failure, celiac disease, psoriasis, rheumatoid arthritis, systemic lupus erythematosus, Sjogren's syndrome, polymyalgia rheumatica, temporal arthritis, chronic active hepatitis, biliary cirrhosis, and systemic sclerosis may also be associated with chronic autoimmune thyroiditis *(72)*.

In patients with chronic autoimmune thyroiditis, the prevalence of primary lymphomas of the thyroid is 80 times greater than expected *(168)*. The lymphomas are mainly non-Hodgkin B-cell type and occur more frequently in older women. Despite this increased incidence, thyroid lymphoma remains a rare occurrence.

Diagnosis

Positive circulating thyroid autoantibodies and a hypoecogenic pattern at ultrasound are the two hallmarks that identify chronic autoimmune thyroiditis and differentiate the autoimmune from other forms of hypothyroidism *(169)*. These include previous treatments of thyroid diseases, other causes of permanent thyroid damage and rare cases of isolated hyperthyrotropinemia, in which TSH rises because of partially inactivating mutations of the TSHR or other defects *(1)*.

LABORATORY INVESTIGATION

As previously reported, TPO and Tg autoantibodies are extremely common in chronic autoimmune thyroiditis. The finding of elevated TPO autoantibodies despite negative Tg autoantibodies is not unusual, whereas the opposite is rare. In comparison with

Tg autoantibodies, TPO autoantibodies are more strictly associated with lymphocytic infiltration of the thyroid *(170)* and correlate directly with the rate of development of hypothyroidism *(6,12)*. Therefore, Tg autoantibody measurement is indicated only when chronic autoimmune is suspected despite negative TPO autoantibodies. Low titers of TPO autoantibodies and Tg autoantibodies can be detected in other thyroid diseases, particularly in goiter and in thyroid cancer, as well as in normal population.

Determination of TSHR autoantibodies by radioreceptor assay is not recommended routinely because only 15% of patients with chronic autoimmune thyroiditis are TBI positive *(96)*. By bioassays, TSHR-B autoantibodies are present in up to 20% of patients with the atrophic and less frequently in those with the goitrous form of chronic autoimmune hypothyroidism *(97,98)*. However, bioassays are available in specialized centers only. High TBI titers and positive TSHR-B autoantibodies in the third trimester of pregnancy in women with chronic autoimmune thyroiditis predict the occurrence of transient neonatal hypothyroidism *(142,171)*. The diagnosis of congenital transient autoimmune hypothyroidism because of maternal autoantibodies crossing the placenta is confirmed by the transitory presence of circulating TSHR (TSHR-B) autoantibodies in neonates.

In juvenile thyroiditis, thyroid autoantibodies are more frequently negative or at lower titers than in adults, and thyroid ultrasound shows a heterogeneous echogenicity *(172)*.

The consequence of thyroid hormone therapy on the levels of thyroid autoantibodies has been controversial, with some authors showing a reduction of their levels *(173)* and others reporting no effect *(174,175)*. A later longitudinal study demonstrated that levo-thyroxine (L-T4) therapy reduces the levels of thyroid autoantibodies in hypothyroid patients from idiopathic myxedema and Hashimoto's thyroiditis and that this reduction is associated with a decrease of TSH levels; no change was observed in treated and untreated patients with euthyroid Hashimoto's thyroiditis *(176)*.

THYROID IMAGING AND OTHER TESTS

The homogeneous thyroid hypoecogenicity at ultrasound, which is typical of chronic autoimmune thyroiditis and Graves' diseases, indicates a diffuse autoimmune involvement. This pattern correlates significantly with the levels of circulating thyroid autoantibodies and is associated with or predicts the occurrence of hypothyroidism in patients with chronic autoimmune thyroiditis *(177)*.

Fine needle thyroid biopsy, which shows typical lymphocytic infiltration and oxiphilic changes of thyroid cells, is not routinely advised but can be useful for the diagnosis of chronic autoimmune thyroiditis in presence of negative circulating thyroid autoantibodies.

TREATMENT

With the exception of some cases of PPT and painless thyroiditis, autoimmune hypothyroidism requires a lifelong treatment.

Treatment with Levo-Thyroxine

Since its availability, synthetic L-T4 has gradually replaced animal thyroid extracts for the treatment of hypothyroidism. During infancy, rapid restoration of euthyroidism is essential. A full replacement dose of 50–75 μg/day should be given as starting dose. In children and adolescent, replacement can be less aggressive, and the starting dose should be 25 μg/day for children and 50 μg/day for adolescent, respectively. The dose should be increased by 25-increments at 4- to 8-week intervals until a normal circulating TSH level is obtained. Starting daily dose of L-T4 in patients under 40 years should be 50–75 μg, with a reassessment of TSH and FT4 levels in 2–3 months. In patients over 40 years, the starting daily dose should be 25–50 μg, with increments of 25 μg every 3–4 weeks. In elderly patients, particularly with known or suspected coronary heart disease, the initial dose of L-T4 should be very small (even 12.5–25 μg/day) and should be increased of 12.5–25 μg every 4–6 weeks, to reach the replacement dose in 3–4 months. Thyroid hormone treatment aims to restore euthyroidism, thus removing symptoms of hypothyroidism without inducing thyrotoxicosis. Normalization of circulating FT4 and TSH should be achieved *(178)*, with a target range for TSH of 0.5–2.0 mIU/L. Low TSH levels should be avoided, particularly in older patients, in whom they are associated with and increased risk of atrial fibrillation *(179)* and with hip and vertebral fractures in women *(180)*. After restoration of euthyroidism with L-T4 treatment, patients should be followed up at intervals of 6–24 months, with a careful monitoring of FT4 and TSH values. The full replacement dose of L-T4 for autoimmune hypothyroidism is 5 μg/kg/day for children 1–5 years old, 4 μg/kg/day for children 6–12 years old, 3 μg/kg/day for adolescents, and 1.6 μg/kg/day for young adults. The dose decreases with aging, paralleling the age-dependent reduction of lean body mass, which is its main determinant *(181)*. In the presence of angina, coronary artery bypass surgery and angioplasty are considered safe even before euthyroidism has been restored by treatment. However, a higher mortality rate in insufficiently replaced hypothyroid patients undergoing coronary artery bypass has been reported *(182)*. Women starting oral estrogen replacement therapy may need to increase L-T4 dose *(183)*. The replacement dose can augment because of treatment with drugs that increase L-T4 metabolism or with drugs and dietary supplements that reduce L-T4 absorption. Impaired acid secretion *(184)* and small bowel disease that induce malabsorption have similar effects. Difference in L-T4 preparation can also modify the required dose.

Association of Liothyronine with Thyroxine

Current guidelines recommend L-T4 monotherapy for the treatment of hypothyroidism because T4 is converted to its biologically active form, T3, in peripheral tissues. Oral L-T4 administration ensures that T3 serum concentrations remain constant and avoids the non-physiological T3 surge and short effect that follow L-T3 ingestion. These are the main considerations that provide the rationale for the preference of L-T4 monotherapy over the combined treatment with L-T4 and L-T3.

However, the question is still open to debate, and some considerations should be taken into account *(185)*. First, although the large majority of T3 originates from the peripheral monodeiodination of T4, at least 20% of circulating T3 in normal individuals is secreted by the thyroid. Second, normalization of plasma TSH and tissue T3 in hypothyroid animals can be obtained by continuous subcutaneous infusion of L-T4 plus L-T3 and not of L-T4 alone (reviewed in ref. *186*). By inference, it may be conceived that, in hypothyroid humans, monotherapy with L-T4 might not provide the right amount of T3 to all tissues. Third, in some L-T4 treated patients, normal serum TSH values can be obtained only by maintaining elevated free T4:T3 serum ratio and serum FT4 values close to the upper limit of its normal range or frankly elevated. This condition probably results in thyreotoxicosis in some organs. Finally, incomplete recovery has been reported by some hypothyroid patients treated with L-T4, despite normal hormonal profiles and lack of signs of thyroid hormone deficiency. On these grounds, the combined treatment would seem logical. It was proposed in the 1960s *(187)*, but abruptly abandoned because of the adverse effects *(188)*, which were mainly induced by the excessive doses of L-T4 and L-T3 used (reviewed in ref. *186*).

More recently, combined treatment has been reported to be more effective than L-T4 alone for the control of psychiatric symptoms of hypothyroidism in athyreotic *(189)* but not in autoimmune hypothyroid patients. Other authors have failed to demonstrate such a benefit *(190–193)*. Some of the discrepancies of the results have been attributed to differences in the ratio of L-T4 and L-T3 used in combination therapy. However, a recent paper evaluating two different ratios of L-T4 and L-T3 treatment showed that they were not superior to monotherapy in improving outcome measures *(194)*. Partial substitution of L-T4 with L-T3 in the treatment of hypothyroid patients might improve their perception of wellbeing, and indeed, some recent studies reported that patients preferred combined treatment to monotherapy *(186,194)*. This could be caused by an overcompensation of thyroid hormone deficiency in the tissues, resulting from transient surge of serum T3 after oral administration of L-T3. Thus, a pharmacologic effect of supraphysiological active hormone concentrations in tissues rather than that of the optimization of the thyroid status could be responsible for this effect *(185)*. In addition, adverse cardiac and skeletal side effects might result from mild thyrotoxicosis if the treatment were prolonged. No controlled studies on the consequences of long-term combined treatment are available to exclude this possibility.

In conclusion, current evidences indicate that combined treatment should not be recommended as a treatment of choice for hypothyroid patients until safety has been definitively proven.

It has been proposed that sustained-release L-T3 preparations would avoid non-physiological serum T3 peak. These preparations are not commercially available as yet.

Treatment of Myxedema Coma

For treatment of myxedema coma, an intravenous bolus of 500 µg of L-T4, followed by a daily maintenance dose of 50–100 µg, is required. Before starting L-T4 treatment, coexistent adrenal insufficiency must be ruled out and treated when present. In addition, hypoglycemia and hyponatremia need adequate treatments.

Treatment in Pregnancy

A correct treatment during pregnancy is required to avoid the consequence of fetal hypothyroidism. In hypothyroid women of childbearing age who plan pregnancy, L-T4 treatment should be adjusted to maintain a TSH value <2.5 mIU/L. The need for additional L-T4 replacement therapy during pregnancy has been established *(195)*. The increment of dosage depends on the etiology; an increment of L-T4 dosage is required in at least 50% of women with autoimmune hypothyroidism (mean increment of about 25%, corresponding to 28 µg/day) but probably only in few patients with subclinical hypothyroidism (reviewed in ref. *196*). The required daily dosage in overt hypothyroidism first diagnosed during pregnancy is usually 1.8–2.0 μg/kg/day. In all hypothyroid pregnant women treated with L-T4, serum TSH levels should be monitored every 6–8 weeks and more frequently after a dosage change. However, during pregnancy, serum TSH falls, as a consequence of human chorionic gonadotrophin (hCG) secretion, and normal trimester-specific serum TSH concentrations are not available at the moment. During the first trimester of pregnancy, maternal FT4 surges, and this increase is probably crucial for fetal neurodevelopment (reviewed in ref. *197*). Therefore, substitutive treatment should be adjusted to maintain FT4 close to its upper normal limit, particularly during the first trimester of pregnancy. After delivery, the required dose usually returns to pre-gestational levels, although the need for a higher dose has been reported in patients with autoimmune hypothyroidism *(198)*.

Treatment of Subclinical Hypothyroidism

Although the need of treatment of clinical hypothyroidism is unanimously accepted, that of subclinical hypothyroidism is under discussion (Table 5). The role of the "evidence-based medicine" approach in managing subclinical hypothyroidism is debated. On the basis of the consideration that large randomized control trials showing benefit of treatment are lacking, a consensus panel has recently recommended against treatment of patients with subclinical hypothyroidism with serum TSH levels of 4.5–10 mIU/L *(158)*. These conclusions were challenged in a Consensus Statement from the American Association of Clinical Endocrinologists (AACE), the American Thyroid Association (ATA), and the Endocrine Society (TES), which considered that these recommendations were based on "the lack of evidence for benefit rather than on evidence for a lack of benefit" *(199,200)*.

There are indeed a number of observations that favor the opportunity to recognize and actively treat subclinical hypothyroidism. As serum TSH values are directly correlated with total and LDL cholesterol levels *(5,201)*, serum TSH determination is recommended when circulating cholesterol is elevated *(202)*. Although optimal total and LDL cholesterol ranges are still uncertain *(203)*, an aggressive control of LDL cholesterol levels is advisable, particularly in the presence of coronary heart disease or its risk equivalents *(202)*. Effectiveness of treatment of subclinical hypothyroidism in normalizing total and/or LDL cholesterol levels and other lipid abnormalities has been reported in many *(201,204–206)* although not all studies *(207,208)*. Similar results have been reported for other abnormalities associated with subclinical hypothyroidism, namely non-specific symptoms, cardiovascular dysfunctions, and vascular impairments *(148,151,153,154,206,209,210)*. Although still debated *(158,208,211)*, based on clinical judgment, it would appear that treatment of subclinical hypothyroidism should be supported or at least not discouraged *(1,199,200,212,213)*.

Management of isolated hyperthyrotropinemia is still uncertain *(1)*.

Treatment of Thyroid Autoimmunity Associated with Recurrent Abortion

Treatment with heparin, aspirin, or intravenous Ig to prevent miscarriage in patients with recurrent abortion and positive thyroid autoantibodies has been proposed. These approaches have been suggested on the basis of the efficacy of treatment with heparin

Table 5
Treatment of Subclinical Hypothyroidism: Pros and Cons

Pros	References
Subclinical hypothyroidism is associated with:	
Neuromuscular symptoms	(148)
Increased cholesterol levels and other lipid abnormalities	(5,149,150,201,202)
Cardiac alterations	(151,152)
Vascular impairments	(153,154)
Subclinical hypothyroidism is a risk factor for:	
Atherosclerosis and myocardial infarction	(155,156)
Treatment of subclinical hypothyroidism is effective in:	
Normalizing total and/or LDL cholesterol levels and other lipid abnormalities	(201,204–206)
Ameliorating non-specific symptoms	(148)
Improving cardiovascular dysfunction	(151,209,210)
Ameliorating vascular impairments	(153,154)
Available data do not advise against and generally favor treatment of subclinical hypothyroidism	(1,200)

Cons	
Subclinical hypothyroidism does not alter mortality rate	(157)
Treatment of hypothyroidism is not effective in	
Normalizing total and/or LDL cholesterol levels and other lipid abnormalities	(207,208)
Available data do not meet the "evidence-based medicine" criteria required to advise treatment of subclinical hypothyroidism	(158,211)

Caveats	
Variations of FT4 in individuals are narrower than variations within the reference range of populations	(159)
Should the upper limit of TSH be reduced to 2.5 mIU/L ?	
Yes	(160)
No	(161)
A mildly elevated TSH may normalize over time	(162)

and/or aspirin in women with recurrent abortion and circulating cardiolipin antibody, but confirmation by larger studies is required (reviewed in ref. *214*).

SCREENING

The need and the extension of screening for thyroid diseases in the adult is debated, and different recommendations have been proposed by different institutions.

The relatively high frequency of subclinical thyroid disease, the vague clinical presentation of hypothyroidism, the progression to overt hypothyroidism and the likely benefit of treatment in many patients have prompted the ATA to favor screening for thyroid disease beginning at age 35 and every 5 years thereafter (*199,200,215*). AACE recommends screening older patients, especially women (*216*). However, the recommendations of other associations diverge largely and the US Preventive Service Task Force has recently recommended against routine screening for thyroid disease in adults *(217)*. Nevertheless, screening or aggressive case finding for mild hypothyroidism and thyroid autoimmunity in fertile women antenatally or during the first trimester of pregnancy is unanimously advised *(158,218)*. TSH measurement is recommended before pregnancy, whereas FT4 is more useful in pregnant women *(219)*. A better definition of cutoff values of thyroid hormone in early pregnancy is awaited *(197)*.

FUTURE DEVELOPMENTS

Identification of genes involved in the predisposition to chronic autoimmune thyroiditis and of endogenous and exogenous factors involved in the evolution from euthyroidism to hypothyroidism would provide precious insights into the etiology of autoimmune hypothyroidism. Elucidation of immunological mechanisms would add invaluable information on the pathogenesis. Treatment of hypothyroidism would probably benefit from a sustained release T3 preparation. Large clinical trials are needed to confirm the utility of treatment of subclinical hypothyroidism and the efficacy of screening for subclinical thyroid disease. A better definition of normal values of serum TSH and of thyroid hormone in pregnancy is required to ameliorate the management of hypothyroidism in this critical period.

ACKNOWLEDGMENTS

This work is supported in part by the grant "Rientro dei cervelli" n. 311 from MIUR and University of Pisa to Francesco Latrofa and an unrestricted grant from Bracco to Aldo Pinchera.

REFERENCES

1. Pinchera A. Subclinical thyroid disease: to treat or not to treat? *Thyroid* 2005; 15(1):1–2.
2. Williams ED, Doniach I. The post-mortem incidence of focal thyroiditis. *J Pathol Bacteriol* 1962; 83:255–264.
3. Bastenie PA, Bonnyns M, Neve P, Vanhaelst L, Chailly M. Clinical and pathological significance of asymptomatic atrophic thyroiditis. A condition of latent hypothyroidism. *Lancet* 1967; 1(7496): 915–918.
4. Tunbridge WM, Evered DC, Hall R, Appleton D, Brewis M, Clark F, et al. The spectrum of thyroid disease in a community: the Whickham survey. *Clin Endocrinol (Oxf)* 1977; 7(6):481–493.
5. Canaris GJ, Manowitz NR, Mayor G, Ridgway EC. The Colorado thyroid disease prevalence study. *Arch Intern Med* 2000; 160(4):526–534.
6. Hollowell JG, Staehling NW, Flanders WD, Hannon WH, Gunter EW, Spencer CA, et al. Serum TSH, T(4), and thyroid antibodies in the United States population (1988 to 1994): National Health and Nutrition Examination Survey (NHANES III). *J Clin Endocrinol Metab* 2002; 87(2):489–499.
7. Mariotti S, Sansoni P, Barbesino G, Caturegli P, Monti D, Cossarizza A, et al. Thyroid and other organ-specific autoantibodies in healthy centenarians. *Lancet* 1992; 339(8808):1506–1508.
8. Pinchera A, Mariotti S, Barbesino G, Bechi R, Sansoni P, Fagiolo U, et al. Thyroid autoimmunity and ageing. *Horm Res* 1995; 43(1–3):64–68.
9. Mariotti S, Franceschi C, Cossarizza A, Pinchera A. The aging thyroid. *Endocr Rev* 1995; 16(6):686–715.

10. Aghini-Lombardi F, Antonangeli L, Martino E, Vitti P, Maccherini D, Leoli F, et al. The spectrum of thyroid disorders in an iodine-deficient community: the Pescopagano survey. *J Clin Endocrinol Metab* 1999; 84(2):561–566.

11. Bulow P, I, Knudsen N, Jorgensen T, Perrild H, Ovesen L, Laurberg P. Large differences in incidences of overt hyper- and hypothyroidism associated with a small difference in iodine intake: a prospective comparative register-based population survey. *J Clin Endocrinol Metab* 2002; 87(10):4462–4469.

12. Vanderpump MP, Tunbridge WM, French JM, Appleton D, Bates D, Clark F, et al. The incidence of thyroid disorders in the community: a twenty-year follow-up of the Whickham Survey. *Clin Endocrinol (Oxf)* 1995; 43(1):55–68.

13. Rallison ML, Dobyns BM, Meikle AW, Bishop M, Lyon JL, Stevens W. Natural history of thyroid abnormalities: prevalence, incidence, and regression of thyroid diseases in adolescents and young adults. *Am J Med* 1991; 91(4):363–370.

14. Brix TH, Kyvik KO, Hegedus L. A population-based study of chronic autoimmune hypothyroidism in Danish twins. *J Clin Endocrinol Metab* 2000; 85(2):536–539.

15. Barbesino G, Chiovato L. The genetics of Hashimoto's disease. *Endocrinol Metab Clin North Am* 2000; 29(2):357–374.

16. Dayan CM, Daniels GH. Chronic autoimmune thyroiditis. *N Engl J Med* 1996; 335(2):99–107.

17. Chopra IJ, Solomon DH, Chopra U, Yoshihara E, Terasaki PI, Smith F. Abnormalities in thyroid function in relatives of patients with Graves' disease and Hashimoto's thyroiditis: lack of correlation with inheritance of HLA-B8. *J Clin Endocrinol Metab* 1977; 45(1):45–54.

18. Phillips D, Prentice L, Upadhyaya M, Lunt P, Chamberlain S, Roberts DF, et al. Autosomal dominant inheritance of autoantibodies to thyroid peroxidase and thyroglobulin–studies in families not selected for autoimmune thyroid disease. *J Clin Endocrinol Metab* 1991; 72(5):973–975.

19. Roman SH, Greenberg D, Rubinstein P, Wallenstein S, Davies TF. Genetics of autoimmune thyroid disease: lack of evidence for linkage to HLA within families. *J Clin Endocrinol Metab* 1992; 74(3):496–503.

20. Tomer Y, Davies TF. Searching for the autoimmune thyroid disease susceptibility genes: from gene mapping to gene function. *Endocr Rev* 2003; 24(5):694–717.

21. Jaume JC, Guo J, Pauls DL, Zakarija M, McKenzie JM, Egeland JA, et al. Evidence for genetic transmission of thyroid peroxidase autoantibody epitopic "fingerprints". *J Clin Endocrinol Metab* 1999; 84(4):1424–1431.

22. Pirro MT, De F, V, Di Cerbo A, Scillitani A, Liuzzi A, Tassi V. Thyroperoxidase microsatellite polymorphism in thyroid diseases. *Thyroid* 1995; 5(6):461–464.

23. Ban Y, Greenberg DA, Concepcion ES, Tomer Y. A germline single nucleotide polymorphism at the intracellular domain of the human thyrotropin receptor does not have a major effect on the development of Graves' disease. *Thyroid* 2002; 12:1079–1083.

24. Ban Y, Greenberg DA, Concepcion E, Skrabanek L, Villanueva R, Tomer Y. Amino acid substitutions in the thyroglobulin gene are associated with susceptibility to human and murine autoimmune thyroid disease. *Proc Natl Acad Sci USA* 2003; 100(25):15119–15124.

25. Vallotton MB, Forbes AP. Autoimmunity in gonadal dysgenesis and Klinefelter's syndrome. *Lancet* 1967; 1(7491):648–651.

26. McHardy-Young S, Doniach D, Polani PE. Thyroid function in Turner's syndrome and allied conditions. *Lancet* 1970; 2:1161–1164.

27. Friedman DL, Kastner T, Pond WS, O'Brien DR. Thyroid dysfunction in individuals with Down syndrome. *Arch Intern Med* 1989; 149(9):1990–1993.

28. Kennedy RL, Jones TH, Cuckle HS. Down's syndrome and the thyroid. *Clin Endocrinol (Oxf)* 1992; 37(6):471–476.

29. Loudon MM, Day RE, Duke EM. Thyroid dysfunction in Down's syndrome. *Arch Dis Child* 1985; 60(12):1149–1151.

30. Bottazzo GF, Mirakian R, Drexhage HA. Adrenalitis, oophoritis and autoimmune polyglandular disease. In: Rich RR, Fleischer TA, Schwartz DB, Shearer WT, Strober W, editors. *Clinical immunology, principles and practice*. St. Louis: Mosby, 1996: 1523–1536.

31. Olsen NJ, Kovacs WJ. Gonadal steroids and immunity. *Endocr Rev* 1996; 17(4):369–384.

32. Chiovato L, Lapi P, Fiore E, Tonacchera M, Pinchera A. Thyroid autoimmunity and female gender. *J Endocrinol Invest* 1993; 16(5):384–391.

33. Nalbandian G, Kovats S. Understanding sex biases in immunity: effects of estrogen on the differentiation and function of antigen-presenting cells. *Immunol Res* 2005; 31(2):91–106.

34. Chiovato L, Vitti P, Cucchi P, Mammoli C, Carajon P, Pinchera A. The expression of the microsomal/peroxidase autoantigen in human thyroid cells is thyrotrophin-dependent. *Clin Exp Immunol* 1989; 76(1):47–53.

35. Wick G, Brezinschek HP, Hala K, Dietrich H, Wolf H, Kroemer G. The obese strain of chickens: an animal model with spontaneous autoimmune thyroiditis. In *Advances in Immunology*. Academic Press, Inc., Burlington, MA 1989: 433–500.

36. Phillips DI, Osmond C, Baird J, Huckle A, Rees-Smith B. Is birthweight associated with thyroid autoimmunity? A study in twins. *Thyroid* 2002; 12(5):377–380.

37. Clarke WL, Shaver KA, Bright GM, Rogol AD, Nance WE. Autoimmunity in congenital rubella syndrome. *J Pediatr* 1984; 104(3):370–373.

38. Metcalfe RA, Ball G, Kudesia G, Weetman AP. Failure to find an association between hepatitis C virus and thyroid autoimmunity. *Thyroid* 1997; 7(3):421–424.

39. Harach HR, Escalante DA, Onativia A, Lederer OJ, Saravia DE, Williams ED. Thyroid carcinoma and thyroiditis in an endemic goitre region before and after iodine prophylaxis. *Acta Endocrinol (Copenh)* 1985; 108(1):55–60.

40. Braverman LE, Ingbar SH, Vagenakis AG, Adams L, Maalof F. Enhanced susceptibility to iodide myxedema in patients with Hashimoto's disease. *J Clin Endocrinol Metab* 1971; 32:515–521.

41. Martino E, Safran M, Aghini-Lombardi F, Rajatanavin R, Lenziardi M, Fay M, et al. Environmental iodine intake and thyroid dysfunction during chronic amiodarone therapy. *Ann Intern Med* 1984; 101(1):28–34.

42. Trip MD, Wiersinga W, Plomp TA. Incidence, predictability, and pathogenesis of amiodarone-induced thyrotoxicosis and hypothyroidism. *Am J Med* 1991; 91(5):507–511.

43. Martino E, Aghini-Lombardi F, Mariotti S, Bartalena L, Lenziardi M, Ceccarelli C, et al. Amiodarone iodine-induced hypothyroidism: risk factors and follow-up in 28 cases. *Clin Endocrinol (Oxf)* 1987; 26(2):227–237.

44. Martino E, Bartalena L, Bogazzi F, Braverman LE. The effects of amiodarone on the thyroid. *Endocr Rev* 2001; 22(2):240–254.

45. Bocchetta A, Mossa P, Velluzzi F, Mariotti S, Zompo MD, Loviselli A. Ten-year follow-up of thyroid function in lithium patients. *J Clin Psychopharmacol* 2001; 21(6):594–598.

46. Imagawa A, Itoh N, Hanafusa T, Oda Y, Waguri M, Miyagawa J, et al. Autoimmune endocrine disease induced by recombinant interferon-alpha therapy for chronic active type C hepatitis. *J Clin Endocrinol Metab* 1995; 80(3):922–926.

47. Atkins MB, Mier JW, Parkinson DR, Gould JA, Berkman EM, Kaplan MM. Hypothyroidism after treatment with interleukin-2 and lymphokine-activated killer cells. *N Engl J Med* 1988; 318(24):1557–1563.

48. van Liessum PA, de Mulder PH, Mattijssen EJ, Corstens FH, Wagener DJ. Hypothyroidism and goitre during interleukin-2 therapy without LAK cells. *Lancet* 1989; 1(8631):224.

49. Hoekman K, von Blomberg-van der Flier BM, Wagstaff J, Drexhage HA, Pinedo HM. Reversible thyroid dysfunction during treatment with GM-CSF. *Lancet* 1991; 338(8766):541–542.

50. Marazuela M, Garcia-Buey L, Gonzalez-Fernandez B, Garcia-Monzon C, Arranz A, Borque MJ, et al. Thyroid autoimmune disorders in patients with chronic hepatitis C before and during interferon-alpha therapy. *Clin Endocrinol (Oxf)* 1996; 44(6):635–642.

51. Eheman CR, Garbe P, Tuttle RM. Autoimmune thyroid disease associated with environmental thyroidal irradiation. *Thyroid* 2003; 13(5):453–464.

52. Larsen PR, Conard RA, Knudsen KD, Robbins J, Wolff J, Rall JE, et al. Thyroid hypofunction after exposure to fallout from a hydrogen bomb explosion. *JAMA* 1982; 247(11):1571–1575.

53. Pacini F, Vorontsova T, Molinaro E, Kuchinskaya E, Agate L, Shavrova E, et al. Prevalence of thyroid autoantibodies in children and adolescents from Belarus exposed to the Chernobyl radioactive fallout. *Lancet* 1998; 352(9130):763–766.

54. Davis S, Kopecky KJ, Hamilton TE, Onstad L. Thyroid neoplasia, autoimmune thyroiditis, and hypothyroidism in persons exposed to iodine 131 from the hanford nuclear site. *JAMA* 2004; 292(21):2600–2613.

55. Nagataki S, Shibata Y, Inoue S, Yokoyama N, Izumi M, Shimaoka K. Thyroid diseases among atomic bomb survivors in Nagasaki. *JAMA* 1994; 272(5):364–370.

56. Imaizumi M, Usa T, Tominaga T, Neriishi K, Akahoshi M, Nakashima E, et al. Radiation dose-response relationships for thyroid nodules and autoimmune thyroid diseases in Hiroshima and Nagasaki atomic bomb survivors 55-58 years after radiation exposure. *JAMA* 2006; 295(9): 1011–1022.

57. Volzke H, Werner A, Wallaschofski H, Friedrich N, Robinson DM, Kindler S, et al. Occupational exposure to ionizing radiation is associated with autoimmune thyroid disease. *J Clin Endocrinol Metab* 2005; 90(8):4587–4592.

58. Spitalnik PF, Straus FH. Patterns of human thyroid parenchymal reaction following low-dose childhood irradiation. *Cancer* 1978; 41(3):1098–1105.

59. Kaplan MM, Boice JD, Jr., Ames DB, Rosenstein M. Thyroid, parathyroid, and salivary gland evaluations in patients exposed to multiple fluoroscopic examinations during tuberculosis therapy: a pilot study. *J Clin Endocrinol Metab* 1988; 66(2):376–382.

60. Hancock SL, Cox RS, McDougall IR. Thyroid diseases after treatment of Hodgkin's disease. *N Engl J Med* 1991; 325(9):599–605.

61. Pinchera A, Liberti P, Martino E, Fenzi GF, Grasso L, Rovis L, et al. Effects of antithyroid therapy on the long-acting thyroid stimulator and the antithyroglobulin antibodies. *J Clin Endocrinol Metab* 1969; 29(2):231–238.

62. Chiovato L, Santini F, Vitti P, Bendinelli G, Pinchera A. Appearance of thyroid stimulating antibody and Graves' disease after radioiodine therapy for toxic nodular goitre. *Clin Endocrinol (Oxf)* 1994; 40(6):803–806.

63. Nygaard B, Knudsen JH, Hegedus L, Scient AVC, Molholm Hansen JE. Thyrotropin receptor antibodies and Graves' disease, a side-effect of 131I treatment in patients with nontoxic goiter. *J Clin Endocrinol Metab* 1997; 82(9):2926–2930.

64. Fukata S, Kuma K, Sugawara M. Relationship between cigarette smoking and hypothyroidism in patients with Hashimoto's thyroiditis. *J Endocrinol Invest* 1996; 19(9):607–612.

65. Pujo-Borrell R, Hanafusa T, Chiovato L, Bottazzo GF. Lectin-induced expression of DR antigen on human cultured follicular thyroid cells. *Nature* 1983; 304(5921):71–73.

66. Hanafusa T, Pujol-Borrell R, Chiovato L, Russell RC, Doniach D, Bottazzo GF. Aberrant expression of HLA-DR antigen on thyrocytes in Graves' disease: relevance for autoimmunity. *Lancet* 1983; 2(8359):1111–1115.

67. Chiovato L, Lapi P, Mariotti S, Del Prete G, De Carli M, Pinchera A. Simultaneous expression of thyroid peroxidase and human leukocyte antigen-DR by human thyroid cells: modulation by thyrotropin, thyroid-stimulating antibody, and interferon-gamma. *J Clin Endocrinol Metab* 1994; 79(2):653–656.

68. Zheng RQ, Abney ER, Grubeck-Loebenstein B, Dayan C, Maini RN, Feldmann M. Expression of intercellular adhesion molecule-1 and lymphocyte function-associated antigen-3 on human thyroid epithelial cells in Graves' and Hashimoto's diseases. *J Autoimmun* 1990; 3(6):727–736.

69. Faure GC, Bensoussan-Lejzerowicz D, Bene MC, Aubert V, Leclere J. Coexpression of CD40 and class II antigen HLA-DR in Graves' disease thyroid epithelial cells. *Clin Immunol Immunopathol* 1997; 84(2):212–215.

70. Metcalfe RA, McIntosh RS, Marelli-Berg F, Lombardi G, Lechler R, Weetman AP. Detection of CD40 on human thyroid follicular cells: analysis of expression and function. *J Clin Endocrinol Metab* 1998; 83(4):1268–1274.

71. Battifora M, Pesce G, Paolieri F, Fiorino N, Giordano C, Riccio AM, et al. B7.1 costimulatory molecule is expressed on thyroid follicular cells in Hashimoto's thyroiditis, but not in Graves' disease. *J Clin Endocrinol Metab* 1998; 83(11):4130–4139.

72. Weetman AP. Chronic autoimmune thyroiditis. In: Braverman LE, Utiger RD, editors. *Werner & Ingbar's The Thyroid: A Fundamental and Clinical Text*. Philadelphia: Lippincott Williams & Wilkins, 2005: 701–713.

73. Quaratino S, Feldmann M, Dayan CM, Acuto O, Londei M. Human self-reactive T cell clones expressing identical T cell receptor beta chains differ in their ability to recognize a cryptic self-epitope. *J Exp Med* 1996; 183(2):349–358.

74. Quaratino S, Duddy LP, Londei M. Fully competent dendritic cells as inducers of T cell anergy in autoimmunity. *Proc Natl Acad Sci USA* 2000; 97(20):10911–10916.

75. Quaratino S, Badami E, Pang YY, Bartok I, Dyson J, Kioussis D, et al. Degenerate self-reactive human T-cell receptor causes spontaneous autoimmune disease in mice. *Nat Med* 2004; 10(9): 920–926.

76. Davies TF, Martin A, Concepcion ES, Graves P, Lahat N, Cohen WL, et al. Evidence for selective accumulation of intrathyroidal T lymphocytes in human autoimmune thyroid disease based on T cell receptor V gene usage. *J Clin Invest* 1992; 89(1):157–162.

77. McIntosh RS, Tandon N, Pickerill AP, Davies R, Barnett D, Weetman AP. IL-2 receptor-positive intrathyroidal lymphocytes in Graves' disease. Analysis of V alpha transcript microheterogeneity. *J Immunol* 1993; 151(7):3884–3893.

78. Ueda H, Howson JM, Esposito L, Heward J, Snook H, Chamberlain G, et al. Association of the T-cell regulatory gene CTLA4 with susceptibility to autoimmune disease. *Nature* 2003; 423(6939):506–511.

79. Marcocci C, Marino M. Thyroid-directed antibodies. In: Braverman LE, Utiger RD, editors. *Werner & Ingbar's The Thyroid: A Fundamental and Clinical Text*. Philadelphia: Lippincott Williams & Wilkins, 2005: 360–372.

80. Mariotti S, Pisani S, Russova A, Pinchera A. A new solid-phase immunoradiometric assay for anti-thyroglobulin autoantibody. *J Endocrinol Invest* 1982; 5(4):227–233.

81. Mariotti S, Caturegli P, Piccolo P, Barbesino G, Pinchera A. Antithyroid peroxidase autoantibodies in thyroid diseases. *J Clin Endocrinol Metab* 1990; 71(3):661–669.

82. Mariotti S, Barbesino G, Caturegli P, Atzeni F, Manetti L, Marino M, et al. False negative results observed in anti-thyroid peroxidase autoantibody determination by competitive radioimmunoassays using monoclonal antibodies. *Eur J Endocrinol* 1994; 130(6):552–558.

83. Latrofa F, Pichurin P, Guo J, Rapoport B, McLachlan SM. Thyroglobulin-thyroperoxidase autoantibodies are polyreactive, not bispecific: analysis using human monoclonal autoantibodies. *J Clin Endocrinol Metab* 2003; 88(1):371–378.

84. Caturegli P, Kuppers RC, Mariotti S, Burek CL, Pinchera A, Ladenson PW, et al. IgG subclass distribution of thyroglobulin antibodies in patients with thyroid disease. *Clin Exp Immunol* 1994; 98(3):464–469.

85. McLachlan SM, Rapoport B. Why measure thyroglobulin autoantibodies rather than thyroid peroxidase autoantibodies? *Thyroid* 2004; 14(7):510–520.

86. McLachlan SM, Rapoport B. Autoimmune response to the thyroid in humans: thyroid peroxidase–the common autoantigenic denominator. *Int Rev Immunol* 2000; 19(6):587–618.

87. Saboori AM, Rose NR, Burek CL. Iodination of human thyroglobulin (Tg) alters its immunoreactivity. II. Fine specificity of a monoclonal antibody that recognizes iodinated Tg. *Clin Exp Immunol* 1998; 113(2):303–308.

88. Dai YD, Rao VP, Carayanniotis G. Enhanced iodination of thyroglobulin facilitates processing and presentation of a cryptic pathogenic peptide. *J Immunol* 2002; 168(11):5907–5911.

89. Latrofa F, Phillips M, Rapoport B, McLachlan SM. Human monoclonal thyroglobulin autoantibodies: epitopes and immunoglobulin genes. *J Clin Endocrinol Metab* 2004; 89(10):5116–5123.

90. Prentice L, Kiso Y, Fukuma N, Horimoto M, Petersen V, Grennan F, et al. Monoclonal thyroglobulin autoantibodies: variable region analysis and epitope recognition. *J Clin Endocrinol Metab* 1995; 80(3):977–986.

91. Caturegli P, Mariotti S, Kuppers RC, Burek CL, Pinchera A, Rose NR. Epitopes on thyroglobulin: a study of patients with thyroid disease. *Autoimmunity* 1994; 18(1):41–49.

92. Kohno Y, Naito N, Hiyama Y, Shimojo N, Suzuki N, Tarutani O, et al. Thyroglobulin and thyroid peroxidase share common epitopes recognized by autoantibodies in patients with chronic autoimmune thyroiditis. *J Clin Endocrinol Metab* 1988; 67(5):899–907.

93. Ruf J, Ferrand M, Durand-Gorde JM, Carayon P. Immunopurification and characterization of thyroid autoantibodies with dual specificity for thyroglobulin and thyroperoxidase. *Autoimmunity* 1992; 11(3):179–188.

94. Ruf J, Carayon P. The molecular recognition theory applied to bispecific antibodies. *Nat Med* 1995; 1(12):1222.

95. Vitti P, Elisei R, Tonacchera M, Chiovato L, Mancusi F, Rago T, et al. Detection of thyroid-stimulating antibody using Chinese hamster ovary cells transfected with cloned human thyrotropin receptor. *J Clin Endocrinol Metab* 1993; 76(2):499–503.

96. Costagliola S, Morgenthaler NG, Hoermann R, Badenhoop K, Struck J, Freitag D, et al. Second generation assay for thyrotropin receptor antibodies has superior diagnostic sensitivity for Graves' disease. *J Clin Endocrinol Metab* 1999; 84(1):90–97.

97. Chiovato L, Vitti P, Santini F, Lopez G, Mammoli C, Bassi P, et al. Incidence of antibodies blocking thyrotropin effect in vitro in patients with euthyroid or hypothyroid autoimmune thyroiditis. *J Clin Endocrinol Metab* 1990; 71(1):40–45.

98. Tamaki H, Amino N, Kimura M, Hidaka Y, Takeoka K, Miyai K. Low prevalence of thyrotropin receptor antibody in primary hypothyroidism in Japan. *J Clin Endocrinol Metab* 1990; 71(5): 1382–1386.

99. Weetman AP, Yateman ME, Ealey PA, Black CM, Reimer CB, Williams RC, Jr., et al. Thyroid-stimulating antibody activity between different immunoglobulin G subclasses. *J Clin Invest* 1990; 86(3):723–727.

100. Latrofa F, Chazenbalk GD, Pichurin P, Chen CR, McLachlan SM, Rapoport B. Affinity-enrichment of thyrotropin receptor autoantibodies from Graves' patients and normal individuals provides insight into their properties and possible origin from natural antibodies. *J Clin Endocrinol Metab* 2004; 89(9):4734–4745.

101. Tokuda Y, Kasagi K, Iida Y, Hatabu H, Misaki T, Arai K, et al. Inhibition of thyrotropin-stimulated iodide uptake in FRTL-5 thyroid cells by crude immunoglobulin fractions from patients with goitrous and atrophic autoimmune thyroiditis. *J Clin Endocrinol Metab* 1988; 67(2):251–258.

102. Rapoport B, Chazenbalk GD, Jaume JC, McLachlan SM. The thyrotropin (TSH) receptor: interaction with TSH and autoantibodies. *Endocr Rev* 1998; 19(6):673–716.

103. Schwarz-Lauer L, Chazenbalk GD, McLachlan SM, Ochi Y, Nagayama Y, Rapoport B. Evidence for a simplified view of autoantibody interactions with the thyrotropin receptor. *Thyroid* 2002; 12(2):115–120.

104. Chen CR, Pichurin P, Nagayama Y, Latrofa F, Rapoport B, McLachlan SM. The thyrotropin receptor autoantigen in Graves disease is the culprit as well as the victim. *J Clin Invest* 2003; 111(12):1897–1904.

105. Chazenbalk GD, Pichurin P, Chen CR, Latrofa F, Johnstone AP, McLachlan SM, et al. Thyroid-stimulating autoantibodies in Graves disease preferentially recognize the free A subunit, not the thyrotropin holoreceptor. *J Clin Invest* 2002; 110(2):209–217.

106. Chiovato L, Latrofa F, Braverman LE, Pacini F, Capezzone M, Masserini L, et al. Disappearance of humoral thyroid autoimmunity after complete removal of thyroid antigens. *Ann Intern Med* 2003; 139(5 Pt 1):346–351.

107. Lisi S, Pinchera A, McCluskey RT, Willnow TE, Refetoff S, Marcocci C, et al. Preferential megalin-mediated transcytosis of low-hormonogenic thyroglobulin: a control mechanism for thyroid hormone release. *Proc Natl Acad Sci USA* 2003; 100(25):14858–14863.

108. Marino M, Chiovato L, Friedlander JA, Latrofa F, Pinchera A, McCluskey RT. Serum antibodies against megalin (GP330) in patients with autoimmune thyroiditis. *J Clin Endocrinol Metab* 1999; 84(7):2468–2474.

109. Sakata S, Nakamura S, Miura K. Autoantibodies against thyroid hormones or iodothyronine. Implications in diagnosis, thyroid function, treatment, and pathogenesis. *Ann Intern Med* 1985; 103(4):579–589.

110. Raspe E, Costagliola S, Ruf J, Mariotti S, Dumont JE, Ludgate M. Identification of the thyroid Na+/I− cotransporter as a potential autoantigen in thyroid autoimmune disease. *Eur J Endocrinol* 1995; 132(4):399–405.

111. Endo T, Kogai T, Nakazato M, Saito T, Kaneshige M, Onaya T. Autoantibody against Na+/I−Symporter in the Sera of Patients with Autoimmune Thyroid Disease. *Biochem Biophys Res Commun* 1996; 224(1):92–95.

112. Chin HS, Chin DK, Morgenthaler NG, Vassart G, Costagliola S. Rarity of anti-Na+/I− symporter (NIS) antibody with iodide uptake inhibiting activity in autoimmune thyroid diseases (AITD). *J Clin Endocrinol Metab* 2000; 85(10):3937–3940.

113. Tonacchera M, Agretti P, Ceccarini G, Lenza R, Refetoff S, Santini F, et al. Autoantibodies from patients with autoimmune thyroid disease do not interfere with the activity of the human iodide symporter gene stably transfected in CHO cells. *Eur J Endocrinol* 2001; 144(6):611–618.

114. Seissler J, Wagner S, Schott M, Lettmann M, Feldkamp J, Scherbaum WA, et al. Low frequency of autoantibodies to the human Na(+)/I(−) symporter in patients with autoimmune thyroid disease. *J Clin Endocrinol Metab* 2000; 85(12):4630–4634.

115. Giordano C, Stassi G, De Maria R, Todaro M, Richiusa P, Papoff G, et al. Potential involvement of Fas and its ligand in the pathogenesis of Hashimoto's thyroiditis. *Science* 1997; 275(5302):960–963.

116. Stokes TA, Rymaszewski M, Arscott PL, Wang SH, Bretz JD, Bartron J, et al. Constitutive expression of FasL in thyrocytes. *Science* 1998; 279:2015a.

117. Fiedler P, Schaetzlein CE, Eibel H. Constitutive expression of FasL in thyrocytes. *Science* 1998; 279:2015a.

118. Chiovato L, Bassi P, Santini F, Mammoli C, Lapi P, Carayon P, et al. Antibodies producing complement-mediated thyroid cytotoxicity in patients with atrophic or goitrous autoimmune thyroiditis. *J Clin Endocrinol Metab* 1993; 77(6):1700–1705.

119. Zimmer KP, Scheumann GF, Bramswig J, Bocker W, Harms E, Schmid KW. Ultrastructural localization of IgG and TPO in autoimmune thyrocytes referring to the transcytosis of IgG and the antigen presentation of TPO. *Histochem Cell Biol* 1997; 107(2):115–120.

120. Guo J, Jaume JC, Rapoport B, McLachlan SM. Recombinant thyroid peroxidase-specific Fab converted to immunoglobulin G (IgG) molecules: evidence for thyroid cell damage by IgG1, but not IgG4, autoantibodies. *J Clin Endocrinol Metab* 1997; 82(3):925–931.

121. Brostoff SW, Howell MD. T cell receptors, immunoregulation, and autoimmunity. *Clin Immunol Immunopathol* 1992; 62(1 Pt 1):1–7.

122. Wenzel BE, Chow A, Baur R, Schleusener H, Wall JR. Natural killer cell activity in patients with Graves' disease and Hashimoto's thyroiditis. *Thyroid* 1998; 8(11):1019–1022.

123. Okamoto Y, Hamada N, Saito H, Ohno M, Noh J, Ito K, et al. Thyroid peroxidase activity-inhibiting immunoglobulins in patients with autoimmune thyroid disease. *J Clin Endocrinol Metab* 1989; 68(4):730–734.

124. Saller B, Hormann R, Mann K. Heterogeneity of autoantibodies against thyroid peroxidase in autoimmune thyroid disease: evidence against antibodies directly inhibiting peroxidase activity as regulatory factors in thyroid hormone metabolism. *J Clin Endocrinol Metab* 1991; 72(1):188–195.

125. Nishikawa T, Jaume JC, McLachlan SM, Rapoport B. Human monoclonal autoantibodies against the immunodominant region on thyroid peroxidase: lack of cross-reactivity with related peroxidases or thyroglobulin and inability to inhibit thyroid peroxidase enzymatic activity. *J Clin Endocrinol Metab* 1995; 80(4):1461–1466.

126. Matsuura N, Yamada Y, Nohara Y, Konishi J, Kasagi K, Endo K, et al. Familial neonatal transient hypothyroidism due to maternal TSH-binding inhibitor immunoglobulins. *N Engl J Med* 1980; 303(13):738–741.

127. Zakarija M, McKenzie JM, Eidson MS. Transient neonatal hypothyroidism: characterization of maternal antibodies to the thyrotropin receptor. *J Clin Endocrinol Metab* 1990; 70(5):1239–1246.

128. Boyages SC, Halpern JP, Maberly GF, Eastman CJ, Chen J, Wang ZH, et al. Endemic cretinism: possible role for thyroid autoimmunity. *Lancet* 1989; 2(8662):529–532.

129. Chiovato L, Vitti P, Bendinelli G, Santini F, Fiore E, Tonacchera M, et al. Humoral thyroid autoimmunity is not involved in the pathogenesis of myxedematous endemic cretinism. *J Clin Endocrinol Metab* 1995; 80(5):1509–1514.

130. Michelangeli VP, Poon C, Topliss DJ, Colman PG. Specific effects of radioiodine treatment on TSAb and TBAb levels in patients with Graves' disease. *Thyroid* 1995; 5(3):171–176.

131. Chiovato L, Fiore E, Vitti P, Rocchi R, Rago T, Dokic D, et al. Outcome of thyroid function in Graves' patients treated with radioiodine: role of thyroid-stimulating and thyrotropin-blocking antibodies and of radioiodine-induced thyroid damage. *J Clin Endocrinol Metab* 1998; 83(1):40–46.

132. Baloch ZW, Livolsi VA. Pathology. In: Braverman LE, Utiger RD, editors. *Werner & Ingbar's The Thyroid: A Fundamental and Clinical Text.* Philadelphia: Lippincott Williams & Wilkins, 2005.

133. Muller AF, Drexhage HA, Berghout A. Postpartum thyroiditis and autoimmune thyroiditis in women of childbearing age: recent insights and consequences for antenatal and postnatal care. *Endocr Rev* 2001; 22(5):605–630.

134. Klintschar M, Schwaiger P, Mannweiler S, Regauer S, Kleiber M. Evidence of fetal microchimerism in Hashimoto's thyroiditis. *J Clin Endocrinol Metab* 2001; 86(6):2494–2498.

135. Srivatsa B, Srivatsa S, Jhonson KL, Samura O, Lee SL, Bianchi DW. Microchimerism of presumed fetal origin in thyroid specimens from women: a case-control study. *Lancet* 2001; 358:2034–2038.

136. Billewicz WZ, Chapman RS, Crooks J, Day ME, Gossage J, Wayne E, et al. Statistical methods applied to the diagnosis of hypothyroidism. *Q J Med* 1969; 38(150):255–266.

137. Zulewski H, Muller B, Exer P, Miserez AR, Staub JJ. Estimation of tissue hypothyroidism by a new clinical score: evaluation of patients with various grades of hypothyroidism and controls. *J Clin Endocrinol Metab* 1997; 82(3):771–776.

138. Huber G, Staub JJ, Meier C, Mitrache C, Guglielmetti M, Huber P, et al. Prospective study of the spontaneous course of subclinical hypothyroidism: prognostic value of thyrotropin, thyroid reserve, and thyroid antibodies. *J Clin Endocrinol Metab* 2002; 87(7):3221–3226.

139. Tonacchera M, Chiovato L, Pinchera A. Clinical Assessment and systemic manifestations of hypothyroidism. In: Wass JAH, Shale SM, editors. *Oxford Textbook of Endocrinology and Diabetes.* Oxford, New York: Oxford University Press Inc., 2002: 491–502.

140. Krassas GE, Pontikides N, Kaltsas T, Papadopoulou P, Paunkovic J, Paunkovic N, et al. Disturbances of menstruation in hypothyroidism 2. *Clin Endocrinol (Oxf)* 1999; 50(5):655–659.

141. Sutherland JM, Esselborn VM, Burket RL, Skillman TB, Benson JT. Familial nongoitrous cretinism apparently due to maternal antithyroid antibody. Report of a family. *N Engl J Med* 1960; 263: 336–341.

142. Brown RS, Bellisario RL, Botero D, Fournier L, Abrams CA, Cowger ML, et al. Incidence of transient congenital hypothyroidism due to maternal thyrotropin receptor-blocking antibodies in over one million babies. *J Clin Endocrinol Metab* 1996; 81(3):1147–1151.

143. Foley TP, Abbassi V, Copeland KC, Draznin MB. Hypothyroidism caused by chronic autoimmune thyroiditis in very young infants. *N Engl J Med* 1994; 330(7):466–468.

144. Latrofa F, Pinchera A. Aging and the thyroid. Hot thyroidology (www.hotthyroidology.com) 2005; July(1).

145. Pop VJ, Kuijpens JL, van Baar AL, Verkerk G, van Son MM, de Vijlder JJ, et al. Low maternal free thyroxine concentrations during early pregnancy are associated with impaired psychomotor development in infancy. *Clin Endocrinol (Oxf)* 1999; 50(2):149–155.

146. Haddow JE, Palomaki GE, Allan WC, Williams JR, Knight GJ, Gagnon J, et al. Maternal thyroid deficiency during pregnancy and subsequent neuropsychological development of the child. *N Engl J Med* 1999; 341(8):549–555.

147. Burrow GN, Fisher DA, Larsen PR. Maternal and fetal thyroid function. *N Engl J Med* 1994; 331(16):1072–1078.

148. Monzani F, Caraccio N, Del Guerra P, Casolaro A, Ferrannini E. Neuromuscular symptoms and dysfunction in subclinical hypothyroid patients: beneficial effect of L-T4 replacement therapy. *Clin Endocrinol (Oxf)* 1999; 51(2):237–242.

149. Bindels AJ, Westendorp RG, Frolich M, Seidell JC, Blokstra A, Smelt AH. The prevalence of subclinical hypothyroidism at different total plasma cholesterol levels in middle aged men and women: a need for case-finding? *Clin Endocrinol (Oxf)* 1999; 50(2):217–220.

150. Kanaya AM, Harris F, Volpato S, Perez-Stable EJ, Harris T, Bauer DC. Association between thyroid dysfunction and total cholesterol level in an older biracial population: the health, aging and body composition study. *Arch Intern Med* 2002; 162(7):773–779.

151. Vitale G, Galderisi M, Lupoli GA, Celentano A, Pietropaolo I, Parenti N, et al. Left ventricular myocardial impairment in subclinical hypothyroidism assessed by a new ultrasound tool: pulsed tissue Doppler. *J Clin Endocrinol Metab* 2002; 87(9):4350–4355.

152. Biondi B, Palmieri EA, Lombardi G, Fazio S. Effects of subclinical thyroid dysfunction on the heart. *Ann Intern Med* 2002; 137(11):904–914.

153. Faber J, Petersen L, Wiinberg N, Schifter S, Mehlsen J. Hemodynamic changes after levothyroxine treatment in subclinical hypothyroidism. *Thyroid* 2002; 12(4):319–324.

154. Taddei S, Caraccio N, Virdis A, Dardano A, Versari D, Ghiadoni L, et al. Impaired endothelium-dependent vasodilatation in subclinical hypothyroidism: beneficial effect of levothyroxine therapy. *J Clin Endocrinol Metab* 2003; 88(8):3731–3737.

155. Hak AE, Pols HA, Visser TJ, Drexhage HA, Hofman A, Witteman JC. Subclinical hypothyroidism is an independent risk factor for atherosclerosis and myocardial infarction in elderly women: the Rotterdam Study. *Ann Intern Med* 2000; 132(4):270–278.

156. Imaizumi M, Akahoshi M, Ichimaru S, Nakashima E, Hida A, Soda M, et al. Risk for ischemic heart disease and all-cause mortality in subclinical hypothyroidism. *J Clin Endocrinol Metab* 2004; 89(7):3365–3370.

157. Parle JV, Maisonneuve P, Sheppard MC, Boyle P, Franklyn JA. Prediction of all-cause and cardiovascular mortality in elderly people from one low serum thyrotropin result: a 10-year cohort study. *Lancet* 2001; 358(9285):861–865.

158. Surks MI, Ortiz E, Daniels GH, Sawin CT, Col NF, Cobin RH, et al. Subclinical thyroid disease: scientific review and guidelines for diagnosis and management. *JAMA* 2004; 291(2):228–238.

159. Andersen S, Pedersen KM, Bruun NH, Laurberg P. Narrow individual variations in serum T(4) and T(3) in normal subjects: a clue to the understanding of subclinical thyroid disease. *J Clin Endocrinol Metab* 2002; 87(3):1068–1072.

160. Wartofsky L, Dickey RA. The evidence for a narrower thyrotropin reference range is compelling. *J Clin Endocrinol Metab* 2005; 90(9):5483–5488.

161. Surks MI, Goswami G, Daniels GH. The thyrotropin reference range should remain unchanged. *J Clin Endocrinol Metab* 2005; 90(9):5489–5496.

162. Diez JJ, Iglesias P, Burman KD. Spontaneous normalization of thyrotropin concentrations in patients with subclinical hypothyroidism. *J Clin Endocrinol Metab* 2005; 90(7):4124–4127.

163. Stagnaro-Green A, Roman SH, Cobin RH, el Harazy E, Alvarez-Marfany M, Davies TF. Detection of at-risk pregnancy by means of highly sensitive assays for thyroid autoantibodies. *JAMA* 1990; 264(11):1422–1425.

164. Glinoer D, Soto MF, Bourdoux P, Lejeune B, Delange F, Lemone M, et al. Pregnancy in patients with mild thyroid abnormalities: maternal and neonatal repercussions. *J Clin Endocrinol Metab* 1991; 73(2):421–427.

165. Poppe K, Velkeniers B. Female infertility and the thyroid. *Best Pract Res Clin Endocrinol Metab* 2004; 18(2):153–165.

166. Poppe K, Glinoer D, Tournaye H, Devroey P, van Steirteghem A, Kaufman L, et al. Assisted reproduction and thyroid autoimmunity: an unfortunate combination? *J Clin Endocrinol Metab* 2003; 88(9):4149–4152.

167. Betterle C, Volpato M, Rees SB, Furmaniak J, Chen S, Zanchetta R, et al. II. Adrenal cortex and steroid 21-hydroxylase autoantibodies in children with organ-specific autoimmune diseases: markers of high progression to clinical Addison's disease. *J Clin Endocrinol Metab* 1997; 82(3): 939–942.

168. Kato I, Tajima K, Suchi T, Aozasa K, Matsuzuka F, Kuma K, et al. Chronic thyroiditis as a risk factor of B-cell lymphoma in the thyroid gland. *Jpn J Cancer Res* 1985; 76(11):1085–1090.

169. Santini F, Pinchera A. Causes and laboratory investigation of hypothyroidism. In: Wass JAH, Shale SM, editors. *Oxford textbook of endocrinology and diabetes*. Oxford, New York: Oxford University Press Inc., 2006: 502–510.

170. Yoshida H, Amino N, Yagawa K, Uemura K, Satoh M, Miyai K, et al. Association of serum antithyroid antibodies with lymphocytic infiltration of the thyroid gland: studies of seventy autopsied cases. *J Clin Endocrinol Metab* 1978; 46:859–862.

171. McKenzie JM, Zakarija M. Clinical review 3: The clinical use of thyrotropin receptor antibody measurements. *J Clin Endocrinol Metab* 1989; 69(6):1093–1096.

172. Set PA, Oleszczuk-Raschke K, von Lengerke JH, Bramswig J. Sonographic features of Hashimoto thyroiditis in childhood. *Clin Radiol* 1996; 51(3):167–169.

173. Jansson R, Karlsson A, Dahlberg PA. Thyroxine, methimazole, and thyroid microsomal autoantibody titres in hypothyroid Hashimoto's thyroiditis. *Br Med J (Clin Res Ed)* 1985; 290(6461):11–12.

174. Hayashi Y, Tamai H, Fukata S, Hirota Y, Katayama S, Kuma K, et al. A long term clinical, immunological, and histological follow-up study of patients with goitrous chronic lymphocytic thyroiditis. *J Clin Endocrinol Metab* 1985; 61(6):1172–1178.

175. Papapetrou PD, Lazarus JM, McSween RNM, Harden RM. Long-term treatment of Hashimoto's thyroiditis with thyroxine. *Lancet* 1972; 2(7786):1045–1048.

176. Chiovato L, Marcocci C, Mariotti S, Mori A, Pinchera A. L-thyroxine therapy induces a fall of thyroid microsomal and thyroglobulin antibodies in idiopathic myxedema and in hypothyroid, but not in euthyroid Hashimoto's thyroiditis. *J Endocrinol Invest* 1986; 9(4):299–305.

177. Marcocci C, Vitti P, Cetani F, Catalano F, Concetti R, Pinchera A. Thyroid ultrasonography helps to identify patients with diffuse lymphocytic thyroiditis who are prone to develop hypothyroidism. *J Clin Endocrinol Metab* 1991; 72(1):209–213.

178. Surks MI, Chopra IJ, Mariash CN, Nicoloff JT, Solomon DH. American Thyroid Association guidelines for use of laboratory tests in thyroid disorders. *JAMA* 1990; 263(11):1529–1532.

179. Sawin CT, Geller A, Wolf PA, Belanger AJ, Baker E, Bacharach P, et al. Low serum thyrotropin concentrations as a risk factor for atrial fibrillation in older persons. *N Engl J Med* 1994; 331(19):1249–1252.

180. Bauer DC, Ettinger B, Nevitt MC, Stone KL. Risk for fracture in women with low serum levels of thyroid-stimulating hormone. *Ann Intern Med* 2001; 134(7):561–568.

181. Santini F, Pinchera A, Marsili A, Ceccarini G, Castagna MG, Valeriano R, et al. Lean body mass is a major determinant of levothyroxine dosage in the treatment of thyroid diseases. *J Clin Endocrinol Metab* 2005; 90(1):124–127.

182. Zindrou D, Taylor KM, Bagger JP. Excess coronary artery bypass graft mortality among women with hypothyroidism. *Ann Thorac Surg* 2002; 74(6):2121–2125.

183. Arafah BM. Increased need for thyroxine in women with hypothyroidism during estrogen therapy. *N Engl J Med* 2001; 344(23):1743–1749.

184. Centanni M, Gargano L, Canettieri G, Viceconti N, Franchi A, Delle FG, et al. Thyroxine in goiter, Helicobacter pylori infection, and chronic gastritis. *N Engl J Med* 2006; 354(17):1787–1795.

185. Pinchera A, Santini F. Is combined therapy with levothyroxine and liothyronine effective in patients with primary hypothyroidism? *Nat Clin Pract Endocrinol Metab* 2005; 1(1):19.

186. Escobar-Morreale HF, Botella-Carretero JI, del Rey FE, de Escobar GM. Treatment of hypothyroidism with combinations of levothyroxine plus liothyronine. *J Clin Endocrinol Metab* 2005; 90(8):4946–4954.

187. Taylor S, Kapur M, Adie R. Combined thyroxine and triiodothyronine for thyroid replacement therapy. *Br Med J* 1970; 1(704):270–271.

188. Smith RN, Taylor SA, Massey JC. Controlled clinical trial of combined triiodothyronine and thyroxine in the treatment of hypothyroidism. *Br Med J* 1970; 4(728):145–148.

189. Bunevicius R, Kazanavicius G, Zalinkevicius R, Prange AJ. Effects of thyroxine as compared with thyroxine plus triiodothyronine in patients with hypothyroidism. *N Engl J Med* 1999; 340(6): 424–429.

190. Walsh JP, Shiels L, Lim EM, Bhagat CI, Ward LC, Stuckey BGA, et al. Combined thyroxine/liothyronine treatment does not improve well-being, quality of life, or cognitive function compared to thyroxine alone: a randomized controlled trial in patients with primary hypothyroidism. *J Clin Endocrinol Metab* 2003; 88(10):4543–4550.

191. Sawka AM, Gerstein HC, Marriott MJ, MacQueen GM, Joffe RT. Does a combination regimen of thyroxine (t4) and 3,5,3'-triiodothyronine improve depressive symptoms better than t4 alone in patients with hypothyroidism? Results of a Double-Blind, Randomized, Controlled Trial. *J Clin Endocrinol Metab* 2003; 88(10):4551–4555.

192. Clyde PW, Harari AE, Getka EJ, Shakir KM. Combined levothyroxine plus liothyronine compared with levothyroxine alone in primary hypothyroidism: a randomized controlled trial. *JAMA* 2003; 290(22):2952–2958.

193. Saravanan P, Simmons DJ, Greenwood R, Peters TJ, Dayan CM. Partial substitution of thyroxine (T4) with tri-iodothyronine in patients on T4 replacement therapy: results of a large community-based randomized controlled trial. *J Clin Endocrinol Metab* 2005; 90(2):805–812.

194. Appelhof BC, Fliers E, Wekking EM, Schene AH, Huyser J, Tijssen JGP, et al. Combined therapy with levothyroxine and liothyronine in two ratios, compared with levothyroxine monotherapy in primary hypothyroidism: a Double-Blind, Randomized, Controlled Clinical Trial. *J Clin Endocrinol Metab* 2005; 90(5):2666–2674.

195. Mandel SJ, Larsen PR, Seely EW, Brent GA. Increased need for thyroxine during pregnancy in women with primary hypothyroidism. *N Engl J Med* 1990; 323(2):91–96.

196. Mandel SJ. Hypothyroidism and chronic autoimmune thyroiditis in the pregnant state: maternal aspects. *Best Pract Res Clin Endocrinol Metab* 2004; 18(2):213–224.

197. Escobar GMd, Obregon MJ, del Rey FEd. Maternal thyroid hormones early in pregnancy and fetal brain development. *Best Pract Res Clin Endocrinol Metab* 2004; 18(2):225–248.

198. Caixas A, Albareda M, Garcia-Patterson A, Rodriguez-Espinosa J, de Leiva A, Corcoy R. Postpartum thyroiditis in women with hypothyroidism antedating pregnancy? *J Clin Endocrinol Metab* 1999; 84(11):4000–4005.

199. Gharib H, Tuttle RM, Baskin HJ, Fish LH, Singer PA, McDermott MT. Subclinical thyroid dysfunction: a joint statement on management from the American Association of Clinical Endocrinologists, the american thyroid association, and the endocrine society. *Thyroid* 2005; 15(1):24–28.

200. Gharib H, Tuttle RM, Baskin HJ, Fish LH, Singer PA, McDermott MT. Subclinical thyroid dysfunction: a joint statement on management from the American Association of Clinical Endocrinologists, the American Thyroid Association, and the Endocrine Society. *J Clin Endocrinol Metab* 2005; 90(1):581–585.

201. Caraccio N, Ferrannini E, Monzani F. Lipoprotein profile in subclinical hypothyroidism: response to levothyroxine replacement, a randomized placebo-controlled study. *J Clin Endocrinol Metab* 2002; 87(4):1533–1538.

202. Expert Panel on Detection EaToHBCiA. Executive Summary of the Third Report of the National Cholesterol Education Program (NCEP) Expert Panel on Detection, Evaluation, and Treatment of High Blood Cholesterol in Adults (Adult Treatment Panel III). *JAMA* 2001; 285(19):2486–2497.

203. O'Keefe JH, Jr., Cordain L, Harris WH, Moe RM, Vogel R. Optimal low-density lipoprotein is 50 to 70 mg/dl: lower is better and physiologically normal. *J Am Coll Cardiol* 2004; 43(11):2142–2146.

204. Tanis BC, Westendorp GJ, Smelt HM. Effect of thyroid substitution on hypercholesterolaemia in patients with subclinical hypothyroidism: a reanalysis of intervention studies. *Clin Endocrinol (Oxf)* 1996; 44(6):643–649.

205. Danese MD, Ladenson PW, Meinert CL, Powe NR. Clinical review 115: effect of thyroxine therapy on serum lipoproteins in patients with mild thyroid failure: a quantitative review of the literature. *J Clin Endocrinol Metab* 2000; 85(9):2993–3001.

206. Meier C, Staub JJ, Roth CB, Guglielmetti M, Kunz M, Miserez AR, et al. TSH-controlled L-thyroxine therapy reduces cholesterol levels and clinical symptoms in subclinical hypothyroidism: a double blind, placebo-controlled trial (Basel Thyroid Study). *J Clin Endocrinol Metab* 2001; 86(10):4860–4866.

207. Efstathiadou Z, Bitsis S, Milionis HJ, Kukuvitis A, Bairaktari ET, Elisaf MS, et al. Lipid profile in subclinical hypothyroidism: is L-thyroxine substitution beneficial? *Eur J Endocrinol* 2001; 145(6):705–710.

208. Kong WM, Sheikh MH, Lumb PJ, Naoumova RP, Freedman DB, Crook M, et al. A 6-month randomized trial of thyroxine treatment in women with mild subclinical hypothyroidism. *Am J Med* 2002; 112(5):348–354.

209. Biondi B, Fazio S, Palmieri EA, Carella C, Panza N, Cittadini A, et al. Left ventricular diastolic dysfunction in patients with subclinical hypothyroidism. *J Clin Endocrinol Metab* 1999; 84(6):2064–2067.

210. Aghini-Lombardi F, Di Bello V, Talini E, Di Cori A, Monzani F, Antonangeli L, et al. Early textural and functional alterations of left ventricula myocardium in mild hypothyroidism. *Eur J Endocrinol* 2006; 155:3–9.

211. Vanderpump M. Subclinical hypothyroidism: the case against treatment. *Trends Endocrinol Metab* 2003; 14(6):262–266.

212. McDermott MT, Ridgway EC. Subclinical hypothyroidism is mild thyroid failure and should be treated. *J Clin Endocrinol Metab* 2001; 86(10):4585–4590.

213. Owen PJ, Lazarus JH. Subclinical hypothyroidism: the case for treatment. *Trends Endocrinol Metab* 2003; 14(6):257–261.

214. Stagnaro-Green A, Glinoer D. Thyroid autoimmunity and the risk of miscarriage. *Best Pract Res Clin Endocrinol Metab* 2004; 18(2):167–181.

215. Ladenson PW, Singer PA, Ain KB, Bagchi N, Bigos ST, Levy EG, et al. American Thyroid Association guidelines for detection of thyroid dysfunction. *Arch Intern Med* 2000; 160(11): 1573–1575.

216. AACE Thyroid Task Force. American Association of Clinical Endocrinologists medical guidelines for clinical practice for the evaluation and treatment of hyperthyroidism and hypothyroidism. *Endocr Pract* 2002; 8:457–469.

217. U.S. Preventive Service Task Force. Screening for thyroid disease: recommendation statement. *Ann Intern Med* 2004; 140(2):125–127.

218. Vanderpump MP, Tunbridge WM. Epidemiology and prevention of clinical and subclinical hypothyroidism. *Thyroid* 2002; 12(10):839–847.

219. Morreale de Escobar G, Jesus Obregon M, Escobar del Rey F. Is neuropsychological development related to maternal hypothyroidism or to maternal hypothyroxinemia? *J Clin Endocrinol Metab* 2000; 85(11):3975–3987.

8

Postpartum Thyroiditis

John H. Lazarus, MA, MD, FRCP, FACE,
FRCOG, *and L. D. K. E. Premawardhana,*
MBBS, FRCP

Summary

Postpartum thyroiditis occurs in 5–9% of women and is strongly associated with positive thyroid peroxidase antibodies (TPOAb positive) as determined around 14 weeks gestation. Postpartum thyroid dysfunction (PPTD) occurs in 50% of TPOAb-positive women (measured at 14 weeks gestation) and presents as transient hyperthyroidism (median onset 13 weeks postpartum) followed by transient hypothyroidism (median onset 19 weeks postpartum); the latter will develop into permanent hypothyroidism in up to 30% of women. Women who then remain euthyroid after transient thyroid dysfunction have a 75% chance of PPTD in a subsequent pregnancy and a 50% risk of permanent hypothyroidism after 7 years. The hyperthyroid phase is relatively asymptomatic, but the hypothyroid phase may be very clinically evident and require levothyroxine treatment.

Key Words: Postpartum thyroiditis, immune, hyperthyroidism, hypothyroidism, antibodies, cellular immunity, screening, incidence.

INTRODUCTION

In addition to changes in circulating thyroid hormone concentrations observed during gestation *(1)*, pronounced alterations in the immune system are evident *(2)*. The cellular changes consist of a change from the so-called Th1 state to a predominance of cytokines such as IL-4 consistent with a Th2 status *(3)*. On the humoral side, the titer of anti-thyroid peroxidase antibodies (anti-TPOAb), found in 10% of pregnant women at

From: *Contemporary Endocrinology: Autoimmune Diseases in Endocrinology*
Edited by: A. P. Weetman © Humana Press, Totowa, NJ

14–16 weeks gestation, decreases markedly during the second and third trimesters. At birth, the Th2 status abruptly reverts back to the non-pregnant Th1 position, and this is accompanied by a dramatic rebound in the titer of anti-TPOAb, which reaches a maximum between 3 and 6 months postpartum (immune rebound phenomenon). If thyrotropin receptor stimulating antibodies (TSHRAb) are present in early pregnancy, they behave in a similar manner through gestation and the postpartum period. These immunological changes at delivery and the postpartum *(4)* set the scene for the development of postpartum thyroid dysfunction (PPTD). Various types of clinical thyroid dysfunction may arise following delivery (Fig. 1). The changes in PPTD may be transient or permanent and may be because of destructive or stimulating disease.

In 1948, H.E.W. Roberton *(6)*, a general practitioner in New Zealand, described the occurrence of lassitude and other symptoms of hypothyroidism relating to the postpartum period. These complaints were treated successfully with thyroid extract. The syndrome remained generally unrecognized until the 1970s when reports from Japan *(7)* and Canada *(8)* rediscovered the existence of postpartum thyroiditis (PPT) and recognized the immune nature of the condition (*see* reviews refs. *9–12*). PPT is essentially sporadic thyroiditis in the postpartum period. The term PPT relates to destructive thyroiditis occurring during the first 12 months postpartum and not to Graves' disease, although the two conditions may be seen concurrently.

Postpartum thyroiditis with thyroid dysfunction (i.e., PPTD) is characterized by an episode of transient thyrotoxicosis followed by transient hypothyroidism. The former presents at about 14 weeks postpartum followed by transient hypothyroidism at a median of 19 weeks. Very occasionally, the hypothyroid state is seen before the thyrotoxicosis. The thyroid dysfunction that occurs in up to 50% of TPO antibody-positive women ascertained around 14 weeks gestation comprises 19% with thyrotoxicosis alone, 49% hypothyroidism alone and the remaining 32% thyrotoxicosis followed by hypothyroidism (i.e., biphasic). Not all women manifest both thyroid states, and the thyrotoxic episode may escape detection as it may be of short duration. PPTD is usually associated with the presence of anti-thyroid antibodies, usually anti-TPO antibodies, which rise in titer after 6 weeks postpartum. Anti-Tg antibody occurs in about 15% and is the sole antibody in <5%. However, PPTD has been described in small numbers of women who have not been shown to have circulating thyroid antibodies *(13)*. Although the clinical manifestations of the thyrotoxic state are not usually severe, lack of energy and irritability are particularly prominent even in thyroid antibody-positive women who do not develop

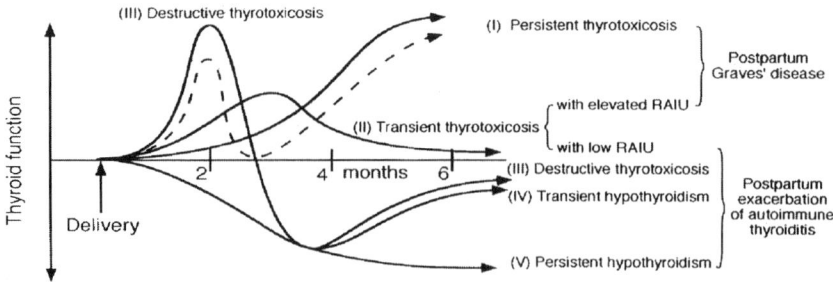

Fig. 1. Thyroid dysfunction occurring after pregnancy (from Amino et al. [*5*]). Illustration of various types of thyroid dysfunction that can occur after delivery. Note that the thyrotoxicosis may be persistent or transient, and the hypothyroidism may also be persistent or transient.

thyroid dysfunction. In contrast, the symptomatology of the hypothyroid phase may be profound. Many classic hypothyroid symptoms occur before the onset of thyroid hormone reduction and persist even when recovery is seen in hormone levels *(14)*. PPT can also occur in women receiving T4 therapy before pregnancy *(15)* and after miscarriage *(16)*. Quantitative evaluation of postpartum depression has shown an increase of mild to moderate symptomatology in thyroid antibody-positive women even when they remain euthyroid during the postpartum period compared with antibody negative controls, and this may present as early as 6 weeks postpartum *(17)*. This increase in depressive symptomatology has not been observed by all groups *(18)*.

EPIDEMIOLOGY

Owing to wide variations in the number of women studied, the frequency of thyroid assessment postpartum, diagnostic criteria employed and differences in hormone assay methodology, a variable incidence (from 3 to 17%) has been reported worldwide (Table 1). The data in the table are also approximate as the calculations have been performed on different proportions of the base population. However, there is a general

Table 1
Worldwide Epidemiology of Postpartum Thyroiditis (PPT)

Country	Year	Base population	% PPT	Reference
Japan	1982	507	5.5	*(19)*
Sweden	1984	644	6.5	*(20)*
USA	1986	216	1.9	*(21)*
Denmark	1987	694	3.9	*(22)*
USA	1987	238	6.7	*(23)*
USA	1988	1034	3.3	*(24)*
USA	1988	261	21.1	*(25)*
UK	1988	901	16.7	*(26)*
Thailand	1990	812	1.1	*(27)*
Denmark	1990	1163	3.3	*(28)*
Italy	1991	372	8.7	*(29)*
Canada	1992	1376	5.9	*(30)*
USA	1992	552	8.8	*(31)*
UK	1992	1248	5.0	*(17)*
Netherlands	1993	382	7.2	*(32)*
Netherlands	1998	448	5.2	*(13)*
Australia	1999	1816	10.3	*(18)*
Spain	2000	757	7.5	*(33)*
Brazil	2000	830	14.6	*(34)*
Japan	2000	4072	6.5	*(35)*
Iran	2001	1040	11.4	*(36)*
Turkey	2001	876	5.5	*(37)*
Czech	2002	650	2.8	*(38)*
India	2002	120	7	*(39)*
Greece	2002	1594	2.4	*(40)*
China	2003	119	5.6–23.1	*(41)*

consensus that the disease occurs in 5–9% of unselected postpartum women, and the clinical characteristics of PPT are similar in different areas with different prevalence for example Brazil *(34)*, Turkey *(37)*, and Greece *(40)*. Women with type 1 diabetes mellitus have a threefold incidence of PPT compared with non-diabetics *(42)*. PPT is also more likely to occur in a woman who has had a previous episode *(43)*. One population-based case–control study in Kuwait found that women who have had PPT were at an increased risk of developing thyroid cancer (odds ratio 10.2) *(44)*. This finding requires confirmation in other areas.

GENETIC AND ENVIRONMENTAL FACTORS

Initially, no association between HLA-A or -B phenotypes and PPT could be found *(45)*. Subsequently, a higher incidence of HLA-A26, -BW46 and -BW67 together with a significantly lower frequency of HLA-BW62 and -CW7 and an increased frequency of HLA-A1 and -B8 in women with this condition were reported *(46)*. In relation to HLA class II, increased frequencies of HLA-DR3 *(46,47)*, DR4 *(48–50)*, and DR5 *(25,47,51,52)* have been reported in patients with PPT. This variation between studies may reflect ethnic differences as well as variations in sample number and methodology. A negative association between PPT and DR2 together with the increased frequency of DR3 was observed *(46,53)*. The frequency of HLA-DQ7 is also raised in PPT probably because of the increase in DR5, because both DR11 and DR12 are in linkage disequilibrium with DQ7 *(52)*.

In view of the impact of iodide on thyroid autoimmunity *(54)*, it might be expected that the development of PPT may be related to the ambient iodine concentration. Initially, it was suggested that iodine intake affected the severity of the thyrotoxic and hypothyroid phases of the condition *(51)*, and iodide administration was shown to aggravate the disease in certain women *(55)*, but a large study of PPT suggested that iodine intake is unlikely to affect the prevalence of the condition *(56)*. Nevertheless, some studies have concluded that the incidence of PPT may be related to iodine deficiency *(41)* and possibly to the transition from low to adequate iodine status *(36)*. Many studies have shown no effect of ambient iodine concentration. For example, in the Kashmir valley, the iodine deficient status of the population does not alter the incidence of PPT significantly *(39,57)*. Administration of iodide to postpartum women did not affect the expression of PPT *(58)*, and this has been confirmed by a randomized placebo-controlled double-blind trial in Denmark *(59)*. The overall conclusion is that although some data suggest moderate alterations in incidence related to iodine status, the majority of studies do not show any effect of administered iodine or ambient iodine concentration. The Danish study has confirmed that iodine supplementation in gestation does not change the incidence of PPT in a moderate iodine-deficient population. This is important in underpinning the strategy of iodine supplementation in pregnancy to benefit the fetus *(60)*.

IMMUNOPATHOGENESIS

There is abundant evidence that PPT is an immunologically related disease *(9)*. Biopsy of the thyroid in this syndrome shows lymphocytic infiltration similar to that seen in Hashimoto's thyroiditis *(61)*. There is also evidence from immunogenetic data in addition to humoral and cellular studies in this condition.

As well as the inference of an immune etiology from examination of class I and II HLA genetic data (*see* Genetic and Environmental Factors), it is known that the class III area of the MHC contains the coding for several proteins, which are important in the pathogenesis of the autoimmune diseases (namely tumor necrosis factor-α, HSP70, complement). The allotype frequency of three complement proteins Bf, C4A, and C4B showed significant differences in frequency distribution in women with PPT *(62)*. These findings are similar to those reported by Ratanachaiavong et al. *(63)* in Graves' disease, an autoimmune thyroid disease, which is also associated with an increased frequency of HLA-DR3. This may indicate linkage disequilibrium with candidate genes in the class III region but could also be related to the pathogenesis of PPT, which is known to be linked to activation of the complement system *(64)*.

Amino et al. *(5)* first documented the association of PPT with high titers of antithyroid antibodies and the dramatic rise of anti-microsomal antibody titer after delivery was confirmed *(26)*. There is also a rise in postpartum thyroglobulin antibody titer in women who have been found to be TgAb-positive in early pregnancy. TgAb is less prevalent than TPOAb in PPT, being present in only around 15% of cases: however, it has been noted to be the only antibody present in 2% of patients. Furthermore, gestation and the postpartum period are characterized by fluctuations in the immune response, and the postpartum increase appears to be a reflection of a general enhancement of immunoglobulin synthesis. This pattern of transient antibody increase in microsomal antibody levels was observed also for serum total immunoglobulin (Ig)G and IgG subclass levels but not for IgM, IgA, or IgE or indeed against viral and bacterial antigens *(65)*.

Various methodologies for the measurement of IgG subclass distribution of the microsomal antibodies have produced conflicting results. For example, IgG-1 and IgG-4 were the dominant subclasses with only minor contributions from IgG-2 and IgG-3 in one study *(66)*, whereas significant IgG-2 and IgG-3 microsomal antibodies were found in women who developed a biphasic thyroid dysfunction *(67)*. No variation in IgG subclass-associated microsomal antibody activity was found between euthyroid and thyroid dysfunctional women during the postpartum year in one study *(68)*, whereas a fourfold increase in IgG1 activity in the PPT group over 12 months postpartum (IgG-3 being low during this time, IgG-2 elevated and IgG-4 constant) was observed in another *(69)*. What is clear is that, despite marked postpartum fluctuations in TPO antibody concentration, the epitopic fingerprint is constant, presumably because of inheritance of this characteristic *(70)*. Although the antibody response is dramatic, its precise role in the immunopathogenesis of the condition remains to be determined. Probably the antibody titer is merely a marker of disease, and the immunological damage is mediated by lymphocyte and complement-associated mechanisms.

Postpartum thyroiditis does not usually occur in women in the absence of elevated thyroid autoantibodies at any time during the postpartum year. However, only some 50% of TPOAb-positive women become symptomatic. Studies on antibody functional affinity *(68)* and IgG subclass distribution *(69)* in PPT suggest that, as in other autoimmune diseases, activation of the complement system may have a role in pathogenesis.

Using tests of complement fixation and complement activation *(71,72)*, it has been shown that there is activation of the complement system by thyroid-directed

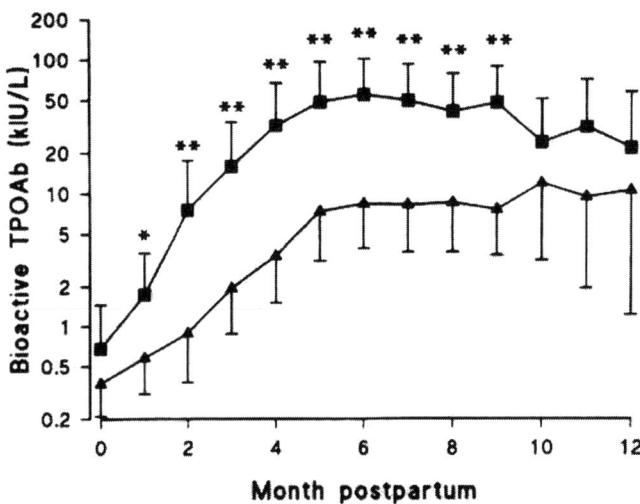

Fig. 2. Bioactive thyroid peroxidase (TPO) antibody in postpartum thyroiditis. Bioactive TPO antibody levels in women euthyroid during the postpartum period (diamonds) compared to levels in women who developed postpartum thyroid function during the postpartum year (filled boxes) $^*p = 0.05$, $^{**}p < 0.001$ (from ref. 64).

autoantibodies (64) (Fig. 2); in addition, complement activation is related to the extent of the thyroiditis (73) and correlates with the severity of the thyroid dysfunction (74).

An antibody-directed sublethal complement attack on nucleated cells can result in an increase in cellular metabolic activity through a number of mechanisms, including a rapid rise in both intracellular Ca^{++} ions (75) and cAMP. In thyroid cells, these metabolic changes could mimic the action of thyroid-stimulating hormone (TSH) leading to the upregulation of thyroid peroxidase (76) and secretion of thyroid hormones into the circulation with a consequent hyperthyroidism. A more severe complement-mediated attack leads to destruction of thyroid follicular architecture, resulting in loss of thyroid function and subsequent hypothyroidism. Complement has been shown to be involved in the pathogenesis of autoimmune thyroid disease by the demonstration of terminal complement complexes (TCC) around thyroid follicles in such patients (77). However, despite the presence of circulating bioactive TPOAbs, the extent of complement activation is inadequate to cause detectable increases in peripheral blood TCC, suggesting that the complement system may not play a major role in the pathogenesis of PPT (78).

During pregnancy, maternal immune reactions are regulated to prevent rejection of the fetal allograft such that the cytokine profile is a T helper (Th) 2 pattern, which switches back to the Th1 state postpartum (3,4). As well as the Th2 status in pregnancy, it is known that hormones such as estradiol, progesterone, and cortisol are in high concentration and have immunological effects designed to maintain the developing fetus and ensure adequate duration of gestation (79).

Early postpartum (within 3 months) changes in T-cell subsets have been described similar to those seen in Hashimoto's thyroiditis (9). The peripheral T-lymphocyte subset ratio CD4/CD8 has been shown to be higher in TPOAb-positive women who developed PPT compared with similar antibody-positive women who did not (31).

Study of lymphocyte populations during and after pregnancy has shown a generalized activation of immune activity at 36 weeks gestation in TPOAb-positive women who went on to develop PPTD compared to those who did not; furthermore, the former group had lower plasma cortisol concentrations pre-delivery (Fig. 3) *(80)*. These data suggest that there may be less immunological suppression at 36 weeks in TPOAb-positive women destined to develop PPTD possibly because of lower levels of cortisol at this time. Thus, the immunological determinants of PPTD may in part occur antenatally, although the mechanisms for this are still unclear.

The immunological effects of microchimerism also require consideration. Leakage of fetal cells into the maternal circulation occurs through the syncytiotrophoblast layer, and it has been suggested that this phenomenon may be of immunopathogenetic importance in scleroderma *(81)* and other connective tissue diseases *(82)*. The presence of activated fetal cells in maternal tissues may trigger susceptible women to develop autoimmune disorders due in part to the continued exposure of the maternal immune system to a paternal antigen *(83)*. Intrathyroidal fetal microchimerism has been observed in human Graves' disease and Hashimoto thyroid glands *(84,85)* as well as in a newborn thyroid *(86)*. The influence of these fetal cells on the expression of PPT in humans and in an animal model requires further investigation *(83,87)*.

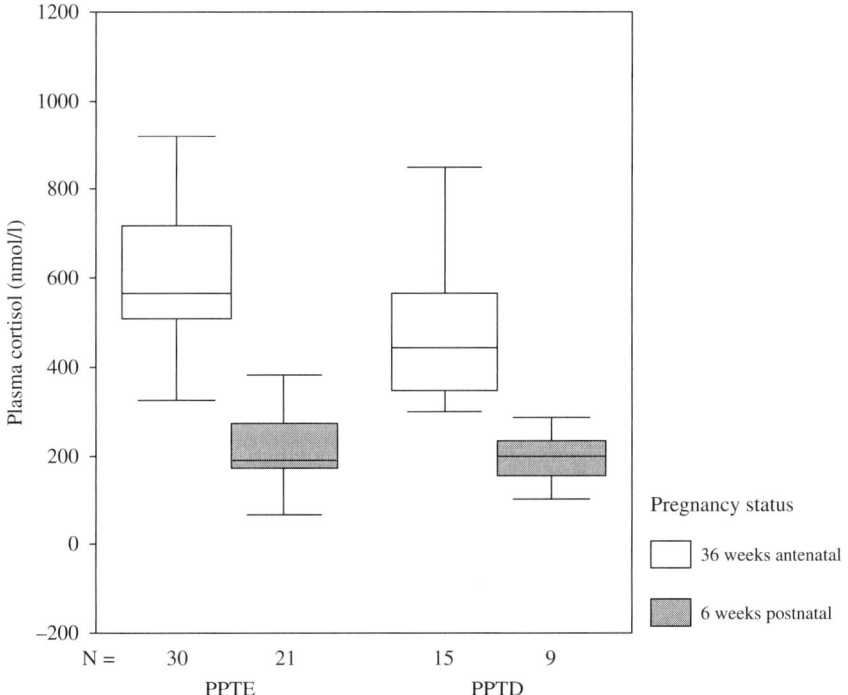

Fig. 3. Median, 25/75 centiles, and range of plasma cortisol levels in the postpartum euthyroid (PPTE) and postpartum thyroid dysfunction (PPTD) groups of patients at 36 weeks antepartum and 6 weeks postpartum. Although there was no significant difference between the two groups at 6 weeks postpartum, the cortisol levels in the PPTE group was significantly higher than those in the PPTD groups at 36 weeks antepartum ($p < 0.022$; Mann–Witney U test). The number (n) of patients in each group is shown at the bottom of the figure (from ref. *80* with permission).

DIAGNOSIS

Thyrotoxicosis in the postpartum period may be because of a recurrence or the development of new Graves' disease or to the destructive, thyrotoxic phase of PPT. Symptoms of thyrotoxicosis are much more evident in Graves' disease.

As postpartum thyrotoxicosis is a destructive process, radioiodine uptake will be very low at early and late times after isotope administration. TSH receptor antibodies are not seen unless there is coexisting Graves' disease. Thyrotoxicosis because of PPT is diagnosed by a suppressed TSH together with an elevated FT4 or FT3, or elevated FT3 and FT4, with either set of criteria occurring on more that one occasion. If possible, a normal range of thyroid hormone concentrations should be derived in the postpartum period as they fall into a narrower range than the general population. Antibodies to thyroxine and T3 may cause confusion in diagnosis, but they are infrequent *(88)*.

Hypothyroidism in the postpartum period occurs at a median of 19 weeks but has been observed as late as 36–40 weeks after birth. The symptoms are often dramatic and may develop before the decrease in thyroid function is noted. The most frequent symptoms have been found to be lack of energy, aches and pains, poor memory, dry skin, and cold intolerance *(14)*.

Hypothyroidism may be defined as TSH >3.6 mU/L together with FT4 <8 pmol/L or FT3 <4.2 pmol/L or TSH >10 mU/L on one or more occasion. The use of thyroid ultrasonography has demonstrated diffuse or multifocal echogenicity, reflecting the abnormal thyroid morphology and consistent with the known lymphocytic infiltration of the thyroid *(89)*. The destructive nature of the thyroiditis is also shown by the increase in urinary iodine excretion in the thyrotoxic as well as the hypothyroid phase of the illness *(56)*. In addition, there is evidence that an early rise in serum thyroglobulin (a further indicator of thyroid destruction) may help in the identification of those women at risk of PPT *(90)*, but it is also raised in other thyroid conditions (e.g., Graves' disease). IL-6 is elevated in Graves' disease and other thyroid destructive processes *(91,92)* but not in PPT *(93)*. Despite the inflammatory nature of PPT, high sensitivity C-reactive protein is also unhelpful in the diagnosis of the condition *(94)*.

MANAGEMENT

The thyrotoxic phase is relatively asymptomatic and usually requires no specific therapy. If symptoms of tachycardia and palpitations are troublesome or if other symptoms such as sweating or anxiety are present, then beta adrenoreceptor-blocking agents may be used. Propanolol is the drug of choice, but if nightmares develop, a more cardioselective β-blocker may be used. If this class of drug is contraindicated, verapamil may be effective for cardiac symptoms. Anti-thyroid drugs are not indicated as the condition is a destructive thyroiditis. In contrast, patients experience persistent and troublesome symptoms related to the hypothyroid period, and treatment with levothyroxine should be given starting with 0.1 mg per day increasing as necessary. At this stage, it will not be clear whether the patient has developed transient or permanent hypothyroidism. In this instance, it is reasonable to treat with thyroxine for up to 1 year postpartum and then review the patient to determine the thyroxine requirement. This will normally mean that the patient should stop the therapy for 4–6 weeks and then have a thyroid function test. Patients who have been known to have transient PPTD should be checked at least annually as 50% of them will develop hypothyroidism after 7 years. This is in contrast to TPOAb-positive women who have not experienced any thyroid dysfunction postpartum whose rate of hypothyroidism at 7 years follow-up is only 5% (95). Clearly, these patients require less intensive surveillance.

Although the thyrotoxicosis of PPT always resolves, several long-term studies have documented persistence of hypothyroidism in 20–30% of cases (53,96). Assessment of anti-TPO-positive women (at 16 weeks gestation) 7 years later showed that the rate of development of hypothyroidism was significantly greater (48 vs 8%) in those who had had PPT compared with those who were euthyroid antibody-positive (95). Recurrence of transient PPT has been observed in small numbers of patients, and a recurrence rate as high as 30–40% has been noted (reviewed in ref. 97). In women studied in two pregnancies, there was a 70% chance of developing recurrent PPT after a first attack and a 25% risk even if the woman was only anti-TPO-positive without thyroid dysfunction during the first postpartum period (43).

FUTURE DEVELOPMENTS

In our opinion, PPT represents a unique experiment of nature where the development of an autoimmune syndrome may be observed during a relatively short time period. Moreover, in many cases, the immune peturbations resolve, and the patient remains euthyroid. Although there have been advances in our understanding of the humoral and cellular immune changes during and after pregnancy, the complete immunopathological picture is not yet available. We need to know more about the immunogenetics as well as appreciating the effects of pregnancy hormones on the immune response during gestation. As suggested (80), it is possible that PPT is actually a disease of dysimmunoregulation of the immune system with its origins during gestation. We need answers as to the role of all currently known cytokines (the role of TGF-β1 has recently been described in PPT (98). These studies may be difficult in patients and normal pregnant women because of ethical considerations, but the opportunity should be taken to perform further studies on appropriate animal models. The phenomenon of microchimerism has been mentioned, but more understanding of this process in regard to PPT is required (99). A tentative pictorial representation of the development of PPT is presented in Fig. 4. Although it is logical to suggest that pregnancy may result in thyroid deficiency in predisposed women, there is no evidence that multiple pregnancy leads to more thyroid disease (100,101).

In view of the high incidence of PPT together with the accompanying medical and psychiatric symptomatology, it would seem logical that an appropriate screening program should exist. The presence of thyroid antibodies in early pregnancy at least alerts the clinician to the possibility of the condition even if their presence is only a 50% predictor of thyroid dysfunction at best. Further clinical features are required to improve the predictive power of TPO antibodies in this setting. For example, the measurement of serum thyroglobulin and biologically active TPO antibody may improve the prediction of thyroid dysfunction perhaps to 75–80%. Proponents of screening for PPTD justify it on the basis that it is relatively common, causes significant morbidity, and can be diagnosed with freely available tests that are inexpensive. Effective treatment is available if required. Screening may also be pertinent in view of the high incidence of long-term thyroid dysfunction in these women. However,

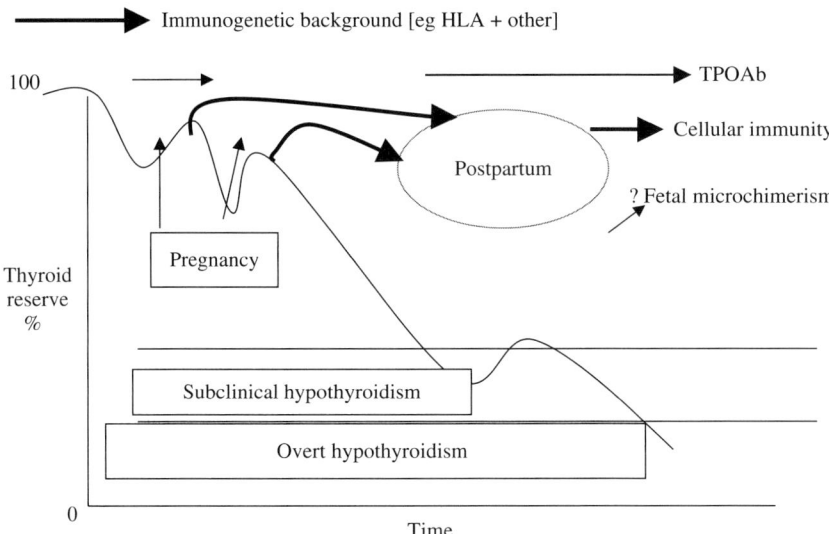

Fig. 4. The development of autoimmune thyroid disease postpartum. Diagram to illustrate a proposed development of hypothyroidism in relation to pregnancy (adapted from Muller et al. [9]).

there is a lack of consensus about the timing of screening or the screening test for PPTD prediction. TPOAb or TSH have all been suggested as possible screening tools. Opponents of screening cite the lack of good prospective cost-benefit analyses to support their view. A review of published data on PPTD prediction using thyroid antibodies in different population groups reveals several reasons for this lack of consensus such as variability of the antibody measured (microsomal or TPOAb), variations in assay methodology, as well as different times of screening during pregnancy and the postpartum period. However, the influence of disease definition and the effects of variability of genetic predisposition, frequency of blood testing, and study design should not be ignored, although TPOAb remains the leading candidate for PPTD screening. The sensitivity, specificity, and positive predictive value of TPOAb in PPTD prediction are highly variable and are dependent to some extent upon the above factors (Table 1). Further refinements to the screening strategy have been suggested to improve its positive predictive value. A variable degree of enthusiasm for screening of this condition has been expressed *(102)* and a compromise would seem to be targeted screening of individuals at the highest risk of developing PPTD, such as subjects with previous PPTD and type 1 diabetes mellitus. The cost of testing is relatively high, but new assay techniques may reduce this *(103,104)*. The high incidence of the disease suggests that a significant reduction in postpartum morbidity will be derived from this strategy.

REFERENCES

1. Glinoer D. The regulation of thyroid function in pregnancy: pathways of endocrine adaptation from physiology to pathology. *Endocr Rev* 1997;18:404–433.
2. Weetman AP. The immunology of pregnancy. *Thyroid* 1999;9:643–646.

3. Wegmann TG, Lin H, Guilbert L, Mosmann TR. Bidirectional cytokine interactions in the maternal-fetal relationship: is successful pregnancy a Th2 phenomenon? *Immunol Today* 1993;14:353–356.

4. Davies TF. The thyroid immunology of the postpartum period. *Thyroid* 1999;9:675–684.

5. Amino N, Tada H, Hidaka Y. Thyroid disease after pregnancy: post-partum thyroiditis. In: Wass JAH, Shalet SM (eds), *Oxford Textbook of Endocrinology and Diabetes*. Oxford, UK: Oxford University Press, 2002:527–532.

6. Roberton HEW. Lassitude, coldness, and hair changes following pregnancy, and their response to treatment with thyroid extract. *Br Med J* 1948;2:93–94.

7. Amino N, Miyai KJ, Onishi T, et al. Transient hypothyroidism after delivery in autoimmune thyroiditis. *J Clin Endocinol Metab* 1976;42:296–301.

8. Ginsberg J, Walfish PG. Postpartum transient thyrotoxicosis with painless thyroiditis. *Lancet* 1977;1:1125–1128.

9. Muller AF, Drexhage HA, Berghout A. Postpartum thyroiditis and autoimmune thyroiditis in women of childbearing age: recent insights and consequences for antenatal and postnatal care. *Endocr Rev* 2001;22:605–630.

10. Lazarus JH, Premawardhana LDKE, Parkes AB. Postpartum thyroiditis. *Autoimmunity* 2002;35:169–173.

11. Stagnaro-Green A. Postpartum thyroiditis. *Best Pract Res Clin Endocrinol Metab* 2004;18:303–316.

12. Lazarus JH. Sporadic and postpartum thyroiditis. In: Braverman LE, Utiger RD (eds), *The Thyroid: A Fundamental and Clinical Text*. 9th edn. New York: Lippincott Williams and Wilkins, 2005:524–535.

13. Kuijpens JL, De Hann-Meulman M, Vader HL, Pop VJ, Wiersinga WM, Drexhage HA. Cell-mediated immunity and postpartum thyroid dysfunction: a possibility for the prediction of disease? *J Clin Endocrinol Metab* 1998;83: 1959–1966.

14. Lazarus JH, Hall R, Othman S, Parkes AB, Richards CJ, McCulloch B, Harris B. The clinical spectrum of postpartum thyroid disease. *Quart J Med* 1996;89:429–435.

15. Caixas A, Albareda M, Garcia-Patterson A, et al. Postpartum thyroiditis in women with hypothyroidism antedating pregnancy. *J Clin Endocrinol Metab* 1999;84:4000–4005.

16. Marqusee E, Hill JA, Mandel SJ. Thyroiditis after pregnancy loss. *J Clin Endocrinol Metab* 1997;82:2455–2457.

17. Harris B, Othman S, Davies JA, et al. Association between postpartum thyroid dysfunction and thyroid antibodies and depression. *BMJ* 1992;305:152–156.

18. Kent GN, Stuckey BG, Allen JR, Lambert T, Gee V. Postpartum thyroid dysfunction: clinical assessment and relationship to psychiatric affective morbidity. *Clin Endocrinol (Oxf)* 1999;51:429–438.

19. Amino N, Mori H, Iwatani Y, et al. High prevalence of transient post-partum thyrotoxicosis and hypothyroidism. *N Engl J Med* 1982;306:849–852.

20. Jansson R, Bernander S, Karlsson A, Levin K, Milsson G. Autoimmune thyroid dysfunction in the post partum period. *J Clin Endocrinol Metab* 1984;58:681–687.

21. Freeman R, Rosen H, Thysen B. Incidence of thyroid dysfunction in an unselected postpartum population. *Arch Intern Med* 1986;146:1361–1364.

22. Lervang HH, Pryds O, Ostergaard Kristensen HP. Thyroid dysfunction after delivery: incidence and clinical course. *Acta Med Scand* 1987;222:369–374.

23. Nikolai TF, Turney SL, Roberts RC. Postpartum lymphocytic thyroiditis. Prevalence, clinical course and long-term follow-up. *Arch Intern Med* 1987;221–224.

24. Hayslip CC, Fein HG, O'Donnell CM, Friedman DS, Klein TA, Smallridge RC. The value of serum antimicrosomal antibody testing in screening for symptomatic postpartum thyroid dysfunction. *Am J Obstet* 1988;159:203–209.

25. Vargas MT, Briones-Urbina R, Gladman D, Papsin FR, Walfish PG. Antithyroid microsomal autoantibodies and HLA-DR5 are associated with postpartum thyroid dysfunction: evidence supporting an autoimmune pathogenesis. *J Clin Endocrinol Metab* 1988;67:327–333.

26. Fung HY, Kologlu M, Collison K, John R, Richards CJ, Hall R, McGregor AM. Postpartum thyroid dysfunction in Mid Glamorgan. *BMJ* 1988;296:241–244.

27. Rajatanavin R, Chailurkit LO, Tirarungsikul K, Chalayondeja W, Jittivanich U, Puapradit W. Postpartum thyroid dysfunction in Bangkok: a geographical variation in the prevalence. *Acta Endocrinol (Copenh)* 1990;122:283–287.

28. Rasmussen NG, Hornnes PJ, Hoier-Madsen M, Feldt-Rasmussen U, Hegedus L. Thyroid size and function in healthy pregnant women with thyroid autoantibodies. Relation to development of postpartum thyroiditis. *Acta Endocrinol (Copenh)* 1990;123:395–401.

29. Roti E, Bianconi L, Gardini E, et al. Postpartum thyroid dysfunction in an Italian population residing in an area of mild iodine deficiency. *J Endocrinol Invest* 1991;14:669–674.

30. Walfish PG, Meyerson J, Provias JP, Vargas MT, Papsin FR. Prevalence and characteristics of post-partum thyroid dysfunction: results of a survey from Toronto, Canada. *J Endocrinol Invest* 1992;15:265–272.

31. Stagnaro-Green A, Roman SH, Cobin RH, el Harazy E, Wallenstein S, Davies TF. A prospective study of lymphocyte-initiated immunosuppression in normal pregnancy: evidence of a T-cell etiology for postpartum thyroid dysfunction. *J Clin Endocrinol Metab* 1992;74:645–653.

32. Pop VJ, de Rooy HA, Vader HL, van der HD, van Son MM, Komproe IH. Microsomal antibodies during gestation in relation to postpartum thyroid dysfunction and depression. *Acta Endocrinol (Copenh)* 1993;129:26–30.

33. Lucas A, Pizarro E, Granada ML, Salinas I, Fox M, Sanmarti A. Postpartum thyroiditis: epidemiology and clinical evolution in a nonselected population. *Thyroid* 2000;10:71–77.

34. Barca MF, Knobel M, Romimori E, Cardia MS, Medeiros-Neto G. Prevalence and characteristics of postpartum thyroid dysfunction in Sao Paulo, Brazil. *Clin Endocrinol (Oxf)* 2000;53:21–31.

35. Sakaihara M, Yamada H, Kato EH, et al. Postpartum thyroid dysfunction in women with normal thyroid function during pregnancy. *Clin Endocrinol (Oxf)* 2000;53:487–492.

36. Shahbazian HB, Sarvghadi F, Azizi F. Prevalence and characteristics of postpartum thyroid dysfunction in Tehran. *Eur J Endocrinol* 2001;145:397–401.

37. Bagis T, Gokeel A, Saygili ES. Autoimmune thyroid disease in pregnancy and the postpartum period: relationship to spontaneous abortion. *Thyroid* 2001;11:1049–1053.

38. Hauerova D, Pikner R, Topolcan O, Mrazova D, Holubee L Jr, Pecen L. Thyroid Disease in pregnant women and its development after childbirth. *Vnitr Lek* 2002;48:1060–1064.

39. Zargar AH, Shah IH, Masoodi SR, Laway BA, Salahuddin M, Bhat IA. Postpartum thyroiditis in India: prevalence of postpartum thyroiditis in Kashmir Valley of Indian sub-continent. *Exp Clin Endocrinol Diabetes* 2002;110:171–175.

40. Kita M, Goulis DG, Avramides A. Post-partum thyroiditis in a Mediterranean population: a prospective study of a large cohort of thyroid antibody positive women at the time of delivery. *J Endocrinol Invest* 2002;25:513–519.

41. Li D, Li CY, Teng WP. Prevalence of postpartum thyroiditis in three different iodine intake areas. *Zhonghua Fu Chan Ke Za Zhi* 2003;38:216–218.

42. Gerstein HC. Incidence of postpartum thyroid dysfunction in patients with type I diabetes mellitus. *Ann Intern Med* 1993;118:419–423.

43. Lazarus JH, Ammari F, Oretti R, Parkes AB, Richards CJ, Harris B. Clinical aspects of recurrent postpartum thyroiditis. *Br J Gen Pract* 1997;47:305–308

44. Memon A, Radovanovic Z, Suresh A. Epidemiological evidence for a link between postpartum thyroiditis and thyroid cancer. *Eur J Epidemiol* 2004;19:607–609.

45. Jenkins H, Farid NR. Subacute thyroiditis like syndrome sin relation to HLA. *Tissue Antigens* 1979;13:167–169.

46. Kologlu M, Fung H, Darke C, Richards CF, Hall R, McGregor AM. Postpartum thyroid dysfunction and HLA status. *Eur J Clin Invest* 1990;20:56–60.

47. Farid NR, Hawe BS, Walfish PG. Increased frequency of HLA-DR3 and 5 in the syndromes of painless thyroiditis with transient thyrotoxicosis: evidence for an autoimmune etiology. *Clin Endocrinol* 1983;19:699–704.

48. Thompson P, Farid NR. Post-partum thyroiditis and goitrous (Hashimoto's) thyroiditis are associated with HLA-DR4. *Immunol Lett* 1985;11:301–303.

49. Lervang HH, Pryds O, Kristensen HPO, Jakobsen BK, Svejgaard A. Post-partum autoimmune thyroid disorder associated with HLA-DR4? *Tissue Antigens* 1984;23:2500–2502.

50. Jansson R, Safwenberg J, Hahlberg PA. Influence of the HLA-DR4 antigen and iodine status on the development of autoimmune postpartum thyroiditis. *J Clin Endocrinol Metab* 1985;60:168–173.

51. Pryds O, Lervang H-H, Ostergaard Kristensen HP, Jakobsen BK, Svejgaard A. HLA-DR factors associated with postpartum hypothyroidism: an early manifestation of Hashimoto's thyroiditis? *Tissue Antigens* 1987;30:34–37.

52. Parkes AB, Darke C, Othman S, et al. MHC class II and complement polymorphism in postpartum thyroiditis. *Eur J Endocrinol* 1996;134:449–453.

53. Tachi J, Amino N, Tamaki H, et al. Long term follow-up and HLA association in patients with postpartum hypothyroidism. *J Clin Endocrinol Metab* 1988;66:480–484.

54. Lazarus JH. Impact of iodide on thyroid autoimmunity. *Curr Opin Endocrinol Diabetes* 2004;11;205–208.

55. Kampe O, Jansson R, Karlsson FA. Effects of L-thyroxine and iodide on the development of autoimmune postpartum thyroiditis. *J Clin Endocrinol Metab* 1990;70:1014–1018.

56. Othman S, Phillips DIW, Lazarus JH, Parkes AB, Richards C, Hall R. Iodine metabolism in postpartum thyroiditis. *Thyroid* 1992;2:107–111.

57. Triggiani V, Ciampolillo A, Guastamacchia E, et al. Prospective study of post-partum thyroid immune dysfunctions in type 1 diabetic women and in a healthy control group living in a mild iodine deficient area. *Immunopharmacol Immunotoxicol* 2004;26:215–224.

58. Reinhardt W, Kohl S, Hollmann D, et al. Efficacy and safety of iodine in the postpartum period in an area of mild iodine deficiency. *Eur J Med Res* 1998;3:203–210.

59. Nohr SB, Jorgensen A, Pedersen KM, Laurberg P. Postpartum thyroid dysfunction in pregnant thyroid peroxidase antibody-positive women living in an area with mild to moderate iodine deficiency: is iodine supplementation safe? *J Clin Endocrinol Metab* 2000;85:3191–3198.

60. Lazarus JH. Iodine and Brain Function. In: Lieberman HR, Kanarek RB, Prasad C (eds), *Nutritional Neuroscience*. Boca Raton, FL: CRC Press, 2005:261–274.

61. Mizukami Y, Michigishi T, Nonomura A, et al. Postpartum thyroiditis – a clinical, histological and immunologic study of 15 cases. *Am J Clin Pathol* 1993;100:200–205.

62. Parkes AB, Darke C, Othman S, Thomas M, Young N, Richards CJ, Hall R, Lazarus JH. Major histocompatibility complex class II and complement polymorphism in postpartum thyroiditis. *Eur J Endocrinol* 1996;134: 449–453.

63. Ratanachaiavong S, Memaine AG, Campbell RD, McGregor AM. Heath shock protein 70 (HSP70) and complement C4 genotypes in patients with hyperthyroid Graves' disease. *Clin Exp Immunol* 1991;84:48–52.

64. Parkes AB, Othman S, Hall R, John R, Richards CJ, Lazarus JH. The role of complement in the pathogenesis of postpartum thyroiditis. *J Clin Endocrinol Metab* 1994;79:395–400.

65. Jansson R, Karlsson FA, Linde A, Sjoberg O. Postpartum activation of autoimmunity: transient increase of total IgG levels in normal women and in women with autoimmune thyroiditis. *Clin Exp Immunol* 1987;70:68–73.

66. Jansson R, Thompson PM, Clark F, McLachlan SM. Association between thyroid microsomal antibodies of subclass IgG-1 and hypothyroidism in autoimmune postpartum thyroiditis. *Clin Exp Immunol* 1986;63:80–86.

67. Hall R, Fund M, Kologu M et al. Postpartum thyroid dysfunction. In: Pinchera A, Ingbar SH, McKenzie JM, Fenzi GF (eds), *Thyroid Autoimmunity*. New York: Plenum Press, 1987:211–219.

68. Weetman AP, Fung HYM, Richards CJ, McGregor AM. IgG subclass distribution and relative functional affinity of thyroid microsomal antibodies in postpartum thyroiditis. *Eur J Clin Invest* 1990;20:133–136.

69. Briones-Urbina R, Parkes AB, Bogner U, Mariotti S, Walfish PG. Increase in antimicrosomal antibody related IgG1, IgG2 and IgG3 and titres of antithyroid peroxidase antibodies, but not antibody dependent cell mediated cytotoxicity in post-partum thyroiditis with transient hyperthyroidism. *J Endocrinol Invest* 1990;13:879–886.

70. Jaume JC, Parkes AB, Lazarus JH, Hall R, Costantes G, McLachlan SM, Rapoport B. Thyroid peroxidase autoantibody fingerprints. II. A longitudinal study in postpartum thyroididis. *J Clin Endocrinol Metab* 1995;80:1000–1005.

71. Parkes AB, Williams S, Howells RD, Harris R, Lazarus JH, Waters JS, Hall R. The measurement of complement fixation by autoantibodies directed against thyroid membrane antigens. *J Clin Lab Immunol* 1991;35:1–7.

72. Carney DF, Lang JT, Shin ML. Multiple signal messengers generated by terminal complement complexes and their role in terminal complement complex elimination. *J Immunol* 1990;145:623–629.

73. Parkes AB, Adams H, Othman S, Hall R, John R, Lazarus JH. The role of complement in the pathogenesis of postpartum thyroiditis. Ultrasound echogenicity and the degree of complement induced thyroid damage. *Thyroid* 1996;6:177–182.

74. Parkes AB, Othman S, Hall R, John R, Lazarus JH. The role of complement in the pathogenesis of postpartum thyroiditis: relationship between complement activation and disease presentation and progression. *Eur J Endorinol* 1995;133:210–215.

75. Morgan BP, Campbell AK. The recovery of human polymorphonuclear leucocytes from sublytic complement attack is mediated by intracellular calcium. *Biochem J* 1985;231:205–208.

76. Mower J, Rickards CR, Parkes AB, Wynford Thomas D. Thyroid peroxidase expression in the transformed thyroid cell line 'HTOR13' is TSH and cyclic AMP dependent. *J Endocrinol Invest* 1992;15:101.

77. Weetman AP, Cohen SB, Oleesky DA, Morgan BP. Terminal complement complexes and C1/C1 inhibitor complexes in autoimmune thyroid disease. *Clin Exp Immunol* 1989;77:25–30.

78. Okosieme OE, Parkes AB, McCullough B, Doukidis D, Morgan BP, Richards CJ, Lazarus JH. Complement activation in postpartum thyroiditis. *Quart J Med* 2002;95:173–179.

79. Elenkov IJ, Wilder RL, Bakalov VK, Link AA, Dimitrov MA, Fisher S, Crane M, Kanik KS, Chrousos GP. IL-12, TNF-α, and hormonal changes during late pregnancy and early postpartum: implications for autoimmune disease activity during these times. *J Clin Endocrinol Metab* 2001;86:4933–4938.

80. Kokandi AA, Parkes AB, Premawardhana LDKE, John R, Lazarus JH. Association of postpartum thyroid dysfunction with antepartum hormonal and immunological changes. *J Clin Endocrinol Metab* 2003;88:1126–1132.

81. Evans PC, Lambert N, Maloney S, Furst DE, Moore JM, Nelson JL. Long-term fetal microchimerism in peripheral blood mononuclear cell subsets in healthy women and women with scleroderma. *Blood* 1999;93:2033–2037.

82. Gannage M, Amoura Z, Lantz O, Piette JC, Caillat-Zucman S. Feto-maternal microchimerism in connective tissue diseases. *Eur J Immunol* 2002;32:3405–3413.

83. Ando T, Davies TF. Self-recognition and the role of fetal microchimerism. *Best Pract Res Clin Endocrinol Metab* 2004;18:197–211.

84. Ando T, Imaizumi M, Graves P, et al. Fetal microchimerism in human Graves' disease. *J Clin Endocrinol Metab* 2002;87:3315–3320.

85. Klintschar M, Schwaiger P, Mannweiler S, et al. Evidence of fetal microchimerism in Hashimoto's thyroiditis. *J Clin Endocrinol Metab* 2001;86:2494–2498.

86. Srivatsa B, Srivatsa S, Johnson KL, et al. Microchimerism of presumed fetal origin in thyroid specimens from women: a case-control study. *Lancet* 2001;358:2034–2038.

87. Badenhoop K. Intrathyroidal microchimerism in Graves' disease or Hashimoto's thyroiditis: regulation of tolerance or alloimmunity by fetal-maternal immune interactions? *Eur J Endocrinol* 2004;150:421–423.

88. John R, Othman S, Parkes AB, Lazarus JH, Hall R. Interference in thyroid function tests in postpartum thyroiditis. *Clin Chem* 1991;37:1397–1400.

89. Adams H, Jones MC, Othman S, Lazarus JH, Parkes AB, Hall R, Phillips DIW, Richards CJ. The sonographic appearances in postpartum thyroiditis. *Clin Radiol* 1992;45:311–318.

90. Parkes AB, Black EG, Adams H, John R, Richards CJ, Hall R, Lazarus JH. Serum thyroglobulin – an early indicator of autoimmune postpartum thyroiditis. *Clin Endocrinol* 1994;41:9–14.

91. Salvi M, Girasole G, Pedrazzoni M, Passeri M, Guiliani N, Minelli R, Braverman LE, Roti E. Increased serum concentrations of interleukin-6 (IL-6) and soluble Il-6 receptor in patients with Graves' disease. *J Clin Endocrinol Metab* 1996;81:2976–2979.

92. Bartalena L, Brogioni S, Grasso L, Rago T, Vitti P, Pinchera A, Martino E. Interleukin-6: a marker of thyroid destructive processes? *J Clin Endocrinol Metab* 1994;79:1424–1427.

93. Ahmad L, Parkes A, Lazarus JH, Bartalena L, Martino E, Diamond E, Stagnaro-Green A. Interleukin-6 levels are not increased in women with postpartum thyroid dysfunction. *Thyroid* 1998;8:371–375.

94. Pearce EN, Bogazzi F, Martino E, Brogioni S, Pardini E, Pellegrini G, Parkes AB, Lazarus JH, Pinchera A, Braverman LE. The prevalence of elevated serum C-reactive protein levels in inflammatory and noninflammatory thyroid disease. *Thyroid* 2003;13;643–648.

95. Premawardhana LDKE, Parkes AB, Ammari F, John R, Darke C, Adams H, Lazarus JH. Postpartum thyroiditis and long-term thyroid status: prognostic influence of thyroid peroxidase antibodies and ultrasound echogenicity. *J Clin Endocrinol Metab* 2000;85:71–75.

96. Othman S, Phillips DIW, Parkes AB, Richards CJ, Harris B, Fung H, Darke C, John R, Hall R, Lazarus JH. Long term follow-up of post-partum thyroiditis. *Clin Endocrinol* 1990;32:550–564.

97. Lazarus JH, Premawardhana LDKE, Parkes AB. Postpartum thyroiditis. In: Weetman AP (ed.), *Immunology & Medicine Series. Endocrine Autoimmunity and Associated Conditions*, Vol. 27. London: Kluwer Academic Publishers, 1998:83–97.

98. Olivieri A, De Angelis S, Vaccari V, Valensise H, Magnani F, Stazi MA, Cotichini R, Gilardi E, Cordeddu V, Sorcini M, Boirivant M. Postpartum thyroiditis is associated with fluctuations in transforming growth factor-β1 serum levels. *J Clin Endocrinol Metab* 2003;88:1280–1284.

99. Bianchi DW, Romero R. Biological implications of bi-directional fetomaternal cell traffic: a summary of a National Institute of Child Health and Human Development-sponsored conference. *J Matern Fetal Neonatal Med* 2003;14:123–129.

100. Phillips DIW, Lazarus JH, Butland BK. Influence of pregnancy and reproductive span on the occurrence of autoimmune thyroiditis. *Clin Endocrinol* 1990;32:301–306.

101. Walsh JP, Bremner AP, Bulsara MK, O'Leary P, Leedman PJ, Feddema P, Michelangeli V. Parity and the risk of autoimmune thyroid disease: a community-based study. *J Clin Endocrinol Metab* 2005;90:5309–5312.

102. Amino N, Tada Hidaka Y, Crapo LW, Stagnaro-Green A. Therapeutic controversy: screening for postpartum thyroiditis. *J Clin Endocrinol Metab* 1999;84:1813–1821.

103. Hofman LF, Foley TP, Henry JJ, Naylor EW. The use of filter paper-dried blood spots for thyroid-antibody screening in adults. *J Lab Clin Med* 2004;144:307–312.
104. Burne P, Mitchell S, Rees Smith B. Point-of-care assays for autoantibodies to thyroid peroxidase and to thyroglobulin. *Thyroid* 2005;15:1005–1010.

9

Thyroid-Associated Ophthalmopathy and Dermopathy

Wilmar M. Wiersinga, MD, PhD

Contents

Summary

Graves' ophthalmopathy (thyroid-associated ophthalmopathy [TAO]) and dermopathy (thyroid-associated dermopathy [TAD]) are extrathyroidal manifestations of Graves' disease, which should be viewed as a multisystem autoimmune disease involving thyrocytes but also orbital and pretibial fibroblasts. Smoking is a risk factor for TAO, and cessation of smoking is useful in the primary, secondary, and tertiary prevention of TAO. The immunopathogenesis of TAO and TAD looks very similar. Fibroblasts expressing functional thyroid-stimulating hormone (TSH) receptors have been identified as the target cells of the autoimmune attack. T cells sensitized to thyroid antigens (or TSH receptor stimulating antibodies, TSAb, in later stages) may recognize shared antigens on fibroblasts, inducing release of cytokines. This results in the production of hydrophylic glycosaminoglycans, causing tissue swelling. Recent findings point to the insulin-like growth factor-1 receptor on fibroblasts as another likely autoantigen. TAO appears to be primarily a Th1-cell-mediated disease. Intravenous methylprednisolone pulses are now recommended as the treatment of choice in severe active TAO and topical corticosteroids under occlusive dressings for TAD. Rehabilitative surgery for TAO should wait until the disease has become inactive. Promising new but still experimental treatment modalities involve monoclonal antibodies against particular cytokines or T-cell surface molecules.

Key Words: Thyroid eye disease, pretibial myxoedema, immunopathogenesis, thyrotropin receptor, IGF-1 receptor, treatment, smoking.

From: *Contemporary Endocrinology: Autoimmune Diseases in Endocrinology*
Edited by: A. P. Weetman © Humana Press, Totowa, NJ

INTRODUCTION

Graves' disease is primarily characterized by hyperthyroidism caused by thyroid-stimulating hormone (TSH) receptor stimulating antibodies (TSAb). Because the autoimmune reaction is directed against the TSH receptor (TSHR) in the thyroid gland, Graves' disease has been considered as the prime example of an organ-specific autoimmune disease. This view, however, seems to be too restricted as it does not take into account the three extrathyroidal manifestations of Graves' disease: thyroid-associated ophthalmopathy (TAO), thyroid-associated dermopathy (TAD), and acropachy. The extrathyroidal phenotypes of Graves' disease cannot be explained by thyroid hormone excess itself. It is doubtful—as will be argued next—whether TSAb can be held fully responsible for the phenotypic variation, although the concentration of serum TSAb in general is higher in TAO and even more so in TAD than in Graves' hyperthyroidism without extrathyroidal manifestations (1). These kinds of considerations have led some authors to view Graves' disease as a multisystem autoimmune disease, in which the autoimmune attack is directed not only toward thyrocytes but also against fibroblasts in the orbit and the dermis (2).

The present review is limited to TAO (also known as thyroid eye disease, Graves' ophthalmopathy, or Graves' orbitopathy) and TAD (also known as pretibial or localized myxoedema), focusing on advances in knowledge obtained since 1990. Considerable progress in understanding the nature of these conditions has been made, but it is fair to say that TAO and TAD are still one of the remaining enigmas of autoimmune thyroid diseases (AITD) with respect to their immunopathogenesis as well as to their management. This is the more worrisome as the burden of disease of these conditions can be substantial: the health-related quality of life in TAO patients is indeed markedly decreased and lower than that of patients with diabetes mellitus, emphysema, or heart failure (3). A short look at the appearance of extrathyroidal manifestations of Graves' disease suffices to understand how the cosmetically disfiguring and the functionally invalidating changes can have a serious impact on the patient's daily life. The NO SPECS classification of eye changes (Table 1) serves as a mnemonic in the examination of the ophthalmopathy.

EPIDEMIOLOGY

A population-based cohort study in Olmsted Country, Minnesota, reports an overall age-adjusted incidence rate of TAO of 16.0 women and 2.9 men per 100,000 inhabitants per year (4). The incidence rate exhibits an apparent bimodal peak in the fifth and the seventh decade of life. Seventy-four percent of the cases had minor eye changes not requiring specific treatment other than supportive measures. Smoking greatly increases the risk for TAO (odds ratio 7.7, 95% confidence interval [CI] 4.3–13.7), and smokers have more severe eye disease than non-smokers (5). A trend toward a lower incidence rate of TAO has been observed since 1990. In a questionnaire survey among thyroidologists from 15 European countries in 1998, 43% of the respondents thought TAO was decreasing in frequency, 42% thought it unchanged, and 12% thought it to be increasing (6). In this respect, it is noteworthy that all responders from Hungary and Poland, where the population of smokers in the general population had increased since 1990, indicated an increased incidence of TAO. The overall trend toward a lower

Table 1

The NO SPECS Classification of Eye Changes in Thyroid-Associated Ophthalmopathy

Class	Description	Signs and symptoms	Immediate cause	Assessment
0	No signs or symptoms			
1	Only signs, no symptoms	Lid retraction, stare, lid lag	Hyperadrenergic tone of thyrotoxicosis. Infiltration of superior rectus/levator complex	Lid aperture in mm
2	Soft tissue involvement	Swelling and redness of eyelids, conjunctiva, and caruncle. Photophobia, lacrimation, grittiness, orbital pain	Impairment of venous drainage; herniation of fat through orbital septum	Color slides, clinical activity score
3	Proptosis	Exophthalmos	Increased retrobulbar pressure pushes globe forward	Hertel exophthalmometry in mm
4	Extraocular muscle involvement	Restricted eye muscle motility; Diplopia (intermittent: at awakening or when tired; inconstant: only at extremes of gaze; constant: in primary gaze or reading position)	Swelling of eye muscles impairs muscle relaxation	Range of motion in various direction of gaze; field of single binocular vision
5	Corneal improvement	Keratitis, corneal ulcer	Overexposure of cornea; disrupted tear film	Rose bengal or fluorescein
6	Sight loss because of optic nerve involvement	Decreased visual acuity; disturbed color vision; visual field defects	Pressure on optic nerve	Visual acuity, color vision, visual fields, papillary function, fundoscopy

incidence rate of TAO might therefore be causally linked to a secular decrease in the prevalence of smoking. An alternative explanation could be earlier diagnosis and treatment of hyperthyroidism (because of the introduction of sensitive TSH assays in the late 1980s), which might prevent to some extent the development of eye changes. A study from the United Kingdom reported a declining proportion of patients with TAO among all referred patients with Graves' hyperthyroidism from 57% in 1960 to 35% in 1990; there was also a decline in the prevalence of severe TAO (dipoplia or optic neuropathy) from 30 to 21% *(7)*.

Most cases of TAO (93%) are indeed observed in patients with Graves' hyperthyroidism, but 3% occur in hypothyroid patients and 4% are euthyroid *(8)*. Among the patients with TAO and Graves' hyperthyroidism, the eye disease becomes manifest before the onset of hyperthyroidism in about 20%, concurrent with hyperthyroidism in 40%, and after the onset of hyperthyroidism in 40% *(9)*. It is not unusual that hypothyroid TAO patients proceed to Graves' hyperthyroidism, probably caused by a shift from TSHR-blocking antibodies to TSAb. Euthyroid TAO patients also develop hyperthyroidism in due time in about 20% of cases, but it is unknown why others remain euthyroid although TSAb can be detected in almost everyone *(10)*. AITD (or, more specific, autoimmunity to the TSHR) thus seems to be present in most if not all TAO patients.

Conversely, TAO seems also to be present in most if not all patients with Graves' hyperthyroidism, although more than half of them have no clinically appreciable TAO. Evidence for subclinical TAO is, however, found in most of the patients without apparent eye changes, including a shift to higher proptosis values than in healthy controls, an abnormal increase in intraocular pressure on upgaze in 61% and enlarged extraocular muscles on computerized tomography (CT) scan or ultrasound in 70–100% *(9)*. The data strongly support the view that the eye and thyroid manifestations belong to the same disease entity: Graves' disease.

GENETIC AND ENVIRONMENTAL FACTORS

Graves' disease is generally viewed as a multifactorial disease in which the autoimmune reaction to thyroidal antigens arises against a certain genetic background, probably provoked by environmental factors. Despite many efforts including wide genome screening the genes involved remain largely unknown. There is consensus on three genes contributing (albeit to a modest degree) to the susceptibility for Graves' disease: *HLA-DR3, CTLA-4*, and *PTPN22*. Here, we address the question whether the phenotypic variation in Graves' disease is related to different genotypes; in other words, is there a difference in the frequency of polymorphisms of particular genes between TAO and non-TAO patients within the population of patients with Graves' hyperthyroidism? So far, the answer is predominantly negative *(11)*. Only human leukocyte antigen (HLA)-DPB1*201 appears to be slightly protective for TAO. The report that the biallelic polymorphism cytotoxic T-lymphocyte-associated antigen (CTLA)-4 A/G at codon 17 confers susceptibility to TAO (in which the strength of the association of the G allele with GO increased with the severity of the eye disease) *(12)* has not been confirmed in subsequent studies *(13,14)*. Non-genetic factors seem more likely to promote the phenotype TAO than genetic ones.

Indeed, among patients with Graves' hyperthyroidism, smoking carries a risk for the development of TAO with an odds ratio of 2.18 (95% CI 1.51–3.14) for current smokers *(15)*. The effect of smoking is further illustrated by a recent European questionnaire study on childhood TAO: TAO was observed in 37% of patients with juvenile Graves' hyperthyroidism, and its prevalence was higher in countries with a higher prevalence of smoking among teenagers *(16)*. Among TAO children in countries with a smoking prevalence of <25% among teenagers, about 20% were ≤10 years old and 80% were 11–18 years; in contrast, in countries with a smoking prevalence of ≥25% the distribution among the two age groups was roughly 50 and 50%. As it is unlikely that children below the age of 10 years are all smokers, the overrepresentation of TAO in children below 10 years living in an environment in which 25% or more of their peers smoke might be because of passive smoking *(16)*.

Another intriguing recent finding is that smoking seems to protect against the development of thyroid peroxidase antibodies (TPO-Ab) and elevated TSH *(17)*. In this respect, it is relevant to note that, in a population of patients with Graves' hyperthyroidism, the absence of TPO-Ab was an independent predictor of TAO *(18)*, suggesting that TPO-Ab confer moderate protection against TAO.

Which mechanisms cause these divergent effects of smoking remains largely obscure. Does smoke really gets into the eyes? Orbital fibroblasts (OF) produce more glycosaminoglycans (GAGs) when cultured under hypoxic conditions; tobacco glycoprotein enhances the production of interleukin (IL)-1, which also stimulates the secretion of GAGs *(19)*.

A combination of nicotin and tar with interferon (IFN)-γ led to upregulation of HLA-DR in OF *(20)*. Smoking enhances the generation of superoxide radicals and reduces the formation of antioxidants *(21)*. Systemic effects of smoking include B- and T-cell polyclonal activation with the resultant production of costimulatory cytokines *(22)*. Cytokines, adhesion molecules, and heat-shock proteins are all involved in the immunopathogenesis of TAO, and differences in the serum concentrations of some of these molecules have been observed between smokers and non-smokers and between TAO and non-TAO patients *(23,24)*. These differences may reflect to some extent what is going on in the orbit but may also just indicate more severe eye disease in smokers than in non-smokers *(11)*. Smoke exposure may lead to inflammation, lymphocyte recruitment, increased adhesion molecule expression and as a result more cell adhesion to vessel walls.

IMMUNOPATHOGENESIS

Pathology

The hallmark of TAO is an increased volume of orbital fatty/connective tissues and extraocular muscles *(25)*. The expanded tissue volume is because of adipose tissue expansion and accumulation of GAGs in the fatty/connective tissue compartments, and inflammation, edema, and GAG accumulation in the endomysial connective tissues. The muscle fibres themselves are intact and widely separated by edema; only in the later stages of the disease, the extraocular muscles may become fibrotic and atrophic. Orbital connective tissue GAGs amount to 254 µg/g wet tissue in TAO patients and 150 µg/g in controls; the higher GAG content in TAO is largely because of an excess of chondroitin sulfate and hyaluronic acid *(26)*. GAGs are large hydrophylic polyanionic compounds, which osmotically attract and bind large amounts of water, thus contributing to volume expansion. The increase in orbital contents and the resulting increase in intraorbital pressure (because of the constraints of the bony walls of the orbit) do explain in a mechanistic sense the eye changes in TAO (Table 1) *(27,28)*.

With regard to the immunopathogenesis of TAO, the most likely sequence of events is that T cells infiltrate the orbit and recognize an orbital autoantigen that is identical to or crossreactive with a thyroid autoantigen. The subsequent release of cytokines induces OF to secrete excessive amounts of GAGs, causing edema and swelling (Fig. 1) *(28)*.

Lymphocytic Infiltrate

A diffuse infiltration of lymphocytes is seen in orbital fatty/connective tissue and extraocular muscle interstitial tissue of TAO patients, composed mostly of T lymphocytes and macrophages with sparse B lymphocytes *(25)*. Both helper/inducer (CD4+) and suppressor/cytotoxic (CD8+) T lymphocytes are present; a substantial proportion of T cells are activated memory cells (CD45RO+), suggesting that TAO involves a T-mediated autoimmune response *(29–31)*.

Several studies have evaluated whether infiltrating T cells are primarily involved in cell-mediated (Th1) or humoral-mediated (Th2) immune responses. On the basis of the cytokine profile secreted by orbital T cell clones of TAO patients, it appears that both Th1 cells (IFN-γ) and Th2 cells (IL-4) are present as well as Th0 cells (producing both Th1 and Th2 cytokines), but Th1 cells are seen more frequently *(32–34)*. Another study reports predominance of the Th1 clones in cultures from patients with recent onset TAO (<2 years), and Th2 clones in patients with longer duration of TAO *(35)*. T-cell receptor V region gene usage is restricted in orbital tissue of active inflammatory TAO, but not longer so in longstanding inactive TAO presumably because of epitope spreading *(25, 36)*. The available data suggest that cell-mediated immunity by infiltrating T cells plays

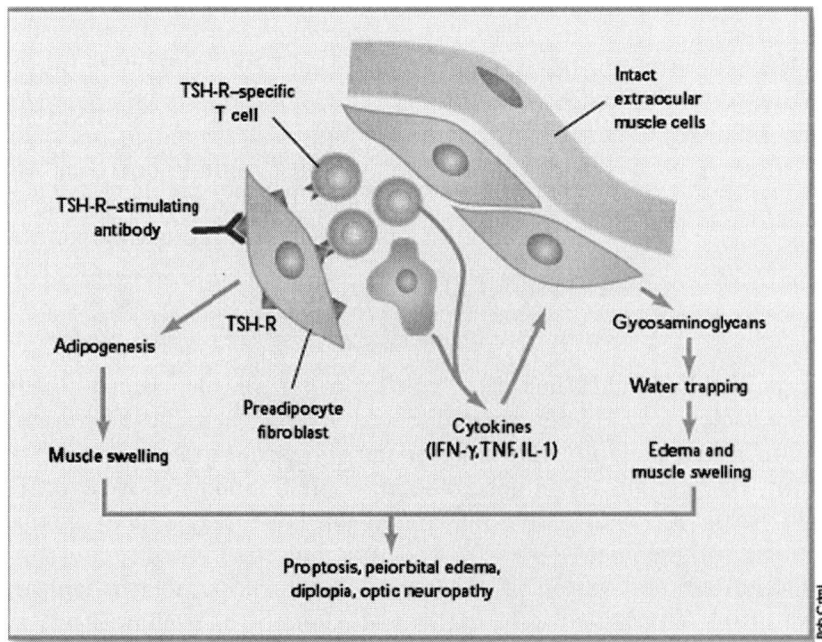

Fig. 1. Pathogenesis of TAO (reproduced with permission from ref. *28*).

a primary role in the immunopathogenesis of TAO. This view is in agreement with the absence of TAO in neonatal hyperthyroidism (caused by transplacental passage of TSHR antibodies), because T cells do not cross the placenta.

Recruitment of T cells to retrobulbar tissues requires attachment to endothelial cells and transendothelial migration, a process involving cytokine-induced expression of adhesion molecules on endothelial cells and lymphocytes. Adhesion molecules (intercellular adhesion molecule [ICAM]-1, vascular intercellular adhesion molecule [VCAM]-1, and endothelium intercellular adhesion molecule [ECAM]-1) are highly expressed in vascular endothelium in retrobulbar tissues of active TAO patients, but much less in inactive TAO (37). Infiltrating lymphocytes also express an increased number of adhesion molecules of the integrin family. Further recruitment of T cells may be facilitated by HLA-DR expression on endothelial cells and OF (29,31,37); the latter cells—upon exposure to Graves' immunoglobulin (Ig)G—produce the T-cell chemoattractants IL-16 and RANTES (38).

T-cell activation requires antigen presentation together with costimulatory signals. The number of macrophages infiltrating retrobulbar tissues is significantly increased in early TAO but less so in longstanding disease (29,50). Retrobulbar macrophages likely are able to activate T cells through antigen presentation and provision of costimulatory signals and by secreting proinflammatory cytokines such as IL-1β, tumour necrosis factor (TNF)-α, and IL-10 (39,40). For efficient activation of T-cell effector functions, it appears necessary that the cell surface receptor CD40 on antigen-presenting cells binds to the CD40 ligand (CD40L, a member of the TNF-α cytokine family) on T cells. Recent findings indicate an active CD40–CD40L pathway in OF. OF express CD40 and activation by CD40L induces hyaluronan synthesis, IL-6 and IL-8, and Cox-2 and PGE2 (41,42). The CD40–CD40L is thus one potential pathway by which T cells can activate fibroblasts.

Orbital Fibroblasts: The Target Cells

Retrobulbar T cells from TAO patients recognize autologous OF (but not eye muscle extracts) in a major histocompatibility complex (MHC) class I restricted manner and proliferate in response to TSHR antigen (43,44). Conversely, OF from TAO patients proliferate in response to autologous T lymphocytes, dependent on MHC class II and CD40–CD40L signaling (45). The data strongly suggest that OF are the target cells of the autoimmune attack in TAO. This view is strengthened by the finding that OF express the full-length TSHR, which is also functional as evident from an increase in cAMP in response to TSH (25,46,47). Interestingly, a subpopulation of OF called preadipocytes can differentiate in vitro into adipocytes; this process of adipogenesis is associated with increased TSHR expression and is—at least in vitro—stimulated by IL-6 and inhibited by TNF-α, IFN-γ, and transforming growth factor-β (TGF-β) (48,49). Evidence for enhanced adipogenesis in vivo is obtained from increased mRNA expression of leptin, adiponectin, PPARγ, and TSHR in TAO compared with normal orbital adipose tissue samples, with positive correlation in TAO tissues between TSHR and leptin and adiponectin and PPARγ (peroxisome proliferator-activated receptor γ) (50).

To further investigate the link between adipogenesis and TSHR expression, TAO-derived OF in culture were treated with rosiglitazone, a thiazolidinedione agonist of the PPARγ receptor that stimulates adipocyte differentiation; the drug stimulated

TSHR and PPARγ expression as well as differentiation into mature lipid-laden adipocytes *(51)*. The use of thiazolidinediones through induction of orbital fat expansion could thus be dangerous in TAO patients; indeed, exacerbation of TAO has been witnessed in a diabetic patient upon prescription of pioglitazone *(52)*. More genes are likely involved; one is secreted frizzled-related protein-1, which is unregulated in orbital adipose tissue of TAO patients and enhances adipogenesis and TSHR expression in cultured OF *(53)*. Differentiation of OF into adipocytes does not occur in fibroblasts displaying the surface glycoprotein Thy-1; in this respect, it is noteworthy that orbital fatty/connective tissue contains both Thy-1+ and Thy-1– OF but that perimysial OF in contrast express only Thy-1 uniformly *(54)*.

OF apparently differ from dermal fibroblasts *(55)*. In particular, the magnitude of cellular responses in OF to proinflammatory cytokines is far greater than that found in dermal fibroblasts. OF express high levels of PGE2 (prostaglandin E_2) when activated by proinflammatory cytokines *(25)*. Upon exposure to cytokines such as IL-1β, OF synthesize IL-6, IL-8, IL-16, and RANTES *(41,56)*, thereby activating and attracting T cells. As well as promoting adipogenesis, IL-6 may also activate B cells locally. When exposed to proinflammatory cytokines, OF synthesize high levels of hyaluronan, whereas the effect is limited or absent in dermal fibroblasts. The induction is dependent on *de novo* protein synthesis and can be inhibited by glucocorticoids *(25)*. Hyaluronan synthesis is catalysed by hyaluronan synthases, which in OF are upregulated by IL-1 and leukoregulin *(57)*. Degradation of GAGs is governed by hyaluronidase, which in contrast to dermal fibroblasts is not expressed by OF in culture *(25)*. The functional heterogeneity of fibroblasts at different anatomical sites may explain why activation of fibroblasts in Graves' disease remains restricted to the orbit (and sometimes to local areas in the dermis when under mechanical pressure as in pretibial myxedema) *(27)*.

The Nature of the Autoantigen

TSH RECEPTOR

The presence of a functional TSHR on OF strongly suggests that the TSHR is indeed the long sought after shared antigen between the orbit and the thyroid. After all, TSAbs are the immediate cause of hyperthyroidism in Graves' disease, and the occurrence of TSHR outside the thyroid gland might explain the various phenotypic appearances of Graves' disease. In patients with untreated Graves' hyperthyroidism, the prevalence of TAO increases indeed with increasing TSAb levels *(18)*, and in TAO patients who had been euthyroid for at least 2 months, serum TSAbs are directly related to proptosis and the clinical activity score (CAS) *(58)*. In line with these data is the finding that TSHR expression in orbital fatty/connective tissue of TAO patients is much higher in the active than in the inactive stage of the disease and in direct relationship to local IL-1β mRNA levels *(34)*. Autoreactive T cells specific for the TSHR may recognize the orbital TSHR upon contact with macrophages presenting the autoantigenic peptides; TSAb could accelerate the immune response in the eye *(39)*. This issue, however, is far from being resolved: we do not really understand—apart from the role of smoking—why the majority of patients with Graves' hyperthyroidism despite high TSAb levels never develop overt ophthalmopathy. Animal experiments involving TSHR immunization so far also have failed to produce TAO *(59)* *(see* Chap. 4).

INSULIN-LIKE GROWTH FACTOR-1 RECEPTOR

It has been known for a long time that in vitro insulin-like growth factor (IGF)-1 stimulates the secretion of collagen and GAGs by OF *(27)*. Weightman et al. *(60)* demonstrated that [125I] IGF-1 binding to OF was displaced by Graves' IgG, suggesting the presence of IGF-1 receptor (IGF-1R) antibodies. Recent studies by Smith et al. *(61,62)* indicate that Graves' IgG (like IGF-1) recognizes the IGF-1R on OF, and by activating that receptor induce IL-16, RANTES and hyaluronan synthesis in these OF. The effects can be abolished by glucocorticoids and by specific IGF-1R-blocking monoclonal antibodies. The effects are not seen in non-TAO OF or in dermal fibroblasts. The data strongly suggest the possibility of IGF-1R as another relevant autoantigen in TAO. Any autoimmunity against IGF-1R, however, does not affect serum concentrations of free and total IGF-1 or IGF-binding proteins, which are completely normal in euthyroid patients with active TAO *(63)*.

OTHER AUTOANTIGENS

A number of antibodies against eye muscle antigens have been observed in the serum of TAO patients, but they do not seem to play a primary role in the immunopathogenesis of TAO. Most likely, the eye muscle antibodies are secondary to cytotoxic T-cell reactions in TAO *(64)*. Antibodies to thyroglobulin occur frequently in Graves' disease but are likely irrelevant in TAO in view of the poor binding of thyroglobulin to OF *(65)*.

Cytokine Profile

Cytokines are produced by inflammatory cells infiltrating the orbit as well as by OF. Locally produced cytokines stimulate proliferation and GAG production of OF; they also localize and augment the immune response by increasing the expression of MHC class II, adhesion molecules, heat-shock protein, CD40, and prostaglandin (Table 2) *(66)*. The listed functional effects of cytokines have been obtained from in

Table 2
Functional Effects of Cytokines in the Orbit in TAO[a]

	Increase
GAG synthesis	IL-1, IFN-γ, TGF-β
Cell proliferation	IL-1, IL-4, TGF-β
Class II expression[b]	IL-1, IFN-γ, TNF-α
Adhesion molecules expression	IL-1, IFN-γ, TNF-α
Heat shock proteins expression	IL-1, IL-6, IFN-γ, TNF-α, TGF-β
Metalloproteinase inhibitors	IL-1, IFNγ, TNF-α, TGF-β
TSHR expression[c]	IL-4, IL-6
CD 40 expression	IL-1, IFN-γ
Prostaglandin E2	IL-1, IL-4

IL, interleukin; IFN, interferon; TGF, transforming growth factor; TNF, tumor necrosis factor.

[a]From ref. *66* with some modifications.

[b]Decreased by IL-6.

[c]Decreased by IFNγ, TNFα, TGFβ.

vitro studies and may not necessarily reflect the in vivo effects. Cytokine profiles of orbital tissue samples have been made *(32–35,40)*, but proper interpretation requires knowledge about the duration and activity of TAO (early inflammatory or late fibrotic stage), any previous treatment (such as glucocorticoids and retrobulbar irradiation) and the cell types producing the cytokines. Activated T cells produce IFN-γ and IL-4, whereas antigen-presenting cells and T-cell activated macrophages produce IL-1β and TGF-β *(39)*. All four cytokines enhance inflammation and stimulate hyaluronan production. IL-1β especially is highly expressed in active TAO *(34,67)*.

DIAGNOSIS

The diagnosis of TAO is based on (1) evaluation of eye changes, (2) evidence of coexisting thyroid autoimmunity, and (3) imaging to exclude an alternative diagnosis. Usually the diagnosis is straightforward when a patient with known Graves' hyperthyroidism presents with bilateral fairly symmetrical eye changes. However, none of the eye changes is specific for TAO, and orbital imaging is required especially in unilateral ophthalmopathy.

Eye Changes

Evaluation of eye changes requires assessment of both disease severity and disease activity. Severity is judged by recording the present signs and symptoms of NO SPECS classes 1–6 (Table 1). Soft tissue involvement is most prevalent (75%), followed by proptosis >21 mm (63%), eye muscle motility dysfunction (49%), keratopathy (16%), and optic nerve involvement (21%) *(8)*. Activity can be judged by various imaging procedures (*see* "Orbital Imaging") but most easily by the CAS. One point is given for each of the following items if present: spontaneous retrobulbar pain; pain on attempted up, side, or down gaze; redness of eyelids; redness of conjunctiva; chemosis; swelling of the caruncle; eyelid edema or fullness. The maximum score is 7 *(68)*. A very useful detailed protocol with comparative photographs for objective assessment has been published *(69)*.

Ocular torticollis is present in 7%, lagophthalmos in 25%, and unilateral eye disease in 5%. TAO is the most frequent cause of unilateral ophthalmopathy. Usually, imaging reveals already some extraocular muscle enlargement in the fellow-eye, and bilateral TAO may develop shortly. Some cases, however, remain strictly unilateral for unknown reasons.

In TAO patients, about 75% are females, 40% are smokers, 14% have glaucoma or cataract, 9% have diabetes, and 9% have dermopathy (TAO) *(8)*.

Thyroid Autoimmunity

Associated hyperthyroidism or hypothyroidism because of AITD increases substantially the chance the eye changes are caused by TAO. In euthyroid patients, one should search for TPO-Ab, and especially for TSAb, which are present in most euthyroid TAO patients *(10)*. Higher TSAb are associated with more severe TAO *(18,70)*. Euthyroid TAO patients frequently develop hyperthyroidism with time, but some always remain euthyroid for unknown reasons.

Orbital Imaging

Orbital imaging by CT or magnetic resonance imaging (MRI) may not be necessary in most TAO patients because the diagnosis is self-evident. It is, however, indicated in unilateral ophthalmopathy (to exclude an alternative diagnosis), in suspected optic neuropathy (crowding of muscles in the apex of the orbit increases the risk on loss of visual functions) and before decompressive surgery (by CT to judge the bony surroundings of the orbit).

Increased size of both eye muscles and orbital fat is found in 46% of TAO-patients; 8% of patients have only increased size of the fat compartment *(71)*. The determinants of this differential involvement of orbital muscles and fat are unknown. Inferior (60%) and medial (50%) rectus muscles are most frequently enlarged, followed by the superior rectus/levator muscle complex (40%); why the lateral rectus muscle is enlarged only in 22% again is unclear *(9)*. In TAO, the muscle swelling is typically most prominent in the muscle belly, sparing the tendons. This is an important sign in the differential diagnosis with orbital myositis, in which the muscle tendons are thickened as well.

Various imaging procedures have been used as indicators of disease activity in TAO *(68,72)*. Active TAO is likely to be present in case of eye muscle reflectivity of <40% on A-mode ultrasonography, a prolonged T2 relaxation time MRI or a high orbital uptake on octreoscan. Interestingly, recombinant human TSH induced significant orbital uptake on octreoscan in a patient with inactive TAO and a negative scan before recombinant TSH *(73)*, further supporting involvement of TSHR in the pathogenesis of TAO. Recent developments are orbital scanning with ^{99m}Tc-P829 (depreotide, a peptide binding to somatostatin receptors 2, 3, and 5) *(74,75)* or ^{67}Gallium *(76)* and blood flow parameters in orbital vessels by Doppler sonography *(77)*. All these measurements have a good direct relationship with CAS and are helpful in predicting the response to immunosuppressive treatment of TAO. These techniques, however, are technically demanding and require considerable expertise; presently, they are performed in a few specialized centers. For day-to-day practice, the CAS may suffice despite its subjective nature, as the scoring is easy to do in a few minutes and inexpensive.

TREATMENT

TAO patients are best treated in a multidisciplinary setting of combined thyroid-eye clinics *(78)*. The management plan should be tailored according to the needs of the individual patient. Schematically, each plan should consider (1) cessation of smoking, (2) restoration and maintenance of euthyroidism, and (3) specific eye treatment.

Cessation of Smoking

There is good circumstantial evidence that refraining from smoking is effective in the primary, secondary, and tertiary prevention of TAO *(79)*. Current smokers consuming >20 cigarettes daily have a RR of 7.0 (95% CI 3.0–16.5) for developing diplopia; in heavy smokers who had quit their habit to smoke >20 cigarettes per day, the RR decreases to 1.9 (95% CI 0.5–7.7) *(80)*. Secondary prevention of TAO refers to patients with Graves' hyperthyroidism but without TAO: to stop smoking at this stage is sensible as recurrent hyperthyroidism (with the associated risk of TAO) after a course of antithyroid drugs is more frequent in smokers than in non-smokers *(81)*.

Tertiary prevention refers to measures that can be taken to inhibit further progression of TAO that already has become manifest. To stop smoking should still be beneficial because the response rate to immunosuppression is clearly lower in smokers than in non-smokers *(82,83)*.

Thyroid Treatment

Restoration and maintenance of a normal thyroid function is important for the eyes: eye changes are more severe in TAO patients who still have abnormal thyroid function and improve slightly (especially NO SPECS classes 2 and 4) upon achieving euthyroidism *(84)*. It has been a matter of debate if it matters for the eyes how the patient is rendered euthyroid (with antithyroid drugs, ^{131}I, or subtotal thyroidectomy). It seems that neither antithyroid drug treatment nor total thyroidectomy affect the natural course of TAO, whereas ^{131}I treatment may cause development or worsening of eye changes in about 15% *(68,85,86)*. The postradioiodine eye changes occur a few months after treatment but fortunately are mostly transient and can be prevented by a course of prednisone starting at the time of ^{131}I therapy *(86)*. It seems prudent to restrict prednisone treatment to those patients with Graves' hyperthyroidism who are at risk for TAO; identified risk factors are severe Graves' hyperthyroidism (plasma T3 > 5 nmol/l, pre-existent (active) ophthalmopathy, smoking, high TSAb and high TSH postradioiodine *(87)*. [131]I therapy in inactive TAO patients is not associated with deterioration of TAO provided postradioiodine hypothyroidism is prevented *(88)*.

If one accepts the view that autoimmunity to thyroid antigens (like the TSHR) is involved in the immunopathogenesis of TAO, it makes sense to get rid of all thyroid antigens by complete ablation of the thyroid gland. A case–control study, however, failed to demonstrate a greater benefit of near-total thyroidectomy as compared to antithyroid drugs with respect to the course of TAO *(89)*. A randomized clinical trial comparing total with subtotal thyroidectomy in patients with active TAO likewise did not find a better outcome of TAO after total thyroidectomy, which was moreover associated with a higher surgical complication rate *(90)*. A retrospective follow-up study in TAO patients reports that TAO becomes more often inactive after thyroidectomy plus ^{131}I ablation than after thyroidectomy alone *(91)*. The results of an ongoing Italian randomized trial comparing near-total thyroidectomy plus ^{131}I ablation with near-total thyroidectomy alone are eargerly awaited.

Eye Treatment

Treatment of eye changes involves general measures, which should be taken in any stage of the disease, and specific measures according to the severity and activity of TAO (Table 3). General measures include dark glasses against photophobia, prisms to alleviate diplopia, eye ointments, and occlusive eye pads at night in case of lagophthalmos and especially artificial tears that should be used liberally to protect the cornea. Specific measures depend primarily on the severity of TAO. Very severe cases (dysthyroid optic neuropathy [DON]) require immediate treatment. Mild TAO (only soft tissue involvement and/or slight proptosis and some restriction of eye muscle motility—mostly in elevation—with or without diplopia) may warrant a wait-and-see policy in view of the tendency to spontaneous improvement of eye changes in the natural course of the disease. Moderately severe TAO (marked proptosis and eye

Table 3
Specific Eye Treatment of TAO

In any stage	Local measures (dark glasses, eye ointments, prisms, and artificial tears)
In very severe TAO (optic neuropathy)	iv methylprednisolone pulses; if no improvement after 2 weeks, urgent surgical decompression
In moderate severe TAO	
If active	iv methylprednisolone pulses; in case of insufficient response: low dose oral prednisone with either retrobulbar irradiation or cyclosporin
If inactive	Rehabilitative surgery (orbital decompression, eye muscle, and eyelid surgery in this order as required)
In mild TAO	"Wait-and-see" policy; retrobulbar irradiation

muscle disturbances usually with diplopia but no optic neuropathy) may benefit from immunosuppressive treatment if the disease is still in its early active inflammatory stage but not in the late inactive fibrotic stage (Fig. 2) *(92)*. Rehabilitative surgery should wait until TAO has reached its inactive stage.

VERY SEVERE TAO (OPTIC NEUROPATHY)

Dysthyroid optic neuropathy (also called malignant exopthalmos) is the most severe expression of TAO. Affected patients are relatively older and more often males and heavy smokers. Usually, there is significant comorbidity, especially diabetes mellitus in which the outcome of DON is worse than in non-diabetics *(93)*. A recent randomized controlled trial—albeit of a limited sample size—indicates that immediate decompressive surgery does not result in a better outcome than methylprednisolone pulse therapy *(94)*. Therefore, it is recommended to start with 1-g methylprednisolone given

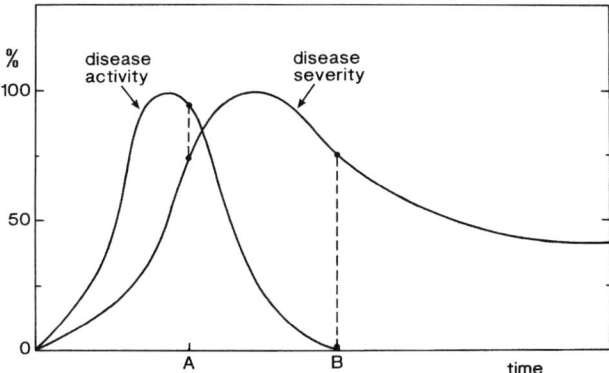

Fig. 2. Relationship between disease activity and disease severity in the natural history of TAO. The curve depicting disease severity reflects the tendency to spontaneous improvement. Immunosuppressive treatment is likely more effective when given in the early active stage (time A) than in the late inactive stage (time B) of the disease (reproduced with permission from ref. *92*).

intravenously on each of three successive days of the first week, to be repeated in the second week. If visual function improves after 2 weeks, one should continue with oral prednisone; if not, urgent surgical decompression of the orbit is indicated.

MILD TAO

Although mild TAO is not considered as mild by the patients themselves as evident from quality-of-life measurements *(95)*, most physicians will be reluctant to prescribe steroids at this stage in view of its side effects and the possibility of spontaneous improvement. Retrobulbar irradiation by virtue of its good tolerability is an option, as it has proven to be effective in mild TAO: in a randomized controlled trial, the outcome was successful in 52% of irradiated vs 27% of sham-irradiated patients ($p = 0.02$) *(96)*. Radiotherapy specifically improved eye muscle motility and decreased the severity of diplopia and orbital pain. It also decreased the proportion of patients requiring further treatment (66 vs 84% after sham-irradiation). On the contrary, radiotherapy did not prevent worsening of TAO ($\sim$15%), and the improvement in quality-of-life was also similar in both groups.

The efficacy of retrobulbar irradiation has also been proven in moderately severe TAO in one randomized trial *(97)* but not in another *(98)*. The latter, however, seems to be biased by for example pretreatment with glucocorticoids in 45%.

Retrobulbar irradiation is usually given in a dose of 20 Gy, administered in 10 daily doses of 2 Gy in 2 weeks. Lower doses might be equally effective: randomized controlled trials did not observe different outcomes between 10 Gy and 20 Gy *(99)* or between 2.4 Gy and 16 Gy *(100)*. Concern has been expressed on the safety of radiotherapy, but long-term follow-up studies so far have neither identified a single case of radiation-induced tumors nor an increased rate of cataract formation *(101–103)*. Retinal micro-aneurysms occur more often in irradiated than in non-irradiated patients, but they are few in number (<5), not associated with lower visual acuity and consequently without clinical significance *(103,104)*. Clear retinopathy after radiotherapy may develop in diabetic patients (RR 21, 95% CI 3–179) *(103)*. Diabetes and possibly hypertensive retinopathy are therefore contraindications for retrobulbar irradiation.

MODERATELY SEVERE TAO

Oral prednisone, retrobulbar irradiation, and intravenous immunoglobulins are all effective in moderately severe TAO, more so in improving soft tissue changes and eye muscle motility than in decreasing proptosis *(68)*. In general, one-third of patients do not respond, most likely because they were in the late inactive stage of TAO (Fig. 2). Restriction of immunosuppressive treatment to patients with active TAO will increase the response rate and save non-responders from its expense and side effects. Discrimination between active and inactive TAO is not always easy. Prognostic score charts using a number of disease activity parameters are able to predict accurately the outcome of immunosuppression in 89% but are not always feasible and await confirmation *(105)*. For daily practice, patients with a duration of TAO of <18 months and a CAS > 3 are likely to be still in the active stage.

Oral prednisone in combination with radiotherapy is more effective than prednisone alone, but two recent randomized clinical trials report that equally high response rates can be reached by using intravenous pulses of methylprednisolone: responders to iv pulses or oral steroids were 88 and 63%, respectively, in an Italian study *(106)* and 77 and 55% in an German study *(107)*; side effects were fewer in both studies after iv pulses than during oral medication. However, acute severe liver damage associated with iv pulse therapy has been observed by the Italian group in about 0.8%, leading to death in three patients *(108)*. This serious side effect remains incompletely understood but might be related to direct damage of hepatocytes and pre-existing liver steatosis, to precipitation of a virus-induced hepatitis or autoimmune hepatitis *(108,109)*. It is thus prudent to monitor liver function but also to assess before pulse therapy hepatitis serology, antinuclear antibodies and liver steatosis by ultrasound. Acute liver failure has not been observed in the German study, which applied a cumulative dose of 4.5 g steroids, much lower than that of about 10 g in the Italian study. Our current recommendation is therefore 500 mg methylprednisolone as a 2-h intravenous infusion every week for 6 weeks, followed by weekly 250 mg methylprednisolone infusions for another 6 weeks *(107)*.

In patients with a flare-up of TAO after discontinuation of steroids, the combination of a low dose of oral prednisone (20 mg daily) with either radiotherapy or cyclosporin might be beneficial *(68)*. Octreotide treatment in two placebo-controlled trials has no significant therapeutic effect on TAO *(110,111)*.

In patients with stable eye changes for about 6 months, who have reached the inactive stage of TAO, rehabilitative surgery can be done as required.

FUTURE PERSPECTIVES

Progress in unraveling the immunopathogenesis of TAO will take in all likelihood many more years but should ultimately provide clues to appopriate treatment. One can speculate that interfering with the expression of orbital TSHRs might be useful. It could be advantageous to identify at an early stage those patients with Graves' hyperthyroidism, who will progress to develop clinically overt TAO; treatment of such subjects with antioxidants *(112)* or pentoxifylline *(113)* might prevent TAO. For immunosuppressive treatment of TAO, we need drug regimens with less side effects and greater efficacy. In this respect, we need dose-finding studies for methylprednisolone pulse therapy and trials on combination therapy of steroids and radiotherapy with for example methotrexate. The newly developed somatostatin analogue SOM 230 might be effective in contrast to octreotide. Anticytokine therapy is promising *(114)*, although a pilot on the use of anti-TNF antibodies was disappointing *(115)*. A recent case report describes that rituximab, a monoclonal antibody against the surface antigen CD 20 expressed solely on B lymphocytes, was highly effective in the treatment of recurrent Graves' hyperthyroidism and steroid-resistant TAO *(116)*.

THYROID-ASSOCIATED DERMOPATHY

Thyroid-associated dermopathy resembles TAO in many aspects *(1)*. The female to male ratio of 4:1 and the association with AITD (Graves' hyperthyroidism 91%, hypothyroidism 6%, and euthyroidism 3%) are similar to those in TAO *(117)*. Only 3% have no TAO, and TAD develops usually (in 72%) after TAO. The clinical forms of TAD are non-pitting edema accompanied by typical skin discoloration giving the lesions an orange-peel appearance in 43%, plaque in 27%, nodules in 19%, and elephantiasis in 3%. They occur most frequently in the pretibial area (93%) but may develop in feet and upper extremities. Predilection for involved skin areas has been explained from the effects of gravity and local trauma *(8,118)*. Histology shows lymphocytic infiltration, edema, and accumulation of GAGs (especially hyaluronan) produced by fibroblasts expressing HLA-DR and heat-shock proteins. The TSHR protein is expressed in elongated cells beneath the epidermis resembling fibroblasts but not in control tissues *(119)*. The immunopathogenesis of TAD is therefore likely identical to that of TAO *(27)*. Treatment, if necessary, is generally with topical corticosteroids under occlusion or compressive dressings (nighttime dressing of 0.05–0.1% triamcinolon acetate in cream base for 2–10 weeks). Octreotide has no or minimal effect *(120)*. After a mean follow-up of 7.9 years, 26% of patients have complete remission, 24% have partial remission, and 50% no or minimal improvement *(117)*.

REFERENCES

1. Fatourechi V, Pajouhi M, Fransway AF. Dermopathy of Graves' disease (pretibial myxoedema). Review of 150 cases. *Medicine (Baltimore)* 1994; 73: 1–7.
2. Wall JR. Graves' disease is a multi-system autoimmune disorder in which extraocular muscle damage and connective tissue inflammation are variable. *Thyroid* 2002; 12: 35–36.
3. Gerding MN, Terwee CB, Dekker FW, Koornneef L, Prummel MF, Wiersinga WM. Quality of life in patients with Graves' ophthalmopathy is markedly decreased: measurement by the medical outcomes study instrument. *Thyroid* 1999; 7: 885–889.
4. Bartley GB. The incidence of Graves' ophthalmopathy in Olmsted County, Minnesota. *Am J Ophthalm* 1995; 120: 511–517.
5. Prummel MF, Wiersinga WM. Smoking and risk of Graves' disease. *JAMA* 1993; 269: 479–482.
6. Weetman AP, Wiersinga WM. Current management of thyroid-associated ophthalmopathy in Europe: results of an international survey. *Clin Endocrinol* 1998; 49: 21–28.
7. Perros P, Kendall-Taylor P. Natural history of thyroid eye disease. *Thyroid* 1998; 8: 423–425.
8. Prummel MF, Bakker A, Wiersinga WM, et al. Multi-center study on the characteristics and treatment strategies of patients with Graves' orbitopathy: the first European Group on Graves' orbitopathy experience. *Eur J Endocrinol* 2003; 148: 491–495.
9. Burch HB, Wartofsky L. Graves' ophthalmopathy: current concepts regarding pathogenesis and management. *Endocr Rev* 1993; 14: 747–793.
10. Khoo DH, Eng PH, Ho SC, et al. Graves' ophthalmopathy in the absence of elevated free thyroxine and triiodothyronine levels: prevalence, natural history, and thyrotropin receptor antibody levels. *Thyroid* 2000; 10: 1093–1100.
11. Wiersinga WM. Genetic and environmental contributions to pathogenesis. In: Bahn RS (ed.), *Thyroid Eye Disease*. Kluwer Academic Publishers, Boston/Dordrecht/London 2001, p. 99–118.
12. Vaidya B, Imric H, Perros P, et al. Cytotoxic T lymphocyte antigen-4 (CTLA-4) gene polymorphism confers susceptibility to thyroid associated orbitopathy. *Lancet* 1999; 354: 743–744.
13. Allahabadia A, Heward JM, Nithiyananthan R, et al. MHC class II region, CTLA-4 gene, and ophthalmopathy in patients with Graves' disease. Lancet 2001; 358: 984–985.
14. Bednarczuk T, Hiromatsu Y, Fukutani T, et al. Association of cytotoxic T-lymphocyte-associated antigen-4 (CTLA-4) gene polymorphism and non-genetic factors with Graves' ophthalmopathy in European and Japanese populations. Eur J Endocrinol 2003; 148: 13–18.
15. Vestergaard P. Smoking and thyroid disorders – a meta-analysis. *Eur J Endocrinol* 2002; 146: 153–161.
16. Krassas GE, Segni M, Wiersinga WM. Childhood Graves' ophthalmopathy: results of a European questionnaire study. *Eur J Endocrinol* 2005; 153: 515–520.

17. Belin RM, Astor BC, Powe NR, Ladenson PW. Smoke exposure is associated with a lower prevalence of serum thyroid autoantibodies and thyrotropin concentration elevation and a higher prevalence of mild thyrotropin concentration suppression in the third National Health and Nutrition Examination Survey (NHANES III). *J Clin Endocrinol Metab* 2004; 89: 6077–6086.

18. Khoo DHC, Ho, SC, Seah LL, et al. The combination of absent thyroid peroxidase antibodies and high thyroid-stimulating immunoglobulin levels in Graves'disease identifies a group at markedly increased risk of ophthalmopathy. *Thyroid* 1999; 9: 1175–1180.

19. Metcalfe RA, Weetman AP. Stimulation of extraocular muscle fibroblasts by cytokines and hypoxia: possible role in thyroid-associated ophthalmopathy. *Clin Endocrinol* 1994; 40: 67–72.

20. Mack WP, Stasior GO, Cao HJ, et al. The effect of cigarette smoke constituents in the expression of HLA-DR in orbital fibroblasts derived from patients with Graves' ophthalmopathy. *Ophthalmic Plastic Reconstructive Surgery* 1999; 15: 260–271.

21. Bartalena L, Tanda ML, Piantanida E, et al. Oxidative stress and Graves' ophthalmopathy: in vitro studies and therapeutic implications. *Biofactors* 2003; 19: 155–163.

22. George J, Levy Y, Schoenfeld Y. Smoking and immunity: an additional player in the mosaic of autoimmunity. *Scand J Immunol* 1997; 45: 1–6

23. Wakelkamp IMMJ, Gerding MN, Meer JWC van der, Prummel MF, Wiersinga WM. Both Th1 and Th2-derived cytokines in serum are elevated in Graves' ophthalmopathy. *Clin Exp Immunol* 2000; 121: 453–457.

24. Wakelkamp IMMJ, Gerding MN, Meer JWC van der, Prummel MF, Wiersinga WM. Smoking and disease severity are independent determinants of serum adhesion molecules in Graves' ophthalmopathy. *Clin Exp Immunol* 2002; 127: 316–320.

25. Prabhakar BS, Bahn RS, Smith TJ. Current perspective on the pathogenesis of Graves' disease and ophthalmopathy. *Endocr Rev* 2003; 24: 802–835.

26. Hansen C, Rouhi R, Förster G, Kahaly GJ. Increased sulfatation of orbital glycosaminoglycans in Graves' ophthalmopathy. *J Clin Endocrinol Metab* 1999; 84: 1409–1413.

27. Bahn RS. Pathophysiology of Graves' ophthalmopathy: the cycle of disease. *J Clin Endocrinol Metab* 2003; 88: 1939–1946.

28. Weetman AP. Determinants of autoimmune thyroid disease. *Nat Immunol* 2001; 2: 769–770.

29. Pappa A, Lawson JM, Calder V, Fells P, Lightman S. T cells and fibroblasts in affected extraocular muscles in early and late thyroid associated ophthalmopathy. *Br J Ophthalmol* 2000; 84: 517–522.

30. Eckstein AK, Quadbeck B, Tews S, et al. Thyroid-associated ophthalmopathy: evidence for CD4+ γδ T cells: de novo differentiation of RED7+ macrophages, but not of RFD1+ dendritic cells; and loss of γδ and αβ T cell receptor expression. *Br J Ophthalmol* 2004; 88: 803–808.

31. Avanduk AM, Avanduk MC, Pazarli H, et al. Immunohistochemical analysis of orbital connective tissue specimens of patients with active Graves' ophthalmopathy. *Curr Eye Res* 2005; 70: 631–638.

32. de Carli M, D'Elios M, Mariotti S, et al. Cytolytic T cells with Th-1 like cytokine profile predominate in retroorbital lymphocytic infiltrates of Graves' ophthalmopathy. *J Clin Endocrinol Metab* 1993; 77: 1120–1124.

33. Hiromatsu Y, Yang D, Bednarczuk T, Miyaki I, Nonaka K, Inoue Y. Cytokine profiles in eye muscle tissue and orbital fat tissue from patients with thyroid-associated ophthalmopathy. *J Clin Endocrinol Metab* 2000; 85: 1194–1199.

34. Wakelkamp IMMJ, Bakker O, Baldeschi L, Wiersinga WM, Prummel MF. TSH-R expression and cytokine profile in orbital tissue of active vs inactive Graves' ophthalmopathy patients. *Clin Endocrinol* 2003; 58: 280–287.

35. Aniszewski JP, Valyasevi RW, Bahn RS. Relationship between disease duration and predominant orbital T cell subset in Graves' ophthalmopathy. *J Clin Endocrinol Metab* 2000; 85: 776–780.

36. Heufelder AE, Wenzel BE, Scriba PC. Antigen receptor variable region repertoires expressed by T cells infiltrating thyroid, retroorbital and pretibial tissue in Graves' disease. *J Clin Endocrinol Metab* 1996; 81: 3733–3739.

37. Pappa A, Calder V, Fells P, Lightman S. Adhesion molecule expression in vivo on extraocular muscles (EOM) in thyroid-associated ophthalmopathy (TAO). *Clin Exp Immunol* 1997; 108: 309–313.

38. Pritchard J, Horst N, Cruikshank W, Smith TJ. IgGs from patients with Graves' disease induce the expression of T cell chemoattractants in their fibroblasts. *J Immunol* 2002; 168: 942–950.

39. Drexhage HA. Are there more than antibodies to the TSH receptor that meet the eye in Graves' disease? *Endocrinology* 2006; 147: 9–12.

40. Kumaz S, Bahn RS. Relative overexpression of macrophage-derived cytokines in orbital adipose tissue from patients with Graves' ophthalmopathy. *J Clin Endocrinol Metab* 2003; 88: 4246–4250.

41. Sempowski G, Rozenblat J, Smith T, Phipps R. Human orbital fibroblasts are activated through CD40 to induce proinflammatory cytokine production. *Am J Physiol* 1998; 274: C707–C714.

42. Cao HJ, Wang HS, Zhang Y, Lin HY, Phipps RP, Smith TJ. Activation of human orbital fibroblasts through CD40 engagement results in a dramatic induction of hyaluronan synthesis and prostaglandin endoperoxide H synthase-2 expression: insights into potential pathogenic mechanisms of thyroid-associated ophthalmopathy. *J Biol Chem* 1998; 273: 29615–29625.

43. Grubeck-Loebenstein B, Trieb K, Sztankay A, Holter W, Anderl H, Wiek G. Retrobulbar T cells from patients with Graves' ophthalmopathy are CD8+ and specifically recognize autologous fibroblasts. *J Clin Invest* 1994; 3: 2738–2743.

44. Otto EA, Ochs K, Hansen C, Wall JR, Kahaly GJ. Orbital tissue-derived T lymphocytes from patients with Graves' ophthalmopathy recognize autologous orbital antigens. *J Clin Endocrinol Metab* 1996; 81: 3045–3050.

45. Feldon SE, Park DJJ, O'Loughlin CW, et al. Autologous T-lymphocytes stimulate proliferation of orbital fibroblasts derived from patients with Graves' ophthalmopathy. *Invest Ophthal Vis Sci* 2005; 46: 3913–3921.

46. Starkey KJ, Janezic A, Jones G. Jordan N, Baker G, Ludgate M. Adipose thyrotrophin receptor expression is elevated in Graves' and thyroid eye diseases ex vivo and indicates adipogenesis in progress in vivo. *J Mol Endocrinol* 2003; 30: 369–380.

47. Valyasevi RW, Erickson DZ, Harteneck DA, et al. Differentiation of human orbital preadipocyte fibroblasts induces expression of functional thyrotropin receptor. *J Clin Endocrinol Metab* 1999; 84: 2557–2562.

48. Valyasevi RW, Jyonouchi SC, Dutton CM, Munsakul N, Bahn RS. Effect of TNFα, IFNγ, and TGFβ on adipogenesis and expression of thyrotropin receptor in human orbital preadiocyte fibroblasts. *J Clin Endocrinol Metab* 2001; 86: 903–908.

49. Jyonouchi SC, Valyasevi RW, Harteneck D, Dutton CM, Bahn RS. Interleukin-6 stimulates thyrotropin receptor expression in human orbital preadipocyte fibroblasts from patients with Graves' ophthalmopathy. *Thyroid* 2001; 11: 929–935.

50. Kumar S, Coenen MJ, Scherer PE, Bahn RS. Evidence for enhanced adipogenesis in the orbits of patients with Graves' ophthalmopathy. *J Clin Endocrinol Metab* 2004; 89: 930–935.

51. Valyasevi RW, Harteneck DA, Dutton CM, Bahn RS. Stimulation of adipogenesis, PPARγ, and thyrotropin receptor by PPARγ agonist in human orbital preadipocyte fibroblasts. *J Clin Endocrinol Metab* 2002; 87: 2352–2358.

52. Starkey K, Heufelder A, Baker G, et al. Peroxisome proliferator-activated receptor-γ in thyroid eye disease: contraindication for thiazolidinedione use? *J Clin Endocrinol Metab* 2003; 88: 55–59.

53. Kumar S, Leontovich A, Coenen MJ, Bahn RS. Gene expression profiling of orbital adipose tissue from patients with Graves'ophthalmopathy: a potential role for secreted frizzled-related protein-1 in orbital adipogenesis. *J Clin Endocrinol Metab* 2005; 90: 4730–4735.

54. Smith TJ, Koumas L, Gagnon A, et al. Orbital fibroblast heterogeneity may determine the clinical presentation of thyroid-associated ophthalmopathy. *J Clin Endocrinol Metab* 2002; 87: 385–392.

55. Smith TJ. Novel aspects of orbital fibroblast pathology. *J Endocrinol Invest* 2004; 27: 246–253.

56. Sciaky D, Brazer W, Center DM, Cruikshank WW, Smith TJ. Cultured human fibroblasts express constitutive IL-16 mRNA: cytokine induction of active IL-16 protein synthesis through a caspase-3-dependent mechanism. *J Immunol* 2000; 164: 3806–3814.

57. Kaback LA, Smith TJ. Expression of hyaluronan synthase mRNA's and their induction by interleukin-1β in human orbital fibroblasts: potential insight into the molecular pathogenesis of thyroid-associated ophthalmopathy. *J Clin Endocrinol Metab* 1999; 84: 4079–4084.

58. Gerding MN, Meer JWC van der, Broenink M, et al. Association of thyrotropin receptor antibodies with the clinical features of Graves' ophthalmopathy. *Clin Endocrinol* 2000; 52: 267–271.

59. Baker G, Mazziotti G, von Ruhland C, Ludgate M. Reevaluating thyrotropin receptor-induced mouse models of Graves' disease and ophthalmopathy. *Endocrinology* 2005; 146: 835–844.

60. Weightman DR, Perros P, Sherif IH, Kendall-Taylor P. Autoantibodies to IGF-1 binding sites in the thyroid associated ophthalmopathy. *Autoimmunity* 1993; 16: 251–257.

61. Pritchard J, Han R, Horst N, Cruikshank WW, Smith TJ. Immunoglobulin activation of T cell chemoattractant expression in fibroblasts from patients with Graves' disease is mediated through the IGF-1 receptor pathway. *J Immunol* 2003; 170: 6348–6354.

62. Smith TJ. Hoa N. Immunoglobulins from patients with Graves' disease induce hyaluronan synthesis in their orbital fibroblasts through the self-antigen, insulin-like growth factor-1 receptor. *J Clin Endocrinol Metab* 2004; 89: 5076–5080.

63. Krassas GE, Pontikides N, Kaltsas T, et al. Free and total IGF-I, -II, and IGF binding protein-1, -2, and -3 serum levels in patients with active thyroid eye disease. *J Clin Endocrinol Metab* 2003; 88: 132–135.

64. Mizokami T, Salvi M, Wall JR. Eye muscle antibodies in Graves' ophthalmopathy: pathogenic or secondary epiphenomenon? *J Endocrinol Invest* 2004; 27: 221–229.

65. Lisi S, Botta R, Agretti P, et al. Poorly specific binding of thyroglobulin to orbital fibroblasts from patients with Graves' ophthalmopathy. *J Endocrinol Invest* 2005; 28: 420–424.

66. Ajjan RA, Weetman AP. New understanding of the role of cytokines in the pathogenesis of Graves' ophthalmopathy. *J Endocrinol Invest* 2004; 27: 237–245.

67. Lantz M, Vondrichova T, Parikh H, et al. Overexpression of immediate early genes in active Graves' ophthalmopathy. *J Clin Endocrinol Metab* 2005; 90: 4784–4791.

68. Bartalena L, Pichera A, Marcocci C. Management of Graves' ophthalmopathy: reality and perspectives. *Endocr Rev* 2000; 21: 168–199.

69. Dickinson AJ, Perros P. Controversies in the clinical evaluation of active thyroid-associated orbitopathy: use of a detailed protocol with comparative photographs for objective assessment. *Clin Endocrinol* 2001; 55: 283–303.

70. Eckstein AK, Plicht M, Lax H, et al. Clinical results of anti-inflammatory therapy in Graves' ophthalmopathy and association with thyroidal antibodies. *Clin Endocrinol* 2004; 61: 612–618.

71. Forbes G, Gorman CA, Brennan MD, Gehring DG, Ilstrup DM, Earnest F. Ophthalmopathy of Graves' disease: computerized volume measurements of the orbital fat and muscle. *Am J Neuroradiol* 1986; 7: 651–656.

72. Kahaly G. Recent developments in Graves' ophthalmopathy imaging. *J Endocrinol Invest* 2004; 27: 254–258.

73. Savastano S, Pivonello R, Acampa W, et al. Recombinant thyrotropin-induced orbital uptake of [111In-diethylenetriamine-pentacetic acid-D-The1]octreotide in a patient with inactive Graves' ophthalmopathy. *J Clin Endocrinol Metab* 2005; 90: 2440–2444.

74. Galuska L, Leovey A, Szues-Farkas Z, et al. SPECT using 99mTc-DTPA for the assessment of disease activity in Graves' ophthalmopathy: comparison with the results of MRI. *Nucl Med Commun* 2002; 23: 1211–1216.

75. Burggasser G, Hurth I, Hauff W, et al. Orbital scintigraphy with the somatostatin receptor tracer 99mTc-P829 in patients with Graves' disease. *J Nucl Med* 2003; 44: 1547–1558.

76. Konuk O, Atasever T, Ũnal M, et al. Orbital Gallium-67 scintigraphy in Graves'ophthalmopathy. *Thyroid* 2002; 12: 603–608.

77. Yanik B, Conkbayir I, Acaroglu G, Hekimoglu B. Graves' ophthalmopathy: comparison of the Doppler sonography parameters with the clinical activity score. *J Clin Ultrasound* 2005; 33: 375–380.

78. Wiersinga WM. The philosophy of Graves' ophthalmopathy. Orbit 2005; 24: 165–171.

79. Wiersinga WM, Bartalena L. Preventing Graves'ophthalmopathy. *Thyroid* 2002; 12: 855–860.

80. Pfeilschiffer J, Ziegler R. Smoking and endocrine ophthalmopathy: impact of smoking severity and current vs lifetime cigarette consumption. *Clin Endocrinol* 1996; 45: 477–481.

81. Glinoer D, de Nayer P, Bex M, et al. Effects of L-thyroxine administration, TSH-receptor antibodies and smoking on the risk of recurrence in Graves' hyperthyroidism treated with antithyroid drugs. *Eur J Endocrinol* 2001; 144: 475–483.

82. Bartalena L, Marcocci C, Tanda ML, et al. Cigarette smoking and treatment outcomes in Graves' ophthalmopathy. *Ann Int Med* 1998; 129: 632–635.

83. Eckstein A, Quadbeck B, Mueller G, et al. Impact of smoking on the response to treatment of thyroid associated ophthalmopathy. *Br J Ophthalmol* 2003; 87: 773–776.

84. Prummel MF, Wiersinga WM, Mourits M Ph, et al. Effect of abnormal thyroid function on the severity of Graves' ophthalmopathy. *Arch Int Med* 1990; 150: 1098–1101.

85. Tallstedt L, Lundell G, Torring O, et al. Occurrence of ophthalmopathy after treatment for Graves' hyperthyroidism. *N Engl J Med* 1992; 326: 1733–1738.

86. Bartalena L, Marcocci C, Bogazzi F, et al. Relation between therapy for hyperthyroidism and the course of Graves' ophthalmopathy. *N Engl J Med* 1998; 338: 73–78.

87. Wiersinga WM, Preventing Graves' ophthalmopathy. *N Engl J Med* 1998; 338: 121–122.

88. Perros P, Kendall-Taylor P, Neoh C, Frewin S, Dickinson J. A prospective study of the effects of radioiodine therapy for hyperthyroidism in patients with minimally active Graves'ophthalmopathy. *J Clin Endocrinol Metab* 2005; 90: 5321–5323.

89. Marcocci C, Bruno-Bossio G, Manetti L, et al. The course of Graves' ophthalmopathy is not influenced by near-total thyroidectomy: a case-control study. *Clin Endocrinol* 1999; 51: 503–506.

90. Järhult J, Rudberg C, Larsson E, et al. Graves' disease with moderate-severe endocrine ophthalmopathy – long term results of a prospective, randomized study of total or subtotal thyroid resection. *Thyroid* 2005; 15: 1157–1164.

91. Moleti M, Mattina F, Salamone I, et al. Effects of thyroidectomy alone or followed by radioiodine ablation of thyroid remnants on the outcome of Graves' ophthalmopathy. *Thyroid* 2003; 13: 653–658.

92. Wiersinga WM, Prummel MF. Retrobulbar radiation in Graves' ophthalmopathy. *J Clin Endocrinol Metab* 1995; 80: 345–347.

93. Kalmann R, Mourits M Ph. Diabetes mellitus: a risk factor in patients with Graves' orbitopathy. *Br J Ophthalmol* 1999; 83: 463–465.

94. Wakelkamp IMMJ, Baldeschi L, Saeed P, Mourits M Ph, Prummel MF, Wiersinga WM. Surgical or medical decompression as a first-line treatment of optic neuropathy in Graves' ophthalmopathy? A randomized controlled trial. *Clin Endocrinol* 2005; 63: 323–328.

95. Terwee CB, Gerding MN, Dekker FW, Prummel MF, Wiersinga WM. Development of a disease-specific quality of life questionnaire for patients with Graves' ophthalmopathy. *Br J Ophthalmol* 1998; 82: 773–779.

96. Prummel MF, Terwee CB, Gerding MN, et al. A randomized controlled trial of orbital radiotherapy versus sham irradiation in patients with mild Graves' ophthalmopathy. *J Clin Endocrinol Metab* 2004; 89: 15–20.

97. Mourits M Ph, van Kempen-Harteveld ML, Garcia MBG, Koppeschaar HPF, Tick L, Terwee CB. Radiotherapy for Graves' orbitopathy: randomized placebo-controlled study. *Lancet* 2000; 355:105–109.

98. Gorman CA, Garrity JA, Fatourechi V, et al. A prospective, randomized, double-blind, placebo-controlled study of orbital radiotherapy for Graves' ophthalmopathy. *Ophthalmology* 2001; 108: 1523–1534.

99. Kahaly GJ, Rösler HP, Pitz S, et al. Low- versus high-dose radiotherapy for Graves' ophthalmopathy: a randomized, single-blind trial. *J Clin Endocrinol Metab* 2000; 85: 102–108.

100. Gerling J, Kommerell G, Henne K, et al. Retrobulbar irradation for thyroid-associated orbitopathy: double-blind comparison between 2.4 and 16 Gy. *Int J Radiat Oncol Biol Phys* 2003; 55: 182–189.

101. Schaefer U, Hesselmann S, Micke O, et al. A long-term follow-up study after retro-orbital irradiation for Graves' ophthalmopathy. *Int J Radiat Oncol Biol Phys* 2002; 52: 192–197.

102. Marcocci C, Bartalena L, Rocchi R, et al. Long-term safety of orbital radiotherapy for Graves' ophthalmopathy. *J Clin Endocrinol Metab* 2003; 88: 3561–3566.

103. Wakelkamp, IMMJ, Tan H, Saeed P, et al. Orbital irridiation for Graves' ophthalmopathy. Is it safe? A long-term follow-up study. *Ophthalmology* 2004; 111: 1557–1562.

104. Robertson DM, Buettner H, Gorman CA, et al. Retinal microvascular abnormalities in patients treated with external radiation for Graves' ophthalmopathy. *Arch Ophthalmol* 2003; 121: 652–657.

105. Terwee CB, Prummel MF, Gerding MN, Kahaly GJ, Dekker FW, Wiersinga WM. Measuring disease activity to predict therapeutic outcome in Graves' ophthalmopathy. *Clin Endocrinol* 2005; 62: 145–155.

106. Marcocci C, Bartalena L, Tanda ML, et al. Comparison of the effectiveness and tolerability of intravenous or oral glucocorticoids associated with orbital radiotherapy in the management of severe Graves'ophthalmopathy: results of a prospective, single-blind, randomized study. *J Clin Endocrinol Metab* 2001; 86: 3652–3657.

107. Kahaly GJ, Pitz S, Hommel G, Dittmar M. Randomized, single-blind trial of intravenous versus oral steroid monotherapy in Graves' orbitopathy. *J Clin Endocrinol Metab* 2005; 90: 5234–5240.

108. Marino M, Morabito E, Brunetto MR, et al. Acute and severe liver damage associated with intravenous glucocorticoid pulse therapy in patients with Graves' ophthalmopathy. *Thyroid* 2004; 14: 403–406.

109. Salvi M, Vannuchi G, Sbrozzi F, et al. Onset of autoimmune hepatitis during intravenous steroid therapy for thyroid-associated ophthalmopathy in a patient with Hashimoto's thyroiditis: a case report. *Thyroid* 2004; 14: 631–634.

110. Dickinson JA, Vaidya B, Miller B, et al. Double-blind, placebo-controlled trial of octreotide long-acting repeatable (LAR) in thyroid associated ophthalmopathy. *J Clin Endocrinol Metab* 2004; 89: 5910–5915.

111. Wémeau JL, Caron P, Beckers A, et al. Octreotide (long-acting release formulation) treatment in patients with Graves' orbitopathy: clinical results of a four-month, randomized, placebo-controlled, double-blind study. *J Clin Endocrinol Metab* 2005; 90: 840–848.

112. Bouzas EA, Karadimas P, Mastorakos G, Koutras D. Anti-oxidant agents in the treatment of Graves' ophthalmopathy. *Am J Ophthalmol* 2000; 129: 618–622.

113. Balazs Cs, Kiss E, Vamos A, Molnar I, Farid NR. Beneficial effect of pentoxifylline on thyroid associated ophthalmopathy: a pilot study. *J Clin Endocrinol Metab* 1997; 82: 1999–2002.

114. Bahn RS. Cytokines in thyroid eye-disease: potential for anticytokine therapy. *Thyroid* 1998; 8: 415–418.

115. Paridaens D, van den Bosch WA, van der Loos TL, Krenning EP, van Hagen PM. The effect of etanercept on Graves' ophthalmopathy: a pilot study. *Eye* 2005; 19: 1286–1289.

116. El Fassi D, Nielsen CH, Hasselbalck HC, Hegedüs L. Successful B lymphocyte depletion with rituximab in a patient with recurrent Graves' disease and severe ophthalmopathy (abstract). *Thyroid* 2005; 15 (Suppl 1): S28.

117. Schwartz KM, Fatourechi V, Ahmed DDF, Pond GR. Dermopathy of Graves' disease (pretibial myxoedema): long-term outcome. *J Clin Endocrinol Metab* 2002; 87: 438–446.

118. Rapoport B, Alsabek R, Aftergood D, McLachlan S. Elephantiasic pretibial myxoedema: insight into and a hypothesis regarding the pathogenesis of the extrathyroidal manifestations of Graves' disease. *Thyroid* 2000; 10: 685–692.

119. Daumerie C, Ludgate M, Costagliola S, Many MC. Evidence for thyrotropin receptor immunore-activity in pretibial connective tissue from patients with thyroid-associated dermopathy. *Eur J Endocrinol* 2002; 146: 35–38.

120. Rotman-Pikielny P, Brucker-Davis F, Turner ML, Sarlis NJ, Skarulis MC. Lack of effect of long-term octreotide therapy in severe thyroid-associated dermopathy. *Thyroid* 2003; 13: 465–470.

III TYPE 1 DIABETES MELLITUS

10 Animal Models of Type 1 Diabetes Mellitus

Lucienne Chatenoud, MD, PhD

Summary

Type 1 diabetes (T1D) or insulin-dependent diabetes is an autoimmune disease caused by the selective destruction of insulin secreting β cells in the pancreas by autoreactive $CD4^+$ and $CD8^+$ T lymphocytes. Animal models of the spontaneous disease as well as genetically modified models have contributed significantly to our understanding of both the pathogenesis and the pathophysiology of the disease. In particular, animal models have allowed a better approach to the complex problem of genetic and environmental factors that are important not only for disease predisposition but also for disease protection. The molecular characterization of triggering autoantigens has also been facilitated by the study of animal models. Although various molecules expressed by β cells are well-recognized targets of the autoimmune response, the use of particular genetically modified mouse models has recently pointed to proinsulin/insulin as the primary autoantigen. Last but not least, when used adequately, animal models of T1D have also been helpful in preclinical studies to search for new immunointervention strategies applicable to the clinic. The overall conclusion of >30 years of studies conducted using animal models of T1D is that they recapitulate quite satisfactorily the human situation. In analyzing the data, it is, however, essential to consider that each of the mouse or rat strains used is genetically identical. In fact, they represent multiple copies of a single individual which is of course not the case for the clinical situation.

Key Words: Type 1 diabetes mellitus, animal models, insulitis, NOD mouse, BB rat, transgenic mice.

INTRODUCTION

Diabetes mellitus is a clinical syndrome mainly characterized by chronic hyperglycemia. Quite recently, in the 1970s, it became apparent that this definition included two totally distinct physiopathological entities namely, Type 1 (T1D) and Type 2 (T2D)

From: *Contemporary Endocrinology: Autoimmune Diseases in Endocrinology*
Edited by: A. P. Weetman © Humana Press, Totowa, NJ

diabetes. Compelling evidence was accumulated to show that T1D is an autoimmune disease because of progressive and selective destruction of insulin-producing β cells of the islets of Langerhans. This explains the absolute requirement for chronic administration of exogenous insulin in patients with overt T1D, also termed insulin-dependent diabetes, to maintain an adequate metabolic control. On the contrary, T2D, or non-insulin-dependent diabetes, is a metabolic disease often associated and/or exacerbated by weight excess and obesity. Here, the abnormal glucose control is not because of deficient insulin production by β cells but due to an aberrant sensitivity of peripheral tissues to the effect of the hormone, a state defined as insulin resistance, which impairs their capacity to handle glucose. Thus, treatment of T2D is not based on insulin replacement therapy but rather on the use of drugs that counteract insulin resistance. The two diseases are genetically controlled and are polygenic. Interestingly, 5–15% of patients diagnosed as T2D present in fact slow-progressing autoimmune T1D. They are now defined as late autoimmune diabetes of the adult (LADA) patients.

In humans, the autoimmune origin of T1D was suspected when Botazzo and Doniach first demonstrated that sera from T1D patients contained autoantibodies to pancreatic islet cells, as assessed by conventional immunofluorescence using sections of normal human pancreas (1). However, the difficulties of having access to the target organ greatly hampered a more in-depth analysis of the disease. This explains why spontaneous models of T1D in rodents, which rapidly became available, constituted invaluable tools not only to address the physiopathology and the genetics of the disease but also to test for immunointervention strategies aimed at both preventing and reversing established T1D.

The aim here will be to provide a critical review of these models, trying to highlight the data that help addressing the main question, namely which lessons may be drawn from the study of these animal models that translate in a better diagnosis, monitoring, and treatment of the disease in humans. Available models fall into two main categories, namely rats or mice that spontaneously develop T1D and genetically engineered autoimmune-prone or non-autoimmune-prone mice.

SPONTANEOUS MODELS OF TYPE 1 DIABETES

The Bio-Breeding Rat

GENERAL CHARACTERISTICS

The bio–breeding (BB) rat was first described in Canada in the 1970s where it was derived from outbred Wistar rats (2). This model was instrumental for Rossini and his team (3) in Worcester (MA, USA), to provide the first robust evidence that autoimmune T1D was a T-cell-mediated disease. BB diabetes prone (DP) rats express the $RT1^u$ major histocompatibility complex (MHC) haplotype, and diabetes develops in 90% of males and females between 2 and 4 months of age. Overt disease is preceded by an infiltration of the islets of Langerhans of the pancreas by mononuclear cells, that is, insulitis that starts 2–3 weeks before the advent of overt hyperglycemia and glycosuria, and is present also in the few BB-DP rats that never develop full-blown disease. Disease incidence is higher under pathogen-free conditions. However, infection with Kilham virus significantly accelerates disease onset (4). Another line of BB rats expressing the same MHC has also been derived the BB diabetes resistant (DR) rats that do not develop T1D and thus represent ideal controls for BB-DP rats (3,5).

BB-DP rats are unique in that they are congenitally lymphopenic *(6,7)*. This lymphopenia mainly involves a subset of immunoregulatory T lymphocytes, expressing the RT6 alloantigen *(6,7)*. Injecting depleting antibodies to RT6 to BB-DR rats that are not lymphopenic, and which exhibit normal proportions of RT6[+] T cells at the same time as they are protected from disease, triggers acute diabetes *(8)*. Moreover, diabetes in BB-DP rats is prevented by the transfer of syngeneic RT6[+] T cells *(9)*. According to new terminology, the RT6 alloantigen is now termed ART2 and is a cell surface adenosine diphosphate-ribosyltransferase. Interestingly, the peripheral lymphopenia in BB-DP rats is not because of defective thymic selection. The thymus of BB-DP rats is normal in terms of cell numbers, but recent thymic emigrants, already Thy1[+] but not yet RT6 (ART2)[+], are very short lived *(5,10)*. This population includes a majority of CD4[+] CD25[+] regulatory T cells *(11)*. More generally, further stressing the fundamental role of RT6 (ART2)[+] regulatory T cells in the control of T1D are the data showing that T-cell-mediated autoimmune T1D may be induced in susceptible rats (expressing the *RT1[u]* haplotype) following thymectomy and γ irradiation, a treatment that promotes lymphopenia. In such animals, T1D is effectively prevented by the transfer of CD4[+] RT6[+] cells, also staining T-cell receptor (TCR)αβ[+] Thy1[+] OX40[+] CD45RC[low] from syngeneic untreated animals *(12)*.

GENETICS

Type 1 diabetes is a polygenic disease, and extensive studies have been devoted to the characterization both in spontaneous experimental models of the disease and in patients of predisposing genes that are termed "insulin-dependent diabetes susceptibility" genes and abbreviated *Iddm, Idd*, and *IDDM* in the rat, mouse, and human, respectively. In all species, MHC alleles play a major role among predisposing genes. In the rat, four other non-MHC susceptibility loci have been identified.

Major histocompatibility complex class II alleles encoded by the *RT1[u]* haplotype are essential for diabetogenesis *(13–15)*; the requirement for the RT1-D[u]/B[u] alleles (the *Iddm2* alleles) at the two class II loci is well established. Sequence analysis of RT1-B[u], the rat DQ homolog, showed that it differed from both the mouse (H2-Ab[g7]) and the human (HLA-DQβ) susceptibility alleles in that residue 57 is an aspartic acid and not a non-asp substitution *(16)*.

Iddm1 is a recessive mutation located on chromosome 4 driving lymphopenia in BB-DP rats and initially termed *Lyp (14)*. Recently, it was demonstrated that *Lyp* is in fact a (Ian)-related gene I-A*n4 (17,18)* that is a GTP-binding protein known to regulate T-cell apoptosis through mechanisms that are as yet undefined.

Iddm4 is a locus apparently involved in insulitis *(19)*. Three other susceptibility loci *Iddm3, Iddm5*, and *Iddm6* have also been reported that still await a more precise characterization *(20)*.

Spontaneously Diabetic Non-Lymphopenic Rats

One major criticism made to the BB-DP rat model was that it did not reflect the human situation because of the lymphopenia, which is not observed in patients with T1D. Two other rat strains have been reported, which are KDP and LEW-*iddm* rats. Although studies using these animals are still limited, they are worth mentioning, because both of them develop spontaneous T1D but, at variance with BB-DP rats, are not lymphopenic *(20–23)*. Both KDP and LEW-*iddm* rats express the susceptibility MHC class II alleles encoded by the *RT1ᵘ* haplotype; overt disease appears by 2–4 months of age both in females and males and is associated with destructive insulitis. KDP rats, at variance with BB-DP and LEW.1AR1-*iddm* rats, but like non-obese diabetic NOD mice (*see* "The Non-Obese Diabetic Mouse; General Characteristics") develop extra-pancreatic autoimmune manifestations (Sjögren's syndrome) *(22)*.

The Non-Obese Diabetic Mouse

GENERAL CHARACTERISTICS

The NOD mouse model of autoimmune diabetes was discovered in Japan some 25 years ago as a novel phenotype in a breeding colony of Jcl:ICR progenitors while screening for T2D *(24)*. A wide number of NOD colonies were rapidly developed in various laboratories, which, quite interestingly, showed a high variability in disease incidence. The initial interpretation of genetic variations among substrains was invalidated by reports showing that the pathogen environment plays a major role in disease development; high disease incidence is only observed under very "clean" specific pathogen-free (SPF) conditions *(25,26)*. Under SPF conditions, disease incidence is higher in females as compared with males (90–95% vs 40–50% by 45 weeks of age). Aside from T1D, NOD mice present other autoimmune manifestations: they often exhibit thyroiditis and sialitis *(27–29)*, they may develop autoimmune hemolytic anemia *(30)*, they produce anti-nuclear antibodies *(31)*, and are prone to lupus-like syndrome following particular treatments *(32)*.

Overt T1D appears by 3 months of age and is preceded by progressive insulitis, including mononuclear cells, which evolves in distinct stages. The first infiltrating cells appear by 3–4 weeks of age *(33,34)*. Up to 8–10 weeks of age, the insulitis progresses in terms of cell numbers but remains mostly confined to the periphery of the islets. This quite long phase of "benign autoreactivity" during which, despite clear evidence for a break in self-tolerance, there is no evidence for massive β-cell destruction. This is generally defined as pre-diabetes. Then, quite abruptly, by 10–14 weeks of age, the infiltrate invades the islets (i.e., invasive/destructive insulitis), β-cell destruction occurs, and overt disease appears. Disease is caused by pathogenic T cells. This was clearly demonstrated by the capacity of "diabetogenic" T cells from the spleen of diabetic NOD mice to transfer disease into syngeneic immunoincompetent recipients (NOD neonates, adult irradiated NOD mice, and NOD SCID mice) *(35–38)*. Importantly, when using polyclonal pathogenic cells, both CD4 and CD8 T lymphocytes are needed to transfer disease; each subset alone would not suffice *(35–38)*. This is at variance with what is observed when using transgenic CD4⁺ or CD8⁺ T cells expressing a clonotypic TCR specific for a cognate autoantigen peptide (*see* Transgenic Expression of TCR Targeting β-Cell Autoantigens). Pathogenic T cells recognize various β-cell antigens including insulin *(39–41)*, proinsulin *(42,43)*, glutamic acid decarboxylase (GAD) *(44–47)*, a β-cell-specific protein phosphatase I-A2 *(48–51)*, a peptide (p277) of heat-shock protein 60 (hsp60) *(52–54)*, and the islet-specific glucose-6-phosphatase catalytic subunit–related protein (IGRP) *(55)*. This latter antigen was characterized as being a preferential target of a significant proportion of pathogenic CD8⁺ T cells from infiltrated NOD islets *(56)*.

Neither B lymphocytes nor islet-reactive autoantibodies also found in NOD mice (albeit detected in lower amounts as compared to T1D patients) are pathogenic.

However, disease development is B-cell-dependent as B-cell-depleted NOD mice are disease free *(57)*. B lymphocytes appear in this setting as in other autoimmune diseases to play a crucial role in autoantigen presentation *(58,59)*.

There is very compelling evidence to show that in NOD mice, as also discussed above for the BB-DP rat, progression to overt disease is tightly controlled by T-cell-mediated immunoregulatory circuits. T-cell depletion that follows thymectomy at 3 weeks of age (i.e., weaning) accelerates disease onset *(60)*. Acceleration of diabetes is also observed within 2 weeks following treatment of both young pre-diabetic NOD mouse females and males with cyclophosphamide *(61–64)*, an alkylating agent that selectively affects T-cell dependent regulation; it enhances delayed-type hypersensitivity *(65)* and exacerbates experimental allergic encephalomyelitis (EAE) *(66,67)*.

Adoptive transfer models provide direct demonstration for the in vivo regulatory function of CD4$^+$ T cells from young pre-diabetic NOD mice *(68)*. Thus, diabetes transfer by pathogenic cells is prevented by co-injection of CD4$^+$ T cells from the spleen or the thymus of young pre-diabetic mice *(68,69)*. At the periphery, spleen cells mediating effective protection from diabetes transfer include not only thymic-derived "natural suppressive" CD4$^+$ CD25$^+$ T cells, initially described by Sakaguchi's group *(70,71)*, but also a CD4$^+$CD25$^-$CD62L$^+$ T-cell subset. CD62-L (L-selectin) is a very interesting marker in the NOD mouse model. It was the first to allow the separation of pathogenic from regulatory T cells. Indeed, in both pre-diabetic and diabetic mice, diabetogenic T cells affording disease transfer are all included within the CD62L$^-$ subset (CD4$^+$ and CD8$^+$) *(72,73)*. Conversely, CD62L$^+$-enriched CD4$^+$ thymocytes *(69)* or spleen cells *(73,74)* protect in the co-transfer model.

A last important point to discuss is that, at variance with what initially thought at the time of overt T1D, all β cells are not destroyed: the residual β-cell mass is quite significant and represents about 30% of normal values *(75)*. In fact in recently diabetic NOD mice, insulin secretion is reduced to a greater degree than β cell mass. This strongly suggests that the physical destruction of β cells is preceded by a phase of functional impairment (that translates into incapacity to release insulin in response to conventional stimulations) because of the immune-mediated inflammation. Thus, heavily infiltrated pancreatic islets from non-diabetic 13-week-old female NOD mouse do not secrete insulin in response to glucose stimulation if examined immediately after the isolation. However, this inhibition is fully reversed on clearing of the immune cell infiltrate after 7 days of in vitro culture *(76)*. Similarly, in vivo administration of agents that rapidly clear insulitis (polyclonal [77] or monoclonal antibodies to T cells: anti-TCR [78] anti-CD3 [79]), within the first 2–7 days of overt diabetes onset, induces complete normalization of glycemia within a few days.

GENETICS

As for BB rats, NOD mice have been crossed with a number of non-autoimmune-prone lines, and the segregation of the diabetic trait or of partial phenotype (such as the cell infiltration of the islets and of other glandular tissues) has been studied in correlation with polymorphic microsatellite markers. In the NOD mouse, these studies that were largely performed by the groups of Todd and Wicker have been far more extensive than in the rat. Presently, about 30 susceptibility loci on 17 chromosomes have been reported, the number of which of course poses the crucial problem of the relative impact of each of these in determining disease risk *(80,81)*.

As already mentioned for the rat model, among all identified loci, those having the major predisposing role are in the MHC (*Idd1*). The NOD mouse $H2^{g7}$ MHC includes common class I alleles (K^d and D^b), a unique class II A^{g7}, and lacks class II *E*. Although the data point to multiple loci in the extended haplotype conferring disease susceptibility *(20)*, the A^{g7} molecule is a special class II molecule, which contributes a significant part of the effect. At variance with other mouse I-A molecules, its β chain does not show an aspartic acid residue at position 57, an interesting property, because it is in keeping with what described in human T1D patients for the DQβ chain *(82,83)*. X-ray crystallography studies and biochemical studies showed that the A^{g7} molecule is also unique in terms of its peptide-binding capacities: it appears more "promiscuous" as compared with normal class II molecules *(84–86)*. Thus, A^{g7} may bind a wider range of peptides but with lower affinity, which, according to certain authors, could provide the basis for abnormal negative selection of diabetogenic cells.

Among the important non-MHC susceptibility genes are *Idd3, Idd5.1*. *Idd3* is the interleukin (*IL*)-2 gene *(87)*. Its homolog in man has not yet been implicated as a major susceptibility locus *(88)*. The *Idd5.1* interval includes the *Ctla4* locus which human homologous *IDDM12* region is a susceptibility locus *(88,89)*. The human *IDDM2* region has been identified in various studies as a major susceptibility loci that translates into polymorphisms in a variable no tandem repeat (VNTR) upstream of the human insulin gene *(88,90,91)*. In the mouse such an association has not been described, even though several results point to proinsulin/insulin as the primary autoantigen in T1D, at least in NOD mice *(92,93)*. This may be explained by the fact that mice express two non-allelic insulin genes (*Ins1* and *Ins2*). *Ins2* is the murine homolog of the human insulin gene and is located on mouse chromosome 7. *Ins1* is thought to be the result of gene duplication; it lacks the second intron of the *Ins2* gene and is located on mouse chromosome 19.

Finally, further complicating the interpretation of segregation analysis is the existence of "protective" genes, which counterbalance the effects of susceptibility genes. Such genes exist in NOD mice as illustrated by the case of the *FcgrII* gene, which is protective and is responsible for the defective expression of this Fcγ receptor on NOD macrophages *(94)*.

MODELS OF TYPE 1 DIABETES IN GENETICALLY MODIFIED MICE

Genetically Modified Non-Autoimmune Strains

The advent of transgenic technology allowing the expression of a given molecule under the control of a tissue-specific promoter was a major breakthrough that provided a whole variety of new models of T1D. These models were instrumental in helping to understand first how the pathogenic autoimmune response to β-cell antigens develops and second what are the mechanisms that render β-cell response chronic.

The pioneering studies of Hanahan's group launched this field by showing that β-cell directed expression of transgenes in relatively high amounts was easily achieved *(95)* using the rat insulin promoter (RIP). These transgenic animals were used as such or after crossing with another transgenic line expressing a particular immunological feature (i.e., a TCR transgene) to create the best conditions for the development of overt diabetes so as to dissect the various underlying steps.

β-Cell Overexpression of Cognate Antigens that Model "Autoantigen" Expression

In these first experiments, the transgene was the SV40 oncogene, which induced the β-cell-specific expression of the SV40 T antigen. When the SV40 T transgene was expressed very early in ontogeny, transgenic mice were tolerant to it (because the transgene was "seen" by the developing immune system as an autoantigen), and an insulinoma developed because of the oncogenic potential of SV40. In contrast, when the transgene was expressed later, tolerance was not observed, and the mice showed insulitis but no overt disease.

Two other interesting models were extensively used, which expressed transgenic viral antigens from lymphocytic choriomeningitis murine virus (LCMV) or influenza virus on β cells that are the RIP-LCMV (96–98) and the RIP influenza virus hemagglutinin (HA) models, respectively (99,100). In the former case, two viral proteins were used as transgenes, the LCMV nucleoprotein (NP) or glycoprotein (GP) (96–98). The viral transgenes were expressed very early in ontogeny, and the encoded antigens could be thus considered as "self-antigens." In both cases, the mice were tolerant to the β-cell-expressed antigens because neither insulitis nor diabetes developed. However, this immune tolerance was not because of complete negative selection in the thymus. All LCMV mouse lines harbor LCMV-reactive cytotoxic T cells of variable affinity. Importantly, even when crossing RIP-LCMV mice with transgenic mice expressing the clonotypic TCR specific to the viral antigen overexpressed on β cells, the resulting double transgenic animals remained disease free (98).

These experiments using either the single or the double transgenic mice became a classic in support of the concept of "immunological indifference" directly proving that immunological self-tolerance was not broken, and neither insulitis nor diabetes appeared, despite the coexistence in the host of a highly expressed β-cell antigen and an overwhelming number of T cells specific to that β-cell antigen. Something more was needed to trigger disease, which turned out to be the infection with the corresponding virus (97,98). The initial interpretation of these results was that self-tolerance through immunological indifference was based on the fact that β cells express class I MHC molecules but not MHC class II or, more importantly, costimulatory molecules (B7.1, B7.2) to provide the adequate second signals to activate autoreactive effectors. Following viral infection, the antigens can be presented by conventional antigen-presenting cells that effectively activate autoreactive effectors, which then migrate to the pancreatic islets where they encounter the target and rapidly destroy it. This conclusion was also supported by results, showing that diabetes was observed, in absence of viral infection, when RIP-LCMV GP mice were crossed with transgenic mice overexpressing B7.1 on their β cells (101).

Unfortunately, things are in fact more complex. If immunological indifference was simply because of lack of adequate costimulation, injecting tolerant transgenic or double transgenic mice with the cognate peptide or with professional antigen-presenting cells pulsed with the corresponding "autoantigenic" peptide would be an efficient way to replace for the viral infection. It turned out that such results were extremely difficult to produce and, in the very few occasions where they did work, to reproduce.

Two different sets of recent data shed new light into this problem. First, using the double transgenic mouse model (RIP-LCMV GP × TCR Tg GP) Lang et al. (102)

showed that overt disease was triggered when the cognate peptide was administered in association with Toll-like receptor ligands. These data point to the importance not only of an adequate/professional antigen presentation but also of a certain degree of "inflammation," triggered by the viral infection or the direct delivery of Toll-like receptor agonists, to trigger overt autoimmunity. Such inflammation is then a key element favoring epitope spreading. This is a phenomenon initially described by Sercarz's group *(103)* and describes the diversification of the autoimmune response, which starts from a self-directed immune response induced by a single peptide (or epitope) and then spreads to include other peptides (or epitopes) of the same autoantigen (i.e., intramolecular spreading) or of other self-molecules clustered in close vicinity within the target cell (i.e., intermolecular spreading) *(104–106)*. Second, data from O'Garra's group *(107)* showed that immunological indifference may not just be the matter of inadequate activation of T-cell effectors but also depends on regulatory T cells. Thus, these authors directly show that, to break immunological indifference, one must adequately activate T-cell effectors and in addition properly downregulate physiological T-cell-mediated regulation, which is highly effective at dampening immune responses to autoantigens *(107)*.

SOME INTERESTING SPECIFIC FEATURES OF THE RIP-LCMV TRANSGENIC MODEL

There are essentially two different types of RIP-LCMV mouse lines *(97)*. RIP-LCMV GP mice only express the viral transgene in the islets of the pancreas and develop rapid-onset T1D by 10–14 days after the viral infection. Here, the disease is dependent on CD8$^+$ cytotoxic T lymphocytes; in vivo depletion of CD8 T cells prevents disease, whereas deletion of CD4 T cells does not *(97)*. In this case, the lack of thymic expression of the transgene explains why high-affinity cytotoxic T cells are not deleted but are exported to the periphery where they rapidly activate and differentiate into mature cytotoxic effectors once they encounter the cognate antigen in an adequate form.

In contrast, RIP-LCMV NP mice that express the viral transgene not only in the islets but also in the thymus develop slow-onset T1D that develops over 1–6 months following the viral infection depending on the MHC haplotype *(97)*. Here, thymic expression of the transgene leads to deletion of high-affinity autoreactive CD8$^+$ cytotoxic T cells but low-affinity CD8$^+$ lymphocytes migrate to the periphery. Development of disease is dependent not only on these NP-specific low-affinity CD8$^+$ cytotoxic T cells, which participate to initiation of β-cell destruction, but also on CD4$^+$ T-cell help as well as interferon (IFN)γ *(108)*.

Thus, the RIP-LCMV models are interesting because of the different kinetics of T1D progression, which may, at least in part, recapitulate some of the features that, in the clinical setting, lead to various clinical patterns observed, ranging from the rapidly progressing forms of childhood diabetes up to the very slow progressing forms observed in the adult.

β-CELL OVEREXPRESSION OF MHC MOLECULES, CYTOKINES, AND COSTIMULATORY MOLECULES

In the early 1980s, Feldman and Botazzo *(109)* proposed the hypothesis that aberrant expression of MHC class II molecules was an essential triggering factor in autoimmune diseases in general and autoimmune endocrine diseases in particular. A direct example was apparently provided in patients with Graves' disease in whom aberrant expression of HLA-DR was demonstrated on thyrocytes *(110)*. Comparable observations were never reported in T1D. However, this hypothesis stimulated interest in establishing transgenic mice overexpressing class I or II MHC molecules on β cells to analyze whether it could impact on the development of autoimmunity *(111–114)*. In these models, autoimmune diabetes did not develop. However, in some cases, glucose metabolic dysfunction was observed, which was interpreted as the result of a β-cell dysfunction due to the transgene expression *(111)*.

Interestingly, in normal non-autoimmune-prone mice, β-cell overexpression of costimulatory molecules such as B7.1 is not on its own sufficient to trigger autoimmunity *(115)*. However, if these mice are crossed with other transgenic lines overexpressing proinflammatory cytokines such as tumor necrosis factor (TNF) or IL-2, then overt disease develops *(116,117)*.

The group of Sarvetnik has been extremely productive in generating a large panel of mice whose β cells overexpressed different cytokines under the control of RIP. One first important observation was that RIP-IFNγ transgenic mice developed full-blown insulitis that could extend to normal islets grafted in the transgenic hosts *(118)*. Although the fine mechanisms underlying this effect were never fully unravelled, they did involve an upregulation of MHC class molecules on β cell that appears more "physiological" than that just discussed following transgenic expression. β-Cell overexpression of IFNγ was also reported to trigger both insulitis and diabetes *(119)*. β-Cell-driven expression of IL-2 induced also promotes pancreatic infiltration *(120)* or diabetes *(121)* and, as previously mentioned, combined overexpression with B7.1 costimulatory molecules exacerbates the process *(117,120)*. Quite unexpectedly, β-cell overexpression of IL-10, which is recognized as an anti-inflammatory cytokine, whose production in different models protects from autoimmunity, promoted fulminant diabetes *(122)*. However, it is important to stress that, in this case, the histological analysis disclosed a pattern that was not that of the typical autoimmune islet infiltration but rather of a pancreatitis with a massive infiltration also involving the exocrine pancreas.

Mice overexpressing TNF in β cells were also constructed by different groups. The results were concordant in showing the presence of insulitis but no overt diabetes *(116, 123,124)*.

Genetically Modified NOD Mice

A large number of genetically modified NOD mice have been characterized, which fall into two main categories, namely transgenic NOD mice overexpressing particular molecules under the control of various promoters, driving the expression to different cell types including antigen-presenting cells, pancreatic β cells or different subsets of T lymphocytes and NOD mice with knockouts for particular genes, taking advantage of the homologous recombination technology.

TRANSGENIC NOD MICE

Transgenic Expression of Candidate Autoantigens in the Thymus. As previously discussed, many candidate autoantigens have been characterized in autoimmune diabetes. Using transgenic NOD mice overexpressing each of these candidate molecules on thymic antigen-presenting cells driving thymocyte selection, various groups explored which among the candidate autoantigens could be primary (if indeed there was one). The rationale is that, although artificial, such "forced" thymic negative selection of autoreactive T cells specific for a key target β-cell autoantigen should lead to full disease protection with no evidence for β-cell-immune response in the hosts. For a very long time, the question was totally open. We shall see how very recent data appear to provide a more definite answer.

Full protection from both insulitis and diabetes was obtained by French et al. *(42)* in proinsulin 2 transgenic mice. Interestingly, these animals did not harbor any T cell reactive to the other key β-cell autoantigen IGRP *(92)*. These data strongly arguing for proinsulin/insulin being the primary autoantigen were challenged by another report describing that tolerance to transgenically expressed pre-proinsulin 2 greatly reduced but did not totally prevent the onset of T1D *(125)*.

In other cases (i.e., mice with thymic expression of GAD, hsp60, or IGRP transgenes), incomplete or no protection from disease was obtained associated with variable degrees of insulitis and/or T-cell responses to the cognate autoantigen *(92,126–128)*. Especially for GAD, despite successful recessive tolerance being induced on expression of a modified form of the enzyme under the control of the invariant chain promoter, insulitis and diabetes occurred just as in wild-type NOD mice *(127)*.

It is important to conclude on this issue by adding that proinsulin has always represented an ideal "primary" candidate for triggering autoimmune diabetes, considering its highly restricted expression in pancreatic β cells. However, for quite a long time, only indirect evidence had accumulated in favor of such a conclusion. The recent data from Eisenbarth's group is the first direct demonstration that, in NOD mice, part of the sequence of the B insulin chain is a primary target of the immune response. Thus, NOD mice lacking native insulin genes and carrying a mutated proinsulin transgene do not develop insulin autoantibodies, insulitis, or diabetes *(129)*. In contrast, autoimmunity develops in mice carrying even a single copy of the native insulin gene *(129)*. Using a totally different approach, the data showing that proinsulin 2 transgenic mice *(42)*, in addition to being insulitis and diabetes-free, do not harbor any T cell reactive to the other key β-cell autoantigen IGRP are also in support of such conclusion *(92)*. In contrast, NOD-IGRP mice (overexpressing IGRP in the thymus) were not protected from disease despite being tolerant to IGRP, as shown by the total absence of IGRP-specific CD8$^+$ cytotoxic T cells. In fact, these animals exhibited an anti-proinsulin autoreactive response, which was identical to that observed in conventional NOD mice *(92)*. The evidence that immune responses to IGRP are downstream to proinsulin-specific ones also points to anti-proinsulin as the primary candidate autoantigen.

Transgenic Expression of Cytokines, Costimulation, and Pro-Apoptotic Molecules in β Cells. Using the RIP promoter, as previously described in non-autoimmune strains, many interesting transgenic NOD lines have been derived. In a few cases, other gene promoters were used to target other cells of the endocrine pancreas such as islet α cells.

Concerning cytokines, substantial prevention of spontaneous disease was observed following overexpression of IL-4 *(130)*, TGF-β *(131,132)*, and TNF *(133)*. In contrast, marked acceleration was noted in NOD mice with high IL-10 expression either on islet β *(134)* or α cells *(135)*. These data that fit with what observed in IL-10 transgenic non-autoimmune-prone mice are puzzling because they contradict the findings showing the protective role of IL-10 in autoimmune diabetes when administered systemically or following gene therapy *(136,137)*. Concerning costimulatory molecules, it is interesting to note that β cell overexpression of B7.1 alone was able to significantly accelerate diabetes onset in NOD mice *(138)*, also at variance with what previously discussed in normal non-autoimmune-prone C57BL/6 mice.

Following the reports describing that Fas-ligand expression explained the protection from immune attack typical of privileged sites, NOD mice overexpressing Fas-ligand in β cell were produced by various groups. Variable results were obtained, probably due at least in part to variable levels of transgene expression *(139)*.

Transgenic Expression of "Protective" MHC Class II Molecules from Non-Autoimmune Haplotypes. The rationale behind this strategy was based on the major diabetes susceptibility effect conferred by NOD class II MHC molecules previously discussed. Transgenes encoding modified I-A molecules or I-E molecules from normal non-autoimmune strains were used. In most cases, disease protection was observed *(140–144)*. This protection was dominant, which is mediated by regulatory T cells, because it was transferable to non-transgenic NOD recipients or could be reversed by cyclophosphamide. It must be mentioned, however, that the interpretation of all these results was questioned by the unexpected observation that "control" transgenic mice overexpressing the susceptibility I-A^{g7} molecule were also protected from disease *(145)*. This may suggest that the simple abnormal overexpression of any MHC class II molecule, including the syngeneic one, is sufficient to block β-cell destruction.

Transgenic Expression of TCR Targeting β-Cell Autoantigens. The rational here has been to clone the TCR from well-characterized pathogenic CD4$^+$ and CD8$^+$ T-cell clones mostly isolated from infiltrated islets in NOD mice. In some cases, the target autoantigens were well-characterized peptides from candidate autoantigens such as the class II-restricted insulin B chain 9-23 peptide for the BDC12-4.1 TCR transgenic mouse *(146)* or the class I-restricted epitope of IGRP for the NOD 8.3 TCR transgenic *(147,148)*. At variance, in one important case (as it happened to be the first TCR transgenic NOD mice reported and very widely used by a number of investigators), namely the BDC 2.5 NOD mouse, the fine structure of the target autoantigen that appears constitutive of β-cell granules was never defined in molecular terms.

Common features of these models are that spontaneous disease develops often very aggressively when the mice exclusively harbor T cells expressing the transgenic TCR. This is the case when they are bred in a NOD background that prevents the recombination of endogenous TCRα chains such as NOD.SCID or NOD.Rag$^{-/-}$ mice. At variance, if the TCR transgene is expressed in the regular NOD background, mice show insulitis but may be totally disease-free because of the presence of T cells whose TCRs express non-transgenic endogenous α chains. Interestingly, there is compelling evidence to show that these non-transgenic T cells express regulatory function and are responsible for disease prevention. Thus, treatment of BDC 2.5 mice with cyclophosphamide or anti-CTLA4, two agents that selectively affect regulatory T cells, precipitates overt disease *(149,150)*.

Transgenic Expression of Human HLA Molecules.   On the basis of the association between particular MHC genes and human T1D, transgenic NOD mice expressing these susceptibility molecules have been produced, which have helped the identification of "naturally" presented autoantigenic peptides. Thus, NOD mice expressing the class II human MHC molecule DR4 have been extensively used for that purpose; proinsulin epitopes were effectively identified *(151,152)*.

Some studies in T1D patients also suggested an association, which remains however to be firmly proven, with some HLA class I molecules (in particular HLA-A*0201), further arguing for the important role of CD8$^+$ T cells in the disease. Transgenic expression in NOD mice of HLA-A*0201, in the absence of murine class I MHC molecules, is sufficient to mediate autoreactive CD8$^+$ T-cell responses contributing to T1D development *(153)*. Interestingly, transgenic CD8$^+$ T cells from these mice are cytotoxic to murine and human HLA-A*0201-positive islet cells *(153)*. As previously mentioned, IGRP is one important candidate autoantigen for pathogenic CD8$^+$ T cells in NOD mice. Using these HLA-A*0201 transgenic mice, some IGRP-derived peptides have been identified that are recognized not only by the transgenic mouse T cells *(153)* but also by some human T cell clones derived from T1D patients (Serreze & Roep, personal communication).

Collectively, these results indicate the utility of humanized HLA expressing NOD mice in the identification of peptide autoantigens of potential relevance to human T1D.

GENETICALLY DEFICIENT NOD MICE

The generation of NOD mice knocked out for a number of different genes has been informative, even though often disappointing because on several occasions results obtained were in complete contrast with the initially expected ones. Depending on the gene targeted, one could observe acceleration, delay, or no modification in disease progression.

Gene Encoding for Cytokines.   Early studies implicated the balance of the pathogenic and protective cytokines as major regulators of autoimmunity. In NOD mice, blockade of Th1 T-cell development inhibited disease progression *(154,155)*, whereas in some settings, treatments that promoted IL-4 production and Th2 development prevented the development of autoimmune diabetes *(130,156,157)*. Conversely, therapies that inhibited Th2 development promote disease incidence and severity *(158)*.

It was thus quite surprising and unexpected to observe that disease course was totally unaffected following invalidation of IFNγ, IL-12, IL-4, or IL-10 *(159–161)*. As a whole, these data point to the wide redundancy that exists within the cytokine network.

Gene Encoding for Costimulation Molecules.   Blockade of the CD28/B7 pathway through disruption of the CD28 gene expression surprisingly led to an earlier onset, increased incidence, and severity of T1D in NOD mice as compared with their littermate controls *(162)*. Further analyses showed that the islet autoreactive T cells that develop produced Th1 cytokines but not immunoregulatory Th2 cytokines *(162)*. In addition, and quite interestingly, a severe (almost complete) depletion of natural suppressor CD4$^+$ CD25$^+$ FoxP3$^+$ regulatory T cells was shown in NOD mice deficient for either CD28 or B7-1 and B7-2 *(163)*. This provides explanation for the paradoxical exacerbation of T1D observed *(162)*. Indeed, adoptive transfer of purified CD4$^+$ CD25$^+$

T cells into CD28-deficient NOD mice restore the deficit of regulatory T cells and delay or prevent diabetes *(163)*. This is well in keeping with data showing that a 9-day-long treatment of normal mice with CTLA-4Ig that blocks CD28/B7 interaction leads to a specific reduction of 80% of $CD4^+$ $CD25^+$ T cells both in the periphery *(163)* and in the thymus *(164)*. Furthermore, mature $CD4^+$ thymocytes from CTLA4-Ig-treated NOD mice do not protect from diabetes transfer at variance with what regularly observed with thymocytes from untreated NOD *(164)*.

Gene Encoding Generating T-Cell- or B-Cell-Less NOD Mice. Insulitis and diabetes is prevented in NOD mice lacking $CD8^+$ T cells consequent to inhibition of MHC class I molecules expression *(165–167)*. Interestingly, in these mice, insulitis but not disease is restored following expression of the RIP-β *2* microglobulin transgene in MHC class I-deficient NOD ($\beta 2m^{-/-}$) *(168)*. These data stress the role of $CD8^+$ T lymphocytes in the initiation of disease. This is further supported by data showing that transfer of T1D by diabetogenic cells does not occur in MHC class I-deficient recipients, whereas it is efficient when such recipients express the RIP-β2m transgene *(168)*. NOD mice lacking expression of MHC class II molecules because of invalidation of the class II transactivator (CIITA) show insulitis but do not progress to overt disease *(61)*.

As previously discussed, B-cell-depleted mice, carrying a μ chain gene knockout, have been produced and are disease free *(57,169)*. Such a model was extremely useful to unravel the fundamental role B lymphocytes have as antigen-presenting cells in T1D *(58,59,169,170)*.

MAIN LESSONS DRAWN FROM THE STUDY OF ANIMAL MODELS TO BETTER DIAGNOSE, MONITOR, AND TREAT HUMAN T1D

The study of the various experimental models of T1D has contributed very significantly to our understanding of both the pathogenesis and the pathophysiology of the disease. The genetic predisposing and protective factors and the role of microbial environmental factors on disease incidence are highly comparable *(26,88,171)*.

As a whole, genetic studies in the various models of spontaneous T1D have been tremendously informative with some loci, having their homologous counterparts in human T1D patients. One may be disappointed, however, that genetic screening does not yet allow identifying with sufficient sensitivity individuals at risk of developing T1D in the general population. This is because, despite the large number of genetic regions mapped, only a few genes have been directly identified. In addition, we are often not dealing with the mutations of the candidate genes but rather with polymorphisms, which may be widely distributed in the normal population and which determine genetic predisposition only when present in combination with other gene polymorphisms. Furthermore, some of the loci also confer susceptibility for autoimmune diseases other than T1D (i.e., EAE or lupus syndromes). This strongly suggests that we are dealing with two distinct categories of genes: those determining the organ specificity of the autoimmune attack and those encoding for more general immune dysregulation mechanisms, which may be common to different diseases.

Concerning pathophysiology, it is now clear that the clinical onset of T1D is preceded by a long phase of non-aggressive autoimmunity associated to non-destructive insulitis.

Importantly, in the spontaneous models of the disease, both CD4$^+$ and CD8$^+$ T lymphocytes play an essential role in processes leading to target destruction. Although B cells play a key role as antigen-presenting cells, autoantibodies to β-cell antigens are not pathogenic and only serve as good markers for β-cell destruction. The models also have pointed to the essential role of T-cell-mediated immunoregulatory pathways in the control of the autoimmune disease.

As far as triggering autoantigens are concerned, among the various molecules expressed by β cells that are well recognized targets of the autoimmune response, proinsulin/insulin appears to have a major initiating role. The more precise definition of the naturally presented epitopes in patients with T1D has opened the way to the production of class II and class I tetramers to track autoreactive CD4$^+$ and CD8$^+$ T cells in the blood of T1D patients *(172–175)*. It would be a tremendous advance if in the near future these tools could implement the routine tests to allow earlier diagnosis of the immunological disease.

In terms of the preclinical use of animal models, the situation has not been very clear until recently. This was essentially based on the observation that a very large panel of agents were able to prevent the onset of T1D, especially in the NOD mouse *(176,177)*. Two important comments should be made. First, nobody knows whether very early interventions in subjects genetically predisposed to T1D would not prevent the disease using several treatments shown to be efficacious in very young NOD mice (i.e., treatments applied in 3-week-old NOD, 3–4 months before disease onset). To prove or disprove this point, one would need to treat subjects long before onset of islet-specific antibody production, which assesses the beginning of the autoimmune aggression of the islets, something that has not been done so far. In fact, it is impossible to exclude that at such very early stage of the disease process, subtle changes in the immune system are sufficient to reset responses toward maintenance of self-tolerance. Second, the number of methods capable of stopping the progression of established disease is extremely limited, considerably less than those able to prevent disease onset. In fact, anti-lymphocyte serum, CD3- and CD4-specific monoclonal antibodies are essentially those to have such a capacity *(77,178,179)*. This is a major fact because recent data have proven that successful transfer to the clinic was obtained using one of these agents, that is a short CD3 antibody treatment in patients with new onset diabetes. A Phase I open trial using the OKT3γ1 Ala–Ala suggested a favorable therapeutic effect *(180,181)* that was definitively confirmed in a randomized double-blind multicenter Phase II placebo-controlled trial we conducted on 80 patients using the ChAglyCD3 antibody *(182)*. ChAglyCD3 treatment very efficiently preserved β-cell function, maintaining significantly higher levels of endogenous insulin secretion in comparison with placebo at 6, 12, and even 18 months, this also leading to a significant decrease in the insulin needs *(182)*. Importantly, at 18 months within the subset of patients showing a high β-cell mass (higher than the median value of the whole population) at the time of treatment, 75% of patients in the ChAglyCD3 group, versus none in the placebo, received insulin doses ≤0.25 U/kg/day *(182)*.

To conclude, it is important to keep in mind that no matter how good an animal model is in recapitulating the human situation, one will always deal with multiple copies of a single individual belonging to a genetically pure strain while human T1D is a heterogeneous disease resulting from the complex interaction of multiple genetic and environmental factors.

REFERENCES

1. Bottazzo, G.F., A. Florin-christensen, and D. Doniach. 1974. Islet-cell antibodies in diabetes mellitus with autoimmune polyendocrine deficiencies. *Lancet* 2:1279–1283.

2. Nakhooda, A.F., A.A. Like, C.I. Chappel, F.T. Murray, and E.B. Marliss. 1977. The spontaneously diabetic Wistar rat. Metabolic and morphologic studies. *Diabetes* 26:100–112.

3. Crisa, L., J.P. Mordes, and A.A. Rossini. 1992. Autoimmune diabetes mellitus in the BB rat. *Diabetes Metab. Rev.* 8:4–37.

4. Ellerman, K.E., C.A. Richards, D.L. Guberski, W.R. Shek, and A.A. Like. 1996. Kilham rat virus triggers T-cell-dependent autoimmune diabetes in multiple strains of rat. *Diabetes* 45:557–562.

5. Markholst, H., S. Eastman, D. Wilson, B.E. Andreasen, and A. Lernmark. 1991. Diabetes segregates as a single locus in crosses between inbred BB rats prone or resistant to diabetes. *J. Exp. Med.* 174:297–300.

6. Jackson, R., N. Rassi, T. Crump, B. Haynes, and G.S. Eisenbarth. 1981. The BB diabetic rat. Profound T-cell lymphocytopenia. *Diabetes* 30:887–889.

7. Greiner, D.L., E.S. Handler, K. Nakano, J.P. Mordes, and A.A. Rossini. 1986. Absence of the RT-6 T cell subset in diabetes-prone BB/W rats. *J. Immunol.* 136:148–151.

8. Greiner, D.L., J.P. Mordes, E.S. Handler, M. Angelillo, N. Nakamura, and A.A. Rossini. 1987. Depletion of RT6.1+ T lymphocytes induces diabetes in resistant biobreeding/Worcester (BB/W) rats. *J. Exp. Med.* 166:461–475.

9. Rossini, A.A., J.P. Mordes, D.L. Greiner, K. Nakano, M.C. Appel, and E.S. Handler. 1986. Spleen cell transfusion in the bio-breeding/Worcester rat. Prevention of diabetes, major histocompatibility complex restriction, and long-term persistence of transfused cells. *J. Clin. Invest.* 77:1399–1401.

10. Iwakoshi, N.N., I. Goldschneider, F. Tausche, J.P. Mordes, A.A. Rossini, and D.L. Greiner. 1998. High frequency apoptosis of recent thymic emigrants in the liver of lymphopenic diabetes-prone BioBreeding rats. *J. Immunol.* 160:5838–5850.

11. Poussier, P., T. Ning, T. Murphy, D. Dabrowski, and S. Ramanathan. 2005. Impaired post-thymic development of regulatory CD4+25+ T cells contributes to diabetes pathogenesis in BB rats. *J. Immunol.* 174:4081–4089.

12. Fowell, D., and D. Mason. 1993. Evidence that the T cell repertoire of normal rats contains cells with the potential to cause diabetes. Characterization of the CD4+ T cell subset that inhibits this autoimmune potential. *J. Exp. Med.* 177:627–636.

13. Colle, E., S.J. Ono, A. Fuks, R.D. Guttmann, and T.A. Seemayer. 1988. Association of susceptibility to spontaneous diabetes in rat with genes of major histocompatibility complex. *Diabetes* 37:1438–1443.

14. Jacob, H.J., A. Pettersson, D. Wilson, Y. Mao, A. Lernmark, and E.S. Lander. 1992. Genetic dissection of autoimmune type I diabetes in the BB rat. *Nat. Genet.* 2:56–60.

15. Ellerman, K.E., and A.A. Like. 2000. Susceptibility to diabetes is widely distributed in normal classIIu haplotype rats. *Diabetologia* 43:890–898.

16. Chao, N.J., L. Timmerman, H.O. McDevitt, and C.O. Jacob. 1989. Molecular characterization of MHC class II antigens (beta 1 domain) in the BB diabetes-prone and -resistant rat. *Immunogenetics* 29:231–234.

17. Hornum, L., J. Romer, and H. Markholst. 2002. The diabetes-prone BB rat carries a frameshift mutation in Ian4, a positional candidate of Iddm1. *Diabetes* 51:1972–1979.

18. MacMurray, A.J., D.H. Moralejo, A.E. Kwitek, E.A. Rutledge, B. Van Yserloo, P. Gohlke, S.J. Speros, B. Snyder, J. Schaefer, S. Bieg, J. Jiang, R.A. Ettinger, J. Fuller, T.L. Daniels, A. Pettersson, K. Orlebeke, B. Birren, H.J. Jacob, E.S. Lander, and A. Lernmark. 2002. Lymphopenia in the BB rat model of type 1 diabetes is due to a mutation in a novel immune-associated nucleotide (Ian)-related gene. *Genome Res.* 12:1029–1039.

19. Martin, A.M., M.N. Maxson, J. Leif, J.P. Mordes, D.L. Greiner, and E.P. Blankenhorn. 1999. Diabetes-prone and diabetes-resistant BB rats share a common major diabetes susceptibility locus, iddm4: additional evidence for a "universal autoimmunity locus" on rat chromosome 4. *Diabetes* 48:2138–2144.

20. Mathews, C.E. 2005. Utility of murine models for the study of spontaneous autoimmune type 1 diabetes. *Pediatr. Diabetes* 6:165–177.

21. Kawano, K., T. Hirashima, S. Mori, Y. Saitoh, M. Kurosumi, and T. Natori. 1992. Spontaneous long-term hyperglycemic rat with diabetic complications. Otsuka Long-Evans Tokushima Fatty (OLETF) strain. *Diabetes* 41:1422–1428.

22. Kawano, K., T. Hirashima, S. Mori, Y. Saitoh, M. Kurosumi, and T. Natori. 1991. New inbred strain of Long-Evans Tokushima lean rats with IDDM without lymphopenia. *Diabetes* 40:1375–1381.

23. Lenzen, S., M. Tiedge, M. Elsner, S. Lortz, H. Weiss, A. Jorns, G. Kloppel, D. Wedekind, C.M. Prokop, and H.J. Hedrich. 2001. The LEW.1AR1/Ztm-iddm rat: a new model of spontaneous insulin-dependent diabetes mellitus. *Diabetologia* 44:1189–1196.

24. Makino, S., K. Kunimoto, Y. Muraoka, Y. Mizushima, K. Katagiri, and Y. Tochino. 1980. Breeding of a non-obese, diabetic strain of mice. *Exp. Anim.* 29:1–13.

25. Ohsugi, T., and T. Kurosawa. 1994. Increased incidence of diabetes mellitus in specific pathogen-eliminated offspring produced by embryo transfer in NOD mice with low incidence of the disease. *Lab. Anim. Sci.* 44:386–388.

26. Bach, J.F. 2002. The effect of infections on susceptibility to autoimmune and allergic diseases. *N. Engl. J. Med.* 347:911–920.

27. Garchon, H.J., P. Bedossa, L. Eloy, and J.F. Bach. 1991. Identification and mapping to chromosome 1 of a susceptibility locus for periinsulitis in non-obese diabetic mice. *Nature* 353:260–262.

28. Many, M.C., S. Maniratunga, and J.F. Denef. 1996. The non-obese diabetic (NOD) mouse: An animal model for autoimmune thyroiditis. *Exp. Clin. Endocrinol. Diabetes* 104:17–20.

29. Many, M.C., S. Maniratunga, I. Varis, M. Dardenne, H.A. Drexhage, and J.F. Denef. 1995. Two-step development of Hashimoto-like thyroiditis in genetically autoimmune prone non-obese diabetic mice: effects of iodine-induced cell necrosis. *J. Endocrinol.* 147:311–320.

30. Baxter, A.G., and T.E. Mandel. 1991. Hemolytic anemia in non-obese diabetic mice. *Eur. J. Immunol.* 21:2051–2055.

31. Humphreys Beher, M.G., L. Brinkley, K.R. Purushotham, P.L. Wang, Y. Nakagawa, D. Dusek, M. Kerr, N. Chegini, and E.K. Chan. 1993. Characterization of antinuclear autoantibodies present in the serum from nonobese diabetic (NOD) mice. *Clin. Immunol. Immunopathol.* 68: 350–356.

32. Baxter, A.G., A.C. Horsfall, D. Healey, P. Ozegbe, S. Day, D.G. Williams, and A. Cooke. 1994. Mycobacteria precipitate an SLE-like syndrome in diabetes-prone NOD mice. *Immunology* 83:227–231.

33. Fujino-kurihara, H., H. Fujita, A. Hakura, K. Nonaka, and S. Tarui. 1985. Morphological aspects on pancreatic islets of non-obese diabetic (NOD) mice. *Virchows Arch. B. Cell. Pathol. Incl. Mol. Pathol.* 49:107–120.

34. Katz, J.D., B. Wang, K. Haskins, C. Benoist, and D. Mathis. 1993. Following a diabetogenic T cell from genesis through pathogenesis. *Cell* 74:1089–1100.

35. Bendelac, A., C. Carnaud, C. Boitard, and J.F. Bach. 1987. Syngeneic transfer of autoimmune diabetes from diabetic NOD mice to healthy neonates. Requirement for both L3T4+ and Lyt-2+ T cells. *J. Exp. Med.* 166:823–832.

36. Rohane, P.W., A. Shimada, D.T. Kim, C.T. Edwards, B. Charlton, L.D. Shultz, and C.G. Fathman. 1995. Islet-infiltrating lymphocytes from prediabetic NOD mice rapidly transfer diabetes to NOD-scid/scid mice. *Diabetes* 44:550–554.

37. Christianson, S.W., L.D. Shultz, and E.H. Leiter. 1993. Adoptive transfer of diabetes into immunode-ficient NOD-scid/scid mice. Relative contributions of CD4+ and CD8+ T-cells from diabetic versus prediabetic NOD.NON-Thy-1a donors. *Diabetes* 42:44–55.

38. Wicker, L.S., B.J. Miller, and Y. Mullen. 1986. Transfer of autoimmune diabetes mellitus with splenocytes from nonobese diabetic (NOD) mice. *Diabetes* 35:855–860.

39. Daniel, D., R.G. Gill, N. Schloot, and D. Wegmann. 1995. Epitope specificity, cytokine production profile and diabetogenic activity of insulin-specific T cell clones isolated from NOD mice. *Eur. J. Immunol.* 25:1056–1062.

40. Wegmann, D.R. 1996. The immune response to islets in experimental diabetes and insulin-dependent diabetes mellitus. *Curr. Opin. Immunol.* 8:860–864.

41. Wegmann, D.R., M. Norbury-glaser, and D. Daniel. 1994. Insulin-specific T cells are a predominant component of islet infiltrates in pre-diabetic NOD mice. *Eur. J. Immunol.* 24:1853–1857.

42. French, M.B., J. Allison, D.S. Cram, H.E. Thomas, M. Dempsey Collier, A. Silva, H.M. Georgiou, T.W. Kay, L.C. Harrison, and A.M. Lew. 1997. Transgenic expression of mouse proinsulin II prevents diabetes in nonobese diabetic mice. *Diabetes* 46:34–39.

43. Harrison, L.C., M.C. Honeyman, S. Trembleau, S. Gregori, F. Gallazzi, P. Augstein, V. Brusic, J. Hammer, and L. Adorini. 1997. A peptide-binding motif for I-A(g7), the class II major histo-compatibility complex (MHC) molecule of NOD and Biozzi AB/H mice. *J. Exp. Med.* 185: 1013–1021.

44. Baekkeskov, S., H.J. Aanstoot, S. Christgau, A. Reetz, M. Solimena, M. Cascalho, F. Folli, H. Richter-olesen, and P. De Camilli. 1990. Identification of the 64K autoantigen in insulin-dependent diabetes as the GABA-synthesizing enzyme glutamic acid decarboxylase. *Nature* 347:151–156.

45. Honeyman, M.C., D.S. Cram, and L.C. Harrison. 1993. Glutamic acid decarboxylase 67-reactive T cells: a marker of insulin-dependent diabetes. *J. Exp. Med.* 177:535–540.

46. Panina-bordignon, P., R. Lang, P.M. Van Endert, E. Benazzi, A.M. Felix, R.M. Pastore, G.A. Spinas, and F. Sinigaglia. 1995. Cytotoxic T cells specific for glutamic acid decarboxylase in autoimmune diabetes. *J. Exp. Med.* 181:1923–1927.

47. Tisch, R., X.D. Yang, R.S. Liblau, and H.O. Mcdevitt. 1994. Administering glutamic acid decar-boxylase to NOD mice prevents diabetes. *J. Autoimmun.* 7:845–850.

48. Trembleau, S., G. Penna, S. Gregori, M.K. Gately, and L. Adorini. 1997. Deviation of pancreas-infiltrating cells to Th2 by interleukin-12 antagonist administration inhibits autoimmune diabetes. *Eur. J. Immunol.* 27:2330–2339.

49. Hawkes, C.J., C. Wasmeier, M.R. Christie, and J.C. Hutton. 1996. Identification of the 37-kDa antigen in IDDM as a tyrosine phosphatase-like protein (phogrin) related to IA-2. *Diabetes* 45:1187–1192.

50. Dotta, F., S. Dionisi, V. Viglietta, C. Tiberti, M.C. Matteoli, M. Cervoni, C. Bizzarri, G. Marietti, M. Testi, G. Multari, L. Lucentini, and U. Di Mario. 1999. T-cell mediated autoimmunity to the insulinoma-associated protein 2 islet tyrosine phosphatase in type 1 diabetes mellitus. *Eur. J. Endocrinol.* 141:272–278.

51. Lampasona, V., M. Bearzatto, S. Genovese, E. Bosi, M. Ferrari, and E. Bonifacio. 1996. Autoanti-bodies in insulin-dependent diabetes recognize distinct cytoplasmic domains of the protein tyrosine phosphatase-like IA-2 autoantigen. *J. Immunol.* 157:2707–2711.

52. Elias, D., T. Reshef, O.S. Birk, R. Van Der Zee, M.D. Walker, and I.R. Cohen. 1991. Vaccination against autoimmune mouse diabetes with a T-cell epitope of the human 65-kDa heat shock protein. *Proc. Natl. Acad. Sci. U. S. A.* 88:3088–3091.

53. Elias, D., and I.R. Cohen. 1994. Peptide therapy for diabetes in NOD mice. *Lancet* 343:704–706.

54. Elias, D., A. Meilin, V. Ablamunits, O.S. Birk, P. Carmi, S. Konenwaisman, and I.R. Cohen. 1997. Hsp60 peptide therapy of NOD mouse diabetes induces a Th2 cytokine burst and downregulates autoimmunity to various beta-cell antigens. *Diabetes* 46:758–764.

55. Lieberman, S.M., A.M. Evans, B. Han, T. Takaki, Y. Vinnitskaya, J.A. Caldwell, D.V. Serreze, J. Shabanowitz, D.F. Hunt, S.G. Nathenson, P. Santamaria, and T.P. DiLorenzo. 2003. Identification of the beta cell antigen targeted by a prevalent population of pathogenic CD8+ T cells in autoimmune diabetes. *Proc. Natl. Acad. Sci. U. S. A.* 100:8384–8388.

56. Utsugi, T., J.W. Yoon, B.J. Park, M. Imamura, N. Averill, S. Kawazu, and P. Santamaria. 1996. Major histocompatibility complex class I-restricted infiltration and destruction of pancreatic islets by NOD mouse-derived beta-cell cytotoxic CD8(+) T-cell clones in vivo. *Diabetes* 45:1121–1131.

57. Serreze, D.V., H.D. Chapman, D.S. Varnum, M.S. Hanson, P.C. Reifsnyder, S.D. Richard, S.A. Fleming, E.H. Leiter, and L.D. Shultz. 1996. B lymphocytes are essential for the initiation of T cell-mediated autoimmune diabetes: analysis of a new "speed congenic" stock of NOD.Ig mu(null) mice. *J. Exp. Med.* 184:2049–2053.

58. Akashi, T., S. Nagafuchi, K. Anzai, S. Kondo, D. Kitamura, S. Wakana, J. Ono, M. Kikuchi, Y. Niho, and T. Watanabe. 1997. Direct evidence for the contribution of B cells to the progression of insulitis and the development of diabetes in non-obese diabetic mice. *Int. Immunol.* 9:1159–1164.

59. Noorchashm, H., N. Noorchashm, J. Kern, S.Y. Rostami, C.F. Barker, and A. Naji. 1997. B-cells are required for the initiation of insulitis and sialitis in nonobese diabetic mice. *Diabetes* 46:941–946.

60. Dardenne, M., F. Lepault, A. Bendelac, and J.F. Bach. 1989. Acceleration of the onset of diabetes in NOD mice by thymectomy at weaning. *Eur. J. Immunol.* 19:889–895.

61. Yasunami, R., and J.F. Bach. 1988. Anti-suppressor effect of cyclophosphamide on the development of spontaneous diabetes in NOD mice. *Eur. J. Immunol.* 18:481–484.

62. Yasunami, R., M. Debray-sachs, and J.F. Bach. 1990. Ontogeny of regulatory and effector T cells in autoimmune NOD mice. *In* Frontiers in Diabetes Research. Lessons from animal diabetes III. E. Shafrir, editor. Smith-Gordon, London. 88–93.

63. Charlton, B., A. Bacelj, R.M. Slattery, and T.E. Mandel. 1989. Cyclophosphamide-induced diabetes in NOD/WEHI mice. Evidence for suppression in spontaneous autoimmune diabetes mellitus. *Diabetes* 38:441–447.

64. Mahiou, J., U. Walter, F. Lepault, F. Godeau, J.F. Bach, and L. Chatenoud. 2001. In vivo blockade of the fas-fas ligand pathway inhibits cyclophosphamide-induced diabetes in NOD mice. *J. Autoimmun.* 16:431–440.

65. Askenase, P.W., B.J. Hayden, and R.K. Gershon. 1975. Augmentation of delayed-type hyper-sensitivity by doses of cyclophosphamide which do not affect antibody responses. *J. Exp. Med.* 141:697–702.

66. Minagawa, H., A. Takenaka, Y. Itoyama, and R. Mori. 1987. Experimental allergic encephalomyelitis in the Lewis rat. A model of predictable relapse by cyclophosphamide. *J. Neurol. Sci.* 78:225–235.

67. Miyazaki, C., T. Nakamura, K. Kaneko, R. Mori, and H. Shibasaki. 1985. Reinduction of experimental allergic encephalomyelitis in convalescent Lewis rats with cyclophosphamide. *J. Neurol. Sci.* 67:277–284.

68. Boitard, C., R. Yasunami, M. Dardenne, and J.F. Bach. 1989. T cell-mediated inhibition of the transfer of autoimmune diabetes in NOD mice. *J. Exp. Med.* 169:1669–1680.

69. Herbelin, A., J.M. Gombert, F. Lepault, J.F. Bach, and L. Chatenoud. 1998. Mature mainstream TCR alpha beta(+)CD4(+) thymocytes expressing L-selectin mediate "active tolerance" in the nonobese diabetic mouse. *J. Immunol.* 161:2620–2628.

70. Nishizuka, Y., and T. Sakakura. 1969. Thymus and reproduction: sex-linked dysgenesia of the gonad after neonatal thymectomy in mice. *Science* 166:753–755.

71. Asano, M., M. Toda, N. Sakaguchi, and S. Sakaguchi. 1996. Autoimmune disease as a consequence of developmental abnormality of a T cell subpopulation. *J. Exp. Med.* 184:387–396.

72. Lepault, F., M.C. Gagnerault, C. Faveeuw, H. Bazin, and C. Boitard. 1995. Lack of L-selectin expression by cells transferring diabetes in NOD mice: insights into the mechanisms involved in diabetes prevention by Mel-14 antibody treatment. *Eur. J. Immunol.* 25:1502–1507.

73. You, S., M. Belghith, P. Cobbold, M.A. Alyanakian, C. Gouarin, S. Barriot, C. Garcia, H. Waldmann, L. Chatenoud, and J.F. Bach. 2005. Autoimmune diabetes onset results from qualitative rather than quantitative age-dependent changes in pathogenic T cells. *Diabetes* 54:1415–1422.

74. Lepault, F., and M.C. Gagnerault. 2000. Characterization of peripheral regulatory CD4(+) T cells that prevent diabetes onset in nonobese diabetic mice. *J. Immunol.* 164:240–247.

75. Sreenan, S., A.J. Pick, M. Levisetti, A.C. Baldwin, W. Pugh, and K.S. Polonsky. 1999. Increased beta-cell proliferation and reduced mass before diabetes onset in the nonobese diabetic mouse. *Diabetes* 48:989–996.

76. Strandell, E., D.L. Eizirik, and S. Sandler. 1990. Reversal of beta-cell suppression in vitro in pancreatic islets isolated from nonobese diabetic mice during the phase preceding insulin-dependent diabetes mellitus. *J. Clin. Invest.* 85:1944–1950.

77. Maki, T., T. Ichikawa, R. Blanco, and J. Porter. 1992. Long-term abrogation of autoimmune diabetes in nonobese diabetic mice by immunotherapy with anti-lymphocyte serum. *Proc. Natl. Acad. Sci. U. S. A.* 89:3434–3438.

78. Sempe, P., P. Bedossa, M.F. Richard, M.C. Villa, J.F. Bach, and C. Boitard. 1991. Anti-alpha/beta T cell receptor monoclonal antibody provides an efficient therapy for autoimmune diabetes in nonobese diabetic (NOD) mice. *Eur. J. Immunol.* 21:1163–1169.

79. Chatenoud, L., E. Thervet, J. Primo, and J.F. Bach. 1994. Anti-CD3 antibody induces long-term remission of overt autoimmunity in nonobese diabetic mice. *Proc. Natl. Acad. Sci. U. S. A.* 91:123–127.

80. Wicker, L.S., J.A. Todd, and L.B. Peterson. 1995. Genetic control of autoimmune diabetes in the NOD mouse. *Annu. Rev. Immunol.* 13:179–200.

81. Wicker, L.S., J. Clark, H.I. Fraser, V.E. Garner, A. Gonzalez-Munoz, B. Healy, S. Howlett, K. Hunter, D. Rainbow, R.L. Rosa, L.J. Smink, J.A. Todd, and L.B. Peterson. 2005. Type 1 diabetes genes and pathways shared by humans and NOD mice. *J. Autoimmun.* 25 (Suppl):29–33.

82. Acha-orbea, H., and H.O. Mcdevitt. 1987. The first external domain of the nonobese diabetic mouse class II I-A beta chain is unique. *Proc. Natl. Acad. Sci. U. S. A.* 84:2435–2439.

83. Todd, J.A., J.I. Bell, and H.O. Mcdevitt. 1987. HLA-DQ beta gene contributes to susceptibility and resistance to insulin-dependent diabetes mellitus. *Nature* 329:599–604.

84. Corper, A.L., T. Stratmann, V. Apostolopoulos, C.A. Scott, K.C. Garcia, A.S. Kang, I.A. Wilson, and L. Teyton. 2000. A structural framework for deciphering the link between I-Ag7 and autoimmune diabetes. *Science* 288:505–511.

85. Stratmann, T., V. Apostolopoulos, V. Mallet-Designe, A.L. Corper, C.A. Scott, I.A. Wilson, A.S. Kang, and L. Teyton. 2000. The I-Ag7 MHC class II molecule linked to murine diabetes is a promiscuous peptide binder. *J. Immunol.* 165:3214–3225.

86. Carrasco-Marin, E., J. Shimizu, O. Kanagawa, and E.R. Unanue. 1996. The class II MHC I-Ag7 molecules from non-obese diabetic mice are poor peptide binders. *J. Immunol.* 156:450–458.

87. Denny, P., C.J. Lord, N.J. Hill, J.V. Goy, E.R. Levy, P.L. Podolin, L.B. Peterson, L.S. Wicker, J.A. Todd, and P.A. Lyons. 1997. Mapping of the IDDM locus Idd3 to a 0.35-cM interval containing the interleukin-2 gene. *Diabetes* 46:695–700.

88. Concannon, P., H.A. Erlich, C. Julier, G. Morahan, J. Nerup, F. Pociot, J.A. Todd, and S.S. Rich. 2005. Type 1 diabetes: evidence for susceptibility loci from four genome-wide linkage scans in 1,435 multiplex families. *Diabetes* 54:2995–3001.

89. Ueda, H., J.M. Howson, L. Esposito, J. Heward, H. Snook, G. Chamberlain, D.B. Rainbow, K.M. Hunter, A.N. Smith, G. Di Genova, M.H. Herr, I. Dahlman, F. Payne, D. Smyth, C. Lowe, R.C. Twells, S. Howlett, B. Healy, S. Nutland, H.E. Rance, V. Everett, L.J. Smink, A.C. Lam, H.J. Cordell, N.M. Walker, C. Bordin, J. Hulme, C. Motzo, F. Cucca, J.F. Hess, M.L. Metzker, J. Rogers, S. Gregory, A. Allahabadia, R. Nithiyananthan, E. Tuomilehto-Wolf, J. Tuomilehto, P. Bingley, K.M. Gillespie, D.E. Undlien, K.S. Ronningen, C. Guja, C. Ionescu-Tirgoviste, D.A.

Savage, A.P. Maxwell, D.J. Carson, C.C. Patterson, J.A. Franklyn, D.G. Clayton, L.B. Peterson, L.S. Wicker, J.A. Todd, and S.C. Gough. 2003. Association of the T-cell regulatory gene CTLA4 with susceptibility to autoimmune disease. *Nature* 423:506–511.

90. Bain, S.C., J.B. Prins, C.M. Hearne, N.R. Rodrigues, B.R. Rowe, L.E. Pritchard, R.J. Ritchie, J.R. Hall, D.E. Undlien, K.S. Ronningen, D.B. Dunger, A.H. Barnett, and J.A. Todd. 1992. Insulin gene region-encoded susceptibility to type 1 diabetes is not restricted to HLA-DR4-positive individuals. *Nat. Genet.* 2:212–215.

91. Bennett, S.T., A.J. Wilson, F. Cucca, J. Nerup, F. Pociot, P.A. Mckinney, A.H. Barnett, S.C. Bain, and J.A. Todd. 1996. IDDM2-VNTR-encoded susceptibility to type 1 diabetes: dominant protection and parental transmission of alleles of the insulin gene-linked minisatellite locus. *J. Autoimmun.* 9:415–421.

92. Krishnamurthy, B., N.L. Dudek, M.D. McKenzie, A.W. Purcell, A.G. Brooks, S. Gellert, P.G. Colman, L.C. Harrison, A.M. Lew, H.E. Thomas, and T.W.H. Kay. 2006. Responses against islet antigens in NOD mice are prevented by tolerance to proinsulin but not IGRP. *J. Clin. Invest.* 116:3258–3265.

93. Nakayama, M., N. Abiru, H. Moriyama, N. Babaya, E. Liu, D. Miao, L. Yu, D. Wegmann, J.C. Hutton, J.F. Elliott, and G. Eisenbarth. 2005. Prime role for an insulin epitope in the development of type 1 diabetes in NOD mice. *Nature* 435:220–223.

94. Luan, J.J., R.C. Monteiro, C. Sautes, G. Fluteau, L. Eloy, W.H. Fridman, J.F. Bach, and H.J. Garchon. 1996. Defective Fc gamma RII gene expression in macrophages of NOD mice: genetic linkage with up-regulation of IgG1 and IgG2b in serum. *J. Immunol.* 157:4707–4716.

95. Adams, T.E., S. Alpert, and D. Hanahan. 1987. Non-tolerance and autoantibodies to a transgenic self antigen expressed in pancreatic beta cells. *Nature* 325:223–228.

96. Oldstone, M.B., M. Nerenberg, P. Southern, J. Price, and H. Lewicki. 1991. Virus infection triggers insulin-dependent diabetes mellitus in a transgenic model: role of anti-self (virus) immune response. *Cell* 65:319–331.

97. Von Herrath, M.G., J. Dockter, and M.B. Oldstone. 1994. How virus induces a rapid or slow onset insulin-dependent diabetes mellitus in a transgenic model. *Immunity* 1:231–242.

98. Ohashi, P.S., S. Oehen, K. Buerki, H. Pircher, C.T. Ohashi, B. Odermatt, B. Malissen, R.M. Zinkernagel, and H. Hengartner. 1991. Ablation of "tolerance" and induction of diabetes by virus infection in viral antigen transgenic mice. *Cell* 65:305–317.

99. Roman, L.M., L.F. Simons, R.E. Hammer, J.F. Sambrook, and M.J. Gething. 1990. The expression of influenza virus hemagglutinin in the pancreatic beta cells of transgenic mice results in autoimmune diabetes. *Cell* 61:383–396.

100. Sarukhan, A., A. Lanoue, A. Franzke, N. Brousse, J. Buer, and H. Von Boehmer. 1998. Changes in function of antigen-specific lymphocytes correlating with progression towards diabetes in a transgenic model. *EMBO J.* 17:71–80.

101. Von Herrath, M.G., S. Guerder, H. Lewicki, R.A. Flavell, and M.B. Oldstone. 1995. Coexpression of B7-1 and viral ("self") transgenes in pancreatic beta cells can break peripheral ignorance and lead to spontaneous autoimmune diabetes. *Immunity* 3:727–738.

102. Lang, K.S., M. Recher, T. Junt, A.A. Navarini, N.L. Harris, S. Freigang, B. Odermatt, C. Conrad, L.M. Ittner, S. Bauer, S.A. Luther, S. Uematsu, S. Akira, H. Hengartner, and R.M. Zinkernagel. 2005. Toll-like receptor engagement converts T-cell autoreactivity into overt autoimmune disease. *Nat. Med.* 11:138–145.

103. Lehmann, P.V., T. Forsthuber, A. Miller, and E.E. Sercarz. 1992. Spreading of T-cell autoimmunity to cryptic determinants of an autoantigen. *Nature* 358:155–157.

104. Miller, S.D., C.L. Vanderlugt, W.S. Begolka, W. Pao, R.L. Yauch, K.L. Neville, Y. Katz-Levy, A. Carrizosa, and B.S. Kim. 1997. Persistent infection with Theiler's virus leads to CNS autoimmunity via epitope spreading. *Nat. Med.* 3:1133–1136.

105. Tisch, R., X.D. Yang, S.M. Singer, R.S. Liblau, L. Fugger, and H.O. Mcdevitt. 1993. Immune response to glutamic acid decarboxylase correlates with insulitis in non-obese diabetic mice. *Nature* 366:72–75.

106. Kaufman, D.L., M. Clare-salzler, J. Tian, T. Forsthuber, G.S.P. Ting, P. Robinson, M.A. Atkinson, E.E. Sercarz, A.J. Tobin, and P.V. Lehmann. 1993. Spontaneous loss of T-cell tolerance to glutamic acid decarboxylase in murine insulin-dependent diabetes. *Nature* 366:69–72.

107. Neighbors, M., S.B. Hartley, X. Xu, A.G. Castro, D.M. Bouley, and A. O'Garra. 2006. Breakpoints in immunoregulation required for Th1 cells to induce diabetes. *Eur. J. Immunol.* 36: 2315–2323.

108. Vonherrath, M.G., and M.B.A. Oldstone. 1997. Interferon-gamma is essential for destruction of beta cells and development of insulin-dependent diabetes mellitus. *J. Exp. Med.* 185:531–539.

109. Bottazzo, G.F., R. Pujol-borrell, T. Hanafusa, and M. Feldmann. 1983. Role of aberrant HLA-DR expression and antigen presentation in induction of endocrine autoimmunity. *Lancet* 2:1115–1119.

110. Hanafusa, T., R. Pujol-borrell, L. Chiovato, R.C. Russell, D. Doniach, and G.F. Bottazzo. 1983. Aberrant expression of HLA-DR antigen on thyrocytes in Graves' disease: relevance for autoimmunity. *Lancet* 2:1111–1115.

111. Allison, J., I.L. Campbell, G. Morahan, T.E. Mandel, L.C. Harrison, and J.F. Miller. 1988. Diabetes in transgenic mice resulting from over-expression of class I histocompatibility molecules in pancreatic beta cells. *Nature* 333:529–533.

112. Gotz, J., H. Eibel, and G. Kohler. 1990. Non-tolerance and differential susceptibility to diabetes in transgenic mice expressing major histocompatibility class II genes on pancreatic beta cells. *Eur. J. Immunol.* 20:1677–1683.

113. Bohme, J., K. Haskins, P. Stecha, W. Van Ewijk, M. Lemeur, P. Gerlinger, C. Benoistt, and D. Mathis. 1989. Transgenic mice with I-A on islet cells are normoglycemic but immunologically intolerant. *Science* 244:1179–1183.

114. Markmann, J., D. Lo, A. Naji, R.D. Palmiter, R.L. Brinster, and E. Heber-katz. 1988. Antigen presenting function of class II MHC expressing pancreatic beta cells. *Nature* 336:476–479.

115. Green, E.A., and R.A. Flavell. 1999. Tumor necrosis factor-alpha and the progression of diabetes in non-obese diabetic mice. *Immunol. Rev.* 169:11–22.

116. Guerder, S., D.E. Picarella, P.S. Linsley, and R.A. Flavell. 1994. Costimulator B7-1 confers antigen-presenting-cell function to parenchymal tissue and in conjunction with tumor necrosis factor alpha leads to autoimmunity in transgenic mice. *Proc. Natl. Acad. Sci. U. S. A.* 91:5138–5142.

117. Allison, J., L.A. Stephens, T.W. Kay, C. Kurts, W.R. Heath, J.F. Miller, and M.F. Krummel. 1998. The threshold for autoimmune T cell killing is influenced by B7-1. *Eur. J. Immunol.* 28:949–960.

118. Sarvetnick, N., D. Liggitt, S.L. Pitts, S.E. Hansen, and T.A. Stewart. 1988. Insulin-dependent diabetes mellitus induced in transgenic mice by ectopic expression of class II MHC and interferon-gamma. *Cell* 52:773–782.

119. Stewart, T.A., B. Hultgren, X. Huang, S. Pitts-meek, J. Hully, and N.J. Maclachlan. 1993. Induction of type I diabetes by interferon-alpha in transgenic mice. *Science* 260:1942–1946.

120. Allison, J., L. Malcolm, N. Chosich, and J.F. Miller. 1992. Inflammation but not autoimmunity occurs in transgenic mice expressing constitutive levels of interleukin-2 in islet beta cells. *Eur. J. Immunol.* 22:1115–1121.

121. Elliott, E.A., and R.A. Flavell. 1994. Transgenic mice expressing constitutive levels of IL-2 in islet beta cells develop diabetes. *Int. Immunol.* 6:1629–1637.

122. Lee, M.S., R. Mueller, L.S. Wicker, L.B. Peterson, and N. Sarvetnick. 1996. IL-10 is necessary and sufficient for autoimmune diabetes in conjunction with NOD MHC homozygosity. *J. Exp. Med.* 183:2663–2668.

123. Higuchi, Y., P. Herrera, P. Muniesa, J. Huarte, D. Belin, P. Ohashi, P. Aichele, L. Orci, J.D. Vassalli, and P. Vassalli. 1992. Expression of a tumor necrosis factor alpha transgene in murine pancreatic beta cells results in severe and permanent insulitis without evolution towards diabetes. *J. Exp. Med.* 176:1719–1731.

124. Picarella, D.E., A. Kratz, C.B. Li, N.H. Ruddle, and R.A. Flavell. 1993. Transgenic tumor necrosis factor (TNF)-alpha production in pancreatic islets leads to insulitis, not diabetes. Distinct patterns of inflammation in TNF-alpha and TNF-beta transgenic mice. *J. Immunol.* 150:4136–4150.

125. Jaeckel, E., M.A. Lipes, and H. von Boehmer. 2004. Recessive tolerance to preproinsulin 2 reduces but does not abolish type 1 diabetes. *Nat. Immunol.* 5:1028–1035.

126. Geng, L.P., M. Solimena, R.A. Flavell, R.S. Sherwin, and A.C. Hayday. 1998. Widespread expression of an autoantigen-GAD65 transgene does not tolerize non-obese diabetic mice and can exacerbate disease. *Proc. Natl. Acad. Sci. U. S. A.* 95:10055–10060.

127. Jaeckel, E., L. Klein, N. Martin-Orozco, and H. von Boehmer. 2003. Normal incidence of diabetes in NOD mice tolerant to glutamic acid decarboxylase. *J. Exp. Med.* 197:1635–1644.

128. Birk, O.S., D.C. Douek, D. Elias, K. Takacs, H. Dewchand, S.L. Gur, M.D. Walker, R. Van Der Zee, I.R. Cohen, and D.M. Altmann. 1996. A role of hsp60 in autoimmune diabetes: analysis in a transgenic model. *Proc. Natl. Acad. Sci. U. S. A.* 93:1032–1037.

129. Nakayama, M., N. Abiru, H. Moriyama, N. Babaya, E. Liu, D. Miao, L. Yu, D.R. Wegmann, J.C. Hutton, J.F. Elliott, and G.S. Eisenbarth. 2005. Prime role for an insulin epitope in the development of type 1 diabetes in NOD mice. *Nature* 435:220–223.

130. Mueller, R., T. Krahl, and N. Sarvetnick. 1996. Pancreatic expression of interleukin-4 abrogates insulitis and autoimmune diabetes in nonobese diabetic (NOD) mice. *J. Exp. Med.* 184:1093–1099.

131. Moritani, M., K. Yoshimoto, S.F. Wong, C. Tanaka, T. Yamaoka, T. Sano, Y. Komagata, J. Miyazaki, H. Kikutani, and M. Itakura. 1998. Abrogation of autoimmune diabetes in nonobese diabetic mice and protection against effector lymphocytes by transgenic paracrine TGF-beta1. *J. Clin. Invest.* 102:499–506.

132. King, C., J. Davies, R. Mueller, M.S. Lee, T. Krahl, B. Yeung, E. O'connor, and N. Sarvetnick. 1998. TGF-beta1 alters APC preference, polarizing islet antigen responses toward a Th2 phenotype. *Immunity* 8:601–613.

133. Grewal, I.S., K.D. Grewal, F.S. Wong, D.E. Picarella, C.A. Janeway, and R.A. Flavell. 1996. Local expression of transgene encoded TNF alpha in islets prevents autoimmune diabetes in nonobese diabetic (NOD) mice by preventing the development of auto-reactive islet-specific T cells. *J. Exp. Med.* 184:1963–1974.

134. Wogensen, L., M.S. Lee, and N. Sarvetnick. 1994. Production of interleukin 10 by islet cells accelerates immune-mediated destruction of beta cells in nonobese diabetic mice. *J. Exp. Med.* 179: 1379–1384.

135. Moritani, M., K. Yoshimoto, F. Tashiro, C. Hashimoto, J. Miyazaki, S. Ii, E. Kudo, H. Iwahana, Y. Hayashi, T. Sano, and M. Itakura. 1994. Transgenic expression of IL-10 in pancreatic islet A cells accelerates autoimmune insulitis and diabetes in non-obese diabetic mice. *Int. Immunol.* 6:1927–1936.

136. Pennline, K.J., E. Roque-gaffney, and M. Monahan. 1994. Recombinant human IL-10 prevents the onset of diabetes in the nonobese diabetic mouse. *Clin. Immunol. Immunopathol.* 71:169–175.

137. Moritani, M., K. Yoshimoto, S. Ii, M. Kondo, H. Iwahana, T. Yamaoka, T. Sano, N. Nakano, H. Kikutani, and M. Itakura. 1996. Prevention of adoptively transferred diabetes in nonobese diabetic mice with IL-10-transduced islet-specific Th1 lymphocytes. A gene therapy model for autoimmune diabetes. *J. Clin. Invest.* 98:1851–1859.

138. Wong, S., S. Guerder, I. Visintin, E.P. Reich, K.E. Swenson, R.A. Flavell, and C.A. Janeway. 1995. Expression of the co-stimulator molecule B7-1 in pancreatic beta-cells accelerates diabetes in the NOD mouse. *Diabetes* 44:326–329.

139. Chervonsky, A.V., Y. Wang, F.S. Wong, I. Visintin, R.A. Flavell, C.A. Janeway Jr, and L.A. Matis. 1997. The role of Fas in autoimmune diabetes. *Cell* 89:17–24.

140. Lund, T., L. O'reilly, P. Hutchings, O. Kanagawa, E. Simpson, R. Gravely, P. Chandler, J. Dyson, J.K. Picard, A. Edwards, D. Kioussis, and A. Cooke. 1990. Prevention of insulin-dependent diabetes

mellitus in non-obese diabetic mice by transgenes encoding modified I-A beta-chain or normal I-E alpha-chain. *Nature* 345:727–729.

141. Singer, S.M., R. Tisch, X.D. Yang, and H.O. Mcdevitt. 1993. An Abd transgene prevents diabetes in nonobese diabetic mice by inducing regulatory T cells. *Proc. Natl. Acad. Sci. U. S. A.* 90: 9566–9570.

142. Hutchings, P., P. Tonks, and A. Cooke. 1997. Effect of MHC transgene expression on spontaneous insulin autoantibody class switch in nonobese diabetic mice. *Diabetes* 46:779–784.

143. Nishimoto, H., H. Kikutani, K. Yamamura, and T. Kishimoto. 1987. Prevention of autoimmune insulitis by expression of I-E molecules in NOD mice. *Nature* 328:432–434.

144. Bohme, J., B. Schuhbaur, O. Kanagawa, C. Benoist, and D. Mathis. 1990. MHC-linked protection from diabetes dissociated from clonal deletion of T cells. *Science* 249:293–295.

145. Wherrett, D.K., S.M. Singer, and H.O. McDevitt. 1997. Reduction in diabetes incidence in an I-Ag7 transgenic nonobese diabetic mouse line. *Diabetes* 46:1970–1974.

146. Jasinski, J.M., L. Yu, M. Nakayama, M.M. Li, M.A. Lipes, G.S. Eisenbarth, and E. Liu. 2006. Transgenic insulin (B:9-23) T-cell receptor mice develop autoimmune diabetes dependent upon RAG genotype, H-2g7 homozygosity, and insulin 2 gene knockout. *Diabetes* 55:1978–1984.

147. Verdaguer, J., D. Schmidt, A. Amrani, B. Anderson, N. Averill, and P. Santamaria. 1997. Spontaneous autoimmune diabetes in monoclonal T cell nonobese diabetic mice. *J. Exp. Med.* 186:1663–1676.

148. Verdaguer, J., J.W. Yoon, B. Anderson, N. Averill, T. Utsugi, B.J. Park, and P. Santamaria. 1996. Acceleration of spontaneous diabetes in TCR-beta-transgenic nonobese diabetic mice by beta-cell cytotoxic CD8(+) T cells expressing identical endogenous TCR-alpha chains. *J. Immunol.* 157: 4726–4735.

149. Luhder, F., P. Hoglund, J.P. Allison, C. Benoist, and D. Mathis. 1998. Cytotoxic T lymphocyte-associated antigen 4 (CTLA-4) regulates the unfolding of autoimmune diabetes. *J. Exp. Med.* 187: 427–432.

150. Andre-Schmutz, I., C. Hindelang, C. Benoist, and D. Mathis. 1999. Cellular and molecular changes accompanying the progression from insulitis to diabetes. *Eur. J. Immunol.* 29:245–255.

151. Congia, M., S. Patel, A.P. Cope, S. De Virgiliis, and G. Sonderstrup. 1998. T cell epitopes of insulin defined in HLA-DR4 transgenic mice are derived from preproinsulin and proinsulin. *Proc Natl Acad Sci U. S. A.* 95:3833–3838.

152. Sonderstrup, G., A.P. Cope, S. Patel, M. Congia, N. Hain, F.C. Hall, S.L. Parry, L.H. Fugger, S. Michie, and H.O. McDevitt. 1999. HLA class II transgenic mice: models of the human CD4+ T-cell immune response. *Immunol. Rev.* 172:335–343.

153. Takaki, T., M.P. Marron, C.E. Mathews, S.T. Guttmann, R. Bottino, M. Trucco, T.P. DiLorenzo, and D.V. Serreze. 2006. HLA-A*0201-restricted T cells from humanized NOD mice recognize autoantigens of potential clinical relevance to type 1 diabetes. *J. Immunol.* 176:3257–3265.

154. Debray-sachs, M., C. Carnaud, C. Boitard, H. Cohen, I. Gresser, P. Bedossa, and J.F. Bach. 1991. Prevention of diabetes in NOD mice treated with antibody to murine IFN gamma. *J. Autoimmun.* 4:237–248.

155. Wang, B., I. Andre, A. Gonzalez, J.D. Katz, M. Aguet, C. Benoist, and D. Mathis. 1997. Interferon-gamma impacts at multiple points during the progression of autoimmune diabetes. *Proc. Natl. Acad. Sci. U. S. A.* 94:13844–13849.

156. Rapoport, M.J., A. Jaramillo, D. Zipris, A.H. Lazarus, D.V. Serreze, E.H. Leiter, P. Cyopick, J.S. Danska, and T.L. Delovitch. 1993. Interleukin 4 reverses T cell proliferative unresponsiveness and prevents the onset of diabetes in nonobese diabetic mice. *J. Exp. Med.* 178:87–99.

157. Tian, J., M.A. Atkinson, M. Clare Salzler, A. Herschenfeld, T. Forsthuber, P.V. Lehmann, and D.L. Kaufman. 1996. Nasal administration of glutamate decarboxylase (GAD65) peptides induces Th2 responses and prevents murine insulin-dependent diabetes. *J. Exp. Med.* 183:1561–1567.

158. Trembleau, S., G. Penna, E. Bosi, A. Mortara, M.K. Gately, and L. Adorini. 1995. Interleukin 12 administration induces T helper type 1 cells and accelerates autoimmune diabetes in NOD mice. *J. Exp. Med.* 181:817–821.

159. Hultgren, B., X.J. Huang, N. Dybdal, and T.A. Stewart. 1996. Genetic absence of gamma-interferon delays but does not prevent diabetes in NOD mice. *Diabetes* 45:812–817.

160. Trembleau, S., G. Penna, S. Gregori, H.D. Chapman, D.V. Serreze, J. Magram, and L. Adorini. 1999. Pancreas-infiltrating Th1 cells and diabetes develop in IL-12-deficient nonobese diabetic mice. *J. Immunol.* 163:2960–2968.

161. Wang, B., A. Gonzalez, P. Hoglund, J.D. Katz, C. Benoist, and D. Mathis. 1998. Interleukin-4 deficiency does not exacerbate disease in NOD mice. *Diabetes* 47:1207–1211.

162. Lenschow, D.J., K.C. Herold, L. Rhee, B. Patel, A. Koons, H.Y. Qin, E. Fuchs, B. Singh, C.B. Thompson, and J.A. Bluestone. 1996. CD28/B7 regulation of Th1 and Th2 subsets in the development of autoimmune diabetes. *Immunity* 5:285–293.

163. Salomon, B., D.J. Lenschow, L. Rhee, N. Ashourian, B. Singh, A. Sharpe, and J.A. Bluestone. 2000. B7/CD28 Costimulation is essential for the homeostasis of the CD4+CD25+ immunoregulatory T cells that control autoimmune diabetes. *Immunity* 12:431–440.

164. Chatenoud, L., B. Salomon, and J.A. Bluestone. 2001. Suppressor T cells—they're back and critical for regulation of autoimmunity! *Immunol. Rev.* 182:149–163.

165. Wicker, L.S., E.H. Leiter, J.A. Todd, R.J. Renjilian, E. Peterson, P.A. Fischer, P.L. Podolin, M. Zijlstra, R. Jaenisch, and L.B. Peterson. 1994. Beta 2-microglobulin-deficient NOD mice do not develop insulitis or diabetes. *Diabetes* 43:500–504.

166. Katz, J., C. Benoist, and D. Mathis. 1993. Major histocompatibility complex class I molecules are required for the development of insulitis in non-obese diabetic mice. *Eur. J. Immunol.* 23:3358–3360.

167. Sumida, T., M. Furukawa, A. Sakamoto, T. Namekawa, T. Maeda, M. Zijlstra, I. Iwamoto, T. Koike, S. Yoshida, H. Tomioka, et al. 1994. Prevention of insulitis and diabetes in beta 2-microglobulin-deficient non-obese diabetic mice. *Int. Immunol.* 6:1445–1449.

168. Kay, T.W.H., J.L. Parker, L.A. Stephens, H.E. Thomas, and J. Allison. 1996. RIP-beta(2)-microglobulin transgene expression restores insulitis, but not diabetes, in beta(2)-microglobulin(null) nonobese diabetic mice. *J. Immunol.* 157:3688–3693.

169. Serreze, D.V., S.A. Fleming, H.D. Chapman, S.D. Richard, E.H. Leiter, and R.M. Tisch. 1998. B lymphocytes are critical antigen-presenting cells for the initiation of T cell-mediated autoimmune diabetes in nonobese diabetic mice. *J. Immunol.* 161:3912–3918.

170. Falcone, M., J. Lee, G. Patstone, B. Yeung, and N. Sarvetnick. 1998. B lymphocytes are crucial antigen-presenting cells in the pathogenic autoimmune response to GAD65 antigen in nonobese diabetic mice. *J. Immunol.* 161:1163–1168.

171. Maier, L.M., and L.S. Wicker. 2005. Genetic susceptibility to type 1 diabetes. *Curr. Opin. Immunol.* 17:601–608.

172. Reijonen, H., R. Mallone, A.K. Heninger, E.M. Laughlin, S.A. Kochik, B. Falk, W.W. Kwok, C. Greenbaum, and G.T. Nepom. 2004. GAD65-specific CD4+ T-cells with high antigen avidity are prevalent in peripheral blood of patients with type 1 diabetes. *Diabetes* 53:1987–1994.

173. Reijonen, H., W.W. Kwok, and G.T. Nepom. 2003. Detection of CD4+ autoreactive T cells in T1D using HLA class II tetramers. *Ann. N. Y. Acad. Sci.* 1005:82–87.

174. Ouyang, Q., N.E. Standifer, H. Qin, P. Gottlieb, C.B. Verchere, G.T. Nepom, R. Tan, and C. Panagiotopoulos. 2006. Recognition of HLA class I-restricted β-cell epitopes in type 1 diabetes. *Diabetes* 55:3068–3074.

175. Standifer, N.E., Q. Ouyang, C. Panagiotopoulos, C.B. Verchere, R. Tan, C.J. Greenbaum, C. Pihoker, and G.T. Nepom. 2006. Identification of novel HLA-A*0201-restricted epitopes in recent-onset type 1 diabetic subjects and antibody-positive relatives. *Diabetes* 55:3061–3067.

176. Atkinson, M.A., and E.H. Leiter. 1999. The NOD mouse model of type 1 diabetes: as good as it gets? *Nat. Med.* 5:601–604.

177. Roep, B.O., M. Atkinson, and M. von Herrath. 2004. Satisfaction (not) guaranteed: re-evaluating the use of animal models of type 1 diabetes. *Nat. Rev. Immunol.* 4:989–997.

178. Makhlouf, L., S.T. Grey, V. Dong, E. Csizmadia, M.B. Arvelo, H. Auchincloss Jr, C. Ferran, and M.H. Sayegh. 2004. Depleting anti-CD4 monoclonal antibody cures new-onset diabetes, prevents recurrent autoimmune diabetes, and delays allograft rejection in nonobese diabetic mice. *Transplantation* 77:990–997.

179. Shoda, L.K., D.L. Young, S. Ramanujan, C.C. Whiting, M.A. Atkinson, J.A. Bluestone, G.S. Eisenbarth, D. Mathis, A.A. Rossini, S.E. Campbell, R. Kahn, and H.T. Kreuwel. 2005. A Comprehensive Review of Interventions in the NOD Mouse and Implications for Translation. *Immunity* 23:115–126.

180. Herold, K.C., W. Hagopian, J.A. Auger, E. Poumian Ruiz, L. Taylor, D. Donaldson, S.E. Gitelman, D.M. Harlan, D. Xu, R.A. Zivin, and J.A. Bluestone. 2002. Anti-CD3 monoclonal antibody in new-onset type 1 diabetes mellitus. *N. Engl. J. Med.* 346:1692–1698.

181. Herold, K.C., S.E. Gitelman, U. Masharani, W. Hagopian, B. Bisikirska, D. Donaldson, K. Rother, B. Diamond, D.M. Harlan, and J.A. Bluestone. 2005. A single course of anti-CD3 monoclonal antibody hOKT3gamma1(Ala-Ala) results in improvement in C-peptide responses and clinical parameters for at least 2 years after onset of type 1 diabetes. *Diabetes* 54:1763–1769.

182. Keymeulen, B., E. Vandemeulebroucke, A.G. Ziegler, C. Mathieu, L. Kaufman, G. Hale, F. Gorus, M. Goldman, M. Walter, S. Candon, L. Schandene, L. Crenier, C. De Block, J.M. Seigneurin, P. De Pauw, D. Pierard, I. Weets, P. Rebello, P. Bird, E. Berrie, M. Frewin, H. Waldmann, J.F. Bach, D. Pipeleers, and L. Chatenoud. 2005. Insulin needs after CD3-antibody therapy in new-onset type 1 diabetes. *N. Engl. J. Med.* 352:2598–2608.

11 Islet Cell Autoantigens

Anastasia Katsarou, MD, Barbro Holm, PhD, Kristian Lynch, MSc, and Åke Lernmark, PhD

CONTENTS

Summary

Type 1 diabetes (T1D) appears after autoimmune processes have eradicated a large majority of the pancreatic islet β cells. Although patients may also have other organ-specific autoimmune diseases such as thyroiditis or celiac disease (CD), most T1D patients suffer from life-long insulin dependence because only the β cells have been eradicated. The genetic etiology is strongly associated with certain HLA-DQ class II heterodimers, which in part may explain the cell-specific loss as these proteins control antigen processing and presentation. Other etiologies include environmental factors such as virus and environmental or dietary toxins. The pathogenesis is closely associated with a number of autoimmune abnormalities, among them are autoantibodies and T cells to specific autoantigens. Autoantibody assays, standardized in international efforts, are used to identify autoantibodies against the islet autoantigens insulin, GAD65 and islet antigen-2 (IA-2). The presence of autoantibodies to these autoantigens predicts T1D. Other β-cell autoantigens have been reported but have failed confirmation especially because such antigens have failed to predict disease. The possible pathogenic importance of minor candidate autoantigens is typically not pursued. Reproducible and standardized T-cell tests of either CD4- or CD8-positive T cells are yet to be developed. Immunomodulating therapies with insulin and GAD65 are in progress, and preliminary data indicate that it may be possible to alter the T1D pathogenic process.

Key Words: Type 1 diabetes, insulin, glutamic acid decarboxylase, GAD65, GAD67, IA-2.

From: *Contemporary Endocrinology: Autoimmune Diseases in Endocrinology*
Edited by: A. P. Weetman © Humana Press, Totowa, NJ

INTRODUCTION

Type 1 (insulin-dependent) diabetes (T1D) is usually classified as an organ-specific autoimmune disease. It could also be classified as a pancreatic islet β cell-specific autoimmune disease. Although comorbidities such as autoimmune thyroiditis (about 20% among new onset patients) and celiac disease (CD) (about 10% of new onset patients) are common, the majority of newly diagnosed T1D patients have suffered the loss of the β cells only *(1)*. The precision of the cell-specific eradication in T1D is most often not appreciated. In current attempts to fully clarify the genetic as well as environmental etiology of this disease, the remarkable β-cell specificity will have to be taken into account. The final common pathogenic pathway of T1D results in the killing of sufficient β cells to produce hyperglycemia due to the lack of insulin. The fraction of β cells that need to be eradicated is related to the degree of insulin sensitivity to maintain the blood glucose at a normal level *(2)*.

Recent clinical trials in subjects who have been followed because they have had autoantibodies to islet cell autoantigens have established that there is a prodrome of β-cell autoimmunity prior to the clinical onset of the disease *(3–6)*. Sufficient evidence has been obtained also to establish that T1D is a predictable disease (for reviews *see* refs. *7–10)*. The reader is referred to Chapter 12 for a more detailed account on the etiology and pathogenesis of T1D. Other reviews on aspects of T1D etiology and pathogenesis are also recommended *(11,12)*. In this review, the focus will be on islet cell autoantigens that are strongly associated with T1D by virtue of being targets for either autoantibodies, T cells, or both. The great majority of the autoantigens have been identified by using sera from T1D patients in immunoprecipitation experiments with extracts of metabolically labeled human islets.

History

In 1965, Gepts *(13)* reported the rediscovery of insulitis to inspire numerous subsequent investigations to test the hypothesis that T1D or insulin-dependent diabetes is an autoimmune disorder. The demonstration of insulitis was followed by observations that T1D is associated with autoimmune thyroiditis *(14)* and hypersensitivity to pancreatic antigens *(15,16)*. Further support to the hypothesis that T1D is an autoimmune condition was spawned by the association between T1D and HLA alleles *(16,17)* and the detection of islet cell antibodies (ICAs) in patients with polyendocrine autoimmune disease including insulin-dependent diabetes *(18,19)*. The presence of ICAs in newly diagnosed T1D children *(20)* further underscored the importance of autoimmunity in the disease process also to demonstrate that ICAs could be detected in subjects at risk several years before the clinical diagnosis *(21)*.

Although the disease pathogenesis was found to be associated with a loss of β cells, the ICAs in direct immunofluorescence reaction covered all islet cells, which means not only the β cells but also the cells producing glucagon, somatostatin (SST), and pancreatic polypeptide. Although numerous in vitro experiments were carried out to demonstrate the presence of islet cell surface antibodies (ICSAs) *(22)*, no evidence of β-cell specificity was obtained *(23,24)*. Attention was therefore drawn to the use of sera from newly diagnosed diabetes children *(25)* to immunoprecipitate antigen(s) recognized by the patient's own antibodies. The antibodies in this case were immunoglobulin G (IgG) that could bind the autoantigen in detergent extracts of metabolically labeled isolated human *(26)* or rat *(27,28)* pancreatic islets. Another prerequisite was that the IgG–autoantigen complex should be sufficiently stable in the detergent extract to permit capture on protein A-sepharose used to separate antibody-bound from free-labeled antigen. The approach resulted in the detection of a major 64K and a minor 38K antigen *(26)*. Shortly thereafter, 125I-labeled insulin was used in a similar radiobinding assay to demonstrate that about 40% of new onset diabetic children have autoantibodies to insulin *(29)*. This was the first demonstration in T1D of autoantibodies to an isolated and purified protein or peptide.

Although insulin and later proinsulin *(30)* were readily available, it took almost 10 years and thousands of isolated human islets before the 64K protein was identified. A major contribution was the demonstration that the immunoprecipitated 64K protein had glutamic acid decarboxylase (GAD) activity *(31)*. Only one GAD was known in 1990, and it was therefore unexpected when it was discovered that human islets expressed a hitherto unknown isoform, GAD65 *(32)*. Further studies revealed that the GAD65 protein was specifically expressed in human β cells *(33,34)*.

The 38K (37K) antigen was later identified as an isoform of the islet antigen-2 (IA-2) protein *(35–37)*, more specifically I-A2β (also known as phogrin) *(35,38)*. Initially, the data suggested that some sera from new onset T1D patients were able to coimmunoprecipitate GAD65, IA-2, as well as IA-2β. Reproducible assays were standardized rapidly to confirm both the high diagnostic specificity and sensitivity as well as predictive value of autoantibodies against GAD65 and IA-2 *(39,40)*.

In parallel to these developments, T1D patients were found to have autoantibodies to insulin at the time of clinical diagnosis, after making certain that none of the subjects had been exposed to insulin prior to their diagnosis *(29)*. Efforts to standardize assays of insulin autoantibodies (IAAs) *(39,41)* have continued in parallel to GADA and IA-2A as well as to dissect the autoimmune response to these autoantigens not only in humoral but also in cellular terms *(42–45)*.

We will review current research on these three major autoantigens along with studies carried out to find yet other islet autoantigens, their role in the etiology and pathogenesis as well as in recent attempts to use autoantigens in immunomodulating therapy. Animal research will not be immediately considered in this review, and the reader is referred to other excellent and comprehensive accounts on the comparative medicine of T1D *(46–48)*.

DEFINITIONS

Islet cell autoantigens represent specific molecules with preferably known sequence or structure, which are recognized by autoantibodies, T cells, or both, in subjects with T1D or with increased risk of developing this disease. Autoantibodies to islet autoantigens are by definition expected to have a high diagnostic sensitivity and specificity for T1D. The preclinical phase of T1D would therefore also be characterized by the appearance of islet autoantigen-specific autoantibodies. It should eventually be possible to determine the positive predictive value of an islet autoantibody for T1D through prospective studies of subjects at risk for the disease. Controlled clinical trials such as DPT-1 *(4)*, ENDIT *(5)*, and DIPP *(49)* are most important in this regard as they allow an evaluation of predictive power of autoantibodies alone or in combination with HLA and other T1D genetic risk factors. Currently, it appears that no islet cell autoantigen is more important than another for either disease initiation or prediction of clinical onset. In contrast, several studies suggest that the presence of multiple autoantibodies to the three major islet cell autoantigens identifies subjects at high risk for developing the disease *(5,9,50)*.

Attempts have been made to define autoantigens by the use of T-cell tests *(42,45,51)*. However, this approach has not so far been able to establish specific autoantigens. The present review will therefore to a great extent be dependent on studies in which IgG has been utilized to capture autoantigens.

The three most important islet cell autoantigens are the minor isoform of GAD65, the protein-tyrosine phosphatase-like IA-2, and insulin (Table 1). Insulin is a major β cell-specific antigen and up to 10% of the β-cell dry weight is insulin and proinsulin. Insulin is expressed early during development in humans and is present in the peripheral blood at an early stage of development. It is therefore surprising that the immunological tolerance to insulin is easily broken. However, the expression of insulin in the thymus *(52,53)* may be important to the understanding of human immune tolerance induction. The thymic expression, or lack thereof, of insulin may be of importance to the pathogenesis of T1D. It cannot be excluded that similar mechanisms of thymic expression are also important to maintain or lose immunological tolerance to GAD65, IA-2, or other autoantigens.

Other islet cell autoantigens have also been identified (Table 2). These are referred to as minor islet cell autoantigens, as the detection of autoantibodies against them have not shown a diagnostic sensitivity and specificity that is high enough to significantly improve the prediction of T1D (Table 2).

Table 1
The Three Major Islet Cell Autoantigens

	GAD65	*IA-2*	*Insulin*
Amino acids	585	974	51
Molecular weight (Da)	65,000	106,000	6000
Location	Synaptic-like microvesicles of β cells and epithelial cells of the fallopian tube and spermatozoa	Secretory granules of β cells and neuroendocrine cells	Pancreatic β cells
Function	Converts glutamic acid to gamma-amino butyric acid (GABA): inhibitory neurotransmitter	Enzymatically inactive member of protein tyrosine phosphatase (PTP) family	Insulin receptor ligand
Role as marker for diabetes prediction	GADA increases with age	IA-2A highest in younger populations	IAAs appear primarily in young children, less common in young adults
	Predicts insulin requirement in type 2 diabetes patients	More specific marker for type 1 diabetes	

Table 2
Candidate Islet Cell Autoantigens

Autoantigen	Description	Function
ICA69	Protein of 54,600d, found in brain, lung, kidney, and heart but expressed in highest levels in islet cells	Possibly involved in neuroendocrine secretion
ICA12 (SOX-13)	Protein of the SOX family, expressed in pancreas, placenta, and kidney	Key role in organ development
Carboxypeptidase H (CPH)	Glycoprotein and a carboxypeptidase B-like enzyme and expression in human islet cells and brain	Cleaves the COOH terminal ends of hormone precursors, involved in the processing of proinsulin to insulin
Sulfatide	Glycolipid, in the surface and secretory granules of β-cells, central and peripheral nervous system, kidneys, gallbladder, and choroid layers of eyes	Major component of the myelin
Ganglioside GM2-1	Islet monosialo-ganglioside and secretory granules of β cells and non-β cells	Participates in the cell-to-cell interaction and in signal transaction
Imogen 38	Mitochondrial islet antigen of 38 kDa	
GLIMA 38	N-glycated β-cell membrane protein of Mr 38,000, expressed in islets and in islet and neuronal cell lines	
Islet specific glucose-6-phosphatase-related protein (IGRP)	Protein expressed in β-cells of humans and NOD mice	Possible role in β-cell metabolism
Somatostatin receptors (SSTRs)	G-protein-coupled receptors present in pituitary, small intestine, heart, spleen, liver, stomach, kidney, and pancreas as well as T and B lymphocytes	Interacts with somatostatin, possible role in T-cell proliferation

GAD65

Structure

Antibodies in sera from newly diagnosed T1D patients were directed to a human islet cell protein of relative molecular mass (Mr) 64,000 *(26)*. Further studies led to the identification of glutamate decarboxylase (GAD) activity *(31)*, a pyridoxal 5′-phosphate (PLP)-dependent enzyme that is widely distributed among eukaryotic and prokaryotic organisms *(54)*. The 64K protein was, however, found to be a novel GAD isoform, GAD65

(32). These investigators demonstrated that there are two isoforms of GAD (GAD65 and GAD67). GAD65 and GAD67 were shown to be products of separate genes *(32,55).* The genes are probably derived from a common ancestral GAD gene following gene duplication at some point during vertebrate evolution *(56).* GAD65 is encoded by a gene on chromosome 10 *(32)* and GAD67 by a gene on chromosome 2 *(55).* Human GAD65 cDNA encodes a polypeptide of 585 amino acids residues that has a calculated molecular weight of 65,000, whereas the human GAD67 cDNA encodes a molecule consisting of 594 amino acids *(55).* The calculated molecular weight of GAD67 is 67,000. The genes of theses two isoforms of GAD share a similar exon–intron structure *(57).* A total of 65% of the amino acids are identical *(32).* The divergence is at the N-terminal region where only 22% of the amino acids are identical compared to over 90% identity in C-terminal regions *(32,55).* Both GAD isoforms are active at neutral pH as dimers *(54).*

GAD is a common enzyme among living organisms including plants. Pyridoxal 5′-phosphate (PLP) is the cofactor required for enzymatic activity *(58).* Crystallized *Escherichia coli* GAD was used to identify the PLP-binding site -Xaa-His-Lys(PLP)-Xaa as the active site of the enzyme *(58).* The structure–function relationship of GAD is not understood as neither GAD65 nor GAD67 have been crystallized. Other PLP-dependent decarboxylases have been isolated, purified, and crystallized *(59),* and the structural information has been used to generate models of GAD based on homology mapping *(60).* As the accuracy of such methods is questioned, it is noted that the absence of a crystal structure has hampered the understanding not only of GAD65 and GAD67 as enzymes but also of epitopes important to the etiology and pathogenesis of T1D. Using a GAD65 model generated based on the crystal structures of mammalian 3,4-dihydroxy-L-phenylalanine (DOPA) decarboxylase and bacterial GAD, three main domains were recognized in the GAD65 monomer structure *(61).* The large domain (residues 188–464) would contain the PLP cofactor-binding site, consisting of an α/β-fold made of a central seven-stranded mixed β-sheet surrounded by eight α-helices, typical of PLP-dependent enzymes. The small domain (residues 465–585) consists of a four-stranded antiparallel β-sheet with three helices packed against the face opposite the large domain *(60).* The N-terminal domain (residues 103–187) did not, however, represent the true N-terminus. As specific Fab reagents of monoclonal antibodies to GAD65 have been generated for epitope mapping, it will be critical to determine the crystal structure of GAD65 to better understand the autoimmune reaction to the GAD65 autoantigen *(62).*

It has been reported that the two isoforms of GAD have distinctive PLP-binding properties. GAD65 exhibits a lower cofactor-binding constant, whereas GAD67 has higher affinity for PLP, with one active site binding the cofactor more tightly than the other *(63).* However, no amino acid substitutions were found in the specific residues in the active site, so the differences in the PLP-binding behavior between the two isoforms can only be explained by structural differences that affect binding in an indirect way *(60).* The possible role of the GAD65 structure for disease initiation as well as possible pathogenic importance remains to be determined.

Expression—β Cells and Elsewhere

Both GAD isoforms are translated on free ribosomes within the cytoplasm to full-length proteins that are not processed through the ER and Golgi apparatus *(63).* While

GAD67 remains soluble, GAD65 has internal N-terminal amino acid residues that seem to be important for the protein to become anchored to the cytosolic face of Golgi membranes or to synaptic vesicle membranes in GABA containing neuroendocrine cells or islet β cells *(64)*. In addition, although the importance is yet to be clarified, GAD65 is undergoing post-translational modification(s) by lipids within the N-terminal domain *(65,66)*. Site-directed mutagenesis of the amino acid residues important to fatty acid acylation did, however, not affect the docking of GAD65 to internal membranes *(67)*.

In addition to the central and peripheral nervous system and islet β cells, the two isoforms of GAD are synthesized in testes and ovaries. GAD65 is more predominant in the pancreatic β cells in humans compared to rodents *(33)*. In rat cells, GAD65 also predominates in the β cells but is detected in α cells as well *(33)*. GAD67 is expressed at a much reduced level in the human β cells but is detectable in the non-β-cell population. Brain cells commonly express GAD67, whereas GAD65 expression is found in distinct cell types. Moreover, GAD67 but not GAD65 seems to be more highly expressed in mouse pancreatic islets *(34)*. Further studies are needed to better understand the genetic control of cell-specific GAD65 and GAD67 expression as well as of the mechanisms by which the two proteins are subjected to subcellular sorting. It will also be critical to understand the role of the subcellular localization in the relation to the generation of GABA, the product of both GAD65 and GAD67.

Function

GAD65 catalyzes the α-decarboxylation of L-glutamate to γ-aminobutyrate (GABA), which is present in the brain as well as several tissues outside the central nervous system. The functional importance of GAD65 in islet cell function is not fully clarified. The presence of both GAD65 and GAD67 and thereby their product, GABA, within the islet β cells as well as the presence of GABA receptors on these cells suggests that GABA is involved in paracrine signaling in the islet *(68,69)*. It has recently been reported that cAMP generators increase GABA release by β cells through stimulation of GABA synthesis by GAD. This effect is shown to be associated with an increased expression of GAD67. It is unclear to what extent GAD65 contributes to the islet cell GABA content and release *(70)*. GABA release from β cells is regulated by glutamine and glucose. Glucose inhibits glutamine-driven GABA formation and release through increasing GABA-T shunt activity by its cellular metabolism *(70)*.

Autoantibody Detection

The presence of GAD65 autoantibodies (GAD65Ab) has been reported in 70–80% of newly diagnosed T1D patients *(71,72)*. GAD65Ab levels are generally low titer and varies by both gender and age at diagnosis *(73,74)*. While the diagnostic sensitivity is high, the specificity is complicated by the presence of low level autoantibodies. The GAD65 autoantibody binding was inhibited by non-radioactive GAD65 to the 70th percentile in healthy adults *(75)* and was associated with an increased BMI *(75,76)*. The so-called upper level of normal is therefore not always easy to determine. In contrast, the relationship between T1D and GAD was discovered through observations that patients with both Stiff-Mann syndrome (SMS) and T1D *(31,77)* had sera that stained cells in the islets of Langerhans as well as CNS cells known to express GABA *(77)*.

The GAD65Ab in SMS patients, reviewed elsewhere *(78,79)*, have exceptionally high titers, and some SMS patients have GAD65Ab that inhibit the enzyme *(80)*. It is possible that the high affinity, high titer sera contribute to the impaired GABA-secreting neurons in this disease. Epitope mapping also suggests that SMS patients have GAD65Ab that target an epitope contained in the N-terminal first eight amino acids *(81)*. In contrast to T1D, the SMS GAD65Ab detect GAD65 in Western blot suggesting that the autoantibodies are directed to a linear as opposed to a conformational epitope *(81)*.

Several methods were reported for the measurement of autoantibodies to GAD65 and GAD67. They include (i) determination of antibody precipitation of GAD (mix of GAD65 and 67) enzymatic activity; (ii) radioimmunoassays utilizing affinity-purified porcine brain GAD65 that has been labeled with I^{125}; (iii) radioimmunoassays utilizing endogenously labeled GAD produced by in vitro transcription and translation of GAD cDNA; and (iv) enzyme-linked immunosorbent assay (ELISA)-type assays (reviewed in refs. *71,79*).

In the most commonly used assay, GAD65 is synthesized by transcription of cDNA template into mRNA and translation of the mRNA into protein *(82)*. The GAD65 mRNA is translated in the presence of ^{35}S-methionine or 3H- or 14C-labeled amino acids of high specific activity into protein. The recombinant radioactive GAD65 is then added to a small volume (2.5 μL often suffice, and this is important when infants are tested) of serum from healthy subjects or patients. IgG antibodies against GAD65 form immune complexes, and these are captured on protein A-sepharose. After extensive washing to remove free radioactive GAD65, the amount of sepharose-bound radioactivity is determined. Results are expressed as units per milliliter derived from standard curves of counts per minute obtained for the World Health Organization (WHO) standard 97/550 *(40)*. This assay has the best results in the Diabetes Autoantibody Standardization Programme (DASP) workshop *(39)*.

As the N-terminal end of GAD65 makes the protein hydrophobic and difficult to keep in solution for iodination, human GAD65 cDNA was cloned after deleting the bases 4–135 of the GAD65 open reading frame. The modified GAD65 is isolated and purified before being labeled with ^{125}I *(83)*. The labeled GAD65 is added to serum and ensuing immune complexes trapped on protein A-sepharose. This assay has also performed well in the DASP *(39)*, but as the N-terminal end has been truncated the assay may miss GAD65 autoantibodies associated with type 2 or latent autoimmune diabetes in adult (LADA) patients *(84,85)*.

GAD65 is expressed in yeast, and when biotinylated is used in an ELISA assay that depends on the ability of antibodies to act divalently and form a bridge between immobilized GAD65 and liquid-phase biotinylated GAD65 *(86)*. Sera from patients are added to GAD65-coated wells, and after incubation and washing, GAD65 biotin is also added. Biotinylated GAD65 bound to GAD65-trapped IgG is next detected by addition of streptavidin peroxidase and a colorogenic peroxidase substrate *(86)*. The results of the GAD65Ab ELISA correlate well with those obtained in the standardized GAD65 radiobinding assay. In the second DASP, the GAD65Ab ELISA showed higher workshop sensitivity (69%) and specificity (98%) compared to the more commonly used GAD65Ab radiobinding assay. The GAD65Ab ELISA test has been used for large scale population screening to predict T1D *(87)*.

A major problem with GAD65Ab determination is the interlaboratory variation. The IDW *(88)* and DASP *(39)* workshops have indicated that these discrepancies in part can be resolved by the use of the common WHO standard *(40)*. Further standardization efforts are needed to be fully able to rely on GAD65Ab determinations to predict T1D.

Autoantigen Processing and Presentation

The immune response to GAD65 and other β-cell autoantigens is likely to be initiated by antigen-presenting cells (APCs). According to one hypothesis, GAD65 is recognized as non-self because CD4+ T cells react against specific GAD65 peptides presented on HLA class II proteins. Such T cells may be able to transfer insulitis and diabetes although this has not been tested in humans. A second hypothesis suggests that the self antigen contains a peptide sequence homologous with a non-self antigen, so the autoimmune process is driven against the self antigen. The "molecular mimicry" hypothesis is supported by the observed sequence similarity between GAD65 and the P2-C protein of Coxsackie B *(89)*.

When an exogenous virus invades and replicates in the islet cells, the APCs, such as macrophages and dendritic cells initiate the phagocytosis of the damaged cells. APCs express HLA class II molecules. When the APCs are processing the antigen, the HLA class II molecules bind peptides of the antigen, and the peptides are then presented in the trimolecular (HLA alpha chain, peptide, and HLA β chain) complex on the APC surface. The APCs are producing cytokines, such as IL-12 and others that stimulate CD4+ T cells. Unique T-cell receptors (TCRs) on T cells recognize the trimolecular complex on the surface of APCs. CD4+ T cells that engage in an interaction between their TCRs and the trimolecular complex begin to differentiate and produce certain cytokines. Briefly, CD4+ T cells may produce IL-2 and interferon (IFN)-γ, which are often referred to as Th1 cytokines or IL-4 and IL-10, referred to as Th2 cytokines. The Th1 cytokines activate cytotoxic CD8+ T cells as well as macrophages. The latter may release cytokines such as IL-1, tumor necrosis factor (TNF)-α, and IFN-γ that may have a deleterious effect on the β cells *(90)*. In addition to this, cytotoxic T cells recognize peptides presented on HLA class I molecules on the target β cells and can, therefore, initiate β-cell killing. The concept of a Th1 and Th2 response is an oversimplification but illustrates the basic mechanisms by which the immune response reacts toward infections and perhaps, during certain circumstances, the initiation of an autoimmune response.

The autoantibody response is dependent on the CD4+ T cells. These helper cells express CD40 ligand (CD154) that recognize the CD40 receptor on the B lymphocyte surface and stimulates antibody production. Autoantibodies in sera of T1D patients are directed primarily to middle (amino acids 245–449) and C-terminal (amino acids 450–585) regions of the molecule *(62,71,91,92)*. The prevalence of GAD65Ab in T1D patients and first-degree relatives rises with increasing age and is highest in subjects with the HLA-DR3 or DQ2 haplotypes type *(73,93)*. GAD65Ab tend to remain in the sera of T1D patients for many years after the diagnosis *(94)*. GAD67 autoantibodies are found in 10–20% of newly diagnosed T1D patients *(33,95)*, but this is probably due to their cross-reactivity with GAD65 *(33)*. GAD67Ab in GAD65Ab-negative sera have been reported in patients with Graves' disease *(92,96)*.

T-Cell Detection

Autoreactive CD4+ T cells are assumed to be the key cells that regulate the killing of the pancreatic β cells *(97)*. The demonstration of autoantigen-reactive CD8+ T cells could potentially represent a reliable index of progressive β-cell destruction *(9)*. Several investigators have reported proliferation assays in response to recombinant GAD65, or GAD65 peptides indicated that T1D patients had an increased proliferation rate compared to healthy controls *(89,98)*. Subsequent studies suggested that the proliferation rate was not reproducible. Human T cells also proved to be difficult to clone, and T-cell clones specific to certain GAD65 peptides and restricted by HLA-DR or HLA-DQ are yet to be generated and made available for worldwide distribution. Novel approaches such as flow cytometric-assisted cytokine secretion assays (CSAs) restricted to HLA and GAD65 epitopes need to be developed and tested in subjects with or without GAD65 autoantibodies. Recent data suggest that the presence of GAD65 autoantibodies may indeed affect and modulate APCs and thereby the proliferative response to GAD65 *(99,100)*. Whether such responses will be more predictive of T1D remains to be determined.

Phenotyping of T cells utilizing HLA class II tetramers provides a novel approach to characterize the autoimmune response in T1D *(101,102)*. The problem with T-cell tests against specific islet autoantigens is lack of reproducibility and development of standardized assays with low interlaboratory variation *(103)*. Promising results are recently reported in ELISPOT assays with GAD65 and other peptides *(104)*.

Therapy and Future Directions

Preclinical studies in non-obese diabetic (NOD) mice suggest that immunomodulation with the GAD65 autoantigens might alter the course of autoimmune diabetes *(105,106)*. A number of therapeutic approaches using GAD or GAD peptides given by intrathymic, intraperitoneal, oral, or intranasal routes have been shown to prevent diabetes *(48,107)*. Although the mechanisms of this therapy is not yet clear, it has been shown that disease prevention may occur through activation of regulatory T cells *(108)*. The understanding of immunological tolerance is vast in mice but limited in humans *(109)*.

Alum-formulated human recombinant GAD65 has been administered subcutaneously in LADA patients *(110)*. None of the patients showed significant study-related adverse events. Fasting c-peptide levels at 24 weeks were increased compared with placebo with a dose of 20 μg. In addition, both fasting and stimulated c-peptide levels increased from baseline to 24 weeks in the 20-μg dose group. The (CD4+) (CD25+) / (CD4+) (CD25–) cell ratio increased at 24 weeks in the 20 microgram group *(110)*. These positive findings for clinical safety further support the clinical development of alum-formulated GAD65 as a therapeutic to prevent T1D. Future immunomodulation trials will better ascertain high-risk subjects based on HLA genetic risk factors, the level of insulin still produced, or by combining autoantigens with antibodies, so as to induce immune tolerance and a possible protection against the destruction of β cells *(109)*.

IA-2 AND IA-2β

Structure

A β-cell autoantigen, named ICA512, was isolated from an islet cDNA expression library by screening with human T1D sera *(111)*. Independently, a transmembrane protein tyrosine phosphatase (PTP), defined as IA-2, was isolated from a human insulinoma cDNA library by subtracting glucagonoma from insulinoma cDNA *(35)*. Analysis of the ICA512 clone showed that the cDNA sequence was essentially identical to IA-2 within the coding region. The IA-2 gene is located on chromosome 2q35 *(112)*. The product of IA-2 cDNA is a 979-amino acid protein with a Mr of 105,847 daltons *(36)*. The protein sequence consists of an extracellular domain (amino acids 1–576), a transmembrane region (amino acids 577–601), and an intracellular domain (amino acids 602–979). The extracellular domain contains a signal peptide and an unusual cysteine-rich region following the signal peptide. The intracellular cytoplasmic domain contains highly conserved regions similar to the catalytic domains found in members of the PTP family; however, certain amino acids are lacking leaving IA-2 with PTP activity *(35,36)*. The extracellular domain appears to reside within secretory granules, whereas the intracellular domain protrudes into the cytoplasm *(113)*. IA-2 undergoes proteolytic cleavage at its luminal domain, and upon exocytosis of secretory granules, it recycles to the Golgi complex region to be sorted into newly formed secretory granules.

A second novel PTP, IA-2β (phogrin), was cloned *(38)* and helped to explain prior tryptic fragments of the 64K autoantigen *(114)*. The overall length of IA-2β is 986 amino acids (Table 1). It has an extracellular domain (amino acids 1–585) that also contains a signal peptide and a cysteine-rich region next to that a transmembrane domain (amino acids 586–610) and an intracellular domain (amino acids 611–986). The extracellular and intracellular domains of IA-2 and IA-2β are only 27 and 74% identical, respectively.

Expression—β Cells and Elsewhere

Both IA-2 and IA-2β are primarily expressed in neuroendocrine cells. They are found in the islets of Langerhans and in many parts of the central nervous system, such as the hypothalamus. In the peripheral tissues, IA-2 is detectable in autonomic nerve fibers and ganglia, particularly at synaptic contacts. It has also been found that IA-2 mRNA is expressed in neuroendocrine tumors and can, therefore, be a marker for distinguishing neuroendocrine from non-neuroendocrine tumors *(115)*.

Function

Despite IA-2's overall similarity to the PTP family, the protein was found to lack detectable PTPase activity, either when immunoprecipitated from cells or produced recombinantly *(36)*. It has, however, been shown that by replacing aspartic acid with alanine at position 911 and alanine with aspartic acid at position 877, IA-2 becomes enzymatically active *(116)*. Yet, the function of IA-2 has not been resolved. IA-2β is also enzymatically inactive and has the same aspartic substitution in the catalytic domain as IA-2.

Autoantibody Detection

The assay that, so far, has given the best results in terms of detecting the autoantibodies against IA-2 is the use of coupled in vitro transcription translation as described previously for GAD65 *(37,117)*. The IA-2 protein produced by in vitro transcription and translation is typically labeled with ^{35}S-methionine. Serum samples of the patients are incubated in 96-well plates with the labeled IA-2 protein and protein A-sepharose is added. The IgG antibodies against the IA-2 molecule are bound to protein A-sepharose and the amount of precipitated radioactivity is determined. Results are expressed as units per milliliter derived from standard curves of counts per minute obtained for the WHO standard 97/550 *(40)*.

A sensitive ELISA for measurement of IA-2 autoantibodies has also been developed *(87)*. This antibody assay is based on the ability of IA-2 autoantibodies to form a bridge between IA-2 intracellular fragment coated onto ELISA plate wells and liquid-phase IA-2 labeled with biotin. It has been shown that the ELISA assay is suitable to detect IA-2A in the serum of patients with T1D with a similar sensitivity and specificity to the radioligand assay. A combination ELISA for the detection of both GAD65 and IA-2 autoantibodies has also been described and uses plates coated with both IA-2 and GAD65 and a mixture of IA-2 biotin and GAD65 biotin *(87)*.

IA-2 autoantibodies can also be measured by the use of recombinant ^{125}I-labeled IA-2 *(118)*. The intracellular part of IA-2 (IA-2ic) is expressed in *E. coli* as a biotinylated fusion protein and affinity purified on a streptavidin column. This IA-2 fusion protein is labeled with ^{125}I and added to the sera of T1D patients. The amount of autoantibodies that are bound to the ^{125}I-labeled IA-2 is then measured. The *E. coli*-derived IA-2 has the correct immunogenic conformation because it has been shown that it can block the autoantibody reactivity to an in vitro synthesized intracellular IA-2 *(118)*. It can, therefore, be used for the detection of IA-2 autoantibodies with a similar sensitivity and specificity as the radioligand assay.

Recently, a novel time-resolved fluorimetric assay for the detection of IA-2 autoantibodies was described *(119)*. The intracellular part of IA-2 is biotinylated and bound to streptavidin-coated 96-well plates by simultaneous incubation with serum samples and glutathione S-transferase (GST)-IA-2ic fusion protein. GST-IA-2ic captured by autoantibodies in the serum is detected with europium-labeled anti-GST antibody, and the signal is measured in a time-resolved fluorimeter. The time-resolved fluorimetric assay provides a simple, non-radioactive analysis method for the detection of IA-2 autoantibodies with a specificity and a sensitivity comparable to the radioligand method.

Autoantigen Processing and Presentation

Autoantibodies against IA-2 and IA-2β have been found in the sera of many patients with T1D. The antigenic regions of the IA-2 molecule are located in the intracellular domain. Approximately 95% of T1D patients' sera reacts with the carboxyl terminus (amino acids 771–979) and 40% with the amino terminus (amino acids 604–776) in the experiments *(120)*. Moreover, others experiments have shown that the disulfide bonds within the intracellular domain of IA-2 *(115)* as well as the glutamine at position 862 and residues 876–880 of the three amino acids tryptophan (W), proline (P) and aspartic acid (D) (WPD) loop of IA-2 *(121)* are of highest importance for the antigenic role of IA-2. Autoantibodies from patients with T1D also react with the intracellular domain of IA-2β and especially with the carboxy terminus. Approximately between 55–75% and 35–50% of T1D patients have antibodies against IA-2 and IA-2β, respectively *(114)*. However, the frequency of IA-2 antibodies varies accordingly with age and HLA genotype *(73)*. It has been shown that IA-2 autoantibodies are highest in the younger age groups and in T1D patients with HLA-DR4 and HLA-DQA1*0301-DQB1*0302 haplotype *(122,123)*. IA-2A in combination with GADA serves to identify over 95% of newly diagnosed cases with diabetes. IA-2 may represent a less sensitive but more specific marker of T1D.

There are two major hypotheses regarding the pathogenic significance of IA-2 immunity. IA-2 and IA-2β can represent a major target of the autoantibodies that are driven against the insulin-secreting β cells and destroy these cells. Alternatively, the destruction of the insulin-producing cells may release the IA-2 and start the immune response with the formation of IA-2 autoantibodies. The precise series of events that lead to IA-2 autoantibody formation needs to be determined.

T-Cell Detection

Although antibody responses to IA-2, IA-2β, and other autoantigens have been widely studied, relatively little is known about T-cell reactivity against these antigens. T cells in the peripheral blood of T1D patients have been found to preferentially recognize the 831–850 and 841–860 amino acids of IA-2. The overlapping region (amino acids 841–850) may represent an immunodominant T-cell epitope on IA-2 *(124)*. These T cells were stimulated by the use of purified recombinant IA-2. In another study, amino acids 805–820 were reported to form an epitope that elicited the highest T-cell responses in all at-risk relatives of T1D patients *(125)*. This epitope had 56% identity and 100% similarity over nine amino acids with a sequence in VP7, a major immunogenic protein of human rotavirus. It was also found to have 45–75% identity and 64–88% similarity over 8–14 amino acids to sequences in dengue, cytomegalovirus, measles, hepatitis C, canine distemper viruses, and the bacterium *Hemophilus influenzae*. Three other IA-2 epitopes have been shown to have 71–100% similarity over 7–12 amino acids to herpes, rhino-, hanta-, and flaviviruses and two others are 80–82% similar over 10–11 amino acids to sequences in milk, wheat, and bean proteins. It is, therefore, critical to investigate whether the CD4+ T cells are activated against IA-2 epitopes by rotavirus or other viruses. Furthermore, ex vivo ELISPOT analyses revealed in new onset T1D patients the presence of IFN-γ-producing cells *(42,126)*.

Therapy and Future Directions

Previous studies suggest that it is now possible to generate IA-2-specific T-cell responses by using a recombinant IA-2. This method can be used for the detection and recognition of specific CD8+ T cells that participate in the destruction of the β cells in the pancreas of T1D patients. Future directions will include the detection of these cells not only in the peripheral blood but also in the pancreas with the use of high-resolution imaging techniques.

INSULIN

Structure

Insulin was discovered in 1921 by Banting and Best, who extracted insulin from the pancreatic tissue of dogs. Insulin is a 51-amino acid polypeptide consisting of two chains, A and B, with 21 and 30 amino acids, respectively, and a molecular weight of 5800-kDa. The chains are linked by two interchain disulfide bridges that connect A7 to B7 and A20 to B19, whereas an intrachain bridge connects A6 and A11. Insulin is produced as a preprohormone that is processed to pro-insulin and, then, to mature insulin by the removal of the C-peptide. Processing occurs within the β-cell's secretory granules, where insulin is packaged in a crystal form.

It was first synthesized in 1979 in *E. coli* cells by the use of recombinant DNA techniques. Before insulin was synthesized, bovine and porcine insulin were used to treat T1D patients. The structures of the bovine and human insulin are almost identical with only three differences in the amino acids. On the human insulin, threonine replaces alanine in position A8, isoleucine replaces valine in position A10, and threonine replaces alanine in position B30. The last substitution is the only difference that human insulin has in comparison with porcine insulin.

Expression Function

The insulin gene on human chromosome 11p15 is predominantly expressed in the β-cells of the pancreatic islets of Langerhans. Insulin and proinsulin are the only β cell-specific autoantigens within human islets. However, studies in humans have indicated that the insulin gene can also be expressed in the thymus, where higher levels of insulin may promote negative selection (deletion) of insulin-specific T lymphocytes, which play a critical role in the pathogenesis of T1D *(52,53)*.

The secretion of insulin by the β cells is controlled by the blood glucose concentration. Insulin plays a major part in the uptake of glucose by the cells. After each meal, the level of glucose increases. Insulin stimulates the formation of glycogen in the muscles and the liver and suppresses the gluconeogenesis by the liver. Insulin stimulates the synthesis of fatty acids and controls the uptake of valine, leucine, and isoleucine by muscle, which helps further to increase the synthesis of muscle proteins.

Autoantibody Detection

The development of antibodies to insulin was accepted as a fact only in terms of consequence of insulin therapy. Insulin antibodies, detected by the use of ^{125}I-insulin, were common among insulin-treated patients. The presence of IAAs in T1D patients that had not yet been treated with insulin was described in 1983 *(29)*. Antibodies against pro-insulin have also been detected in newly diagnosed T1D patients, but it has been shown that IAAs are a better predictive and more specific marker for the disease *(127)*.

IAAs have also been described in insulin autoimmune syndrome (IAS) that develops primarily in Japanese patients *(128)*. This condition is characterized by reactive hypoglycemia, normal fasting blood glucose, hyperinsulinemia, and the presence of insulin-binding autoantibodies. All patients are positive for HLA-DR4, and further analysis has shown that they have the DRB1*0406/DQA1*0301/DQB1*0302. This syndrome has been reported to these patients in most cases after they receive drugs that contain a sulfhydryl compound. The hypoglycemia usually resolves after the discontinuation of the medication. However, studies have shown that certain polymorphisms of IAAs, identified by their binding site on the insulin molecule, can distinguish between diabetes-related and diabetes-unrelated antibodies (128).

Most studies have shown that IAAs are strongly associated with T1D in children (129), but they can be present for years before the development of the disease. IAAs are present in more than 50% of young children at the time of clinical diagnosis, so IAAs are a particularly important marker for the disease in the young. Furthermore, IAAs were associated with DR4, DQ8, and some DQA1 alleles, such as DQA1*0102, 0201, 0301, 0401 (53).

Current assay formats for IAAs vary although the international workshops for IAA standardization (41,88) have improved assay quality and harmonization. The IAA method most frequently used is a microadaptation using protein A-sepharose to separate free from antibody-bound 125I-insulin (127). Initially, two different assays were used to detect the IAAs in the sera of T1D patients, the fluid phase Radio Immuno Assay (RIA) and the solid phase ELISA. The two assays gave very different results relative to the positive predictive value for the development of T1D. It was then described that the two assays were measuring different antibodies and that the IAAs measured by RIA methodology were more disease related than those measured by ELISA methods (41). IAAs seem to react with a conformational epitope (either A or B chain), and that can explain the fact that it is so difficult to measure IAAs by ELISA or other similar tests. Studies have shown that IAA binding a conformational epitope including the A-chain residues, A8–A13, and the B-chain residues, B1–B3, are T1D associated (130).

Williams et al. recently developed a novel radioligand microassay using serum from the diabetic patients in microtiter plates in duplicates and incubating it with ^{125}I-labeled human insulin (131). After immunoprecipitation of IAA-^{125}I-labeled insulin complexes with protein A-sepharose and removal of the unbound label, the samples were washed, centrifuged, and the precipitate was transferred to tubes for counting in a gamma counter. Results are expressed as percentage binding or related to a IAA-positive serum.

Autoantigen Processing, Presentation, and T-Cell Detection

The 9–23 amino acid region of the insulin B chain (B9–23) is a dominant epitope recognized by pathogenic T lymphocytes in NOD mice, the animal model for T1D (132). Similar (B9–23)-specific T-cell responses in peripheral lymphocytes obtained from patients with recent-onset T1D and from prediabetic subjects at high risk for disease were recently described (133). Use of the highly sensitive cytokine-detection ELISPOT assay revealed that these (B9–23)-specific cells produced the proinflammatory cytokine IFN-γ.

Antibody-blocking experiments with cells from an HLA-DQ8 homozygous patient showed that the insulin B peptide was presented by DQ8, and moreover, Lee et al. determined the three-dimensional structure of the DQ8 in complex with the insulin B peptide (134). The insulin B chain has one of the highest affinities for DQ8 among peptides from islet autoantigens, and it also binds to the major histocompatibility complex (MHC) of the I-A^{g7} subtype in the NOD mouse. The peptide side chain-binding pockets of human DQ8 and DQ2 share chemical and geometric properties with the murine I-A^{g7}, suggesting that diabetes is caused by the same antigen-presentation events in humans and NOD mice *(134)*.

The role of insulin in CTL killing of β-cells requires the expression of insulin peptides on HLA class I molecules. The use of new techniques, such as HLA tetramers, may be useful in identifying the T cells that have receptors which recognize specific insulin peptides *(102)*. The identification of specific peptides of islet autoantigens may be important for the design of antigen-specific immunotherapy for T1D and to protect from CD8+ T cells recognizing insulin *(135)*.

Therapy and Future Directions

The subcutaneous injection of insulin is the first-line treatment of T1D. Different types of insulin are used based on their times of onset and durations of action. Human insulin is less antigenic than previously used animal-derived varieties. Rapid-acting insulins include regular, lispro, and aspart insulin, the only types that can be administered intravenously. Regular insulin is a preparation of zinc insulin crystals in solution. Lispro insulin is regular insulin that has been genetically engineered with the reversal of amino acids lysine and proline in the B chain. Aspart insulin has aspartic acid instead of proline in position 28 of the B chain. Both of these insulins are more quickly absorbed, and therefore they can be administered shortly before eating. Semilente is a slightly slower rapid-acting insulin that contains zinc insulin microcrystals in an acetate buffer.

Intermediate-acting insulins include (i) the neutral protamine Hagedorn (NPH) insulin that contains a mixture of regular and protamine zinc insulin and (ii) the lente insulin that contains 30% semilente insulin and 70% ultralente insulin in an acetate buffer.

Long-acting insulins include (i) the ultralente insulin that contains large zinc insulin crystals in an acetate buffer and (ii) the glargine insulin, a new long-acting insulin that produces a stable level lasting more than 24 h. Both insulins can provide a basal 24-h insulin with a single daily injection. In the event that insulin can be used in immune tolerance induction therapy, it will be important to decide which one of these many insulin preparations are most effective. One such study has been carried out.

In a randomized, controlled, non-blinded clinical trial (Diabetes Prevention Trial-T1D Study Group), first- and second-degree relatives of patients with T1D, positive for ICAs and considered as having high risk to develop the disease were administered low-dose subcutaneous ultralente insulin, twice daily for a total dose of 0.25 unit per kilogram of body weight per day, plus annual 4-day continuous intravenous infusions of insulin *(4)*. Diabetes was diagnosed in 69 subjects in the intervention group and 70 subjects in the observation group. The cumulative incidence of diabetes was similar in the two groups, suggesting that in persons at high risk, insulin administered at this dosage cannot delay or prevent T1D. In a similar trial from the same study group, oral insulin was administered to first- and second-degree relatives of patients with T1D who had high risk for the disease. However, oral insulin did delay the onset of T1D in subjects with high IAA levels *(136)*. More studies are needed to determine the potential role of oral insulin in the prevention and delay of T1D.

STANDARDIZATION

Autoantibody Detection

Concordance of the results obtained from different laboratories for the measurement of antibodies against islet cell antigens is essential for the comparison of studies from different centers, as well as for the recruitment of centers into multicenter studies. The DASP was established in order to evaluate and improve the assay methods and to evaluate the new WHO reference reagent for antibodies to GAD and IA-2 *(40)*. The aim of the first proficiency evaluation in 2003 was to assess and improve the comparability of islet autoantibody measurements between different laboratories and to introduce a common standard to allow laboratories to express antibody results in common units *(39)*.

Sera were obtained from 50 newly diagnosed type 1 diabetic subjects and 50 controls and distributed to 46 laboratories in 13 countries. The evaluation showed a high degree of concordance between laboratories in GADA and IA-2A measurement and only radio-binding assays achieved high sensitivity and specificity for both antibodies. The mean adjusted sensitivity for GADA (45 laboratories) and IA-2A (43 laboratories) was 84 and 58%, respectively. In contrast, there was wide variation between IAA assays and although some sensitive assays were identified, the overall performance of IAA was poor. Most laboratories used the novel radio-binding microassay using protein A precipitation that is described above *(127)*. The mean adjusted sensitivity for IAAs from 23 laboratories was 36%. It was also shown that good interlaboratory concordance was achieved when antibody levels were expressed in WHO units, therefore the Immunology of Diabetes Society recommends that all GADA and IA-2A results be expressed in WHO units/ml *(39)*.

T-Cell Detection

A T-cell workshop was organized by the Immunology of Diabetes Society. Its aim was to appreciate and identify any problems associated with autoreactive T-cell assays in T1D. The First International Workshop for Standardization of T-cell Assays in T1D assessed numerous islet autoantigens preparations for their ability to stimulate peripheral blood T cells *(137)*. This workshop demonstrated that the limitations of current assay technology and the quality of antigen preparations are the two main factors that mostly affect the reliability and the consistency in the detection of islet autoreactive T cells.

The Second International Workshop, two years later, evaluated again the quality of several recombinant preparations of the islet autoantigens GAD65, IA-2 and proinsulin and their ability to stimulate proliferation of a panel of known antigen-specific T-cell clones or T-cell lines *(138)*. It was demonstrated that preparations of GAD65 and IA-2 expressed using baculovirus or obtained from *E. coli* were able to stimulate specific T-cell clones, but the baculovirus GAD65 preparation was shown to be of superior quality. The single proinsulin preparation used was unable to elicit proliferation from an insulin B chain-specific T-cell clone. Preparations of islet autoantigens with high quality and ability to stimulate specific T cells are needed to promote the development of sensitive assays of islet-reactive T cells in patients with T1D or subjects at high risk for the disease *(138)*.

CANDIDATE AUTOANTIGENS

A number of other molecules have been reported to be related to autoimmune diabetes (Table 2).

ICA69

A novel islet peptide termed ICA69 was identified by screening human islet lambda gt11 cDNA expression library with cytoplasmic islet cell antibody-positive sera from relatives of T1D patients who progressed to the overt disease *(139)*. The molecular weight of the protein was found to be 54,600. ICA69 is present in brain, lung, kidney, and heart *(139)*, but the highest levels have been detected in islets and other neuroendocrine tissues *(140,141)*. It has been suggested that ICA69 participates in the process of neuroendocrine secretion through association with the outside of secretory vesicles *(141)*. Anti-ICA69 antibodies are diabetes related, but they have been found to be present also in the sera of patients with rheumatoid arthritis (RA). ICA69 shares two short regions of similarity with bovine serum albumin, one of several cow milk proteins. Epidemiological studies have indicated that the risk for the development of T1D increases with the infant's ingestion of cow's milk.

ICA12 (SOX-13)

ICA12 was identified during the screening of islet expression libraries with T1D patients' antibodies *(111)*. The complete sequence of ICA12 is still not known. ICA12 is the transcription factor SOX13 that plays a key role in organ development. Antibodies against ICA12 have been detected in about 18% of patients with new onset T1D *(142)*, but in most studies, they are found in T1D patients at the same frequency as in patients with rheumatic diseases or healthy control subjects *(143)*. Antibodies to SOX-13 have been detected in patients with primary biliary cirrhosis *(143)*. It has been suggested that SOX13 antibodies may be a non-specific marker of tissue damage associated with chronic hyperglycemia *(144)*. These antibodies would therefore primarily be found among adults, and the contribution to prediction of T1D may be limited.

Carboxypeptidase H

Carboxypeptidase H (CPH) is a glycoprotein and a carboxypeptidase B-like enzyme that is expressed by cells secreting polypeptide hormones and neurotransmitters, in which CPH cleaves the COOH terminal ends of hormone precursors *(145)*. CPH is involved in the processing of proinsulin to insulin. CPH is present in human islet cells and brain and in bovine adrenal, pituitary, and kidney. CPH was cloned from a human islet cDNA library and found to have a strong similarity to the human brain CPH sequence *(145)*. The frequency of T1D patients who have CPH autoantibodies has not been fully investigated. In one study the diagnostic sensitivity was only 3%, which did not differ from the controls *(146)*. The frequency doubled among subjects with GAD65Ab positive LADA patients, and it is possible that CPH autoantibodies may improve the diagnostic sensitivity and specificity among adults.

Sulfatide

Sulfatide is the major acidic glycosphingolipid in myelin in the central and peripheral nervous system. It is also expressed in the islets of Langerhans, both in the surface and in the secretory granules of the insulin-producing cells (for a review *see* ref. *147*). It is also found in kidneys, gallbladder, and the choroid layer of the eyes. Antibodies against the sulfatide have been detected in T1D in a small number of patients *(148)*. Sulfatide antibodies are also found in the sera of patients with Guillain–Barre syndrome *(149)* and peripheral neuropathies *(150)*. It has been suggested that neuronal elements contribute to T1D pathogenesis, and it will be important therefore to analyze whether sulfatide antibodies are associated with HLA types or with other genetic factors associated with T1D.

Ganglioside GM2-1

Gangliosides are amphiphilic molecules containing a hydrophobic portion, the ceramide, and a hydrophilic one, the sialo-oligosaccharide chain, through which they bind to hormones, toxins, and viruses. Within cells, they tend to be associated with plasma membranes and they have been shown to take part in cell-to-cell interaction and in signal transaction. Gangliosides are also expressed in cytosolic membranes of secretory granules in some endocrine cells. GM2-1 was described as pancreatic islet monosialo-ganglioside, equally expressed in β- and non-β cells *(151)* and was mainly localized with the secretory granules *(151)*. GM2-1 has been shown to be the target of IgG autoantibodies strongly correlated with progression to diabetes in ICA-positive relatives of type 1 diabetic subjects, which may explain that occurrence of GM2-1 autoantibodies was significantly correlated with positivity for GAD65 autoantibodies, but not for IAAs or GAD67 autoantibodies *(152)*. There are no recent studies on the role of GM2-1 gangliosides and T1D.

Imogen 38

T cells from new onset T1D patients have been shown to specifically proliferate to β-cell membrane fractions that contain the mitochondrial 38-kDa IA, imogen 38 *(153)*. Imogen 38 is found more frequently in β cells than in α cells, but it is rather broadly distributed as a structural component to all oxidative tissues *(154)*. No humoral response has so far been identified against this antigen. Imogen 38 was thought to be a target for bystander islet autoimmune attack rather than a primary autoantigen.

GLIMA 38

GLIMA 38 is an amphiphilic N-Asp glycated β-cell membrane protein of Mr 38,000, expressed in islets and in islet and neuronal cell lines *(155)*. Antibodies against GLIMA 38 have been detected in about 20% of new onset T1D patients and 15% of prediabetic subjects *(155)*. The GLIMA 38 antibodies were associated with high levels of IA-2A and ICAs, which are considered markers of rapid progression to clinical diabetes *(156)*. The diagnostic sensitivity of GLIMA 38 antibodies in prediabetic subjects was considered lower than that for IAAs, ICAs, IA-2Ab, and GAD65Ab *(156)*. Further studies are needed to explore the contribution of the GLIMA 38 autoimmunity in T1D.

Islet-Specific Glucose-6-Phosphatase-Related Protein

Islet-specific glucose-6-phosphatase-related protein (IGRP) was investigated initially as a key component in a glucose substrate cycle and energy metabolism in the β cells of the pancreas, and it was cloned using a subtractive cDNA expression cloning procedure from mouse insulinoma tissue *(157)*. Recently, IGRP was recognized as an autoantigen targeted by a prevalent population of pathogenic CD8$^+$ T cells in NOD mice *(158)*. This observation was of considerable interest as IGRP would represent yet another intracellular enzyme as a potential target in human islet autoimmunity as well. Furthermore, IGRP was found to be mainly expressed in the islet β cells of humans and NOD mice and, rarely, in the islet α cells. IGRP has a significant role in islet cell metabolism although its overall contribution to the islet β-cell function has not yet been identified.

Although CD8+ and CD4+ T cells targeted against IGRP peptides have been detected in the NOD mouse, it was unclear whether IGRP has a significant role in the human disease pathogenesis. IGRP-specific tetramers were used to evaluate the prevalence of IGRP-reactive T cells in healthy and T1D subjects *(159)*. IGRP-reactive T cells were detected in both T1D and healthy subjects and there were recent reports of other autoreactive T cells detected in healthy subjects. This study rather underlines the prevalence of potentially autoreactive blood T cells in the population than T-cell recognition of an islet-specific autoantigen.

SST Receptors

SST has an inhibitory action on hormone secretion but also cell proliferation. Five SST G-protein-coupled receptors (SSTR1-5) have been identified and cloned from multiple mammalian species. In humans, SSTR1 and 2 are present in pituitary, small intestine, heart, and spleen, whereas SSTR2 predominates in the pancreas, pituitary, and stomach. SSTR3 and 4 are expressed in pituitary, heart, liver, spleen, stomach, small intestine and kidney, whereas SSTR5 is found mostly in the pituitary and is the dominant receptor of SST peptides in pancreatic islet cells. SSTR5 has also been found on T and B lymphocytes (for a review *see* ref. *160*). SSTRs consist of seven transmembrane domains with an extracellular amino terminus, an intracellular carboxy terminus, three extracellular loops, and three intracellular loops *(161)*. Many studies have investigated the potential role in modulating both macrophage and T cells in the immune system and it has been suggested that SST–SSTR interaction in APCs may lead to T-cell proliferation *(162)*. However, the role of SST–SSTR5 in islet cell proliferation and specific antigen presentation during the development of T1D remains speculative *(163)*. Currently, there is no evidence that either SST or any of its receptors are autoantigens.

ANIMAL ISLET CELL AUTOANTIGENS

The NOD mouse is the most studied animal model for T1D, as the pathogenesis of the disease in this animal resembles most of the disease process in humans. As it is well established that both CD4+ and CD8+ T cells play an important role in the pathogenesis of diabetes in the NOD mouse *(47)*, numerous attempts have been made to isolate diabetogenic T cells. The first pathogenic T-cell clone was a CD4+ T lymphocyte that proliferated and produced lymphokines in response to islet cell antigen- and NOD APCs, reviewed in ref. *164*.

Most attempts to isolate pathogenic CD4 T-cell clones have been focused on the already known major islet autoantigens, insulin, and GAD65. T-cell clones autoreactive to insulin, and most specifically to the epitope B9-23 residues of the B chain, have been identified. Attempts to identify autoreactive T-cell clones against GAD have been less successful. However, GAD-reactive CD4+ T-cell clones were isolated from transgenic mice expressing the human HLA class II DQ8 molecule after immunization with GAD peptides *(164)*. Successful studies on the induction of immune tolerance by GAD include the isolation of a GAD65-specific Th2 cell clone that was transferred to NOD mice and that prevented the progression of insulitis and subsequent development of overt T1D *(165)*. Insulin and GAD65 have also been identified as targets for CD8+ T-cell clones.

Reactive T-cell clones to IA-2β (phogrin) were detected in peripheral T cells of NOD mice as young as 4 weeks of age *(166)*. Mapping of T-cell reactivity resulted in the identification of two major epitopes of the polypeptide: the 629–649 residues immediately adjacent to the transmembrane domain and the 755–777 residues lying in the NH(2)-terminal region of the PTP domain *(167)*.

The role of insulin as an autoantigen in NOD mouse autoimmune diabetes is reviewed in detail elsewhere *(47,164)*.

MODIFICATION OF AUTOANTIGENS TO MAKE THEM DIABETOGENIC

In inflammatory responses caused by an infection or other physiological stress-induced states, the levels of oxidative mediators such as nitric oxide, hypochlorous acid, hydrogen peroxide and peroxynitrite anion are often elevated. These mediators may cause a cascade of oxidative events that may result in oxidation of locally expressed proteins. Cytokines produced by islet infiltrating mononuclear cells may also stimulate the b cells to produce nitric oxide and reactive oxygen species (ROS). ROS may denature autoantigens to display neoepitopes, that is, epitopes that have not previously been presented to the immune system. Such post-translational modifications may lead to an immune response that eventually may cross-react with the native protein and thereby cause autoimmunity. It is an enigma why tolerance is broken to GAD65, IA-2, and insulin in T1D. Oxidatively modified aggregates of GAD react with serum antibodies of T1D patients *(168)*. In the following, we will therefore review possible post-translational modifications that may contribute to T1D.

A majority of mammalian proteins are subject to post-translational modifications resulting in neoepitopes. These neoepitopes probably act by generating a new peptide-HLA protein complex to be recognized by T cells with high-affinity TCRs. Examples of post-translational modifications are listed in Table 3. Malondialdehyde (MDA) is a chemical compound used for in vitro aldehydation. It is a three-carbon dialdehyde resulting from lipid peroxidation and forms covalent adducts on primary amino groups, such as the side chain residue of lysine. Recent studies have defined that MDA-aldehydation of the myelin autoantigen myelin oligodendrocyte glycoprotein (MOG) leads to more severe experimental autoimmune encephalomyelitis (EAE), a model of multiple sclerosis (Holm B., personal communication).

In RA patients, antibodies toward citrullinated antigens have been demonstrated, with a higher specificity for RA patients than the otherwise commonly used rheumatoid factor, reviewed in ref. *169*. This has resulted in a new diagnostic tool for RA, where patient sera are tested for antibody positivity against a cyclic citrullinated peptide (CCP). This CCP test is highly specific (<97%) for RA patients. The prognostic

Table 3
Selection of Post-Translational Modifications that Could Occur in vivo and the Affected
Amino Acid or the Expected End Product of Post-Translational Modification

Post-translational modification	Affected amino acid → end product
Aldehydation	Lysine
Citrullination	Arginine → citrulline
Chlorination	Methionine, tryptophan, and tyrosine
Deamidation	Asparagine and glutamine
Deiminiation	Arginine
Glycation (the Maillard reaction)	→ Various advanced glycation end products [pentosidine, crosslines, imidazolones, N^e-(carboxymethyl) lysine (CML), and pyrraline]
N-linked glycosylation	Asparagine
O-linked glycosylation	Lysine and threonine
Hydroxylation	Lysine and proline
Isomerization	Asparagine and aspartic acid
Metal-catalyzed oxidative reaction	Tyrosine → reactive nitrogen species and nitric oxide → Reactive oxygen species (ROS)
Methylation	Arginine: glutamic acid, histidine, and lysine
Phosphorylation	Serine

relevance of this test is also proven, as sera taken from RA patients prior to disease onset are CCP positive *(169)*.

Chlorinated amino acids, that is, methionine, thryptophane, and tyrosine, are reactive oxidants themselves and are more stable than HOCl, thus being able to induce a more persistent oxidative microenvironment. The adaptive immune tolerance toward ubiquitously expressed autoantigens is broken on chlorination *(170)*. Deamidation results in the conversion of an asparagine residue to a mixture of isoaspartate and aspartate. Deamidation of glutamine residues in glutamine-rich gliadin components is thought to be a critical post-translational modification that may trigger CD. Studies on CD patients have demonstrated that gliadin becomes an even more potent (gliadin specific) T-cell activator if deamidated, reviewed in ref. *171*. This is done by the gut enzyme tissue transglutaminase (tTG) that converts glutamine to glutamic acid. It is of considerable interest that autoantibodies against tTG predict CD and yet unexplained why the enzyme responsible for modifying gliadin becomes an autoantigen itself.

Many potential targets for self-reactive T cells are glycoproteins, suggesting that T cells might recognize peptides with glycosylated side chains although not responding to sugars in isolation. Usually, glycosylation is either N-linked or O-linked, depending on which amino acid is affected. In N-linked glycosylation, the oligosaccharides links to the amine group on the side chain of asparagine, whereas in O-linked glycosylation the oligosaccharide links to lysine, serine, or threonine side chain hydroxyl groups. Whether these types of post-translational modifications are important to T1D is yet to be explored.

ROS could be generated in vitro if proteins are treated with iron or copper salts in the presence of peroxide or ascorbic acid (vitamin C), as the proteins undergo specific cleavage or aggregation. The metal-catalyzed Haber–Weiss reaction was used to increase the autoantigenicity of GAD65 by Trigwell and coworkers *(168)*. Oxidative modification has been extensively studied in atherosclerosis, primarily in the oxidation of low-density lipoprotein (LDL) and its role in development of atherosclerotic plaques. Macrophages also seem to engulf oxidized LDL more readily than unmodified LDL, leading to formation of foam cells that are the basis for formation of atherosclerotic lesions as well as to antibodies against ox-LDL *(172)*.

CONCLUSIONS AND FUTURE DIRECTIONS

Research in islet autoantigens since 1981 has resulted in the discovery of three autoantigens that collectively have contributed to the understanding of the etiology and pathogenesis of T1D. The presence of these autoantibodies predicts diabetes to the extent that 50% of triple autoantibody-positive healthy subjects develop T1D within 5 years. Subjects at risk for T1D can be identified and followed to antibody positivity, and antibody-positive individuals can be followed until the clinical onset of diabetes. Intervention trials have been conducted with parenteral insulin or nicotinamide. Although these treatment modalities did not prevent diabetes, other approaches such as immunomodulation with alum-formulated GAD65 or oral insulin are subject to controlled clinical trials. Assays of humoral autoantigen responses are well developed, including autoantibody isotype and subtype analyses and epitope-specific reactivity. International standardization efforts allow a reduction in interlaboratory variation that contributes to advancement in T1D research. Recent attempts also to include a dissection of the cellular autoimmune response may add to a better understanding of trigger events and novel approaches to therapy. As there are sera in very young children and also in adults which are ICA positive but negative for GAD65, IA-2, and insulin antibodies, a fourth antigen lures. A fourth antigen is of importance as it would increase both the diagnostic sensitivity and specificity and perhaps yield yet another target for immune tolerance induction.

ACKNOWLEDGMENTS

Studies in the authors' laboratory were supported by the National Institutes of Health (DK26190, DK53004, DK17047, DK63861, and AI42380), the American Diabetes Association, the Juvenile Diabetes Research Foundation, the Swedish Research Council (72X-14064), the Robert H. Williams Endowment, the Swedish Diabetes Association, the Swedish Childhood Diabetes Fund, and the UMAS Research Fund.

REFERENCES

1. Rahier J, Goebbels RM, Henquin JC. Cellular composition of the human diabetic pancreas. *Diabetologia* 1983;24(5):366–71.
2. Greenbaum CJ, Sears KL, Kahn SE, Palmer JP. Relationship of beta-cell function and autoantibodies to progression and nonprogression of subclinical type 1 diabetes: follow-up of the Seattle Family Study. *Diabetes* 1999;48(1):170–5.
3. Sosenko JM, Palmer JP, Greenbaum CJ, et al. Patterns of metabolic progression to type 1 diabetes in the Diabetes Prevention Trial-Type 1. *Diabetes Care* 2006;29(3):643–9.
4. DPT-1. Effects of insulin in relatives of patients with type 1 diabetes mellitus. *N Engl J Med* 2002;346(22):1685–91.

5. Gale EA, Bingley PJ, Emmett CL, Collier T. European Nicotinamide Diabetes Intervention Trial (ENDIT): a randomised controlled trial of intervention before the onset of type 1 diabetes. *Lancet* 2004;363(9413):925–31.

6. Bingley PJ, Gale EA. Progression to type 1 diabetes in islet cell antibody-positive relatives in the European Nicotinamide Diabetes Intervention Trial: the role of additional immune, genetic and metabolic markers of risk. *Diabetologia* 2006;49(5):881–90.

7. Lernmark A. Type 1 diabetes as a model for prediction and diagnosis. *Autoimmunity* 2004;37(4):341–5.

8. Notkins AL. Type 1 diabetes as a model for autoantibodies as predictors of autoimmune diseases. *Autoimmun Rev* 2004;3(Suppl 1):S7–9.

9. Notkins AL, Lernmark A. Autoimmune type 1 diabetes: resolved and unresolved issues. *J Clin Invest* 2001;108(9):1247–52.

10. Lernmark A. Type 1 diabetes as a model for prediction and diagnosis. *Autoimmunity* 2004;37(4):341–5.

11. Gianani R, Eisenbarth GS. The stages of type 1A diabetes: 2005. *Immunol Rev* 2005;204:232–49.

12. Tsai EB, Sherry NA, Palmer JP, Herold KC. The rise and fall of insulin secretion in type 1 diabetes mellitus. *Diabetologia* 2006;49(2):261–70.

13. Gepts W. Pathologic anatomy of the pancreas in juvenile diabetes mellitus. *Diabetes* 1965;14(10):619–33.

14. Nerup J, Bendixen G, Binder C. Autoimmunity in diabetes mellitus. *Lancet* 1970;2(7673):610–1.

15. Nerup J, Andersen OO, Bendixen G, Egeberg J, Poulsen JE. Anti-pancreatic cellular hypersensitivity in diabetes mellitus. *Diabetes* 1971;20(6):424–7.

16. Singal DP, Blajchman MA. Histocompatibility (HL-A) antigens, lymphocytotoxic antibodies and tissue antibodies in patients with diabetes mellitus. *Diabetes* 1973;22(6):429–32.

17. Nerup J, Platz P, Andersen OO, et al. HL-A antigens and diabetes mellitus. *Lancet* 1974;2(7885):864–6.

18. Bottazzo GF, Florin-Christensen A, Doniach D. Islet-cell antibodies in diabetes mellitus with autoimmune polyendocrine deficiencies. *Lancet* 1974;2(7892):1279–83.

19. MacCuish AC, Irvine WJ, Barnes EW, Duncan LJ. Antibodies to pancreatic islet cells in insulin-dependent diabetics with coexistent autoimmune disease. *Lancet* 1974;2(7896):1529–31.

20. Lendrum R, Walker G, Gamble DR. Islet-cell antibodies in juvenile diabetes mellitus of recent onset. *Lancet* 1975;1(7912):880–2.

21. Gorsuch AN, Spencer KM, Lister J, et al. Evidence for a long prediabetic period in type I (insulin-dependent) diabetes mellitus. *Lancet* 1981;2(8260–61):1363–5.

22. Lernmark A, Sehlin J, Taljedal IB, Kromann H, Nerup J. Possible toxic effects of normal and diabetic patient serum on pancreatic B-cells. *Diabetologia* 1978;14(1):25–31.

23. Lernmark A, Freedman ZR, Hofmann C, et al. Islet-cell-surface antibodies in juvenile diabetes mellitus. *N Engl J Med* 1978;299(8):375–80.

24. Dobersen MJ, Scharff JE, Ginsberg-Fellner F, Notkins AL. Cytotoxic autoantibodies to beta cells in the serum of patients with insulin-dependent diabetes mellitus. *N Engl J Med* 1980;303(26):1493–8.

25. Lernmark A, Baekkeskov S. Islet cell antibodies-theoretical and practical implications. *Diabetologia* 1981;21(5):431–5.

26. Baekkeskov S, Nielsen JH, Marner B, Bilde T, Ludvigsson J, Lernmark A. Autoantibodies in newly diagnosed diabetic children immunoprecipitate human pancreatic islet cell proteins. *Nature* 1982;298(5870):167–9.

27. Gerling I, Baekkeskov S, Lernmark A. Islet cell and 64K autoantibodies are associated with plasma IgG in newly diagnosed insulin-dependent diabetic children. *J Immunol* 1986;137(12):3782–5.

28. Christie M, Landin-Olsson M, Sundkvist G, Dahlquist G, Lernmark A, Baekkeskov S. Antibodies to a Mr-64,000 islet cell protein in Swedish children with newly diagnosed type 1 (insulin-dependent) diabetes. *Diabetologia* 1988;31(8):597–602.

29. Palmer JP, Asplin CM, Clemons P, et al. Insulin antibodies in insulin-dependent diabetics before insulin treatment. *Science* 1983;222(4630):1337–9.

30. Kuglin B, Gries FA, Kolb H. Evidence of IgG autoantibodies against human proinsulin in patients with IDDM before insulin treatment. *Diabetes* 1988;37(1):130–2.

31. Baekkeskov S, Aanstoot HJ, Christgau S, et al. Identification of the 64K autoantigen in insulin-dependent diabetes as the GABA-synthesizing enzyme glutamic acid decarboxylase. *Nature* 1990;347(6289):151–6.

32. Karlsen AE, Hagopian WA, Grubin CE, et al. Cloning and primary structure of a human islet isoform of glutamic acid decarboxylase from chromosome 10. *Proc Natl Acad Sci USA* 1991;88(19): 8337–41.

33. Hagopian WA, Michelsen B, Karlsen AE, et al. Autoantibodies in IDDM primarily recognize the 65,000-M(r) rather than the 67,000-M(r) isoform of glutamic acid decarboxylase. *Diabetes* 1993;42(4):631–6.

34. Kim J, Richter W, Aanstoot HJ, et al. Differential expression of GAD65 and GAD67 in human, rat, and mouse pancreatic islets. *Diabetes* 1993;42(12):1799–808.

35. Lan MS, Lu J, Goto Y, Notkins AL. Molecular cloning and identification of a receptor-type protein tyrosine phosphatase, IA-2, from human insulinoma. *DNA Cell Biol* 1994;13(5):505–14.

36. Lan MS, Wasserfall C, Maclaren NK, Notkins AL. IA-2, a transmembrane protein of the protein tyrosine phosphatase family, is a major autoantigen in insulin-dependent diabetes mellitus. *Proc Natl Acad Sci USA* 1996;93(13):6367–70.

37. Payton MA, Hawkes CJ, Christie MR. Relationship of the 37,000- and 40,000-M(r) tryptic fragments of islet antigens in insulin-dependent diabetes to the protein tyrosine phosphatase-like molecule IA-2 (ICA512). *J Clin Invest* 1995;96(3):1506–11.

38. Wasmeier C, Hutton JC. Molecular cloning of phogrin, a protein-tyrosine phosphatase homologue localized to insulin secretory granule membranes. *J Biol Chem* 1996;271(30):18161–70.

39. Bingley PJ, Bonifacio E, Mueller PW. Diabetes Antibody Standardization Program: first assay proficiency evaluation. *Diabetes* 2003;52(5):1128–36.

40. Mire-Sluis AR, Gaines Das R, Lernmark A. The World Health Organization International Collaborative Study for islet cell antibodies. *Diabetologia* 2000;43(10):1282–92.

41. Greenbaum CJ, Wilkin TJ, Palmer JP. Fifth International Serum Exchange Workshop for Insulin Autoantibody (IAA) Standardization. The Immunology and Diabetes Workshops and participating laboratories. *Diabetologia* 1992;35(8):798–800.

42. Karlsson Faresjo M, Vaarala O, Thuswaldner S, Ilonen J, Hinkkanen A, Ludvigsson J. Diminished IFN-gamma response to diabetes-associated autoantigens in children at diagnosis and during follow up of type 1 diabetes. *Diabetes Metab Res Rev* 2006.

43. Toma A, Haddouk S, Briand JP, et al. Recognition of a subregion of human proinsulin by class I-restricted T cells in type 1 diabetic patients. *Proc Natl Acad Sci USA* 2005;102(30):10581–6.

44. Tree TI, Duinkerken G, Willemen S, de Vries RR, Roep BO. HLA-DQ-regulated T-cell responses to islet cell autoantigens insulin and GAD65. *Diabetes* 2004;53(7):1692–9.

45. Kent SC, Chen Y, Bregoli L, et al. Expanded T cells from pancreatic lymph nodes of type 1 diabetic subjects recognize an insulin epitope. *Nature* 2005;435(7039):224–8.

46. Chatenoud L, Bach JF. Regulatory T cells in the control of autoimmune diabetes: the case of the NOD mouse. *Int Rev Immunol* 2005;24(3–4):247–67.

47. Mathis D, Vence L, Benoist C. beta-Cell death during progression to diabetes. *Nature* 2001;414(6865):792–8.

48. Leiter EH, von Herrath M. Animal models have little to teach us about type 1 diabetes: 2. In opposition to this proposal. *Diabetologia* 2004;47(10):1657–60.

49. Keskinen P, Korhonen S, Kupila A, et al. First-phase insulin response in young healthy children at genetic and immunological risk for Type I diabetes. *Diabetologia* 2002;45(12):1639–48.

50. Krischer JP, Cuthbertson DD, Greenbaum C. Male sex increases the risk of autoimmunity but not type 1 diabetes. *Diabetes Care* 2004;27(8):1985–90.

51. Roep BO, Arden SD, de Vries RR, Hutton JC. T-cell clones from a type-1 diabetes patient respond to insulin secretory granule proteins. *Nature* 1990;345(6276):632–4.

52. Vafiadis P, Ounissi-Benkalha H, Palumbo M, et al. Class III alleles of the variable number of tandem repeat insulin polymorphism associated with silencing of thymic insulin predispose to type 1 diabetes. *J Clin Endocrinol Metab* 2001;86(8):3705–10.

53. Pugliese A, Brown D, Garza D, et al. Self-antigen-presenting cells expressing diabetes-associated autoantigens exist in both thymus and peripheral lymphoid organs. *J Clin Invest* 2001;107(5): 555–64.

54. Ueno H. Enzymatic and structural aspects on glutamate decarboxylase. *J Mol Catal B: Enzymatic* 2000;10:67–79.

55. Bu DF, Erlander MG, Hitz BC, et al. Two human glutamate decarboxylases, 65-kDa GAD and 67-kDa GAD, are each encoded by a single gene. *Proc Natl Acad Sci USA* 1992;89(6):2115–9.

56. Bosma PT, Blazquez M, Collins MA, et al. Multiplicity of glutamic acid decarboxylases (GAD) in vertebrates: molecular phylogeny and evidence for a new GAD paralog. *Mol Biol Evol* 1999;16(3):397–404.

57. Bu DF, Tobin AJ. The exon-intron organization of the genes (GAD1 and GAD2) encoding two human glutamate decarboxylases (GAD67 and GAD65) suggests that they derive from a common ancestral GAD. *Genomics* 1994;21(1):222–8.

58. Strausbauch PH, Fischer EHB. Structure of the binding site of pyridoxal 5'-phosphate to Escherichia coli glutamate decarboxylase. *Biochemistry* 1970;20:233–8.

59. Dutyshev DI, Darii EL, Fomenkova NP, et al. Structure of Escherichia coli glutamate decarboxylase (GADalpha) in complex with glutarate at 2.05 angstroms resolution. *Acta Crystallogr D Biol Crystallogr* 2005;61(Pt 3):230–5.

60. Capitani G, De Biase D, Aurizi C, Gut H, Bossa F, Grutter MG. Crystal structure and functional analysis of Escherichia coli glutamate decarboxylase. *EMBO J* 2003;22(16):4027–37.

61. Schwartz HL, Chandonia JM, Kash SF, et al. High-resolution autoreactive epitope mapping and structural modeling of the 65 kDa form of human glutamic acid decarboxylase. *J Mol Biol* 1999;287(5):983–99.

62. Padoa CJ, Banga JP, Madec AM, et al. Recombinant Fabs of human monoclonal antibodies specific to the middle epitope of GAD65 inhibit type 1 diabetes-specific GAD65Abs. *Diabetes* 2003;52(11):2689–95.

63. Chen CH, Battaglioli G, Martin DL, Hobart SA, Colon W. Distinctive interactions in the holoenzyme formation for two isoforms of glutamate decarboxylase. *Biochim Biophys Acta* 2003;1645(1):63–71.

64. Kanaani J, Lissin D, Kash SF, Baekkeskov S. The hydrophilic isoform of glutamate decarboxylase, GAD67, is targeted to membranes and nerve terminals independent of dimerization with the hydrophobic membrane-anchored isoform, GAD65. *J Biol Chem* 1999;274(52):37200–9.

65. Namchuk M, Lindsay L, Turck CW, Kanaani J, Baekkeskov S. Phosphorylation of serine residues 3, 6, 10, and 13 distinguishes membrane anchored from soluble glutamic acid decarboxylase 65 and is restricted to glutamic acid decarboxylase 65alpha. *J Biol Chem* 1997;272(3):1548–57.

66. Dirkx R, Jr., Thomas A, Li L, et al. Targeting of the 67-kDa isoform of glutamic acid decarboxylase to intracellular organelles is mediated by its interaction with the NH2-terminal region of the 65-kDa isoform of glutamic acid decarboxylase. *J Biol Chem* 1995;270(5):2241–6.

67. Shi Y, Veit B, Baekkeskov S. Amino acid residues 24–31 but not palmitoylation of cysteines 30 and 45 are required for membrane anchoring of glutamic acid decarboxylase, GAD65. *J Cell Biol* 1994;124(6):927–34.

68. Rorsman P, Berggren PO, Bokvist K, et al. Glucose-inhibition of glucagon secretion involves activation of GABAA-receptor chloride channels. *Nature* 1989;341(6239):233–6.

69. Wendt A, Birnir B, Buschard K, et al. Glucose inhibition of glucagon secretion from rat alpha-cells is mediated by GABA released from neighboring beta-cells. *Diabetes* 2004;53(4):1038–45.

70. Wang C, Kerckhofs K, Van de Casteele M, Smolders I, Pipeleers D, Ling Z. Glucose inhibits GABA release by pancreatic beta-cells through an increase in GABA shunt activity. *Am J Physiol Endocrinol Metab* 2006;290(3):E494–9.

71. Hawa MI, Leslie RD. GAD antigen and its significance in type I diabetes. *J Endocrinol Invest* 2002;25(7):576.

72. Pihoker C, Gilliam LK, Hampe CS, Lernmark A. Autoantibodies in diabetes. *Diabetes* 2005;54(Suppl 2):S52–61.

73. Graham J, Hagopian WA, Kockum I, et al. Genetic effects on age-dependent onset and islet cell autoantibody markers in type 1 diabetes. *Diabetes* 2002;51(5):1346–55.

74. Leslie RD, Atkinson MA, Notkins AL. Autoantigens IA-2 and GAD in type I (insulin-dependent) diabetes. *Diabetologia* 1999;42(1):3–14.

75. Rolandsson O, Hagg E, Hampe C, et al. Glutamate decarboxylase (GAD65) and tyrosine phosphatase-like protein (IA-2) autoantibodies index in a regional population is related to glucose intolerance and body mass index. *Diabetologia* 1999;42(5):555–9.

76. Weets I, Van Autreve J, Van der Auwera BJ, et al. Male-to-female excess in diabetes diagnosed in early adulthood is not specific for the immune-mediated form nor is it HLA-DQ restricted: possible relation to increased body mass index. *Diabetologia* 2001;44(1):40–7.

77. Solimena M, Folli F, Aparisi R, Pozza G, De Camilli P. Autoantibodies to GABA-ergic neurons and pancreatic beta cells in stiff-man syndrome. *N Engl J Med* 1990;322(22):1555–60.

78. Murinson BB. Stiff-person syndrome. *Neurologist* 2004;10(3):131–7.

79. Lernmark A. Glutamic acid decarboxylase–gene to antigen to disease. *J Intern Med* 1996;240(5):259–77.

80. Raju R, Foote J, Banga JP, et al. Analysis of GAD65 autoantibodies in Stiff-Person syndrome patients. *J Immunol* 2005;175(11):7755–62.

81. Kim J, Namchuk M, Bugawan T, et al. Higher autoantibody levels and recognition of a linear NH2-terminal epitope in the autoantigen GAD65, distinguish stiff-man syndrome from insulin-dependent diabetes mellitus. *J Exp Med* 1994;180(2):595–606.

82. Grubin CE, Daniels T, Toivola B, et al. A novel radioligand binding assay to determine diagnostic accuracy of isoform-specific glutamic acid decarboxylase antibodies in childhood IDDM. *Diabetologia* 1994;37(4):344–50.

83. Akamine H, Komiya I, Shimabukuro T, et al. High prevalence of GAD65 (and IA-2) antibodies in Japanese IDDM patients by a new immunoprecipitation assay based on recombinant human GAD65. *Diabet Med* 1997;14(9):778–84.

84. Tuomi T, Groop LC, Zimmet PZ, Rowley MJ, Knowles W, Mackay IR. Antibodies to glutamic acid decarboxylase reveal latent autoimmune diabetes mellitus in adults with a non-insulin-dependent onset of disease. *Diabetes* 1993;42(2):359–62.

85. Hagopian WA, Karlsen AE, Gottsater A, et al. Quantitative assay using recombinant human islet glutamic acid decarboxylase (GAD65) shows that 64K autoantibody positivity at onset predicts diabetes type. *J Clin Invest* 1993;91(1):368–74.

86. Brooking H, Ananieva-Jordanova R, Arnold C, et al. A sensitive non-isotopic assay for GAD65 autoantibodies. *Clin Chim Acta* 2003;331(1–2):55–9.

87. Chen S, Willis J, Maclean C, et al. Sensitive non-isotopic assays for autoantibodies to IA-2 and to a combination of both IA-2 and GAD65. *Clin Chim Acta* 2005;357(1):74–83.

88. Verge CF, Stenger D, Bonifacio E, et al. Combined use of autoantibodies (IA-2 autoantibody, GAD autoantibody, insulin autoantibody, cytoplasmic islet cell antibodies) in type 1 diabetes: Combinatorial Islet Autoantibody Workshop. *Diabetes* 1998;47(12):1857–66.

89. Atkinson MA, Bowman MA, Campbell L, Darrow BL, Kaufman DL, Maclaren NK. Cellular immunity to a determinant common to glutamate decarboxylase and coxsackie virus in insulin-dependent diabetes. *J Clin Invest* 1994;94(5):2125–9.

90. Bergholdt R, Heding P, Nielsen K, et al. Type 1 database mellitus: an inflammatory disease of the islet. *Adv Exp Med Biol* 2004;552:129–53.

91. Hampe CS, Hammerle LP, Bekris L, et al. Recognition of glutamic acid decarboxylase (GAD) by autoantibodies from different GAD antibody-positive phenotypes. *J Clin Endocrinol Metab* 2000;85(12):4671–9.

92. Ronkainen MS, Savola K, Knip M. Antibodies to GAD65 epitopes at diagnosis and over the first 10 years of clinical type 1 diabetes mellitus. *Scand J Immunol* 2004;59(3):334–40.

93. Sanjeevi CB, Falorni A, Kockum I, Hagopian WA, Lernmark A. HLA and glutamic acid decarboxylase in human insulin-dependent diabetes mellitus. *Diabet Med* 1996;13(3):209–17.

94. Borg H, Gottsater A, Fernlund P, Sundkvist G. A 12-year prospective study of the relationship between islet antibodies and beta-cell function at and after the diagnosis in patients with adult-onset diabetes. *Diabetes* 2002;51(6):1754–62.

95. Vandewalle CL, Falorni A, Svanholm S, Lernmark A, Pipeleers DG, Gorus FK. High diagnostic sensitivity of glutamate decarboxylase autoantibodies in insulin-dependent diabetes mellitus with clinical onset between age 20 and 40 years. The Belgian Diabetes Registry. *J Clin Endocrinol Metab* 1995;80(3):846–51.

96. Hallengren B, Falorni A, Landin-Olsson M, Lernmark A, Papadopoulos KI, Sundkvist G. Islet cell and glutamic acid decarboxylase antibodies in hyperthyroid patients: at diagnosis and following treatment. *J Intern Med* 1996;239(1):63–8.

97. Ou D, Jonsen LA, Metzger DL, Tingle AJ. CD4+ and CD8+ T-cell clones from congenital rubella syndrome patients with IDDM recognize overlapping GAD65 protein epitopes. Implications for HLA class I and II allelic linkage to disease susceptibility. *Hum Immunol* 1999;60(8):652–64.

98. Kallan AA, Roep BO, Arden SD, Hutton JC, de Vries RR. Beta-cell reactive T-cell clones from type I diabetes patients are not beta cell specific and recognize multiple antigens. *J Autoimmun* 1995;8(6):887–99.

99. Reijonen H, Daniels TL, Lernmark A, Nepom GT. GAD65-specific autoantibodies enhance the presentation of an immunodominant T-cell epitope from GAD65. *Diabetes* 2000;49(10):1621–6.

100. Jaume JC, Parry SL, Madec AM, Sonderstrup G, Baekkeskov S. Suppressive effect of glutamic acid decarboxylase 65-specific autoimmune B lymphocytes on processing of T cell determinants located within the antibody epitope. *J Immunol* 2002;169(2):665–72.

101. Reijonen H, Novak EJ, Kochik S, et al. Detection of GAD65-specific T-cells by major histocompatibility complex class II tetramers in type 1 diabetic patients and at-risk subjects. *Diabetes* 2002;51(5):1375–82.

102. Oling V, Marttila J, Ilonen J, et al. GAD65- and proinsulin-specific CD4+ T-cells detected by MHC class II tetramers in peripheral blood of type 1 diabetes patients and at-risk subjects. *J Autoimmun* 2005;25(3):235–43.

103. Schloot NC, Meierhoff G, Karlsson Faresjo M, et al. Comparison of cytokine ELISpot assay formats for the detection of islet antigen autoreactive T cells. Report of the third immunology of diabetes society T-cell workshop. *J Autoimmun* 2003;21(4):365–76.

104. Nagata M, Kotani R, Moriyama H, Yokono K, Roep BO, Peakman M. Detection of autoreactive T cells in type 1 diabetes using coded autoantigens and an immunoglobulin-free cytokine ELISPOT assay: report from the fourth immunology of diabetes society T cell workshop. *Ann N Y Acad Sci* 2004;1037:10–5.

105. Kaufman DL, Clare-Salzler M, Tian J, et al. Spontaneous loss of T-cell tolerance to glutamic acid decarboxylase in murine insulin-dependent diabetes. *Nature* 1993;366(6450):69–72.

106. Tisch R, Yang XD, Singer SM, Liblau RS, Fugger L, McDevitt HO. Immune response to glutamic acid decarboxylase correlates with insulitis in non-obese diabetic mice. *Nature* 1993;366(6450):72–5.

107. McDevitt H. Specific antigen vaccination to treat autoimmune disease. *Proc Natl Acad Sci USA* 2004;101(Suppl 2):14627–30.

108. Li A, Ojogho O, Franco E, Baron P, Iwaki Y, Escher A. Pro-apoptotic DNA vaccination ameliorates new onset of autoimmune diabetes in NOD mice and induces foxp3+ regulatory T cells in vitro. *Vaccine* 2006;24(23):5036–46.

109. Lernmark A, Agardh CD. Immunomodulation with human recombinant autoantigens. *Trends Immunol* 2005;26(11):608–12.

110. Agardh CD, Cilio CM, Lethagen A, et al. Clinical evidence for the safety of GAD65 immunomodulation in adult-onset autoimmune diabetes. *J Diabetes Complications* 2005;19(4):238–46.

111. Rabin DU, Pleasic SM, Palmer-Crocker R, Shapiro JA. Cloning and expression of IDDM-specific human autoantigens. Diabetes 1992;41(2):183–6.

112. Lan MS, Modi WS, Xie H, Notkins AL. Assignment of the IA-2 gene encoding an autoantigen in IDDM to chromosome 2q35. *Diabetologia* 1996;39(8):1001–2.

113. Dirkx R, Jr., Hermel JM, Rabin DU, Solimena M. ICA 512, a receptor tyrosine phosphatase-like protein, is concentrated in neurosecretory granule membranes. *Adv Pharmacol* 1998;42:243–6.

114. Notkins AL, Lu J, Li Q, et al. IA-2 and IA-2 beta are major autoantigens in IDDM and the precursors of the 40 kDa and 37 kDa tryptic fragments. *J Autoimmun* 1996;9(5):677–82.

115. Xie H, Notkins AL, Lan MS. IA-2, a transmembrane protein tyrosine phosphatase, is expressed in human lung cancer cell lines with neuroendocrine phenotype. *Cancer Res* 1996;56(12):2742–4.

116. Magistrelli G, Toma S, Isacchi A. Substitution of two variant residues in the protein tyrosine phosphatase-like PTP35/IA-2 sequence reconstitutes catalytic activity. *Biochem Biophys Res Commun* 1996;227(2):581–8.

117. Verge CF, Gianani R, Yu L, et al. Late progression to diabetes and evidence for chronic beta-cell autoimmunity in identical twins of patients with type I diabetes. *Diabetes* 1995;44(10):1176–9.

118. Morgenthaler NG, Lobner K, Morgenthaler UY, Christie MR, Seissler J, Scherbaum WA. Recombinant IA-2 expressed in E. coli can be used for the routine detection of autoantibodies in type-I diabetes. *Horm Metab Res* 1998;30(9):559–64.

119. Westerlund A, Ankelo M, Ilonen J, Knip M, Simell O, Hinkkanen AE. Absence of avidity maturation of autoantibodies to the protein tyrosine phosphatase-like IA-2 molecule and glutamic acid decarboxylase (GAD65) during progression to type 1 diabetes. *J Autoimmun* 2005;24(2):153–67.

120. Zhang B, Lan MS, Notkins AL. Autoantibodies to IA-2 in IDDM: location of major antigenic determinants. *Diabetes* 1997;46(1):40–3.

121. Bearzatto M, Lampasona V, Belloni C, Bonifacio E. Fine mapping of diabetes-associated IA-2 specific autoantibodies. *J Autoimmun* 2003;21(4):377–82.

122. Vandewalle CL, Falorni A, Lernmark A, et al. Associations of GAD65- and IA-2-autoantibodies with genetic risk markers in new-onset IDDM patients and their siblings. The Belgian Diabetes Registry. *Diabetes Care* 1997;20(10):1547–52.

123. Genovese S, Bonfanti R, Bazzigaluppi E, et al. Association of IA-2 autoantibodies with HLA DR4 phenotypes in IDDM. *Diabetologia* 1996;39(10):1223–6.

124. Hawkes CJ, Schloot NC, Marks J, et al. T-cell lines reactive to an immunodominant epitope of the tyrosine phosphatase-like autoantigen IA-2 in type 1 diabetes. *Diabetes* 2000;49(3):356–66.

125. Honeyman MC, Stone NL, Harrison LC. T-cell epitopes in type 1 diabetes autoantigen tyrosine phosphatase IA-2: potential for mimicry with rotavirus and other environmental agents. *Mol Med* 1998;4(4):231–9.

126. Herzog BA, Ott PA, Dittrich MT, et al. Increased in vivo frequency of IA-2 peptide-reactive IFNgamma+/IL-4- T cells in type 1 diabetic subjects. *J Autoimmun* 2004;23(1):45–54.

127. Williams AJ, Bingley PJ, Chance RE, Gale EA. Insulin autoantibodies: more specific than proinsulin autoantibodies for prediction of type 1 diabetes. *J Autoimmun* 1999;13(3):357–63.

128. Uchigata Y, Hirata Y. Insulin autoimmune syndrome (IAS, Hirata disease). *Ann Med Interne (Paris)* 1999;150(3):245–53.

129. Hagopian WA, Sanjeevi CB, Kockum I, et al. Glutamate decarboxylase-, insulin-, and islet cell-antibodies and HLA typing to detect diabetes in a general population-based study of Swedish children. *J Clin Invest* 1995;95(4):1505–11.

130. Castano L, Ziegler AG, Ziegler R, Shoelson S, Eisenbarth GS. Characterization of insulin autoantibodies in relatives of patients with type I diabetes. *Diabetes* 1993;42(8):1202–9.

131. Williams AJ, Bingley PJ, Moore WP, Gale EA. Islet autoantibodies, nationality and gender: a multinational screening study in first-degree relatives of patients with Type I diabetes. *Diabetologia* 2002;45(2):217–23.

132. Nakayama M, Abiru N, Moriyama H, et al. Prime role for an insulin epitope in the development of type 1 diabetes in NOD mice. *Nature* 2005;435(7039):220–3.

133. Alleva DG, Crowe PD, Jin L, et al. A disease-associated cellular immune response in type 1 diabetics to an immunodominant epitope of insulin. *J Clin Invest* 2001;107(2):173–80.

134. Lee KH, Wucherpfennig KW, Wiley DC. Structure of a human insulin peptide-HLA-DQ8 complex and susceptibility to type 1 diabetes. *Nat Immunol* 2001;2(6):501–7.

135. Kimura K, Kawamura T, Kadotani S, Inada H, Niihira S, Yamano T. Peptide-specific cytotoxicity of T lymphocytes against glutamic acid decarboxylase and insulin in type 1 diabetes mellitus. *Diabetes Res Clin Pract* 2001;51(3):173–9.

136. Skyler JS, Krischer JP, Wolfsdorf J, et al. Effects of oral insulin in relatives of patients with type 1 diabetes: The Diabetes Prevention Trial–Type 1. *Diabetes Care* 2005;28(5):1068–76.

137. Roep BO, Atkinson MA, van Endert PM, Gottlieb PA, Wilson SB, Sachs JA. Autoreactive T cell responses in insulin-dependent (Type 1) diabetes mellitus. Report of the first international workshop for standardization of T cell assays. *J Autoimmun* 1999;13(2):267–82.

138. Peakman M, Tree TI, Endl J, van Endert P, Atkinson MA, Roep BO. Characterization of preparations of GAD65, proinsulin, and the islet tyrosine phosphatase IA-2 for use in detection of autoreactive T-cells in type 1 diabetes: report of phase II of the Second International Immunology of Diabetes Society Workshop for Standardization of T-cell assays in type 1 diabetes. *Diabetes* 2001;50(8):1749–54.

139. Pietropaolo M, Castano L, Babu S, et al. Islet cell autoantigen 69 kD (ICA69). Molecular cloning and characterization of a novel diabetes-associated autoantigen. *J Clin Invest* 1993;92(1):359–71.

140. Mally MI, Cirulli V, Hayek A, Otonkoski T. ICA69 is expressed equally in the human endocrine and exocrine pancreas. *Diabetologia* 1996;39(4):474–80.

141. Pilon M, Peng XR, Spence AM, Plasterk RH, Dosch HM. The diabetes autoantigen ICA69 and its Caenorhabditis elegans homologue, ric-19, are conserved regulators of neuroendocrine secretion. *Mol Biol Cell* 2000;11(10):3277–88.

142. Kasimiotis H, Fida S, Rowley MJ, et al. Antibodies to SOX13 (ICA12) are associated with type 1 diabetes. *Autoimmunity* 2001;33(2):95–101.

143. Fida S, Myers MA, Whittingham S, Rowley MJ, Ozaki S, Mackay IR. Autoantibodies to the transcriptional factor SOX13 in primary biliary cirrhosis compared with other diseases. *J Autoimmun* 2002;19(4):251–7.

144. Davis TM, Mehta Z, Mackay IR, et al. Autoantibodies to the islet cell antigen SOX-13 are associated with duration but not type of diabetes. *Diabet Med* 2003;20(3):198–204.

145. Alcalde L, Tonacchera M, Costagliola S, Jaraquemada D, Pujol-Borrell R, Ludgate M. Cloning of candidate autoantigen carboxypeptidase H from a human islet library: sequence identity with human brain CPH. *J Autoimmun* 1996;9(4):525–8.

146. Zhou ZG, Yang L, Huang G. Diagnostic value of carboxypeptidase-H autoantibodies in detecting latent autoimmune diabetes in adults. *Hunan Yi Ke Da Xue Xue Bao* 2003;28(6):549–52.

147. Buschard K, Blomqvist M, Osterbye T, Fredman P. Involvement of sulfatide in beta cells and type 1 and type 2 diabetes. *Diabetologia* 2005;48(10):1957–62.

148. Andersson K, Buschard K, Fredman P, et al. Patients with insulin-dependent diabetes but not those with non-insulin-dependent diabetes have anti-sulfatide antibodies as determined with a new ELISA assay. *Autoimmunity* 2002;35(7):463–8.

149. Ilyas AA, Mithen FA, Dalakas MC, et al. Antibodies to sulfated glycolipids in Guillain-Barre syndrome. *J Neurol Sci* 1991;105(1):108–17.

150. Pestronk A, Li F, Griffin J, et al. Polyneuropathy syndromes associated with serum antibodies to sulfatide and myelin-associated glycoprotein. *Neurology* 1991;41(3):357–62.

151. Dotta F, Previti M, Neerman-Arbez M, et al. The GM2–1 ganglioside islet autoantigen in insulin-dependent diabetes mellitus is expressed in secretory granules and is not beta-cell specific. *Endocrinology* 1998;139(1):316–9.

152. Dotta F, Falorni A, Tiberti C, et al. Autoantibodies to the GM2–1 islet ganglioside and to GAD-65 at type 1 diabetes onset. *J Autoimmun* 1997;10(6):585–8.

153. Geluk A, van Meijgaarden KE, Roep BO, Ottenhoff TH. Altered peptide ligands of islet autoantigen Imogen 38 inhibit antigen specific T cell reactivity in human type-1 diabetes. *J Autoimmun* 1998;11(4):353–61.

154. Arden SD, Roep BO, Neophytou PI, et al. Imogen 38: a novel 38-kD islet mitochondrial autoantigen recognized by T cells from a newly diagnosed type 1 diabetic patient. *J Clin Invest* 1996;97(2):551–61.

155. Aanstoot HJ, Kang SM, Kim J, et al. Identification and characterization of glima 38, a glycosylated islet cell membrane antigen, which together with GAD65 and IA2 marks the early phases of autoimmune response in type 1 diabetes. *J Clin Invest* 1996;97(12):2772–83.

156. Winnock F, Christie MR, Batstra MR, et al. Autoantibodies to a 38-kDa glycosylated islet cell membrane-associated antigen in (pre)type 1 diabetes: association with IA-2 and islet cell autoantibodies. *Diabetes Care* 2001;24(7):1181–6.

157. Arden SD, Zahn T, Steegers S, et al. Molecular cloning of a pancreatic islet-specific glucose-6-phosphatase catalytic subunit-related protein. *Diabetes* 1999;48(3):531–42.

158. Lieberman SM, Evans AM, Han B, et al. Identification of the beta cell antigen targeted by a prevalent population of pathogenic CD8+ T cells in autoimmune diabetes. *Proc Natl Acad Sci USA* 2003;100(14):8384–8.

159. Yang J, Danke NA, Berger D, et al. Islet-specific glucose-6-phosphatase catalytic subunit-related protein-reactive CD4+ T cells in human subjects. *J Immunol* 2006;176(5):2781–9.

160. Li M, Fisher WE, Kim HJ, et al. Somatostatin, somatostatin receptors, and pancreatic cancer. *World J Surg* 2005;29(3):293–6.

161. Patel YC, Greenwood MT, Panetta R, Demchyshyn L, Niznik H, Srikant CB. The somatostatin receptor family. *Life Sci* 1995;57(13):1249–65.

162. Krantic S. Peptides as regulators of the immune system: emphasis on somatostatin. *Peptides* 2000;21(12):1941–64.

163. Wang XP, Norman MA, Brunicardi FC. Somatostatin receptors and autoimmune-mediated diabetes. *Diabetes Metab Res Rev* 2005;21(1):15–30.

164. Haskins K. Pathogenic T-cell clones in autoimmune diabetes: more lessons from the NOD mouse. *Adv Immunol* 2005;87:123–62.

165. Tisch R, Wang B, Atkinson MA, Serreze DV, Friedline R. A glutamic acid decarboxylase 65-specific Th2 cell clone immunoregulates autoimmune diabetes in nonobese diabetic mice. *J Immunol* 2001;166(11):6925–36.

166. Achenbach P, Kelemen K, Wegmann DR, Hutton JC. Spontaneous peripheral T-cell responses to the IA-2beta (phogrin) autoantigen in young nonobese diabetic mice. *J Autoimmun* 2002;19(3):111–6.

167. Kelemen K, Wegmann DR, Hutton JC. T-cell epitope analysis on the autoantigen phogrin (IA-2beta) in the nonobese diabetic mouse. *Diabetes* 2001;50(8):1729–34.

168. Trigwell SM, Radford PM, Page SR, et al. Islet glutamic acid decarboxylase modified by reactive oxygen species is recognized by antibodies from patients with type 1 diabetes mellitus. *Clin Exp Immunol* 2001;126(2):242–9.

169. van Gaalen F, Ioan-Facsinay A, Huizinga TW, Toes RE. The devil in the details: the emerging role of anticitrulline autoimmunity in rheumatoid arthritis. *J Immunol* 2005;175(9):5575–80.

170. Westman E, Harris HE. Alteration of an autoantigen by chlorination, a process occurring during inflammation, can overcome adaptive immune tolerance. *Scand J Immunol* 2004;59(5):458–63.

171. Sollid LM. Coeliac disease: dissecting a complex inflammatory disorder. *Nat Rev Immunol* 2002;2(9):647–55.

172. Binder CJ, Shaw PX, Chang MK, et al. The role of natural antibodies in atherogenesis. *J Lipid Res* 2005;46(7):1353–63.

12 Type 1 Diabetes Mellitus

Huriya Beyan, PhD, and R. David G. Leslie, FRCP

Summary

Autoimmune diseases affect 10% or more of the North American and European populations. In organ-specific autoimmune diseases, an organ is targeted by an aggressive immune response, which can damage and even destroy it. Type 1 diabetes mellitus (T1DM), one such organ-specific autoimmune disease, is because of the destruction of the insulin-secreting beta cells in the islets of Langerhans of the pancreas. T1DM is because of the interaction of genetic and non-genetic factors thought to induce an immune response, which destroys insulin secretory cells over months, even years. We present the orthodox position regarding the cause of autoimmune T1DM but also emphasize where that orthodox is not based on a firm footing. We discuss the nature of the disease and how we can predict it with a degree of certainty and how we are now trying to modulate the disease process. Lessons learned from autoimmune diabetes could be relevant to other autoimmune diseases.

Key Words: Diabetes, autoimmunity, HLA genes, autoantibodies, disease prediction, immunomodulation.

INTRODUCTION

Autoimmune diseases afflict 10% or more of the UK population. In organ-specific autoimmune diseases, an organ is targeted by an aggressive immune response, which can damage and even destroy it. Type 1 diabetes mellitus (T1DM), one such organ specific autoimmune disease, is because of the destruction of the insulin secreting beta cells in the islets of Langerhans of the pancreas *(1)*. At the clinical onset of T1DM, about 80% of islets contain no insulin secreting islet cells, and the islets may be infiltrated with mononuclear cells *(2)*, with a predominance of macrophages and

From: *Contemporary Endocrinology: Autoimmune Diseases in Endocrinology*
Edited by: A. P. Weetman © Humana Press, Totowa, NJ

CD8$^+$ T lymphocytes *(3)*. This infiltrate is, directly or indirectly, probably the major cause of the beta-cells destruction. In this review, we will present the orthodox position regarding the cause of autoimmune T1DM but also emphasize where that orthodox is not based on a firm footing. Lessons learned from autoimmune diabetes could be relevant to other autoimmune diseases.

GENETIC FACTORS

Type 1 diabetes mellitus is genetically determined as shown by family, twin, and genetic studies. The frequency of T1DM is higher in siblings of diabetic patients (e.g., in the United Kingdom 6% by age 30) than in the general population (0.4% by age 30) *(4)*. The most important genes implicated in the susceptibility to T1DM are in the histocompatibility (human leukocyte antigen [HLA]) region of chromosome 6 *(4)*. HLA genes predispose to a number of autoimmune diseases including T1DM *(4,5)* as demonstrated in both population and family studies *(5–7)*. Genes encoding HLA molecules and located within the major histocompatibility complex (MHC) on the short arm of chromosome 6 are associated with T1DM. The MHC complex is a polymorphic gene complex in that multiple alleles exist for each genetic locus. The MHC is divided into class I (HLA-A, -B, and -C), class II (HLA-DR, -DQ, and -DP), and class III (genes for complement components). The class I and class II proteins coded by the relevant genes are transmembrane cell surface glycoproteins, which are critically involved in the presentation of both self- and foreign antigens as short peptides to T lymphocytes.

HLA genes are highly polymorphic with a degree of coding region diversity unequalled elsewhere in the genome. Polymorphisms of certain genes probably originated in the selection pressures exerted by environmental factors including epidemics, climatic change, and availability of food. A non-human somatic study of the HLA-DQ beta region suggests that this region has been in balanced polymorphism for 10 or more million years *(8)*. To maintain the extraordinary diversity of HLA types over this time, selection pressures must have been operating; otherwise, most alleles would have been lost through genetic drift. It has been proposed that infectious pathogens are the major cause of HLA diversity. The distribution of sequence variation is clustered in nucleotides that code for amino acids composing the antigen-binding groove. This implies that natural selection must have acted at this binding site to maintain structural diversity for peptide binding. HLA associations with T1DM may therefore operate through susceptibility to certain undefined infections, which could be modern, just as there is an argument that T1DM and other autoimmune diseases are modern diseases. Perhaps even more important, because of the known role of HLA molecules in antigen presentation, the HLA linkage and association supported the hypothesis that T1DM has an autoimmune component.

The evidence is that class II genes are more important than class I genes and that DQ genes are more important than DR genes *(4)*. About 95% of European patients with T1DM have either HLA-DR3 or -DR4 compared with about 60% of the normal population. However, 90% of the HLA-DR4-positive diabetic patients have the DQ allele DQB1 0302 and only 10% have the DQB1 0301 allele, whereas both alleles were equally represented in the normal DR4-positive population. Extended haplotypes identical at the DQB1 loci are associated with very different risks of T1DM, implying that MHC genes outside the DQ region play an important role in determining genetic susceptibility *(4)*. HLA alleles associated with diabetes susceptibility, include HLA-DR3, DQB1*0201 and DR4, DQB1*0302, whereas others are associated with disease protection, for example HLA-DR2, DQB1*0602 haplotype occurs in over 20% of some populations, but <1% of children who develop T1DM express these alleles *(4,9)*. Type 1 diabetic children show an increased prevalence of the heterozygous alleles HLA-DR3, DQB1*0201 and DR4, DQB1*0302, the proportion of heterozygotes declining with age at diagnosis *(9–11)*. Children with the diabetes protective HLA-DR2, DQB1*0602 are unlikely to develop diabetes, whereas in adult-onset diabetes, the same alleles carry less protection *(10–11)*. Patients with HLA-DR4, DQB1*0302 are at particular risk of having insulin autoantibodies, and these HLA alleles and insulin autoantibodies are more prevalent in children with T1DM *(12)*. The extended haplotype could be important because it codes for the overall structure of the molecule that forms the binding groove. Alternatively, it might include other as yet unidentified genes that play a role is disease susceptibility. Certain individual residues confer a particular susceptibility or protection from disease. Thus, disease susceptibility correlates with the expression of a DQ molecule bearing an arginine in the 52 position of the alpha chain and lacking an aspartate at the 57 position of the beta chain *(13)*. A combination of these changes confers a greater risk for disease than either one alone, as has been shown for HLA-DR3 and DR4, implying that two or more genes are important in disease susceptibility. On balance, the evidence suggests that certain amino acid substitutions are important but only within the context of the whole molecule.

Although T1DM is genetically determined, the term heritability reflects gene expression or penetrance in a given environment. The best estimate of heritability can be obtained by determining concordance rates of twins. Both identical and non-identical twins share the same environment in childhood, but only identical twins share the same genes. In the classic twin method, the difference between the concordance rates for identical and non-identical twins is doubled to give an index of heritability. Higher concordance rates, for autoimmune diseases in general and T1DM in particular, in identical compared with non-identical twins is consistent with a genetic influence on these diseases *(14)*. Estimates of heritability can be obtained from studies in Finland and the University of Southern California; in both, the estimates are substantially <100%, which means the disease is unlikely to be autosomal dominant *(7,15)*. However, we cannot make broad statements about the genetics of autoimmune diabetes because it shows substantial disease heterogeneity. Hence, age-related genetic factors influence the risk of T1DM, but also the presence of diabetes-associated autoantibodies, the rate of progression to clinical diabetes, as well as the severity of reduced insulin secretory capacity *(1)*. Not only is the age incidence of T1DM lower in adults than in children, the range of incidence across European countries is also reduced *(16)*. Survival analysis estimated that non-diabetic identical twins of probands diagnosed with T1DM under 25 years of age had, in one study, a 38% probability of developing diabetes compared with only 6% for twins of probands diagnosed later *(6)*. Such a remarkably low twin concordance rate for adult-onset T1DM implies that the genetic impact in adult-onset T1DM is limited and certainly lower than that in childhood-onset disease *(6,7,15)*.

It should be noted that other gene polymorphisms, within the insulin gene upstream promoter region as well as within the cytotoxic T-lymphocyte-associated antigen *(CTLA)-4*, protein tyrosine phosphatase non-receptor *(PTPN)22*, insulin receptor substrate-1 (IRS-1), inducible co-stimulatory molecule (ICOS), and small ubiquitin like modifier 4 (Sumo 4 genes), confer a substantial risk to T1DM with odds ratios (OR) between 1.8 and 2.5 *(17,18)*. Of particular note, the *CTLA-4* gene also plays a role in thyroid autoimmunity and with the HLA region comprises an important molecule in the so-called immunological synapse at the interface of the presentation of an antigen by antigen-presenting cells to immune effector cells.

Thus, there is a hierarchy of genetically determined risk to T1DM ranging from susceptibility at one extreme to protection at the other. Even within families, the pattern of inheritance can be complex because children of fathers with T1DM are at higher risk of developing the disease than children of affected mothers *(19,20)*. This difference may be due, in part, to preferential transmission of diabetic alleles in the HLA complex, but this may not explain why the same HLA allele is associated with a greater disease risk in childhood than in adulthood. To be precise, we do not know at which stage of the disease process the HLA risk operates—is it at the initiation, the activation, or the progression of the destructive immune process? Preliminary data supporting a role for HLA genes in determining the age at the onset of diabetes raises the possibility that such genes operate through promotion or restraint of the destructive effect. For all that we know so much about HLA disease risk, it seems that we know very little about how it interacts with non-genetic events to cause the disease.

ENVIRONMENTAL FACTORS

The incidence of autoimmune diseases has increased, notably over the last three decades *(21)*. The current low selection density and relative stability of HLA polymorphisms indicate that this increasing incidence cannot be because of genetic selection pressures, at least operating through HLA genes, and is most likely the result of non-genetic factors. Non-genetic factors play a major role in causing T1DM as shown by studies of populations that have migrated, of populations with changing disease incidence, and of twins.

Population studies are of limited value in identifying the impact of non-genetic factors because it is difficult to segregate genetic from environmental influences. However, changes in disease incidence within a genetically stable population are important when disease incidence rises rapidly or in migrants *(22,23)*. In the USA, the reported death rates from diabetes in children aged <15 years, by implication the T1DM incidence as this was before insulin therapy, from 1890 to 1920 were 1.3/100,000/year and 3.1/100,000/year respectively *(22)*, rising by 1959–1961 in Erie County, USA, to 11.3/100,000/year, a substantial change within four generations *(23)*. Such changes have been most striking in children diagnosed under 5 years of age as in Switzerland where the incidence rose from 4.5/100,000 in 1965 to 10.5/100,000 in 2000 *(24)*.

Migration studies also support a role for environmental factors influencing disease incidence. T1DM incidence increased in Ethiopian Jews migrating to Israel and in Asian children who migrated to Britain—in the latter, there was an increase from 3.1/100,000 per year in 1978–1981 to 11.7/100,000 per year in 1988–1990, much higher than in their native Karachi (1/100,000 per year) *(25–27)*. There are no comparable studies of adults.

Increases in disease risk in young children could be because of an accelerated progression to T1DM (as set out in the accelerator hypothesis and the early spring harvest hypothesis) or to an increased disease risk or both. In support of an increased disease risk, there has been a recent shift in Finland in the HLA genetic susceptibility to include more cases with low or moderate risk HLA genotypes (28). In support of accelerated disease progression, the disease incidence rose in the young (age 0–14 years) with a coincident fall later up to 39 years of age at diagnosis (29,30). Therefore, both factors could explain the increasing disease incidence in young children. Acceleration of the disease process, or of metabolic decompensation, probably results from non-genetic factors and could result from reduced insulin sensitivity, due to either increased linear growth, which has been linked to diabetes risk, or increased childhood obesity, which has been correlated with age at presentation (31–33).

We have previously argued that these non-genetically determined factors are likely to be environmental factors (1). Certainly there is powerful evidence that immune-mediated diseases are because of environmental factors given that the majority of identical twins with an autoimmune disease have an unaffected twin, that is they are discordant for the disease. Nevertheless, even identical twins can differ genetically: X-chromosome inactivation in females can lead to different patterns of mosaicism; methylation of CpG islands is associated with repression of transcription; somatic rearrangements are involved in the development of T-cell receptors and antibodies. Thus, discordance between identical twins may be determined by non-genetic (epigenetic) factors operating on genetic expression. Studies are underway to establish whether there are epigenetic differences such as differences in gene methylation even between identical twins. Nevertheless, if a somatic mutation of the immune system caused T1DM, the aberrant immune response would probably be monoclonal and not polyclonal as is the case in T1DM (34). We therefore believe, although we cannot be certain, that the disease is because of an environmental agent not a somatic mutation, but we are uncertain about this position; so, we are pursuing epigenetic effects in identical twins discordant for T1DM.

A Critical Event Operates in Early Childhood

Whatever the nature of the non-genetic or environmental factors inducing diabetes, they are likely to be ubiquitous and probably occur in a proportion of cases in early childhood (Table 1). The migration studies, however, argue against an equivalent worldwide environmental effect and suggest that the effect is seen when migrating from non-developing to developed countries but perhaps not when migrating between

Table 1
List of Potential Environmental Agents

General factors	Specific factors
Hygiene	Viruses (e.g., enteroviruses)
Parasites	Bacteria
Coexistent infections (TB or malaria)	Cow's milk (through early exposure)
	Toxins

developed T1DM is similar worldwide: extremely rare before 9 months of age, it has a peak incidence between the ages of 5 and 15 years and declines sharply thereafter, although with a long tail, so that adults can present with it in old age. The consistent and striking decline in disease incidence after puberty could be because of either a loss of a genetic or environmental effect. The latter is most likely. Loss of the genetic effect could result from attrition of the genetically susceptible pool or an increasing impact of protective genes, but we know from twin studies that the majority of genetically susceptible individuals do not develop the disease. Furthermore, data from population studies show that the impact of HLA protective genes falls with age *(10)*. The fall in disease risk is even seen in identical twins of patients with T1DM, at least in those with an index twin under 15 years of age at diagnosis in whom the risk of developing diabetes falls sharply 1 year after the diagnosis of the index twin *(6)*. Such a decline in disease risk in young twins suggests that the non-genetic events leading to T1DM occur within a finite period in early childhood. A disproportionate maternal influence suggests that this event may be very early indeed, perhaps even *in utero*.

Maternal-related events influence diabetes risk and by implication that genetic and particularly non-genetic factors operate *in utero* or on neonates to determine disease risk (Table 2). Children of diabetic mothers are less likely to develop T1DM than children of diabetic fathers, and the risk in mothers is less than the expected risk based on their HLA status *(19–20,36)*. This low risk is confined to offspring of mothers who had become diabetic after the age of 8 years. It remains unclear whether the reduction in transmission rates is because of genetic or non-genetic factors. The risk of offspring developing diabetes increases with maternal age and paternal age also has an effect, but it is smaller than the maternal effect *(37)*. The risk of diabetes is reduced by 15% per child born, so that the firstborn has the highest risk. Blood group incompatibility between a mother and her child may also predispose to T1DM *(36)*, although the nature and implications of this association remain obscure. Group-specific enteroviral immunoglobulin (Ig)G and IgM antibodies during pregnancy are higher in mothers of children who later develop T1DM than in controls *(38)*. Further diabetes-associated autoantibodies may be induced by such infections *(39)*. Finally, the early infant diet may affect T1DM onset in later life. Epidemiological studies have established that the risk of developing T1DM is higher in non-breast-fed children than breast-fed children and that breastfeeding for

Table 2
List of Potential Risk Factors for Diabetes

Increased risk of diabetes in children is associated with
- Being born to diabetic fathers rather than diabetic mothers
- Having a diabetic mother aged <8 years at diagnosis compared with mother diagnosed later
- Increasing maternal age at delivery
- Being firstborn
- ABO incompatibility with the mother
- The season of delivery
- Increasing maternal enterovirus infection rate
- Early cessation of breastfeeding

more than 3 months protects from T1DM. This is possibly because early cessation of breastfeeding is associated with the early introduction of foreign antigens, for example cow's milk proteins *(40)*. These observations implicate specific environmental factors.

Disease Induction by Environmental Factors

Environmental factors may cause autoimmune diseases (Table 1). These factors include temperate climate, increased hygiene and decreased rates of infection, vaccinations and antibiotics, and increasing wealth (possibly all relevant for most autoimmune and atopic diseases), but also for T1DM factors include overcrowding in childhood and virus infections, early exposure to cow's milk, reduced rates or duration of breastfeeding and vitamin D and nitrite consumption *(41–43)*.

The declining T1DM disease risk in childhood-onset, but not adult-onset, diabetes implies that those critical environmental events causing childhood-onset T1DM operate preferentially within a limited period in early childhood. If two events or "hits" widely separated in time led to diabetes, then the longer the time of follow-up, the more likely would susceptible individuals be to encounter both "hits," as happens with cancer in which the disease risk rises with time, in contrast with childhood-onset T1DM after 15 years of age *(44)*. No such claim can be made currently for adult-onset autoimmune diabetes. It is not possible to be sure whether the loss of the non-genetic or environmental effect with age, even in genetically susceptible subjects, is because of lack of exposure or loss of susceptibility. It is difficult to envisage a ubiquitous environmental factor to which only children are exposed.

VIRUSES AND T1DM

It is not known whether T1DM is initiated by single or multiple exposures during the critical period. Diabetes can be produced in animal models using viruses and chemical toxins in combination *(45)*. Cumulative damage, if it were to occur, would probably have to do so over a limited period as previously outlined. In man, viruses may damage the pancreas either generally, as with mumps pancreatitis, or specifically by only damaging the islets. Damage to the islet cells can be found after fatal viral infections involving Coxsackie B, cytomegalovirus, and rubella. The most persuasive evidence that a persistent viral infection can cause human diabetes derives from the studies of patients with congenital rubella syndrome *(46)*. Children infected congenitally may show rubella virus in the pancreas with insulitis and insulin secretory cell destruction. Diabetes is found in about 20% of patients with the congenital rubella syndrome with a latent period of many years and a median age of onset of 13 years *(47)*. Not all cases are dependent on insulin treatment. Those patients with the HLA genetic susceptibility associated with T1DM (HLA-DR3 and DR4) tend to develop diabetes and as with T1DM HLA-DR2 is apparently protective *(46)*. Rubella-induced diabetes is a rare phenomenon and unlikely to account for the generality of patients with T1DM. More convincing evidence for viral involvement derives from the study of a young boy who died from an overwhelming viral infection and diabetic ketoacidosis *(46)*. A Coxsackie B4 virus was isolated from his pancreas, which induced diabetes with islet cell damage in mice susceptible to diabetes. Unfortunately, the evidence supporting a critical role for a virus infection is gleaned from the presence of viral antibodies or viral particles and then usually in the minority of cases. Viruses, being the last refuge of the diagnostically destitute, should remain a speculative cause of T1DM.

TOXINS AS THE CRITICAL FACTORS IN T1DM

A number of structurally diverse agents are diabetogenic in animals and in some cases also in man. Toxins could damage the insulin secretory cell directly or indirectly, for example by inducing endogenous viral replication or an immune reaction against a transformed cell. Of toxins, only N-nitroso derivatives are known to induce acute islet-cell destruction and diabetic ketoacidosis. Alloxan, one such agent, was originally introduced for its toxicity to renal tubular cells *(48,49)*. Indeed, most toxic substances damage tissues other than the islet cell and are therefore unlikely candidates to explain the specific insulin secretory cell targeting in T1DM. The rat poison Vacor, a nitro-phenylurea, can cause neurotoxicity and diabetes in man, and after fatal poisoning, necropsy has shown extensive islet-cell damage *(50)*. As with viruses, it is unlikely that these or other toxins that cause acute cytolytic damage could account for T1DM with its long latency period.

DIETARY FACTORS AND T1DM

Evidence that dietary factors are important in the etiology of T1DM in man derives from studies of infant feeding *(40)*. The low prevalence of T1DM in primitive societies may be worth noting in the context of toxic food additives. The increasing rates of T1DM in certain populations have been attributed to a decline in breastfeeding, and particularly to early exposure to cow's milk or solid food, rather than lack of breastfeeding. A consistent but weak relationship has been established *(40)*. In one American study, the attributable risk, which is the proportion of cases that could be prevented by removal of a risk factor from a population, was 8% for cow's milk and 25% for solid foods if these factors were introduced after the age of 3 months or more *(51)*. This hypothesis fits with the evidence that the immune response leading to T1DM is generated very early in life but does not explain the rapid rise in incidence of the condition unless commercial processing of cow's milk, or of milk-based food products, has in some way increased their antigenicity.

IMMUNOPATHOGENESIS

Autoimmunity is important to the fitness of the organism *(21)*. Most individuals produce autoantibodies and autoreactive T lymphocytes. However, only about 5% of any population develop an autoimmune disease. Control mechanisms must therefore operate to control the development of autoimmune diseases. These control mechanisms remove cytotoxic immune cells in various ways including clonal deletion, clonal energy, and limiting antigen accessibility to the immune system. Antigen accessibility is limited by being processed for presentation to the immune system or by autoreactive T lympho-cytes circulating in an inert state. Breakdown in these control mechanisms could lead to disease. Disease associated with autoimmune phenomena tends to distribute themselves within a spectrum of organ-specific diseases such as T1DM and non-organ-specific diseases such as systemic lupus erythematosus. There may be clustering of diseases at either end of this spectrum; thus, T1DM is more common in patients with thyroiditis or adrenalitis. Autoimmune disease has long been considered a shadow following infectious diseases *(21)*. Epidemiological evidence shows that rheumatic fever follows streptococcal infection and *Trypanosoma cruzi* infection is the instigator of Chagas' disease. There is, however, very little information of the mechanism by which such a train of events is initiated. Autoimmunity, in the form of autoantibodies, is common after many infections and may well result from the mimicking of host proteins by antigens of the infectious agent. There are, however, few if any examples in humans where molecular mimicry gives rise to autoimmune disease. The progression from benign autoimmunity to pathogenic autoimmune disease depends on many factors, probably including the balance of cytokines produced during the inflammatory process accompanying infection *(21)*.

For all the talk that T1DM is an autoimmune disease, we must acknowledge that the evidence is incomplete. Rose and Bona *(52)* defined autoimmune diseases as those that show three features: (1) defined autoantigens and autoantibodies must be present; (2) passive transfer of T-lymphocytes (specific or non-specific) must lead to disease development, and (3) immunomodulation of subjects with disease must ameliorate symptoms. We know that the first of these is true and that the autoantibodies can predict the disease with a degree of certainty. Autoantibodies have been detected in about 90% of newly diagnosed patients with T1DM to three major autoantigens, glutamic acid decarboxylase (GAD), insulinoma-associated antigen (IA)-2, and insulin antibodies (IAA) *(see* Chap. 10). There are two isoforms of GAD, the *GAD65* gene found on chromosome 10p11 encodes a protein of 585 amino acids with a molecular weight of 65 kd *(53)*. The two isoforms are approximately 65% identical and are expressed in neurons and pancreatic islet cells, where GAD65 predominates. GAD65 is involved in the conversion of glutamic acid to γ-aminobutyric acid (GABA), a major inhibitory neurotransmitter. IA-2, also known as islet cell antibody (ICA)512, is an unusual member of the transmembrane PTP family and is located on chromosome 2q35 *(54)*. The molecular weight is 106 kd, and the protein is 979 amino acids in length. It is atypical in that it lacks enzymatic activity because of a critical amino acid substitution at position 911 (Asp for Ala) in the catalytic domain of the molecule. The protein is expressed in neuroendocrine tissues and is found in pancreatic islets. Immunofluorescence studies have localized IA-2 to the secretory vesicles of both endocrine and neuronal cells, but its function is not known. Insulin, the third autoantigen in T1DM *(55)*, is a short protein of 51 amino acids encoded on chromosome 11p15. As with the GAD65- and IA-2-specific autoantibodies, insulin autoantibodies in the sera of type 1 diabetic patients are directed primarily to conformational epitopes. For IAA, these epitopes map to the B chain of human proinsulin or insulin. Unlike the GAD65 and IA-2 autoantibodies, insulin autoantibodies are not useful for confirming the classification of diabetes after insulin replacement therapy has begun, because patients develop antibodies to exogenous insulin.

Deliberate transfer of disease from one person to another is clearly ethically unacceptable, although a single case has been described of apparent transfer of T1DM following a bone marrow transplant from a diabetic donor to a non-diabetic recipient *(56)*. Furthermore, there was rapid destruction of apparently normal islet insulin secretory cells when pancreatic tissue was transplanted from non-diabetic twins to diabetic identical cotwins, indicating that the destructive process must be outside the islet insulin secretory cell specific and must retain its cytotoxic memory *(57)*. The immune system is the obvious candidate for such a specific destructive extra-islet effect. However, we are currently unable to fully immunomodulate this disease, although there is some evidence that the disease process can be modified by immunotherapy.

Thus, subjects with newly diagnosed T1DM given cyclosporine A, a modifier of T-cell activation, are more likely to show a transient improvement in metabolic control in the first 2 years post-diagnosis *(58)*.

Insulin-Dependent Diabetes Need Not Be Autoimmune

If we accept that not all children presenting with insulin-dependent diabetes can be strictly defined as having autoimmune diabetes, then we can also accept that there may be several different causes for insulin-dependent diabetes in children which is not autoimmune. There are at least three conditions in which the insulin secretory cells fail to produce much, if any, insulin because of immaturity, destruction, or dysfunction *(59)*. In Wolfram syndrome, an autosomal-recessive defect of developmental genes, the insulin secretory cells fail to mature, although levels of insulin secretion can vary substantially between individuals; it occurs in association with diabetes insipidus, optic atrophy, and high tone deafness (also called DIDMOAD syndrome). Acute and chronic pancreatitis can be complicated by damage to the islet insulin secretory cells whether induced by viruses, alcohol, or gall stones. A form of diabetes (type 1b diabetes), rare in most of the world but relatively common in Japan, affects young adults and is characterized by the severity of its presentation, marked insulin deficiency, rapid onset with evidence of a short prodrome, insulitis, and raised serum alkaline phosphatase, all consistent with a viral infection, although supportive evidence is lacking *(59,60)*. Finally, inherited defects of the islet potassium ion channels involved in insulin secretion can compromise insulin secretion and present as neonatal diabetes with little or no insulin secretion. Remarkably, these individuals with Kir6.2 mutations, despite being insulin dependent, can discontinue insulin and be controlled using high-dose sulphonylurea tablets *(61)*. Sulphonylureas increase insulin secretion from the pancreatic beta cell by closing ATP-sensitive potassium (K_{ATP}) channels, depolarizing the beta-cell plasma membrane and increasing intracellular calcium concentration. It follows that sulphonylureas are of value when there is insulin secretory deficiency but not when insulin resistance has a major impact as is the case in forms of type 2 diabetes and neonatal diabetes when there is a potassium channel mutation. Functional studies show that the severity of the clinical phenotype is reflected in the functional changes seen in the mutated channel *(61)*.

Autoimmune Diabetes Need Not Be Insulin-Dependent

Autoimmune diabetes may also present in adults (adult-onset T1DM) and may not require insulin treatment initially. The latter group of patients are only identified as having autoimmune diabetes when their blood is checked for diabetes-associated autoantibodies. As their autoimmunity is clinically latent, this form of diabetes has been classified as latent autoimmune diabetes of adults (LADA) *(62,63)*.

Non-insulin requiring autoimmune diabetes developing in adults or LADA is typically diagnosed when the patient is between 30 and 70 years of age, with positive detection of diabetes-associated autoantibodies, and the diabetes remains non-insulin requiring for at least 6 months post-diagnosis *(62,63)*, although the definition is semantic and can vary in terms of the age at diagnosis and the duration of non-insulin requiring diabetes. The epidemiology of LADA is influenced by geography, genetic susceptibility, environmental factors, gender, and age at diagnosis. In Northern

Europe and North America, about 5–10% of newly diagnosed non-insulin requiring diabetes patients have LADA, according to the mode of ascertainment, the sourced population, the age of the patient (frequency is higher in younger age groups) and the definition of the disease *(61,62,64)*. Non-insulin requiring diabetes with diabetes-associated autoantibodies is not confined to the age group 30–70 years, and when found in children is called latent autoimmune diabetes of the young (LADY). The use of ICA in defining LADA or LADY patients further extends the percentage of patients with these clinical conditions as many patients with ICA do not have GAD autoantibodies and that percentage increases with the age at clinical onset of diabetes. The genetics of non-insulin requiring autoimmune diabetes has yet to be well characterized. In classic T1DM, HLA-DR3, DQB1*0201 and DR4, DQB1*0302 are associated with increased disease susceptibility, whereas HLA-DR2, DQB1*0602, DRB1*0403 seem to confer protection *(4,63)*. In a substantial study, LADA was also associated with increased frequencies of HLA-DR3 (28%), DR4 (27%), and DR3/4 (22%), and as with classical T1DM, these risk allele frequencies declined with age at diagnosis *(4,65)*. As with adult-onset T1DM, HLA-DR2 appears to play little role in disease protection. A feature of LADA is that following diagnosis some patients may progress over months or years toward insulin dependence. As we shall discuss, this is not an invariant feature of LADA, but it does reflect the propensity for autoimmune diabetes to show variable rates of disease progression even to insulin-dependence *(66,67)*.

We can summarize the analysis to date of patients with autoimmune diabetes defined solely by the presence of diabetes-associated autoantibodies as those who are insulin dependent at diagnosis or within a short period thereafter (called T1DM), those who are not insulin-dependent initially and for a period of at least 6 months (called LADA or LADY according to age at diagnosis), and those who are not insulin-dependent initially but progress over a variable period to insulin dependence (called LADA, LADY, or slowly progressive insulin-dependent diabetes [SPIDDM]).

Activation and Induction of Autoimmune Diabetes

If the critical event that induces the destructive immune process operates in early childhood, it follows that those diabetes-associated immune changes that reflect that process may also be detected at an early age. Timing of the onset of autoimmunity is a prerequisite for unmasking triggers in the pathogenesis of this disease. At birth, children of diabetic mothers often have ICA, IAA, and GAD autoantibodies. But these autoantibodies can also be found in the maternal serum and are probably placentally transferred to the child because autoantibody specificities are similar in mother and cord blood and are not detected in the infants of mothers without such autoantibodies *(68–70)*. Passively acquired maternal autoantibodies disappear after birth as expected but can subsequently be replaced by the infant's own autoantibodies. The cumulative risk of T1DM in 1353 offspring of diabetic parents was 18% at age 5 years, but the risk was 50% in those with more than one diabetes-associated autoantibody *(68)*. Intriguingly, passively acquired maternal autoantibodies may protect children from later autoimmune diabetes *(71)*.

While cord blood autoantibodies are mainly transplacentally acquired, diabetes-associated autoantibodies can appear at a very young age. For example 85% of New Zealand schoolchildren who seroconverted to ICA did so before 5 years of age *(72)*.

Of 137 children with ICA from a prospective Finnish study of 4590 consecutive newborns with the disease-risk HLA-DQB1, IAA, and GAD autoantibodies usually appeared before ICA, whereas IA-2 autoantibodies usually appeared afterwards *(73)*. Strikingly, 95% of seroconversions to IAA, GAD, or IA-2 autoantibodies occurred in a cluster (−12 to +8 months) around the time of ICA seroconversion. Children at high genetic risk seroconverted steadily at approximately twice the rate of those at moderate risk *(73)*. Thus, induction and activation of diabetes-associated autoantibodies are not confined to early childhood, and seroconversion may be detected up to at least 10 years of age. For all that we know about the induction and activation of the autoimmune response in childhood-onset disease, we know next to nothing about the same induction events in adult-onset autoimmune diabetes.

Taken together, these observations suggest that non-genetic activation of the diabetes-associated immune process, possibly by viruses or dietary factors, can occur in early childhood. However, seroconversion is not confined to early childhood; so, by implication, activation of the diabetes-associated immune response cannot occur in early childhood in all cases of autoimmune diabetes. It remains unclear whether the age at clinical diagnosis is in part dependent on the age at which an environmental event activates the immune response. If this is the case, then the immune process that leads to adult-onset T1DM, and LADA would be induced later than in childhood-onset T1DM (Table 3). Importantly, the precise nature of the destructive immune process also remains unclear, although we assume it is because of adaptive and innate immune effectors.

The Destructive Process Causing Autoimmune Diabetes

Several lines of evidence indicate that T cells play a major role in the pathogenesis of autoimmune diabetes in the non-obese diabetic (NOD) mice (*see* Chap. 10) and men *(74–75)*, although other cells, such as macrophages, dendritic cells, and B cells, are also involved *(76)*. What we know about the pathogenesis of human T1DM comes largely from autopsy specimens obtained from patients who died either close to

Table 3
Distinction Between Childhood-Onset and Adult-Onset Type 1 Diabetes and LADA

	Children	*Adults*	*LADA*
Age at diagnosis	Childhood	Adulthood	Adulthood
Identical twin			
Concordance rate	38%	6%	?
HLADR3/ DR4-risk	Moderate	Low	Low
HLADR2-protection	Moderate	Low	Low
Autoantibodies	IAA GAD IA-2	GAD IA-2	GAD IA-2

IAA, Insulin autoantibodies; GAD, glutamic acid decarboxylase; LADA, late autoimmune diabetes of the adult.
Note that the children, compared with the others, have a higher identical twin concordance rate, frequency of HLA genetic susceptibility heterozygosity and insulin autoantibodies and lower serum insulin levels. Data compiled from different sources *(6,11,65,84,85)*. HLA DR3/4 is found in about 6% of North American and European control populations.

diagnosis from ketoacidosis or late in the course of the disease, as pancreatic biopsies on live patients are considered hazardous. The autopsy findings probably represent a late stage of the disease, many months after the initial triggering event (3,77). Morphological techniques show a marked decrease in insulin secretory cells associated with a chronic inflammation, probably driven by macrophages and lymphocytes that surround and infiltrate the islets. CD8+ T cells seem to predominate, but neither the proportion of CD4+ and CD8+ cells nor the significance of other cell types in the infiltrate (e.g., natural killer cells, macrophages, and dendritic cells) is known. Moreover, the proportion of CD4+ or CD8+ cells specific for diabetes-associated autoantigens is unknown, although insulin-specific cells have been detected in pancreatic draining lymph nodes, albeit using very high doses of antigen (78).

Various cell-mediated immune models have been proposed to explain the autoimmune destruction, but none of these models in man have been verified. It is widely believed that insulin secretory cells express HLA class I alleles in association with selected peptides (epitopes) either from one of the major autoantigens or from environmental triggers (e.g., viruses) that act as targets for destruction by specific cytotoxic CD8+ T cells. The difficulty in identifying such antigen-specific T cells in peripheral blood could be because pathogenic T cells are concentrated in the islets and only sparsely represented in peripheral blood (79). Alternatively, or in addition, inflammatory cells can express cytokines, which can be toxic to human islet cells in vitro (80). Although autoantibodies to IA-2 and GAD65 are primarily of the IgG1 isotype, which argues in favor of a cytotoxic Th1-type immune response, the evidence is indirect and not persuasive (34). In future, ELISPOT or soluble HLA class II tetramer assays might be more valuable in defining the disease process, but until then, we are left with the limited autopsy data on which to base our understanding of the pathogenesis of T1DM.

AUTOIMMUNE DIABETES AS A SPECTRUM OF METABOLIC CHANGES

There is evidence in autoimmune diabetes for a continuum of metabolic changes, predominantly decreased insulin secretory capacity but also insensitivity to insulin. These extend from the severe changes seen in childhood onset T1DM to the relatively minor changes initially detected in LADA, as previously discussed.

Some individuals pass through a "pre-diabetic" stage of impaired glucose tolerance or even non-insulin requiring diabetes before becoming frankly insulin-dependent, and this stage is more prevalent in adults than in children. The Diabetes Prevention Trial of T1DM (DPT-1) detected 585 relatives of T1DM patients who had ICA plus either IAA or low first-phase insulin response to intravenous glucose. Of them, 427 had normal glucose tolerance, 87 had impaired glucose tolerance and 61 were diabetic, yet asymptomatic, on glucose tolerance testing (81). Of these latter, those with impaired fasting glucose were significantly older (mean age 21 years) than those with normal fasting glucose (mean age 12 years). These subjects with asymptomatic autoimmune diabetes resemble LADA, but their age is <30 years precluding the diagnosis. It follows that some patients with autoimmune diabetes pass through a phase of altered glucose levels, including non-insulin requiring diabetes, before becoming insulin-dependent, and the frequency of this phase, to a degree, is age dependent.

The rate of progression to clinical diabetes may be more rapid in patients presenting at <5 years of age than in those presenting much later. Histological evidence supports this contention: islet beta cells tend to be absent within 12 months of diagnosis in patients aged <7 years, but detected for longer periods in older patients *(77)*. Variability in progression to clinical diabetes can even be detected in very young children; for example, of children identified between 1 and 5 years of age with diabetes-associated autoantibodies and subnormal insulin responses; half of them progress rapidly to diabetes, whereas the remainder are free from diabetes up to 4 years later *(82)*. Other studies have noted such variable progression to T1DM, which is more rapid in obese than lean children *(33)* and in children than adults *(83)*. From these observations, it follows that there is a spectrum in the rate of metabolic decompensation during the pre-diabetic period in autoimmune T1DM, but no data are available, as yet, in LADA.

Insulin secretory capacity is less in children than in adults at the onset of T1DM, and following diagnosis deteriorates more rapidly. A study of 235 consecutive cases with newly diagnosed T1DM found that those aged <7 years had the lowest baseline residual insulin secretion and required the highest insulin dose for optimal control, whereas the older the age at diagnosis the higher was the basal C-peptide level *(84)*. Patients with LADA also have reduced fasting and stimulated C-peptide at diagnosis, although the levels of C-peptide are higher than those found in children and similar to those found in adult-onset T1DM *(85)*. However, post-diagnosis, the C-peptide levels fall more rapidly in childhood-onset T1DM than in adult-onset T1DM and in the latter more rapidly than in LADA *(78,86,87)*. In summary, there is a continuous spectrum of loss of insulin secretory capacity, the severity of which is age-related, being more severe in children than adults with T1DM and more severe in the latter than in LADA subjects.

A study of identical twins of patients with T1DM found both reduced insulin secretion and reduced insulin sensitivity relative to levels of insulin secretion in pre-diabetic twins who went on to develop diabetes *(88)*. As changes in identical twins detected in the pre-diabetic period were not found in low disease risk identical twins of patients with T1DM, it is likely that these changes are non-genetically determined. The metabolic decompensation that leads to frank diabetes could result either from increased linear growth, which has been linked to diabetes risk, or from increased childhood obesity, which has been correlated with age at presentation *(31,33)*. Indeed, the normal relationship between insulin sensitivity and insulin secretion is disrupted in those diabetes-associated autoantibody-positive siblings who progress most rapidly to diabetes *(81,89)*.

People with LADA may well have more severe loss of insulin sensitivity than in childhood-onset T1DM. Certainly, the frequency of the metabolic syndrome in LADA, although less prevalent than in type 2 diabetic patients of similar age, is more prevalent than in the general population *(85,90)*. For example, the metabolic syndrome, which is found in approximately 22% of the North American population, was identified in 74% of LADA patients but in 84% of type 2 diabetes subjects *(90)*.

VARIABLE RATE OF DISEASE PROGRESSION

If the critical initiating environmental events were to operate exclusively in childhood, then the subsequent rate of progression to clinical disease would be rapid in patients presenting under 5 years of age and slow in those presenting much later *(1,72)*.

Histological evidence supports this contention; islet beta cells tend to be absent within 12 months of diagnosis in patients aged <7 years but detected for longer periods in older patients *(77)*. Even when immune changes are activated in very young children, there can be variability in the progression to clinical diabetes; remarkably, of children identified between 1 and 5 years of age with diabetes-associated autoantibodies and subnormal insulin responses, half of them progressed rapidly to diabetes, whereas the remainder are not diabetic up to 4 years later *(82)*. This observation implies variable disease progression even among very young children with similar HLA genetic susceptibility, numbers of diabetes-associated autoantibodies and degree of metabolic disturbance. Other studies have emphasized such variable progression, being more rapid in children, in the presence of diabetes-associated autoantibodies, but being independent of autoantibody type and the degree of insulin secretory loss and being more rapid in obese than lean children *(33,91,92)*. Genetic factors also determine when T1DM presents.

Identical twins develop the disease at a similar age, which is for them also at a similar time, with a heritability for age at diagnosis of 74% *(93)*. Family studies comparing affected siblings show a correlation in them with age at diagnosis and not with time of diagnosis *(93)*. Lack of correlation between siblings for time of diagnosis argues against a common environmental exposure precipitating diabetes and favors a distinct environmental event *(93)*. Given clustering in time between siblings for immune activation, as judged by autoantibody seroconversion, as well as clustering by age at the time of diagnosis, the rate of progression of the destructive process during the intervening pre-diabetic period is probably, to a degree, genetically determined in both children and adults.

FACTORS DETERMINING METABOLIC DECOMPENSATION PRE-DIABETES

The metabolic decompensation that leads to frank clinical diabetes could result in part either from increased linear growth, which has been linked to diabetes risk, or from increased childhood obesity, which has been correlated with age at presentation *(33,93–95)*. Indeed, the normal relationship between insulin sensitivity relative to insulin secretion is disrupted in those diabetes-associated autoantibody-positive siblings who progress most rapidly to diabetes *(88,89)*. Although several unifying theories, including the accelerator hypothesis, have sought to explain the loss of glucose tolerance with changes in both insulin sensitivity and insulin secretion in patients with either T1DM or T2DM, there is no reason to suspect a causal link beyond that which describes the interrelationship of these two variables and that relationship should hold irrespective of whether the loss of insulin sensitivity results from reduced insulin secretory cell mass because of either autoimmune factors (as in T1DM) or unknown factors including amyloid deposition (as for T2DM).

FACTORS DETERMINING METABOLIC DECOMPENSATION POST-DIAGNOSIS

Similar variability in disease progression is evident post-diagnosis. Insulin secretory capacity is less in children than in adults at the onset of T1DM and following diagnosis deteriorates more rapidly. A study of 235 consecutive cases with newly diagnosed T1DM found that the older the age at diagnosis the higher was the basal C-peptide level *(84)*. Patients with LADA also have reduced fasting and stimulated C-peptide at diagnosis, although the levels of C-peptide are higher than those found in children and similar to those found in adult-onset T1DM *(85)*. SPIDDM, by definition, is associated with sufficiently reduced insulin secretory capacity to cause insulin dependence *(66,67)*. Post-diagnosis of T1DM, the C-peptide levels falls more rapidly in childhood-onset T1DM than in adult-onset T1DM and in the latter more rapidly than in LADA *(85, 87,96–98)*. Of LADA patients, 94% required insulin treatment by 6 years as compared with only 14% in those initially non-insulin requiring diabetes patients without either GAD autoantibodies or ICA *(64)*. Progression to insulin dependence in LADA patients was more rapid in those aged <45 years than in older cases *(64)*. It follows that patients with autoimmune diabetes, including both T1DM and LADA, are at high risk of progression to insulin dependence but that that risk declines with age at diagnosis. In the same manner, SPIDDM also becomes less common as adult age advances *(66)*.

It is likely, therefore, that within autoimmune diabetes, there is an age-related spectrum of decreasing severity of loss of insulin secretory capacity and increasing severity of insulin insensitivity and metabolic syndrome *(1,84,99,100)*. LADA occupies one end of this spectrum without any clear division between it and other forms of autoimmune T1DM.

PREDICTION OF DIABETES

It is the predictable pattern of diseases, both in their natural history and in their response to therapy, which has been the cornerstone of modern medicine. The early induction of diabetes-associated autoantibodies and the long pre-diabetic period suggested the possibility that autoimmune diabetes could be predicted. Indeed, autoantibodies, which appear in the peripheral blood long before clinical symptoms, are more reliable predictive markers than the presence of high-risk genes, not only in diabetes but also in a substantial number of other autoimmune diseases *(91,101–103)*.

If an autoantibody is used to predict a disease, then three criteria must be fulfilled: first, every non-diseased subject with the autoantibody would eventually develop the disease (high disease-positive predictive value); second, every non-diseased subject with the autoantibody would develop the associated disease and not any other disease (high disease specificity); and third, every subject who developed the disease would have that particular autoantibody (high disease sensitivity). The positive predictive value is higher the greater is the population risk of developing the disease (disease risk). The feasibility of screening for autoantibodies as predictors of disease has been convincingly demonstrated over the last few years in the case of T1DM *(102,103)* (Table 4). International workshops have demonstrated the validity of assays, in terms of consistency and accuracy, for certain antigen-specific autoantibodies. Using these

Table 4
Autoantibodies as Predictors of T1DM

Autoantibodies
- Can appear at an early age, even around the time of birth
- Can precede the clinical onset of diabetes by some years
- Have variable predictive value depending on the autoantigen recognized
- Have increasing positive predictive value with increasing numbers

assays, the positive predictive value for diabetes increases for one, two, or three autoantibodies from approximately 10 to 50 and 80%, respectively, within 5 years and even higher thereafter *(102,103)*.

As before, there is a caveat that our ability to predict autoimmune diabetes in childhood-onset disease has yet to be demonstrated in adult-onset cases. If the immune process associated with the development of T1DM is sometimes initiated later in life, then population screening will have to be performed at different ages to detect induction of diabetes-associated autoantibodies in the pre-diabetic period. Indeed, as autoantibodies to different antigens appear sequentially, and the predictive value of an autoantibody combination varies with age, disease-risk based on autoantibody combinations will require repeated screening with different combinations. Thus, screening strategies will need to be flexible.

TREATMENT AND FUTURE DIRECTIONS

The aim of disease prediction is disease prevention. T1DM could be prevented by avoiding those environmental factors that cause the disease process (primary prevention) or by modulating the destructive process before the onset of clinical diabetes (secondary prevention) or by trying to cure the disease process at the time of diagnosis (tertiary prevention).

Primary Prevention of T1DM

Any such strategy for T1DM requires that critical environmental factors such as diet or viruses are recognized and removed or their effect negated, while remembering that infections could be protective *(104–106)*. Thus, diabetes could theoretically be prevented by vaccination against enterovirus infections or by postponing the introduction of cow's milk beyond 4 months of age *(106)*. Alternatively, maintaining breastfeeding beyond 3 months post-partum could limit the risk of disease because studies suggest that cessation of breastfeeding before that time are associated with an increased diabetes risk *(106)*. A study, the Trial to Reduce the Incidence of diabetes in Genetically at Risk (TRIGR), is now underway to test the hypothesis that late introduction of cow's milk protein prevents T1DM. This multinational study plans to enroll 2400 genetically high-risk babies (identified by HLA alleles) who will be randomized to formula feed containing either cow's milk or casein hydrolysate after breastfeeding in children aged <9 months *(106)*. But if environmental factors causing diabetes can operate later, then these factors might be different and could induce a different type of destructive immune process. In that case, primary and secondary prevention strategies might also differ from those which are used for childhood-onset diabetes *(1)*.

Secondary Prevention of T1DM

Secondary prevention (i.e., after disease induction but before clinical diabetes develops) could prevent autoimmune diabetes by (1) protection of insulin secreting cells, (2) rest of insulin-secreting cells, and (3) immune modulation including antigen-based strategies. The field of study has been hindered by the extensive use of an animal model, the NOD mouse, which can be cured of diabetes in many different ways that offer little of value to modify human autoimmune diabetes *(45)*. A number of studies suggested that nicotinamide could prevent diabetes onset both in NOD mice and in man. Nicotinamide may operate through promoting DNA repair. Two studies that set out to evaluate the potential of nicotinamide to prevent progression to T1DM in high disease-risk children of individuals with T1DM (DENIS and ENDIT) failed to show any benefit *(107,108)*.

An alternative approach, again successful in the NOD mouse, used early and aggressive therapy with insulin therapy before the onset of clinical diabetes to rest the insulin-secreting beta cell, making it less prone to immune attack. As a result, a trial was mounted to determine whether insulin therapy can delay or prevent diabetes in non-diabetic relatives of patients with diabetes (DPT-1); but there was no beneficial effect *(103)*. Alternatively, insulin might modulate the aggressive immune response if that response is targeting insulin as an antigen. In both BB rats and NOD mice, such insulin therapy delayed the development of diabetes and of insulitis, but a study of oral insulin in at-risk children based on such hypothetical immunomodulation also failed to identify a positive benefit *(109)*. Such trial failures have being disappointing but highlight the problem with relying too heavily on an inconsistent animal model. Furthermore, given the differences between childhood-onset and adult-onset autoimmune diabetes, therapy to modify the disease process could also differ; for example, antigen-specific therapy might involve insulin-related compounds in children, whereas in adults, GAD- or IA-2-related strategies could be more relevant. Future strategies may benefit from incorporating the patient's age at diagnosis into the study design.

Tertiary Prevention of T1DM

Tertiary prevention (i.e., in recently diagnosed patients with diabetes) has the ethical advantage that a more aggressive therapy can be considered as the patient already has the disease, but the disadvantage that it may be too late to offer therapy because much of the insulin secretory capacity is already lost. Two approaches have been employed: (1) general immunosuppression and (2) immune modulation including antigen-based strategies.

The first immunosuppression study was started in 1976 using high-dose steroids, azathioprine, anti-lymphocyte globulin, and plasmapheresis over a 1-month period in newly diagnosed men with T1DM *(110)*. No controls were considered necessary because a cure would have been sufficient, and only a cure could have justified such aggressive therapy. No cure was obtained. Subsequently, the goal of immune therapy shifted from a cure to an effect, physicians became more modest in their ambitions seeking improved C-peptide levels, reduction in hypoglycemia or a fall in glycated hemoglobin (an index of blood glucose control). These end-points may well prove beneficial but are some way off the initial grandiose target of a cure. The immunosuppressant cyclosporine A, studied in large randomized multinational trials, could modify the disease process, so that at 2 years post-diagnosis patients in the treatment arm had more C-peptide indicating some preservation of islet beta cell function *(111)*.

Another interesting approach has been the use of anti-CD3 antibodies. In animal models of diabetes, these antibodies can reverse established disease. A small study found some effect of anti-CD3 antibodies in preserving C-peptide response to a mixed-meal challenge in patients with newly diagnosed T1DM *(112,113)*. The mode of action is unclear, but there is some depletion of T cells, which is incomplete and transient. Most likely anti-CD3 antibodies operate, at least in NOD mice, through immunomodulation causing tolerance induction by modifying $CD4^+$ $CD25^+$ T regulatory cells (114). More recently, modified anti-CD3 monoclonal antibody in T1DM patients induced a subset of regulatory $CD8^+$ T cells, and this population of cells stained positive for Foxp3 and CTLA-4 (115).

A more targeted approach uses immune modulation with antigen-based strategies. Heat-shock protein (hsp60) is a stress protein that could be a major target antigen in several inflammatory diseases, including T1DM and rheumatoid arthritis (116). T cells that recognize hsp60 derived from pre-diabetic NOD spleens are capable of adoptively transferring insulitis and hyperglycemia to young pre-diabetic NOD mice, thus demonstrating that the autoimmune response to hsp60 is not an epiphenomenon but plays a role in the pathogenesis of diabetes in NOD mice (116). The diabetogenic T cells were found to recognize a hsp60 epitope corresponding to positions 437-460, called p277. A more stable modified peptide called Diapep277, proved to be a potent inducer of protection from the development of diabetes in the mouse models. One preliminary study in man suggests that Diapep277 injections can preserve endogenous insulin production in patients with recently diagnosed with T1DM, although again it will be important to determine whether this effect is age-related and consistent (117).

As the primary defect in autoimmune diabetes is loss of insulin secretion, treatment should aim to restore islet insulin secretion. Therapy to prevent progression toward insulin dependency could include insulin, or immunomodulation, given the inflammatory nature of the disease process thought to cause insulin secretory cell destruction. The optimal insulin regime is unclear; given the broad loss of insulin secretory capacity, it might be argued that the early introduction of long-acting insulin could be beneficial. Alternatively, the loss of rapid insulin release in LADA patients suggests that replacement with a fast-acting insulin would be more valuable. One study in Japan of patients with LADA compared early treatment with insulin given as multiple injections with sulphonylureas (118). Although of limited power, this study did show a statistically significant persistence of C-peptide in the insulin-treated group as compared with the sulphonylurea group with the proviso that the insulin-treated group had preserved insulin secretory capacity and a high titre of GAD autoantibodies at the start of the study. An alternative interpretation of this study is that sulphonylureas are disadvantageous, in support of which sulphonylureas could theoretically promote apoptosis; apoptosis being one mechanism whereby insulin-secreting cells could be destroyed in autoimmune diabetes.

A pilot phase 2 trial in LADA patients found that a tolerance induction plan using alum formulated whole GAD (Diamyd) had a significant effect on the C-peptide response to a mixed meal consistent with modulation of the aggressive process (119). Another phase 2 trial in TIDM patients used alum formulated GAD and has been completed and showed positive results in protecting residual beta-cell function in recent onset T1DM patients (unpublished observation). Both interventions with GAD and Diapep277 in autoimmune diabetes were promising and led the groups to pursue these therapies in larger Phase 3 studies now underway (http://www.actionlada.org). These immunomodulatory studies pioneer a novel approach toward the maintenance of islet cell function, itself a new field in the management of autoimmune diabetes. However for success, they presuppose that the disease is immune mediated. Even if we are correct in making this presumption, then we must also be realistic, and the reality is that we are a long way from preventing autoimmune diabetes.

ACKNOWLEDGMENTS

We thank the funding agencies involved in our studies, including the Diabetic Twin Research Trust, Juvenile Diabetes Research Foundation International, the Joint Research Board of St Bartholomew's and the Royal London Medical College, European Union and Eli Lilly.

REFERENCES

1. Leslie RD, Delli Castelli M. Age-dependent influences on the origins of autoimmune diabetes: evidence and implications. *Diabetes* 2004; 53:3033–40.
2. Foulis AK, Stewart JA. The pancreas in recent-onset type 1 (insulin-dependent) diabetes mellitus: insulin content of islets, insulitis and associated changes in the exocrine acinar tissue. *Diabetologia* 1984; 26:456–61.
3. Itoh N, Hanafusa T, Miyazaki A, Miyagawa J, Yamagata K, Yamamoto K, Waguri M, Imagawa A, Tamura S, Inada M. Mononuclear cell infiltration and its relation to the expression of major histocompatibility complex antigens and adhesion molecules in pancreas biopsy specimens from newly diagnosed insulin-dependent diabetes mellitus patients. *J Clin Invest* 1993; 92: 2313–22.
4. Field LL: Genetic linkage and association studies of type 1 diabetes: challenges and rewards. *Diabetologia* 2002; 45:21–35.
5. Concannon P, Erlich HA, Julier C, Morahan G, Nerup J, Pociot F, Todd JA, Rich SS. Type 1 diabetes genetic consortium. Type 1 diabetes: evidence for susceptibility loci from four genome-wide linkage scans in 1,435 multiplex families. *Diabetes* 2005; 54:2992–3001.
6. Redondo MJ, Yu L, Hawa M, Mackenzie T, Pyke DA, Eisenbarth GS, Leslie RDG. Heterogeneity of type I diabetes: analysis of monozygotic twins in Great Britain and the United States. *Diabetologia* 2001; 44:354–362.
7. Kumar D, Gemayel NS, Deapen D, Kapadia D, Yamashita PH, Lee M, Dwyer JH, Roy-Burman P, Bray GA, Mach TM: North-American twins with IDDM: genetic, etiological, and clinical significance of disease concordance according to age, zygosity, and the interval after diagnosis in first twin. *Diabetes* 1993; 42:1351–63.
8. Meyer D, Thomson G: How selection shapes variation of the human major histocompatibility complex: a review. *Ann Hum Genet* 2001; 65:1–26.
9. Greenbaum CJ, Schatz DA,Cuthbertson D, Zeidler A, Eisenbarth GS, Krischer JP. Islet cell antibody-positive relatives with human leukocyte antigen DQA1*0102, DQB1*0602: identification by the Diabetes Prevention Trial-type 1. *J Clin Endocrinol Metab* 2000; 85:1255–60.
10. Sabbah E, Savola K, Ebeling T, Kulmala P, Vahasalo P, Ilonen J, Salmela PI, Knip M. Genetic, autoimmune, and clinical characteristics of childhood- and adult-onset type 1 diabetes. *Diabetes Care* 2000; 23:1326–32.
11. Vanderwalle CL, Cecraene T, Schuit FC, De Leeuw IH, Pipeleers DG, Gorus FK, and the Belgian Diabetes Register. Insulin antibodies and high titre islet cell antibodies are preferentially associated with the HLA DQA1*03100-DQB1*0302 haplotype at clinical onset of type 1 (insulin-dependent) diabetes mellitus before age 10 years but not at onset between age 10 and 40 years. *Diabetologia* 1993; 36:1155–62.

12. Hamalanian A-M, Savola K, Kulmala PK, Koskela P, Akerblom HK, Knip M, and the Finnish TRIGR Study Group. Disease-associated autoantibodies during pregnancy and at birth in families affected by type 1 diabetes. *Clin Exp Immunol* 2001; 126:231–6.

13. Wang WY, Barrate BJ, Clayton DG, Todd JA. Genome-wide association studies: theoretical and practical concerns. *Nat Rev Genet* 2005; 6:109–18.

14. Salvetti M, Ristori G, Bomprezzi R, Pozzilli P, Leslie RDG: Twins: mirrors of the immune system. *Immunol Today* 2000; 21:342–7.

15. Hyttinen V, Kaprio J, Kinnunen L, Koskenvuo M, Tuomilehto J. Genetic liability of type 1 diabetes and the onset age among 22,650 young Finnish twin pairs: a nationwide follow-up study. *Diabetes* 2003; 52:1052–5.

16. Kyvick KO, Nystrom L, Gorus F, Songini M, Oestman J, Castell C, Green A, Guyrus E, Ionescu-Tirgoviste C, Mckinney PA, Michalkova D, Ostrauskas R, Raymond NT. The epidemology of type I diabetes mellitus is not the same in young adults as in children. *Diabetologia* 2004; 47:377–84.

17. Baker JM. Type 1 diabetes associated autoimmunity: natural history, genetic associations and screening. *J Clin Endocrinol Metab* 2006; 91:1210–1217.

18. Guo D, Li M, Zhang Y, Yang P, Eckenrode S, Hopkins D, Zheng W, Purohit S, Podolsky RH, Muir A, Wang J, Dong Z, Brusko T, Atkinson M, Pozzilli P, Zeidler A, Raffel LJ, Jacob CO, Park Y, Serrano-Rios M, Larrad MT, Zhang Z, Garchon HJ, Bach JF, Rotter JI, She JX, Wang CY. A functional variant of SUMO4, a new I kappa B alpha modifier, is associated with type 1 diabetes. *Nat Genet* 2004; 36:837–41.

19. Warram JH, Krolewski AS, Gottlieb MS, Kahn CR. Differences in risk of insulin-dependent diabetes in offspring of diabetic mothers and diabetic fathers. *N Engl J Med* 1984; 311:149–52.

20. Bleich D, Polak M, Eisenbarth GS, Jackson RA: Decreased risk of type 1 diabetes in offspring of mothers who acquire diabetes during adrenarchy. *Diabetes* 1993; 42:1433–9.

21. Bach JF. The effect of infections on susceptibility to autoimmune and allergic diseases. *N Engl J Med* 2002; 347:911–20.

22. Joslin EP. The treatment of diabetes mellitus with observations based upon three thousand cases, 3rd edn. Philadelphia and New York, Lea and Febiger, 1923. *Nutr Rev.* 1983; 41:187–9.

23. Sultz HA. Childhood diabetes mellitus. In: *Long-Term Childhood Illness*. Sultz HA Ed. Pittsburg, PA, University of Pittsburg Press, p.223–48, 1972.

24. Schoenle EJ, Lang-Muritano M, Gschwend S, Laimbacher J, Mullis PE, Torresani T, Biason-Lauber A, Molinari L. Epidemiology of type 1 diabetes. *Diabetologia* 2001; 44:286–9.

25. Bodansky HJ, Saines A, Stephenson C, Haigh D, Cartwright R. Evidence for an environmental effect in the aetiology of insulin dependent diabetes in a transmigratory population. *BMJ* 1992; 304:1020–2.

26. Zung A, Elizur MN, Weintrob T. Bistritzer, Hanukoglu A, Zadik Z, Phillip M, Miller K, Koren IC. Brautbar and S Israel. Type 1 diabetes in Jewish Ethiopian immigrants in Israel: HLA class II immunogenetics and contribution of new environment. *Hum Immunol* 2004; 65:1463–8.

27. Staines A, Hanif S, Ahmed S, Mckinney PA, Shera S, Bodansky HJ. Incidence of insulin-dependent diabetes mellitus in Karachi, Pakistan. *Arch Dis Child* 1997; 76:121–3.

28. Hermann R, Knip M, Veijola R, Simell O, Laine AP, Akerblom HK, Groop PH, Forsblom C, Pettersson-Fernholm K, Ilonen J. Temporal changes in the frequencies of HLA genotypes in patients with type 1 diabetes-indication of an increased environmental pressure? *Diabetologia* 2003; 46:420–5.

29. Pundziute-Lycka A, Dahlquist G, Nystrom L, Amqvist H, Bjork E, Blohme G, Bolinder J, Eriksson JW, Sundkvist G, Ostman J, Swedish Chidhood Diabetes Study Group. The incidence of type 1 diabetes has not increased but shifted to a younger age at diagnosis in the 0-34 years group in Sweden 1983-1998. *Diabetologia* 2002; 45:783–91.

30. Weets I, Leeuw IH, Du Caju MV, Rooman R, Keymeulen B, Mathieu C, Rottiers R, Daubresse JC, Rocour-Brumoul D, Pipeleers DG, Gorus FK, Belgian Diabetes Registry. The incidence of type 1 diabetes in the age group 0-39 years has not increased in Antwerp (Belgium) between 1989 and 2000: evidence for earlier disease manifestation. *Diabetes Care* 2002; 25:840–6.

31. Hypponen E, Virtanen SM, Kenward MG, Knip M, Akerblom HK, Childhood Diabetes in Finland Study Group. Obesity, increased linear growth, and risk of type 1 diabetes in children. *Diabetes Care* 2000; 23:1755–60.

32. Bruining GJ. Association between infant growth before onset of juvenile type 1 diabetes and autoantibodies to IA-2. Netherlands Kolibrie study group of childhood diabetes: *Lancet* 2000; 356:655–6.

33. Kibirige M, Metcalf B, Renuka R, Wilkin TJ. Testing the accelerator hypothesis; the relationship between body mass and age at diagnosis of type 1 diabetes. *Diabetes Care* 2003; 26:2865–70.

34. Hawa MI, Fava D, Medici F, Deng YJ, Notkins AL, De Mattia G, Leslie RD. Antibodies to IA-2 and GAD65 in type 1 and type 2 diabetes: isotype restriction and polyclonality. *Diabetes Care* 2000; 23:228–33.

35. Muntoni S, Fonte MT, Stoduto S, Marietti G, Bizzarri C, Crino A, Ciampalini P, Multari G, Suppa MA, Matteoli MC, Lucentini L, Sebastiani LM, Visalli N, Pozzilli P, Boscherini B, Muntoni S. Incidence of insulin-dependent diabetes mellitus among Sardinian-heritage children born in Lazio region, Italy. *Lancet* 1997; 349:160–2.

36. Bingley PJ, Douek IF, Rogers CA, Gale EA. Influence of maternal age at delivery and birth order on risk of type 1 diabetes in childhood: prospective population based family study. *BMJ* 2000; 321:420–4.

37. Dahlquist G, Kallen B: Maternal-child blood group incompatability and other perinatal events increase the risk for early-onset type 1 (insulin-dependent) diabetes mellitus. *Diabetologia* 1992; 35:671–5.

38. Dahlquist G, Ivarsson S, Lindberg B, Forsgren M: Maternal enteroviral infection during pregnancy asa risk factor for childhood IDDM. *Diabetes* 1995; 44:408–13.

39. Viskari H, Ludvigsson J, Uibo R, Salur L, Marciulionyte D, Hermann R, Soltesz G, Fuchtenbusch M, Ziegler AG, Kondrashova A, Romanov A, Kaplan B, Laron Z, Koskela P, Vesikari T, Huhtala H, Knip M, Hyoty H. Relationship between the incidence of type 1 diabetes and maternal enterovirus antibodies: time trends and geographical variation. *Diabetologia* 2005; 48:1280–7.

40. Knip M. Cow's milk and the new trials for prevention of type I diabetes. *J Endocrinol Invest* 2003; 26:265–7.

41. Hypponen E, Laara E, Reunanen A, Jarvelin MR, Virtanen SM. Intake of vitamin D and risk of type 1 diabetes: a birth-cohort study. *Lancet* 2001; 358:1500–3.

42. Dahlquist GG, Blom LG, Persson LA, Sandstrom AI, Wall SG: Dietary factors and the risk of developing insulin dependent diabetes in childhood. *BMJ* 1990; 300:1302–6.

43. Parslow RC, McKinney PA, Law GR, Staines A, Williams R, Bodansky HJ. Incidence of childhood diabetes mellitus in Yorkshire, northern England, is associated with nitrate in drinking water: an ecological analysis. *Diabetologia* 1997; 40:550–6.

44. Bellacosa A. Genetic hits and mutation rate in colorectal tumorigenesis: Versatility of Knudson's theory and implications for cancer prevention. *Genes Chromosomes Cancer* 2003; 38:382–8.

45. Atkinson MA, Leiter EH. The NOD mouse model of type 1 diabetes: as good as it gets? *Nat Med* 1999; 5:601–4.

46. McEvoy RC, Fedun B, Cooper LZ, Thomas NM, Rodriguez de Cordoba S, Rubinstein P, Ginsberg-Fellner F. Children at high risk of diabetes mellitus: New York studies of families with diabetes and of children with congenital rubella syndrome. *Adv Exp Med Biol* 1988; 246:221–7.

47. Yoon JW, Austin M, Onodera T, Notkins AL. Isolation of a virus from the pancreas of a child with diabetic ketoacidosis. *N Engl J Med* 1979; 300:1173–9.

48. Akerblom HK, Vaarala O, Hyoty H, Ilonen J, Knip M. Environmental factors in the etiology of type 1 diabetes. *Am J Med Genet* 2002; 115:18–29.

49. Knip M, Veijola R, Virtanen SM, Hyoty H, Vaarala O, Akerblom HK. Environmental triggers and determinants of type 1 diabetes. *Diabetes*. 2005; 54 (Suppl 2):S125–36.

50. Fears WB. The rat poison Vacor. *N Engl J Med* 1980; 15;302:1147.

51. Gerstein HC, Simpson JR, Atkinson S, Taylor DW, VanderMeulen J. Feasibility and acceptability of a proposed infant feeding intervention trial for the prevention of type I diabetes. *Diabetes Care* 1995; 18:940–2.

52. Rose NR, Bona C. Defining criteria for autoimmune diseases (Witebsky's postulates revisited). *Immunol Today* 1993; 14: 426–30.

53. Baekkeskov S, Aanstoot HJ, Christgau S, Reetz A, Solimena M, Cascalho M, Folli F, Richter-Olesen H, De Camilli P. Identification of the 64K autoantigen in insulin-dependent diabetes as the GABA-synthesizing enzyme glutamic acid decarboxylase. *Nature* 1990; 347:151–6.

54. Lan MS, Wasserfall C, Maclaren NK, Notkins AL. IA-2, a transmembrane protein of the protein tyrosine phosphatase family, is a major autoantigen in insulin-dependent diabetes mellitus. *Proc Natl Acad Sci USA* 1996; 93:6367–70.

55. Palmer JP, Asplin CM, Clemons P, Lyen K, Tatpati O, Raghu PK, Paquette TL. Insulin antibodies in insulin-dependent diabetics before insulin treatment. *Science* 1983; 222:1337–9.

56. Lampeter EF, Homberg M, Quabeck K, Schaefer UW, Wernet P, Bertrams J, Grosse-Wilde H, Gries FA, Kolb H. Transfer of insulin-dependent diabetes between HLA-identical siblings by bone marrow transplantation. *Lancet* 1993; 34: 1243–4.

57. Sibley RK, Sutherland DE, Goetz F, Michael AF. Recurrent diabetes mellitus in the pancreas iso- and allograft. A light and electron microscopic and immunohistochemical analysis of four cases. *Lab Invest* 1985; 53:132–44.

58. Feutren G, Papoz L, Assan R, Vialettes B, Karsenty G, Vexiau P, for the Cyclosporine/Diabetes French Study Group. Cyclosporine increases the rate and length of remissions in insulin dependent diabetes of recent onset: results of a multicentre double-blind trial. *Lancet* 1986; 2: 119–24.

59. World Health Organization. Diagnosis and classification of diabetes mellitus. *Diabetes Care* 2006 (Suppl 1):S43–S48.

60. Imagawa A, Hanafusa T, Miyagawa J, Matsuzawa Y. A novel subtype of type 1 diabetes mellitus characterized by a rapid onset and an absence of diabetes-related antibodies. Osaka IDDM Study Group. *N Engl J Med* 2000; 342:301–7.

61. Proks P, Antcliff JF, Lippiat J, Gloyn AL, Hattersley AT, Ashcroft FM. Molecular basis of Kir6.2 mutations associated with neonatal diabetes or neonatal diabetes plus neurological features. *Proc Natl Acad Sci USA* 2004; 101:17539–44.

62. Fourlanos S, Dotta F, Greenbaum CJ, Palmer JP, Rolandsson O, Colman PG, Harrison LC. Latent autoimmune diabetes in adults (LADA) should be less latent. *Diabetologia* 2005; 48:2206–12.

63. Palmer JP, Hampe CS, Chiu H, Goel A, Brooks-Worrell BM. Is latent autoimmune diabetes in adults distinct from type 1 diabetes or just type 1 diabetes at an older age? *Diabetes* 2005; 54 (Suppl 2):S62–7.

64. Turner R, Stratton I, Horton V, Manley S, Zimmet P, Mackay IR, Shattock M, Bottazzo GF, Holman R. 1997. UKPDS 25: autoantibodies to islet-cell cytoplasm and glutamic acid decarboxylase for prediction of insulin requirement in type 2 diabetes. UK Prospective Diabetes Study Group. *Lancet*; 350:1288–93.

65. Horton V, Stratton I, Bottazzo GF, Shattock M, Mackay I, Zimmet P, Manley S, Holman R, Turner R for the UK Prospective Diabetes Study (UKPDS) Group 1999 Genetic heterogeneity of autoimmune diabetes: age at presentation in adults is influenced by HLA DRB1 and DQB1 genotypes (UKPDS 43). *Diabetologia* 1999; 42:608–16.

66. Ohtsu S, Takubo N, Kazahari M, Nomoto K, Yokota F, Kikuchi N, Koike A, Matsuura N. Yokota F. Slowly progressing form of type 1 diabetes mellitus in children: genetic analysis compared with other forms of diabetes mellitus in Japanese children. *Pediatr Diabetes* 2005; 6:221–9.

67. Kobayashi T, Tanaka S, Okubo M, Nakanishi K, Murase T, Lernmark A. Unique epitopes of glutamic acid decarboxylase autoantibodies in slowly progressive type 1 diabetes. *J Clin Endocrinol Metab* 2003; 88:4768–75.

68. Ziegler AG, Hummel M, Schenker M, Bonifacio E. Autoantibody appearance and risk for development of childhood diabetes in offspring of parents with type 1 diabetes: the 2-year analysis of the German BABYDIAB study. *Diabetes* 1999; 48:460–8.

69. Lindberg B, Ivarsson S-A, Landin-Olsson M, Sundkvist G, Svanberg L, Lernmark A. Islet autoantibodies in cord blood from children who developed type 1 (insulin-dependent) diabetes mellitus before 15 years of age. *Diabetologia* 1999; 42:181–7.

70. Hamalanian A-M, Savola K, Kulmala PK, Koskela P, Akerblom HK, Knip M and the Finnish TRIGR study group. Disease-associated autoantibodies during pregnancy and at birth in families affected by type 1 diabetes. *Clin Exp Immunol* 2001; 126:231–6.

71. Koczwara K, Bonifacio E, Ziegler A-G. Transmission of maternal islet antibodies and risk of autoimmune diabetes in offspring of mothers with type 1 diabetes. *Diabetes* 2004; 53:1–4.

72. Leslie RDG, Elliott RB. Early environmental events as a cause of IDDM. Evidence and implications. *Diabetes* 1994; 43:843–50.

73. Kupila A, Keskinen P, Simell T, Erkkila S, Arvilommi P, Korhonen S, Kimpimaki T, Sjoroos M, Ronkainen M, Ilonen J, Knip M, Simell O. Genetic risk determines the emergence of diabetes-associated autoantibodies in young children. *Diabetes* 2002; 51:646–51.

74. Wong FS, Janeway CA Jr.The role of CD4 and CD8 T cells in type I diabetes in the NOD mouse. *Res Immunol* 1997; 148:327–32.

75. Roep BO. T-cell responses to autoantigens in IDDM. The search for the Holy Grail. *Diabetes* 1996; 45(9):1147–56.

76. Wilson SB, Kent SC, Patton KT, Orban T, Jackson RA, Exley M, Porcelli S, Schatz DA, Atkinson MA, Balk SP, Strominger JL, Hafler DA. Extreme Th1 bias of invariant Valpha24JalphaQ T cells in type 1 diabetes. *Nature* 1998; 391:177–81.

77. Pipeleers D, Ling Z: Pancreatic β cells in insulin-dependent diabetes. *Diabetes Metab Rev* 1992; 8:209–227.

78. Kent SC, Chen Y, Bregoli L, Clemmings SM, Kenyon NS, Ricordi C, Hering BJ, Hafler DA. Expanded T cells from pancreatic lymph nodes of type 1 diabetic subjects recognize an insulin epitope. *Nature* 2005; 435:224–8.

79. Lohmann T, Hawa M, Leslie RD, Lane R, Picard J, Londei M. Immune reactivity to glutamic acid decarboxylase 65 in stiffman syndrome and type 1 diabetes mellitus. *Lancet* 2000; 356:31–5.

80. Mauricio, D., and Mandrup-Poulsen, T. Apoptosis and the pathogenesis of IDDM: a question of life and death. *Diabetes* 1998; 47:1537–43.

81. Greenbaum CJ, Cuthbertson D, Krischer JP, Disease Prevention Trail of Type 1 Diabetes Study Group. Type I diabetes manifested solely by 2-h oral glucose tolerance test criteria. *Diabetes* 2001; 50:470–6.

82. Keskinen P, Korhonen S, Kupila A, Veijola R, Erkkila S, Savolainen H, Arvilommi P, Simell T, Ilonen J, Knip M, Simell O. First-phase insulin response in young healthy children at genetic and immunological risk for Type I diabetes. *Diabetologia* 2002; 45:1639–48.

83. The DCCT Research Group: Effects of age, duration and treatment of insulin-dependent diabetes mellitus on residual beta-cell function: observations during eligibility testing for the Diabetes Control and Complications Trial (DCCT). *J Clin Endocrinol Metab* 1987; 65:30–6.

84. Pozzilli P, Visalli N, Buzzetti R, Cavallo MG, Marietti G, Hawa M, Leslie RD. Metabolic and immune parameters at clinical onset of insulin-dependent diabetes: a population-based study. IMDIAB Study Group. *Immunotherapy Diabetes Metabolism* 1998; 47:1205–1210.

85. Hosszufalusi N, Vatay A, Rajczy K, Prohaszka Z, Pozsonyi E, Horvath L, Grosz A, Gero L, Madacsy L, Romics L, Karadi I, Fust G, Panczel P. Similar genetic features and different islet cell autoantibody pattern of latent autoimmune diabetes in adults (LADA) compared with adult-onset type 1 diabetes with rapid progression. *Diabetes Care* 2003; 26:452–7.

86. The DCCT Research Group. Effects of age, duration and treatment of insulin-dependent diabetes mellitus on residual beta-cell function: observations during eligibility testing for the Diabetes Control and Complications Trial (DCCT). *J Clin Endocrinol Metab* 1987; 65:30–6.

87. Martin S, Pawlowski B, Greulich B, Ziegler AG, Mandrup-Poulsen T, Mahon J. Natural course of remission in IDDM during 1st yr after diagnosis. *Diabetes Care* 1992; 15:66–74.

88. Hawa MI, Bonfanti R, Valeri C, Delli Castelli M, Beyan H, Leslie RD. No evidence for genetically determined alteration in insulin secretion or sensitivity predisposing to type 1 diabetes: a study of identical twins. *Diabetes Care* 2005; 28:1415–8.

89. Fourlanos S, Narendran P, Byrnes GB, Colman PG, Harrison LC. Insulin resistance is a risk factor for progression to type 1 diabetes. *Diabetologia* 2004; 47:1661–7.

90. Zinman B, Kahn SE, Haffner SM, O'Neill MC, Heise MA, Freed MI; ADOPT Study Group. Phenotypic characteristics of GAD antibody-positive recently diagnosed patients with type 2 diabetes in North America and Europe. *Diabetes* 2004; 53:3193–200.

91. Bingley PJ, Bonifacio E, Gale EA. Can we really predict IDDM? *Diabetes* 1993; 42:213–20.

92. Gorus FK. Diabetes registries and early biological markers of insulin-dependent diabetes mellitus. Belgian Diabetes Registry. *Diabetes Metab Rev* 1997; 13:247–74.

93. Fava D, Gardner S, Pyke D, Leslie RD. Evidence that the age at diagnosis of IDDM is genetically determined. *Diabetes Care* 1998; 21:925–9.

94. Bruining GJ: Association between infant growth before onset of juvenile type 1 diabetes and autoantibodies to IA-2. Netherlands Kolibrie study group of childhood diabetes. *Lancet* 2000; 356:655–6.

95. Gale EA. Spring harvest? Reflections on the rise of type 1 diabetes. *Diabetologia* 2005; 48:2445–50.

96. Bonfanti R, Bazzigaluppi E, Calori G, Riva MC, Viscardi M, Bognetti E, Meschi F, Bosi E, Chiumello G, Bonifacio E. Parameters associated with residual insulin secretion during the first year of disease in children and adolescents with Type 1 diabetes mellitus. *Diabet Med* 1998; 15:844–50.

97. Palmer JP, Fleming GA, Greenbaum CJ, Herold KC, Jansa LD, Kolb H, Lachin JM, Polonsky KS, Pozzilli P, Skyler JS, Steffes MW. C-peptide is the appropriate outcome measure for type 1 diabetes clinical trials to preserve beta-cell function: report of an ADA workshop, 21-22 October 2001. *Diabetes* 2004; 53:250–64.

98. Gottsater A, Landin-Olsson M, Fernlund P, Lernmark A, Sundkvist G. Beta-cell function in relation to islet cell antibodies during the first 3 yr after clinical diagnosis of diabetes in type II diabetic patients. *Diabetes Care* 1993; 16:902–10.

99. Carlsson A, Sundkvist G, Groop L, Tuomi T. Insulin and glucagon secretion in patients with slowly progressing autoimmune diabetes (LADA). *J Clin Endocrinol Metab* 2000; 85:76–80.

100. Behme MT, Dupre J, Harris SB, Hramiak IM, Mahon JL.Insulin resistance in latent autoimmune diabetes of adulthood. *Ann N Y Acad Sci* 2003; 1005:374–7.

101. Leslie D, Lipsky P, Notkins AL. Autoantibodies as predictors of disease. *J Clin Invest* 2001; 108:1417–22.

102. Kulmala P, Savola K, Petersen JS, Vahasalo P, Karjalainen J, Lopponen T, Dyrberg T, Akerblom HK, Knip M Prediction of insulin-dependent diabetes mellitus in siblings of children with diabetes. A population-based study. The Childhood Diabetes in Finland Study Group. *J Clin Invest* 1998; 101:327–36.

103. Diabetes Prevention Trial–Type 1 Diabetes Study Group. Effects of insulin in relatives of patients with type 1 diabetes mellitus. *N Engl J Med* 2002; 346:1685–91.

104. Knip M. Cow's milk and the new trials for prevention of type I diabetes. *J Endocrinol Invest* 2003; 26:265–7.

105. Stene LC, Barriga K, Norris JM, Hoffman M, Klingensmith G, Erlich HA, Eisenbarth GS, Rewers M. Symptoms of common maternal infections in pregnancy and risk of islet autoimmunity in early childhood. Diabetes Care 2003; 26:3136–41.

106. Paronen J, Knip M, Savilahti E, Virtanen SM, Ilonen J, Akerblom HK, Vaarala O. Effect of cow's milk exposure and maternal type 1 diabetes on cellular and humoral immunization to dietary insulin in infants at genetic risk for type 1 diabetes. Finnish Trial to Reduce IDDM in the Genetically at Risk Study Group. *Diabetes* 2000; 49:1657–65.

107. Lampeter EF, Klinghammer A, Scherbaum WA, Heinze E, Haastert B, Giani G, Kolb H. The Deutsche Nicotinamide Intervention Study: an attempt to prevent type 1 diabetes. DENIS Group. *Diabetes* 1998; 47:980–4.

108. Gale EA, Bingley PJ, Emmett CL, Collier T; European Nicotinamide Diabetes Intervention Trial (ENDIT) Group. European Nicotinamide Diabetes Intervention Trial (ENDIT): a randomised controlled trial of intervention before the onset of type 1 diabetes. *Lancet* 2004; 363:925–31.

109. Skyler JS, Krischer JP, Wolfsdorf J, Cowie C, Palmer JP, Greenbaum C, Cuthbertson D, Rafkin-Mervis LE, Chase HP, Leschek E. Effects of oral insulin in relatives of patients with type 1 diabetes: The Diabetes Prevention Trial–Type 1. *Diabetes Care* 2005; 28:1068–76.

110. Leslie RDG, Pyke DA, Denman A. Immunosoppressive therapy in diabetes. *Lancet* 1985; 1:516.

111. Feutren G, Papoz L, Assan R, Vialettes B, Karsenty G, Vexiau P, for the Cyclosporine/Diabetes French Study Group. Cyclosporine increases the rate and length of remissions in insulin dependent diabetes of recent onset: results of a multicentre double-blind trial. *Lancet* 1986; 2: 119–24.

112. Herold KC, Hagopian W, Auger JA, Poumian-Ruiz E, Taylor L, Donaldson D, Gitelman SE, Harlan DM, Xu D, Zivin RA, Bluestone JA. Anti-CD3 monoclonal antibody in new onset type 1 diabetes mellitus. *N Engl J Med* 2002; 346:1692–8.

113. Keymeulen B, Vandemeulebroucke E, Ziegler AG, Mathieu C, Kaufman L, Hale G, Gorus F, Goldman M, Walter M, Candon S, Schandene L, Crenier L, De Block C, Seigneurin JM, De Pauw P, Pierard D, Weets I, Rebello P, Bird P, Berrie E, Frewin M, Waldmann H, Bach JF, Pipeleers D, Chatenoud L. Insulin needs after CD3-antibody therapy in new-onset type 1 diabetes. *N Engl J Med* 2005; 352:2598–608.

114. Bisikirska B, Colgan J, Luban J, Bluestone JA, Herold KC.TCR stimulation with modified anti-CD3 mAb expands CD8+ T cell population and induces CD8+CD25+ Tregs. *J Clin Invest* 2005; 115:2904–13.

115. Belghith M, Bluestone JA, Barriot S, Megret J, Bach JF, Chatenoud L.TGF-beta-dependent mechanisms mediate restoration of self-tolerance induced by antibodies to CD3 in overt autoimmune diabetes. *Nat Med* 2003; 9:1202–8.

116. Elias D, Meilin A, Ablamunits V, Birk OS, Carmi P, Konen-Waisman S, Cohen IR. Hsp60 peptide therapy of NOD mouse diabetes induces a Th2 cytokine burst and down-regulates autoimmunity to various beta-cell antigens. *Diabetes* 1997; 46:758–64.

117. Raz I, Elias S, Avron A, Tamir M, Metzger M, Cohen IR. B-cells function in new onset type 1 diabetes and immunomodulation with heat-shock protein peptide (DiaPep277): a randomised, double blind phase II trail. *Lancet* 2001; 358: 1749–53.

118. Kobayashi T, Maruyama T, Shimada A, Kasuga A, Kanatsuka A, Takei I, Tanaka S, Yokoyama J. Insulin intervention to preserve beta cells in slowly progressive insulin-dependent (type 1) diabetes mellitus. *Ann N Y Acad Sci* 2002; 958:117–30.

119. Agardh CD, Cilio CM, Lethagen A, Lynch K, Leslie RD, Palmer M, Harris RA, Robertson JA, Lernmark A. Clinical evidence for the safety of GAD65 immunomodulation in adult-onset autoimmune diabetes. *J Diabetes Complications* 2005; 19:238–46.

IV   OTHER AUTOIMMUNE ENDOCRINOPATHIES

13 | Addison's Disease

Corrado Betterle, MD, Renato Zanchetta, MD, and Fabio Presotto, MD, PhD

CONTENTS

Summary

The adrenal insufficiency, also called Addison's disease (AD) in honor of the physician who first described this disease in 1855, results from the bilateral involvement of the adrenal cortex, together with a deficiency in the production of glucocorticoids, mineralocorticoids, and androgens, associated with high levels of both adrenocorticotropin hormone and plasma renin activity. The prevalence of the disease is 110–140 cases per million, and autoimmune AD represents the most frequent cause in the developed countries. In autoimmune AD, the adrenal glands are infiltrated by lymphocytes and ultimately become very small. Circulating adrenal cortex autoantibodies (ACAs) directed to a cytoplasmic autoantigen common to all the three cell layers of the adrenal cortex have been found. The adrenocortical autoantigen was identified as the 21-hydroxylase (21-OH), and now, it is possible to test 21-OH antibodies (21-OHAb) using cloned antigens. ACAs/21-OHAbs are present at diagnosis in more than 90% of the patients with autoimmune AD. The detection of ACAs/21-OHAbs in subjects without clinical AD may be a useful indicator of future development of adrenal failure. The main clinical manifestations of this disease are usually anorexia, weakness, nausea, vomiting, weight loss, low blood pressure, cutaneous and mucosal hyperpigmentation, abdominal pain, and salt craving. These clinical symptoms do not appear until approximately 90% of the adrenal cortex has been destroyed or when stress events occur, which require an increase in adrenocortical function. Autoimmune AD may be isolated or associated with other autoimmune diseases, mostly organ specific, giving rise to different forms of autoimmune polyglandular syndromes. The substitutive therapy with gluco- and mineral-corticoid for patients with chronic adrenal insufficiency is life saving.

From: *Contemporary Endocrinology: Autoimmune Diseases in Endocrinology*
Edited by: A. P. Weetman © Humana Press, Totowa, NJ

Key Words: Addison's disease, adrenal insufficiency, adrenal cortex antibodies, 21-hydroxylase autoantibodies, autoimmune diseases, autoimmune polyglandular syndromes.

INTRODUCTION

Historical Background

The adrenal glands were first described by Bartolomeo Eustachius in 1564 *(1)* as "glandulae quae renibus incumbent." In 1855, Thomas Addison (1793–1860), a physician at Guy's Hospital in London, proved that the adrenals were very important organs for survival. In his famous monograph "On the Constitutional and Local Effects of Disease of the Suprarenal Capsules," Addison originally described the signs and symptoms of a disease marked by "anemia, general languor and debility, remarkable feebleness of the heart's action, and a peculiar change of colour in the skin, occurring in connexion with a disease condition of the supra-renal capsules," calling this disorder *melasma suprarenale.* Following the post-mortem examination of 11 patients who died with a similar clinical picture, Addison reported that six patients were suffering from adrenal tuberculosis, three had adrenal malignancies, one case had had an adrenal hemorrhage, and one suffered from adrenal fibrosis of an unknown origin. This last case was probably the first description of an autoimmune form of adrenalitis. In this case, Addison reported that "the two adrenals together weighed 49 grains, they appeared exceedingly small and atrophied, so that the diseased condition did not result, as usual, from a deposit either of a strumous or malignant character, but appears to have been occasioned by an actual inflammation, that inflammation having destroyed the integrity of the organs, which finally led to their contraction and atrophy" *(2).* Subsequently, it was proved that bilateral adrenalectomy was invariably and rapidly fatal in animals "because both glands are required in order to detoxify a lethal pigment" *(3).* In 1856, Trousseau named this type of adrenal insufficiency "Addison's disease" (AD), in honour of the scientist who first described the illness *(4).*

Many years later, it was discovered that the adrenal and pituitary functions were regulated by the pituitary and the hypothalamus, respectively *(5).* From 1920 to 1930, adrenal cortical extracts were obtained from animals *(6–8),* and their use allowed for the survival of both the adrenalectomized animals and those patients with an adrenal insufficiency *(6,9).* Both corticosterone and deoxycorticosterone were synthetized in 1937 *(10,11),* and, since 1938, they have been employed in the treatment of AD in humans *(12).*

Anatomy and Physiology of the Adrenal Glands

The cortex of the adrenal glands develops from the embrional mesodermal layer, whereas the medulla arises from the neuroectodermal layer and includes part of the chromaffin system *(13).* The adrenal glands are usually located over the kidneys and their weight, in adults, ranges from 4.0 to $4.2\,g \pm 15\%$ *(14).* Histological studies of the adrenal cortex demonstrate a separation into three layers. The *zona glomerulosa* represents 5–10% of the cortex with discontinuous, subcapsular aggregates of small cells. This zone is less rich in cytoplasm than the other cortical zones and contains the enzymes that synthesize aldosterone and the other mineralocorticoids, under the control of the renin-angiotensin system. The *zona fasciculata,* which is formed by radial cords of large columned cells, with abundant lipid-filled cytoplasms covers 70%

of the cortex. It produces glucocorticoids under the influence of the adrenocorticotropin hormone (ACTH) produced by the pituitary gland. The *zona reticularis,* which amounts to about 20% of the cortex, is composed of cells arranged in cords, with compact, finely granular, eosinophilic cytoplasms, and synthesizes the adrenal androgens (such as dehydroepiandrosterone) *(15).* The adrenal blood supply derives from the three main supra-renal arteries, which pierce the gland surface, dividing into 50–60 small branches and forming a subcapsular plexus, which embraces the cell clusters in the *zona glomerulosa,* and then runs along the cellular cords in the *zona fasciculata.* The capillary branching from the arterial system forms a microvascular network around the zona reticularis, which drains into the medullary sinusoids by means of relatively few small venules, which eventually form a large central vein. This transition from the arterial to the capillary system is so sharp that it forms a sort of functional "vascular dam" *(16).* In addition, the medullary veins show an eccentric musculature, which facilitates the development of pouches of localized stasis when the bundles contract. The vein contraction is also promoted by the high catecholamine concentration at this level.

The homeostasis of the glucocorticoids is regulated by a feedback mechanism; firstly through the hypothalamus by means of a corticotropin-releasing hormone (CRH), then through the pituitary gland by means of ACTH, and last through the adrenal cortex by means of cortisol *(17).* On the contrary, the mineralocorticoids are mainly regulated by the renin-angiotensin system and by certain specific serum electrolytes (potassium and sodium).

Definition of Adrenal Insufficiency

Primary adrenocortical insufficiency, or AD, results from the bilateral involvement of the adrenal cortex, together with a deficiency in the production of glucocorticoids, mineralocorticoids, and androgens, associated with high levels of both ACTH and plasma renin activity (PRA). Secondary adrenocortical insufficiency results from a deficiency in pituitary ACTH secretion, with a secondary insufficiency concerning adrenal cortisol incretion. Tertiary adrenocortical insufficiency results from a reduced or absent secretion of the hypothalamic CRH causing pituitary ACTH deficiency and thus a low glucocorticoid production rate. In contrast to cases of AD, the production of mineralocorticoids is generally normal when an insufficiency of the hypothalamic–hypophyseal axis occurs *(18).*

EPIDEMIOLOGY

Prevalence of AD

In the developed countries, autoimmune AD is now the most frequent form of primary adrenal failure and tuberculosis is the second. In our personal series of 434 patients with AD, the autoimmune form was diagnosed in 353 (81%) patients, the tuberculous in 51 (12%) patients, and the other causes were uncommon and cumulatively accounting for 7% of all the cases (Fig. 1).

In the past, tuberculosis was the most common cause of primary AD worldwide. Of the 11 cases originally described by Thomas Addison, 55% had tuberculosis and only 9% had "idiopathic" or autoimmune AD *(2).* In 1930, Guttman examined 566 autopsied patients with AD and found that 70% of them had tuberculous adrenalitis,

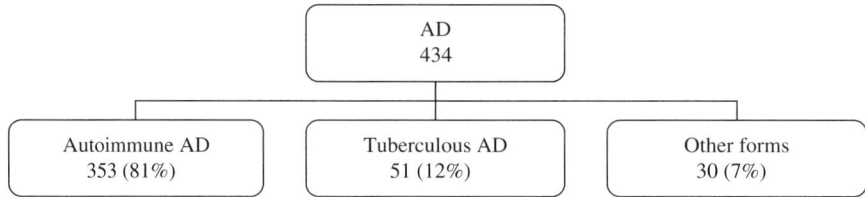

Fig. 1. Causes of Addison's disease (AD) in our personal series.

whereas only 17% showed signs of "idiopathic" adrenal atrophy *(19)*. Similar results on the frequency of tuberculosis (79%) were reported by Dunlop in 1963, who reviewed 86 cases of AD *(20)*. In 1968, in England *(21)*, and in 1974, in Denmark *(22)*, the prevalences of tuberculous AD were reported to be 31 and 17%, respectively. Major and minor causes responsible for the occurrence of AD are summarized in the Table 1.

As far as primary AD is concerned, the prevalence in the general population is undoubtedly low. However, despite the constant decrease in the tuberculous form over the last decades, a parallel increase in the prevalence of AD has been observed, probably because of a subsequent rise in cases of the autoimmune AD *(23)*.

In Europe, it is believed that AD affected 40–70 cases per million of inhabitants during the 1970s *(21,22)*. However, in recent years, the prevalence has been estimated to be 93–140 cases per million *(24–27)*, with an incidence of six new cases per million per year *(27)*. The prevalence of the disease also varies with regard to different geographical areas as, for example, 4.5 cases per million were found in New Zealand *(28)*, 5 in Japan *(29)*, about 50 in the United States *(30)*, and 93–140 in Europe *(26–27)*.

Another uncommon autoimmune-related form of AD is observed in the antiphospholipid syndrome *(31)*, which accounts for less than 0.5% of all the causes of AD (personal data).

IMMUNOPATHOGENESIS OF AUTOIMMUNE AD

Histopathology

In cases of autoimmune adrenalitis, both the adrenal glands are very small, weighing only 1 g, and it is difficult to locate them at autopsy. The capsule is thickened, and the cortex is usually completely destroyed. The remaining adrenocortical cells, disposed in small clusters, are enlarged, with pleomorphism and eosinophilia. A mononuclear cell infiltration is present and is characterized by the presence of lymphocytes, plasma cells, macrophages, and sporadic germinal centers. In general, the remaining cells are surrounded by the heaviest infiltration of lymphocytes, with varying amounts of fibrosis, whereas the adrenal medulla is usually preserved. Most of the cells infiltrating the adrenal cortex are T cells, with a CD4/CD8 ratio of 5–6/1. There is only 5% of B-cells. Almost half of them are positive for class II human leukocyte antigen (HLA) *(14)*. These histological pictures are similar to the histological changes commonly reported in other endocrine autoimmune diseases, such as thyroiditis or insulitis *(32,33)*.

In addition to activated lymphocytes, HLA class II molecules have also been found to be aberrantly expressed on adrenal cells under normal conditions *(34)*. However, an increased expression of these molecules has been reported on adrenocortical cells in autoimmune AD *(35)*, as already demostrated on thyrocytes in autoimmune

Table 1
Causes of Addison's Disease (AD)

	Autoimmune AD	Tubercular infection	Other infections	Primary or secondary cancers	Infiltrative disorders	Adrenal hemorrhage or thrombosis	Bilateral adrenalectomy	Drugs	Genetics
Etiology	Unknown	Mycobacterium tuberculosis	Histoplasmosis Coccidioidomycosis Blastomycosis Cryptococcosis Syphylis Cytomegalovirosis HIV	Adrenal carcinoma Lymphoma Cancers of the •Breast •Lung •Kidney •Stomach •Colon Melanoma	Amyloidosis Hemochromatosis Hemosiderosis Histiocytosis X Sarcoidosis (?) Niemann-Pick disease Wolman disease	Anticoagulant therapy Antiphospholipid syndrome Traumas Systemic lupus erythematosus Panarteritis nodosa	Cushing's syndrome	Fluconazole Ketoconazole Mitotane Aminoglutethimide Metopyrone	Enzymatic defects Adrenoleukodystrophy
Prevalence	75–80%	15–20%	1%	1%	1%	<1%	1%	1%	1%

(?) is unclear if sarcoidosis can induce AD.

thyroiditis *(36,37)*. HLA class II molecules were initially believed to be expressed only on antigen-presenting cells (APC) and the capillary endothelium, and they play an important role in the regulation of the immune reponse by the CD4$^+$ lymphocytes. Therefore, their presence on endocrine cells might constitute a prerequisite for the successful presentation of the self-antigens to the CD4$^+$ cells and for the activation of autoreactive T lymphocytes.

Cellular Immunity

Both the experimental and the clinical findings indicate that a cell-mediated autoimmune response may be the pathogenic mechanism, leading to glandular destruction in autoimmune AD, as is true of many other organ-specific autoimmune diseases *(38–40)*. Early studies, which employed a migration inhibitory factor assay or a skin delayed-type hypersensitivity test by intracutaneous injection of adrenal extracts *(41,42)*, demonstrated the involvement of cell-mediated immunity in affected patients. In the following years, a decrease in T-cell suppressor function was reported *(43)*, together with an increased percentage of activated T lymphocytes expressing HLA-DR (class II) molecule *(44)*. Moreover, an enhanced proliferative T-cell response to an adrenal-specific protein fraction of 18–24 kDa molecular weight has been described *(39)*. A defective suppressor function of the human CD4$^+$/CD25$^+$ regulatory T cells has recently been demonstrated in patients with autoimmune AD in the context of an autoimmune polyglandular syndrome (APS) type 2 but not in patients with isolated autoimmune AD *(45)*. Taken together, all these data strongly support the hypothesis that (abnormalities in) T lymphocytes assume a key role in the developement of autoimmune AD.

Over the last decade, great attention has been paid to the chemokines, which are a large group of cytokines involved in the pathogenesis of both inflammatory and autoimmune diseases *(46,47)*. In several endocrine autoimmune diseases, including AD, the CXC chemokine ligand-10 (CXCL10) has been identified as playing an important role in regulating the recruitment of specific subsets of activated lymphocytes *(46–48)* (*see* Pathogenesis of Autoimmune AD).

Animal Models

An experimentally induced adrenalitis was initially reported in guinea pigs and rabbits, but circulating antibodies to the adrenal cortex were detected only in rabbits *(49–53)*.

In 1968, an adrenalitis characterized by an infiltration of the adrenal cortex by mononuclear cells was induced in rats by means of the injection of adrenal extracts *(54,55)*. These animals also revealed the presence of circulating antibodies against adrenal tissue and eventually developed adrenal cortex insufficiency *(55)*. In the same year, a passive transfer of the so-called "allergic adrenalitis" was induced by lymphoid cells in rats *(56)*. Using the same murine model, in 1992 it was confirmed that repeated immunizations with adrenal extracts results in adrenalitis; it was also demonstrated that the disease can be passively transferred only by spleen cells in syngenic animals *(38)*. These data provide additional evidence of the autoimmune nature of adrenalitis and contribute to its classification in the group of cell-mediated immune diseases.

A spontaneous type of autoimmune AD was also reported in dogs *(57–62)* and in cats *(58,63–65)*, but the presence of adrenal cortex autoantibodies (ACAs) was never described in these animals. Finally, non-obese diabetic (NOD) mice that develop type 1 diabetes mellitus can also present a mononuclear cell infiltrate in the adrenal cortex, in the absence of overt signs of hypoadrenalism. The NOD mice, indeed, have been proposed as a spontaneous model of autoimmune polyendocrine syndrome *(66)*.

Humoral Immunity

THE ADRENAL CORTEX AUTOANTIBODIES

In 1957, Anderson *(67)*, using a conventional complement fixation test with adrenal cortex extracts, first demonstrated the presence of circulating adrenal cortex antibodies (ACAs) in 25% of the patients with "idiopathic" AD. Employing this method, from 1957 to 1970, ACAs were detected in 36% of the patients with autoimmune AD but also in 9% of those with tuberculous AD as reviewed by Betterle *(68)*. In 1963, Blizzard *(69)*, using the classical indirect immunofluorescence technique on animal adrenal sections, demonstrated that the ACAs are present in 51% of patients with autoimmune AD. These antibodies are organ-specific and directed to the cytoplasmic (microsomal) autoantigen(s) common to all three cell layers of the adrenal cortex *(69–71)*. ACAs have also been found to react against the surface of the adrenocortical cells in culture, thus indicating that the microsomal antigen(s) may also be expressed on the cytoplasm membrane of these cells *(72)*.

The mean prevalence of ACAs in various studies performed from 1963 to 2002 by means of indirect immunofluorecence was 61% in patients with autoimmune AD and 6.7% in those with tuberculous AD *(68)*.

THE 21-HYDROXYLASE AUTOANTIBODIES

In 1992, the shared adrenocortical autoantigen was identified as the 21-hydroxylase (21-OH) *(73–75)* (*see* "Adrenal Autoantigens"). After this discovery, an immunopre-cipitation assay using 21-OH labeled with ^{35}S-methionine was developed in 1995 to detect 21-OH antibodies (21-OHAbs) *(76–78)*. Two years later, for detecting these antibodies, a more convenient type of assay was employed, using recombinant human ^{125}I-labelled 21-OH plus the precipitation of the immunocomplexes by a solid-phase protein A *(79)*. These methods improved both the sensitivity and specificity of the autoantibody testing in patients affected by AD. Studies carried out on patients with autoimmune AD demonstrated a positive test for 21-OHAbs in 78% of the cases and only in 1.9% of the patients with tuberculous AD *(68)*.

THE STEROID PRODUCING CELL AUTOANTIBODIES AND ANTIBODIES TO BOTH 17α-HYDROXYLASE (17α-OHABS) AND TO P450 SIDE CHAIN CLEAVAGE (P450SCCABS)

Anderson first reported in 1968 the presence of steroid-producing cell autoanti-bodies (StCAs) in males affected by autoimmune AD but without gonadal failure *(80)*. Subsequently, these autoantibodies were found in almost all the females affected by autoimmune AD associated to premature ovarian failure (POF) with normal karyotype and lymphocytic infiltration of the ovaries (so-called lymphocytic oophoritis) *(71–81)*. These antibodies are rare in males with autoimmune AD and impaired testicular function *(81)*. Conversely, the majority of the patients with a POF and a recognized lymphocytic oophoritis at biopsy was found to be positive for StCAs and, in general, was also affected by adrenal autoimmunity *(81)*. In the search for the detection of the relevant autoantigens in autoimmune AD, some authors identified 17α-hydroxylase (17α-OH) and p450 side chain cleavage enzyme (p450scc) as autoantigens, but this was seen only in the sera of the patients with autoimmune AD in the context of the APS type 1 *(75,82–84)*. Following this discovery, these antigens were cloned, and an immunoprecipitation assay was performed to identify 17α-OHAbs or P450sccAbs *(78)*.

The 17α-OHAbs or P450sccAbs may be present in autoimmune AD and are usually associated to primary gonadal failure positive for StCAs *(81,85)*. These antibodies can sometimes be found in patients with adrenal autoimmunity in the absence of gonadal failure, and in these cases, they may be predictors of future progression to hypergonadotropic hypogonadism *(86,87)*.

AUTOANTIBODIES TO HYDROCORTISONE

The presence of autoantibodies to hormones (e.g., thyroglobulin, triiodothyronine, thyroxine, and insulin) are usually a hallmark of the relevant organ-specific autoimmune diseases *(88)*. Autoantibodies to hydrocortisone have also been described, but these antibodies have never been reported in patients with autoimmune AD but only in those with an Addison's-like syndrome during the course of AIDS *(89)*.

AUTOANTIBODIES TO THE ACTH RECEPTOR

Autoantibodies of immunoglobulin (Ig)G class capable of blocking the ACTH receptor were first described in a patient suffering from autoimmune AD in the context of APS type 1 by using cultured guinea pig adrenal cells *(90)*. This ACTH receptor-blocking activity was then described in 90% of patients with autoimmune AD and in 22% of non-autoimmune adrenal disorders using guinea pig adrenal segments *(91)*. However, this blocking activity was subsequently attributed to non-IgG components present in the bioassay *(92)*.

ANTIPHOSPHOLIPID ANTIBODIES

The immunologic hallmark of AD in the rare antiphospholipid syndrome is the presence of circulating antiphospholipid antibodies (APA), which are a group of auto-antibodies directed against different phospholipids and phospholipid-associated plasma proteins that have been associated with a hypercoagulability state *(56)*.

OTHER AUTOANTIBODIES

Other autoimmune diseases may precede, accompany, or follow the autoimmune AD, and they are usually marked by the presence of the relevant autoantibodies, thus originating different forms of APS. When autoimmune AD occurs as an isolated form, an autoantibody screening (i.e., to thyroid, gastric parietal cells, islet cells, transglutaminase, and so on) is advisable to detect subclinical or latent forms of APS *(93)*.

Adrenal Autoantigens

An important goal of autoimmunity is the identification of the specific autoantigen(s) responsible for the production of autoantibodies. As regards autoimmunity to the adrenal glands, a specific 55-kDa protein obtained from human adrenal microsomes reacting with ACAs was originally described by a group of researchers in Cardiff in 1988 *(94)*. Subsequently, two independent laboratories demonstrated that the 21-OH was the major autoantigen of adrenocortical cells *(73–75)*. This observation was confirmed by means of specific absorption studies with purified human 21-OH, which made use of sera from patients affected by autoimmune AD *(95)*. 21-OH is an adrenal-specific enzyme, formed by a single chain of 494 amino acids, belonging to the cytochrome p450 family of 55 kDa. It is located within a membrane of smooth endoplasmic reticulum and has a key role in the synthesis of steroid hormones because it catalyzes the conversion of progesterone and of 17-hydroxyprogesterone into deoxy-corticosterone and 11-deoxycortisol, respectively. Two genes (*CYP21A* and *CYP21B*) located on the short arm of chromosome 6 in the HLA class III region are involved in the synthesis of this enzyme, but only *CYP21B* is active *(96,97)*.

The domains responsible for targeting and anchoring the molecule to the membrane are situated at the N-terminal fragment of the protein. The domains responsible for the binding sites of substrates associated with 21-OH enzyme activity are located at the C-terminal fragment of the molecule. Studies on 21-OH containing N-terminal, internal, and C-terminal amino acid sequence deletions indicated that both the central and the C-terminal regions of the 21-OH sequence (amino acids 241–494) are important with regard to autoantibody binding *(98–100)* and that these epitopes do not vary in patients with different forms of autoimmune AD *(101)*.

As previously mentioned, some authors identified the 17α-OH and p450scc as an autoantigen in the sera of patients with autoimmune AD in the context of the APS type 1 and not in the other forms of autoimmune AD *(75,82–84)*.

Different Clinical Forms of Autoimune AD

Autoimmune AD may be associated with multiple endocrine insufficiencies or with other autoimmune diseases *(93)*. Additional autoimmune and non-autoimmune diseases have also been observed in first-degree relatives of affected patients. APSs were first classified by Neufeld and Blizzard *(102,103)* and recently revised by Betterle *(93,104)*.

This classification includes four types of APS (Table 2). According to this classification, autoimmune AD can represent one of the major components in the APS type 1, type 2, and type 4. The main clinical forms of autoimmune AD are summarized in the Table 3. In our personal series of 353 patients with autoimmune AD, the frequency of the four different clinical forms is shown in Fig. 2.

Genetic and Environmental Factors

The genetic profile reported in autoimmune AD greatly varies on the basis of the clinical form (Table 3). APS type 1 is associated with mutations in the AutoImmune REgulator (AIRE) gene, which is located on the chromosome 21q22 *(105,106)*. Until 2004, 48 separate mutations associated with APS type 1 have been identified in the AIRE gene *(107)*. The association with HLA-DR5 alleles suggested in Persian Jews and in Italian patients with APS type 1 *(108,109)* needs to be confirmed.

On the contrary, a link with class II HLA genes present in the chromosome 6 was demonstrated in the other forms of autoimmune AD. In particular, an increased frequency of HLA-DR3 and/or DR4 has been found in patients with APS type 2 *(104)*,

Table 2
Classification of the Autoimmune Polyglandular Syndromes (APS)

APS type 1	Chronic candidiasis + chronic hypoparathyroidism + autoimmune Addison's disease (AD)
APS type 2	Autoimmune AD + thyroid autoimmune diseases and/or type 1 diabetes mellitus
APS type 3	Thyroid autoimmune diseases + other autoimmune diseases (excluding autoimmune AD)
APS type 4	Combinations of two or more autoimmune diseases not falling into the above categories

Table 3
The Four Different Clinical Forms of Autoimmune Addison's Disease (AD)

	APS type 1	*APS type 2*	*APS type 4*	*Isolated AD*
Features				
Age at onset of autoimmune AD	~13 years	~36 years	~36 years	~30 years
F/M ratio	F ≥ M	F > M	F > M	M > F
Clinical associations				
Hypoparathyroidism and/or candidiasis	Required	Absent	Absent	Absent
TAD and/or type 1 diabetes	Rare	Required	Absent	Absent
Other diseases (hypergonadotropic hypogonadism, vitiligo, alopecia, atrophic gastritis, pernicious anemia, celiac disease, myasthenia gravis, and so on)	Frequent	Rare	Required	Absent
Ectodermal dystrophy	Yes	Absent	Absent	Absent
Genetic association				
Mutations in the *AIRE* gene	Yes	Absent	Absent	Absent
HLA-DR	DR5 (?)	DR3 and/or DR4	?	DR3
Autoimmunity				
ACAs and/or 21-OHAbs at the onset of AD	>90%	>90%	>90%	~80%
StCAs and/or 17α-OHAbs and/or P450sccAbs	Frequent	Rare	Rare	Rare
Hystopathologic findings				
Lymphocytic adrenalitis	Yes	Yes	Yes	Yes
Adrenal atrophy	Yes	Yes	Yes	Yes
CT or NMR imaging				
Normal or small glands	Yes	Yes	Yes	Yes

ACAs, adrenal cortex autoantibodies; AIRE, autoimmune regulator; APS, autoimmune polyglandular syndrome; CT, computerized tomography; HLA, human leukocyte antigen; NMR, nuclear magnetic resonance; StCAs, steroid-producing cell autoantibodies; TAD, thyroid autoimmune disease; 21-OHAbs, 21-hydroxylase autoantibodies; ?, undefined.

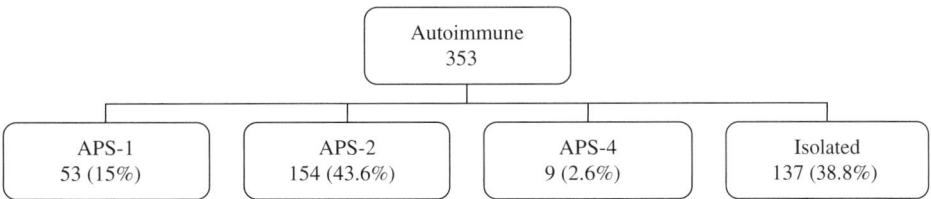

Fig. 2. Subtypes of autoimmune AD in our personal series.

whereas an increased frequency of HLA-DR3 was found in patients with isolated autoimmune AD *(93)*. Regarding the patients with autoimmune AD in the context APS type 4, only a few cases have been studied, and data are not evaluable.

A microsatellite polymorphism of the cytotoxic T-lymphocyte-associated antigen (CTLA)-4 gene can be associated with autoimmune AD, but this was observed only in English and Norwegian patients with isolated autoimmune AD or APS type 2 *(110,111)*.

Although it has long been postulated that infectious processes may underlie or precede autoimmune diseases, these factors have never been demonstrated in the case of autoimmune AD. Therefore, the involvement of environmental factors and their potential role in the natural history of autoimmune AD still remains unknown.

THE NATURAL HISTORY OF AUTOIMMUNE AD

ACAs/21-OHAbs in Euadrenal Subjects

The frequency of ACAs/21-OHAbs in patients without clinical autoimmune AD may vary greatly according to the population studied. Among the 31,379 subjects cumulatively investigated in the literature from 1957 to 2003, only 430 (1.4%) were found to be positive, as reviewed by Betterle *(112)* (Table 4).

Importantly, the highest frequency of these antibodies was shown in patients with hypoparathyroidism and/or POF, where they were detectable in 15–30 and 10% of the respective cases *(87,113–116)*. ACAs and/or 21-OHAbs, detected in subjects without clinical autoimmune AD, may be useful indicators of future development to adrenal failure. Their potential predictive role has been reported since 1963, when was described the first patient, already affected by chronic thyroiditis with both thyroid and ACAs, who developed clinical autoimmune AD several months later *(117)*. Subsequently, Blizzard revealed that 4 of 27 patients with idiopathic hypoparathyroidism were found

Table 4
Frequency of Adrenal Cortex Autoantibodies in Different Cohorts of Subjects without Clinical Addison's Disease

	Number tested	Number positive	Percent	Range (%)
Autoimmune patients	23,480	333	1.4	0–15
Hospitalized patients	1,273	53	4.1	0–5.3
First degree relatives	138	7	5.0	0–8
Healthy controls	6,488	37	0.6	0.09–1.6
All cases	31,379	430	1.4	

to be positive for ACAs and that one of them had a reduced 17-hydroxycorticosteroid response to ACTH *(113)*.

Two studies performed on patients with type 1 diabetes or hospitalized patients with ACAs did not report a progression to the overt disease *(28,118)*. However, in 1982, Scherbaum followed a group of 30 ACAs-positive patients with organ-specific autoimmunity and identified five who had had or had developed a biochemical/subclinical adrenal failure and were then treated with substitutive therapy *(119)*. One year later, we identified four subjects with complement-fixing IgG ACAs, among nine initially euadrenal patients with organ-specific autoimmunity, who developed clinically overt autoimmune AD over 1–31 months of follow-up *(120)*.

Table 5 summarizes the studies performed between 1980 and 2004 to investigate the rate of progression toward clinical AD. Cumulatively, 275 ACAs/21-OHAbs-positive patients were enrolled and 72 of them (28%) developed clinical autoimmune AD. These studies revealed a great variability in the predictive value, which ranged from 0 to 90%, depending on the duration of the follow-up, the age of the patients, the adrenal function at entry the study, the titer of the antibodies, the genetic status, and the pre-existing diseases *(86,114,115,124,125,127)*. A seroconversion for 21-OHAbs has recently been demonstrated in patients with hepatitis C virus (HCV) chronic hepatitis undergoing interferon therapy, but none of them developed clinical autoimmune AD so far *(126)*.

Laboratory Investigations in Euadrenal Subjects with ACAs

In ACAs/21-OHAbs-positive subjects, the best way of evaluating adrenal function is the measurement of the basal plasma levels of ACTH, cortisol, aldosterone, and PRA, followed by the detection of cortisol levels after 60 min from the i.v. injection of high doses (250 μg) of synthetic ACTH (Synacthen®) *(114,115,121,122)*. Using this stimulation test, it is possible to recognize five different stages of adrenal impairment.

Stage 0, also defined as *potential AD*, is characterized only by the positivity for ACAs and/or 21-OHAbs because all of the biochemical parameters are normal. Stage 1, also defined as *subclinical AD*, is indicated by an increase in PRA associated to normal or low levels of aldosterone. Stage 2 is denoted by normal levels of ACTH, cortisol levels in the normal range, and a low cortisol response to ACTH. Stage 3 is marked by an increase in ACTH with low levels of cortisol without response to ACTH. At this stage, overt clinical manifestations are usually absent; skin hyperpigmentation may occur but only many months after the increase in ACTH levels. Finally, Stage 4 is signed by very high levels of ACTH with low levels of cortisol and by the presence of the classical clinical features of the disease (Table 6).

These observations on the natural history in the development of autoimmune AD suggest that the first layer affected by the immune-mediated destruction is usually the mineralocorticoid compartment. This is possibly because of the *zona glomerulosa* is thinner compared with the other layers or, alternatively, is more vulnerable to the autoimmune assault advancing with blood flow. By contrast, the *zona fasciculata* seems to be more resistant because it is thicker or because it protects itself from the autoimmune attack by producing cortisone.

During the subclinical phases of autoimmune AD, any kind of stressful event (i.e., physical traumas, infections, surgery, and pregnancy) requires an increase in cortisol secretion, which may induce the onset of adrenocortical failure. Recently, assuming

Table 5
Follow-Up Studies of ACAs/21-OHAbs-Positive Patients

Authors	Number of patients	Gender (M/F)	Age (year range)	Population studied	Months of follow-up (range)	No. progressed to AD	Predictive value of AD (%)	Annual incidence of AD (%)
Riley (1980) (118)	6	n.d.	11–27	Type 1 DM	24	0	0	n.d.
Eason (1982) (28)	20	3M/17F	1–76	HP	32 (4–76)	0	0	n.d.
Scherbaum (1982) (119)	30	n.d.	n.d.	OSAD	12–42	0[a]	0	n.d.
Betterle (1983) (120)	9	4M/5F	6–64	OSAD	42	4	44	n.d.
Ahonen (1987) (86)	31	8M/23F	2–33.8	CHP	100 (14–145)	23	74	n.d.
Betterle (1988) (121)	17	5M/12F	6–65	OSAD	38 (6–120)	7	41	19
De Bellis (1993) (122)	20	3M/17F	11–32	OSAD	60	2	10	n.d.
Betterle (1997a) (114)	48	3M/45F	17–69	APS-2	50 (3–163)	10	21	4.9
Betterle (1997b) (115)	10	5M/5F	5–12	APS-1	31 (3–121)	9	90	34.6
Peterson (1997) (123)	7	2M/5F	7–15	Type 1 DM	48	0	0	n.d.
Laureti (1998) (124)	19	5M/12F	18–44	OSAD	12–60	8	42	n.d.
Yu (1999) (125)	15	n.d.	8–40	Type 1 DM	0–36	3	20	n.d.
Wesche (2001) (126)	4	n.d.	47	HCV-CH	24–48	0	0	n.d.
Barker (2004) (127)	39	n.d.	n.d.	Type 1 DM	31	6	19	n.d.
All cases	275					72	28 (range 0–90)	

n.d., not defined; DM, diabetes mellitus; HP, hospitalized patients; CHP, chronic hypoparathyroidism; OSAD, organ-specific autoimmune diseases; APS, autoimmune polyglandular syndrome; HCV-CH, chronic hepatitis. Modified from Betterle et al. (112) with permission from Elsevier.
[a]Five patients developed "biochemical" adrenal failure and started substitutive therapy.

Table 6
Adrenal Cortex Function in ACAs/21-OHAbs-Positive Patients Under ACTH-Test

Phases of Addison's disease	Stages	Basal PRA	Basal aldosterone	Basal ACTH	Basal cortisol	Cortisol response	Signs or symptoms
Potential	0	Normal	Normal	Normal	Normal	Normal	Absent
Subclinical	1	High	Normal[a] or Low	Normal	Normal	Normal	Absent
Subclinical	2	High	Low	Normal	Normal	Low	Absent
Subclinical	3	High	Low	High	Normal[a] or Low	Absent	Absent
Clinical	4	High	Low	Very high	Very Low	Absent	Present

ACAs, adrenal cortex autoantibodies; ACTH, adrenocorticotropin hormone; 21-OHAbs, 21-hydroxylase autoantibodies; PRA, plasma renin activity.
[a]In the lower limits of the normal range.

that the conventional high-dose ACTH test might have inadequate sensitivity, a low-dose ACTH test (1 μg) has been proposed. However, the low-dose test did not show any difference in the cortisol response with respect to the response obtained using high doses neither in normal controls nor in patients with ACAs/21-OHAbs *(128)*. Therefore, the two tests may be considered equivalent.

Is the Progression to Clinical AD Inevitable?

Studies have reported a great variability in the advancement towards the overt form of the disease in ACAs-positive subjects. In general, subjects who develop AD pass through all stages of subclinical adrenal failure, and only those in Stage 1 can spontaneously restore the adrenal function. De Bellis et al. *(122)* demonstrated that some patients in Stage 2 of adrenal impairment may recover from their subclinical adrenocortical failure as well and also become negative for ACAs, either spontaneously or after treatment with high doses of corticosteroids (carried out for a concurrent Graves' ophthalmopathy). Subsequently, the same authors reported that, in one case, the remission of the adrenal impairment continued after 100 months of follow-up *(129)*. These studies suggest that in theory, it is, possible to intervene in the natural history of autoimmune AD.

To define whether the risk of developing autoimmune AD can be estimated, we followed a group of 100 Italian subjects with ACAs for a maximum of 20 years. During the follow-up, 14 of the 20 children and 17 of the 80 adults developed clinical AD after a mean period of 3 years (range 3 to 121 months). The cumulative risk of developing the disease was 48.5% (95% confidence intervals, 40.8–56.1) (personal observations). The occurrence of autoimmune AD was found to be independently associated with male gender, presence of chronic hypoparathyroidism and/or mucocutaneous candidiasis, abnormal adrenal function at entry, and high titers of adrenal cortex antibodies. On the basis on these findings, a risk stratification model of progression to hypoadrenalism has been developed in euadrenal subjects with ACAs. In those patients assigned to be at high risk, the adrenal function should be performed most frequently to prevent a life-threatening adrenal crisis by starting early substitutive therapy *(130)*.

PATHOGENESIS OF AUTOIMMUNE AD

Autoimmune AD is related to a combination of endogenous (genetic) and probably to environmental factors capable of inducing a rupture in the immune tolerance and of initiating an autoimmune attack to the adrenal cortex, as has already been speculated concerning other autoimmune diseases *(131)*. The mechanisms by which the adrenal cortex is destroyed remain unclear. The autoantigens that are principally targeted are the p450 cytochrome enzymes involved in steroid synthesis (21-OH, 17α-hydroxylase, and the cholesterol side chain cleaving enzyme), are intracellular, and are located in the endoplasmic reticulum. It can be inferred that immune sensitisation to these autoantigens does not take place because the immunoglobulins are unable to cross the plasma membranes. Thus, the presence of the autoantibodies to these antigens might only be the consequence of adrenal destruction induced by other factors. However, endoplasmic adrenal antigens have also been found to be present on the surface of the plasma membrane of the adrenal cells *(72)*. Therefore, the antibodies may be directly involved in the adrenocortical damage, either by activating the cytolytic complement cascade or by triggering an antibody-dependent cell-mediated cytotoxicity. This hypothesis is supported by the fact that the sera from patients with autoimmune AD can produce a cytotoxic effect by means of complement activation on steroid cell cultures *(132)*.

We found that the ACAs with complement-fixing properties, especially those which activate the complement pathway up to the membrane attack through the C_5–C_9 lytic complex, are strongly associated with the development of autoimmune AD *(120)*. Similar data were also reported regarding the presence of islet cell antibodies in the preclinical or subclinical phases of type 1 diabetes mellitus *(133,134)*. Moreover, it was found that the IgG taken from patients with autoimmune AD who are positive for 21-OHAbs inhibits the activity of 21-OH, in vitro *(135)*. However, this effect was not confirmed in patients with ACAs/21-OHAbs, because their levels of 17-OH-progesterone are not increased, as usually observed in patients with congenital 21-OH deficiency *(136)*. Moreover, the passive transfer from an Addisonian mother to the fetus of ACAs/21-OHAbs of IgG class during pregnancy does not lead to any form of adrenal insufficiency in the newborn, suggesting that these antibodies are not pathogenic in vivo *(137)*. Finally, blocking antibodies that bind to the ACTH receptor might have a pathogenic effect concerning the impairment of the adrenal function, but their existence has never been definitively demonstrated.

In the antiphospholipid syndrome, the anti-phospholipid autoantibodies may play an indirect role leading to hypoadrenalism by inducing thrombosis of the adrenal veins and consequent development of hemorrhagic infarction, which is favored by the peculiar pattern of the adrenal vascular anatomy *(138,139)*.

Concerning cell-mediated immunity, it has been postulated that the aberrant expression of HLA-DR by adenocortical cells may critically be involved in the pathogenesis of autoimmune adrenalitis. Aberrant HLA class II antigen expression could be the effect of the interferon (IFN)-γ produced by the activated T cells as a result of a prior infection. This enhanced expression of the HLA-DR molecules would, in turn, induce the T lymphocytes to react against the putative autoantigen(s) *(36,37)*. However, the consequence of T-cell activation with HLA on the target (adrenal cells) will depend on the costimulation with other membrane proteins. In the absence of a positive costimulatory signal, the binding of the autoantigen with the T-cell receptor on CD4+ lymphocytes remains ineffective. This positive costimulatory signal is provided mainly by the interaction of CD28 with its B7 ligands on APC, while CTLA-4, which binds to the same B7 ligands, delivers inhibitory signals to T-cell activation and expansion (*see* next page). Therefore, the competition between CD28 and CTLA-4 expressed on the surface membrane by T lymphocytes for the B7-binding sites will modulate the autoimmune responses. Although it has long been postulated that infectious processes may underlie or precede autoimmune diseases, these factors have never been demonstrated in the case of autoimmune AD.

Over the last years, the role of the chemokines, a family of cytokines, which directs the normal leukocyte migration and are involved in the signaling of leukocyte development, has been taken into consideration concerning adrenal autoimmunity *(47)*. A significant increase in serum levels of the CXCL10 has been found in patients with autoimmune AD compared with either non-autoimmune AD or healthy subjects *(48)*. It has also been demonstrated that the human *zona fasciculata* cells are capable of producing CXCL10, in vitro, under IFN-γ and TNF-α stimulation *(48)*. For this reason, the presence of activated T cells producing IFN-γ may favor the CXCL10 secretion and, thus, the adrenocortical leukocyte infiltration. Interestingly, either hydro-cortisone or ACTH significantly inhibited cytokine-induced CXCL10 secretion by the human *zona fasciculata* cells *(48)*. This may explain why the involvement of the *zona fasciculata* is subsequent to that of the *zona glomerulosa* regarding the sequence of adrenocortical failure (*see* Laboratory Investigation).

The direct role of the T lymphocytes in the pathogenesis of autoimmune diseases has long been indicated, and CTLA-4, a cell surface receptor molecule expressed on the activated T cell, seems to be crucially involved in the case of endocrine autoimmunity *(140)*. It has been demonstrated that CTLA-4 receptor can intervene by controlling T-cell proliferation, by mediating T-cell apoptosis and by down-regulating T-cell activation *(141)*. Together with CD28, another costimulatory molecule expressed on both resting and activated T cells which mediates T-cell stimulation, CTLA-4 competes with the same ligands B7.1 (CD80) and B7.2 (CD86) on APC and is therefore critical in maintaining the immunologic homeostasis. As defects in T-cell regulation are believed to underlie the pathophysiology of endocrine autoimmunity and defects in apoptosis have been associated with autoimmune diseases *(142)*, it is likely that faulty CTLA-4 expression or activity may confer susceptibility to autoimmunity. Mice that have been engineered to lack the CTLA-4 receptor develop a lethal lymphopro-liferative disease, which is characterized by massive T-lymphocyte infiltration and a multiorgan tissue destruction, which includes the heart, the pancreas, the spleen, and other tissues *(143)*. In this context, it has been found that a microsatellite polymorphism of the CTLA-4 gene can be associated with the development of AD *(110)*.

Recently, three novel costimulatory molecules have also been identified: inducible costimulator (ICOS) providing positive and programmed death (PD)-1 and B- and T-lymphocyte attenuator (BTLA) delivering negative costimulatory signals *(144,145)*, but their role in regulating autoimmunity remains to be elucidated.

Further studies will provide more evidence of how autoantigen expression, as well as immune disregulation, contributes to the development of autoimmune AD.

DIAGNOSIS OF AUTOIMMUNE AD

Clinical Manifestations

Autoimmune AD shows, in general, a long preclinical or clinically silent period marked by the presence of ACAs. The clinical symptoms and signs do not appear until 90%, or more, of the adrenal cortex has been destroyed, but obviously, they depend on the speed of the adrenal cortex destruction and, also, on superimposed stress events.

The main clinical manifestations are usually anorexia, general malaise, weakness, nausea, vomiting, weight loss, low blood pressure with syncope, cutaneous and mucosal hyperpigmentation, abdominal pain, salt craving, and diarrhea *(146)*. Moreover, in patients with autoimmune AD, the clinical manifestations of the other autoimmune diseases (vitiligo, alopecia, type 1 diabetes mellitus, hypogonadism, thyroid dysfunction, malabsorption, and so on) can precede, accompany, or follow the adrenal insufficiency.

Immunologic and Biochemical Tests

At the diagnosis, the vast majority of the patients with autoimmune AD are ACAs and/or 21-OHAbs positive. Patients show a reduction in serum levels of sodium, chloride, and bicarbonate, while the potassium level is elevated. Hyponatremia is usually found in all the patients and is because of a loss of sodium in the urine and to an increase in plasma vasopressin, which impairs free water clearance. The aldosterone deficiency causes hyperkalemia in 50–70% of the patients. For unknown reasons, mild or moderate hypercalcemia is present in 10–20% of patients *(146)*. Anemia is found in 40–50%, with a 10–15% of the patients showing a wild eosinophilia and lymphocytosis. In the case of a suspected antiphospholipid syndrome anti-cardiolipin antibodies or lupus anti-coagulant activity must be identified *(139)*.

In the presence of other clinical autoimmune diseases, the relevant autoantibodies are usually detectable. Furthermore, in patients with clinically isolated autoimmune AD, a screening for the main organ-specific autoantibodies is generally required to unveil those with underlying subclinical or potential autoimmune diseases *(93,104)*.

Hormonal Tests

The determination of the plasma levels of ACTH and cortisol in the morning (8:00 AM) are fundamental tests for the differentiation of primary adrenal failure from both a healthy status and other types of adrenal failure *(147)*. Primary adrenal failure is characterized by an increase in ACTH (normal values, 4–22 pmol/L) and a decrease in basal cortisol levels (normal values, 140–550 nmol/L). By contrast, in secondary adrenal failure, the levels of both ACTH and cortisol are low, and, in general, those of aldosterone and PRA are normal. In the initial phases of primary AD, the PRA increases above the normal range, and the plasma aldosterone is either normal or subnormal. Dehydroepiandrosterone sulfate, the major precursor of the sex steroid hormones, is involved in adrenal failure, causing a pronounced androgen deficiency in women, resulting in the loss of both axillary and pubic hair, dry skin, a reduced libido, and an impairment in wellbeing *(148)*. In cases in which there are no clear clinical manifestations of AD and/or in the presence of ACAs or 21-OHAbs, it may be necessary to perform an ACTH test (*see* Laboratory Investigation). Thyroid-stimulating hormone (TSH) levels are increased in 30% of patients because of the lack of the inhibitory effect exerted by cortisol on TSH secretion or, alternatively, by the presence of a coexisting autoimmune hypothyroidism *(149)*.

Imaging

The use of both computerized tomography (CT) and nuclear magnetic resonance (NMR) greatly facilitates the diagnosis and characterization of adrenal insufficiency, because the adrenal glands can be seen to be bilaterally minuscule and without calcification *(150)*. In the case of the anti-phospholipid syndrome, the imaging usually shows an increased volume in both adrenal glands because of bilateral hemorrhagic infarction *(139)*.

TREATMENT

For patients with chronic adrenal insufficiency, the therapy is life-saving *(146,148, 151)*. Glucocorticoids (20–30 mg of hydrocortisone or 25–50 mg of cortisone acetate) are required in three daily doses. The first dose is administered in the morning, the second in the early afternoon (about 6–8 h after the first), and the third in the late afternoon or early evening (at least 4 h before sleep). The drugs must not be taken with food. A 24-h urinary free cortisol test is considered a good marker for deciding a correct dosage of cortisone *(152,153)*, but measurement of the ACTH level cannot be used for this purpose. A single daily dose of 0.05–0.1 mg of fludrocortisone is usually required for the purposes of mineralocorticoid replacement. Patients should also receive a consistent amount of sodium (3–4 g daily), which can be assessed by the measurement of the blood pressure, the serum electrolytes, and the PRA levels, paying particular attention to a possible onset of hypokalemia, hypertension, sodium retention, or heart disease *(146)*. Complications are rare in this type of therapy. Patients with autoimmune AD should carry a medical identification card, outlining their current therapy and containing advice regarding emergency situations such as febrile illnesses, injury, vomiting, surgical interventions, dental extractions, or pregnancies. In these situations, the intake of glucocorticoids must be doubled or tripled *(18)*.

FUTURE DEVELOPMENTS

The goal in the prevention of organ-specific autoimmune diseases lies in the identification of individuals at high risk of developing clinical dysfunctions over the future. Over the last three decades, significant developments have been done in the discovery of both genetic and immunologic markers conferring disease susceptibility. Currently, subjects at high risk may be more easily recognized and therefore initiate early substitutive therapy to avoid a potentially life-threatening adrenal crisis. Moreover, subjects at high risk are also the ideal group for intervention trials, including immunosuppression, in the attempt to halt, or at least delay, the progression of adrenal cortex destruction and, thus, the clinical onset of the disease.

The identification of the environmental factors involved in the immunological activation of a genetically susceptible individual may enable to interfere in the early phases of autoimmune AD. It can also be envisaged that, in forthcoming years, more susceptibility genes for different complex traits will be identified through high-resolution genetic studies of candidate genes. Therapeutic manipulation of the immune system, involving for instance CTLA-4 molecules expression or felicitation, might be an option in the management of autoimmune endocrine diseases, and the administration of CTLA-4-blocking monoclonal antibodies has already been used in mice. However, pilot trials in humans must be performed with caution on selected subjects identified as being at maximal risk. Hopefully, an international standardization program should be performed for ACAs measurement, similar to that successfully performed for other main autoantibodies.

ACKNOWLEDGMENTS

This work was partially sponsored by FP6-Specific Targeted Research Project of the European Community. Entitled EurAPS: Autoimmune Polyendocrine Syndrome type I-a rare disorder of childhood as a model for autoimmunity. Contract.n° LSHM-CT-2005-005223.

REFERENCES

1. Eustachius B. *Opuscula anatomica de renum structura, efficio et adminstratione*. Venice: V.V. Luchino, 1564.

2. Addison T. *On the constitutional and local effects of disease of the suprarenal capsules*. London: Warren & Son, 1855.

3. Brown-Sequard CE. Recherches experimentales sur la physiologie e la pathologie des capsules surrenales. *Acad Sci Paris* 1856;43:422–425.

4. Trousseau A. Bronze Addison's disease. *Arch Gen Med* 1856;8:478–485.

5. Cushing HW. *The pituitary body and its disorders*. Philadelphia: JB Lippincott, 1912.

6. Hartman FA, MacArthur CJ, Hartman WE. Substances which prolongs life of adrenalectmized cats. *Proc Soc Exp Biol Med* 1927;25:69–70.

7. Stewart GN, Rogoff JM. The influence of extracts of adrenal cortex on the survival period of adrenalectomized dogs and cats. *Am J Physiol* 1929;91:254–264

8. Swingle WW, Pfiffner JJ. Preparation of an active extract of suprarenal cortex. *Anat Rec* 1929;44:225.

9. Rowntree LG, Greene CH, Swingle WW. The treatment of patients with Addison's disease with the "cortical hormone" of Swingle and Pfiffner. *Science* 1930:72:482–483.

10. DeFremery P, Laqueur E, Reichstein T, Spanhoff RW, Uyldert JE. Corticosterone, a cristallized compound with the biological activity of the adrenocortical hormone. *Nature* 1937;139:26–29.

11. Steiger M, Reichstein T. Desoxycorticosterone (21-oxyprogesterone aust-3-oxy-atio cholensaure). *Helv Chem Acta* 1937;20:1164–1179.

12. Simpson SL. The use of synthetic desoxycorticosterone acetate in Addison's disease. *Lancet* 1938;2:557–558

13. Kannan CR. Addison's disease. In: Kannan CR (ed.), *The adrenal gland*. London: Plenum Medical Book Company, 1988:31–96.

14. McNicol AM, Laidler P. The adrenal glands and extra-adrenal paraganglia. In: Lewis PD (ed.), *Endocrine system*. New York: Churchill Livingstone, 1996:59–129.

15. Auchus RJ, Miller WL. The principles, pathways and enzymes of human steroidogenesis. In: DeGroot LJ, Jameson JL (eds), *Endocrinology*, Vol 2. Philadelphia. WB Saunders Company, 2001:1616–1631.

16. Fox B. Venous infarction of the adrenal glands. *J Pathol* 1976;119:65–89.

17. Koch CA. Adrenal cortex physiology, In: Martini L (ed.), *Encyclopedia of endocrine disease*, Elsevier, San Diego, CA: Academic Press, 2004:68–74.

18. Oelkers W. Adrenal insufficiency. *N Engl J Med* 1996;335:1206–1212.

19. Guttman PH. Addison's disease: statistical analysis of 566 cases and study of the pathology. *Arch Pathol* 1930;10:742–895.

20. Dunlop D. Eighty-six cases of Addison's disease. *Br Med J* 1963;3:887–891.

21. Stuart-Mason A, Meade TW, Lee JAH, Morris JN. Epidemiological and clinical picture of Addison's disease. *Lancet* 1968;2:19–30.

22. Nerup J. Addison's disease-clinical studies. A report of 108 cases. *Acta Endocrinol* 1974;76: 127–141.

23. Cooper GS, Stroehla BC. The epidemiology of autoimmune diseases. *Autoimmun Rev* 2002;2: 119–125.

24. Kong MF, Jeffocoate W. Eighty-six cases of Addison's disease. *Clin Endocrinol* 1994;41:757–761.

25. Willis AC, Vince FP. The prevalence of Addison's disease in Coventry, UK. *Postgrad Med J* 1997;73:286–288.

26. Laureti S, Vecchi L, Santeusanio F, Falorni A. Is the prevalence of Addison's disease underestimated? *J Clin Endocrinol Metab* 1999;84:1762.

27. Løvås K, ES Husebye. High prevalence and increasing incidence of Addison's disease in western Norway. *Clin Endocrinol* 2002;56:787–791.

28. Eason RJ, Croxon MS, Perry MC, Somerfield SD. Addison's disease, adrenal autoantibodies and compuerized adrenal tomography. *N Z Med J* 1982;95:569–573.

29. Takayanagi R, Miura K, Nakagawa H, Nawata H. Epidemiological study of adrenal gland disorders in Japan. *Biomed Pharmacother* 2000;54:164–168.

30. Jacobson DL, Gange SJ, Rose NR, Graham NMH. Epidemiology and estimated population burden of selected autoimmune diseases in the United States. *Clin Immunol Immunopathol* 1997;84: 223–243.

31. Levine JS, Ware Branch DW, Rauch J. The antiphospholipid syndrome. *N Engl J Med* 2002; 346:752–763.

32. Li Volsi VA. The pathology of autoimmune thyroid disease: a review. *Thyroid* 1994;4:333–339.

33. Foulis AK, McGill M, Farquaharson MA, Hilton DA. The pathology of the endocrine pancreas in Type 1 (insulin-dependent) diabetes mellitus. *APIMS* 1996;104:161–167.

34. McNicol AM. Class II MHC antigen expression in adrenal cortex. *Lancet* 1986;2:1282.

35. Jackson R, McNicol AM, Farquarson M, Foulis AK. Class II MHC expression in normal adrenal cortex and cortical cell in autoimmune Addison's disease. *J Pathol* 1988;155:113–120.

36. Bottazzo GF, Pujol Borrell R, Hanafusa T, Feldmann M. Hypothesis. Role of aberrant HLA-DR expression and antigen presentation in induction of endocrine autoimmunity. *Lancet* 1983;2: 1115–1119.

37. Hanafusa T, Pujol Borrell R, Chiovato L, Russell RCG, Doniach D, Bottazzo GF. Aberrant expression of HLA-DR antigen on thyrocytes in Graves' disease: relevance for autoimmunity. *Lancet* 1983;2:1111–1115.

38. Fujii Y, Kato N, Kito J, Asai J, Yokochi T. Experimental autoimmune adrenalitis: a murine model for Addison's disease. *Autoimmunity* 1992;12:47–52.

39. Freeman M, Weetman AP. T and B cell reactivity to adrenal antigens in autoimmune Addison's disease. *Clin Exp Immunol* 1992;88:275–279.

40. Volpé R. Autoimmune endocrinopathies: aspects of pathogenesis and the role of immune assays in investigation and management. *Clin Chem* 1994;40:2132–2145.

41. Nerup J, Bendixen G. Anti-adrenal cellular hypersensitivity in Addison's disease. 2. Correlation with clinical and serological findings. *Clin Exp Immunol* 1969;5:341–353.

42. Nerup J, Andersen V, Bendixen G. Antiadrenal cellular hypersensitivity in Addison's disease. IV. In vivo and in vitro investigations of the mitochondrial fraction. *Clin Exp Immunol* 1970;6:733–739.

43. Verghese MV, Ward FE, Eisembarth GS. Decreased suppressor cell activity in patients with polyglandular failure. *Clin Res* 1980;28:270A.

44. Rabinowe SL, Jackson RA, Dluhy RG, Williams GH. Ia-positive T lymphocytes in recently diagnosed idiopathic Addison's disease. *Am J Med* 1984;77:597–601.

45. Krieghel MA, Lohmann T, Gabler C, Blank N, Kalden JR, Lorenz HM. Defective suppressor function of human CD4+ CD25+ regulatory T cells in autoimmune polyglandular syndrome type II. *J Exp Med* 2004;199:1285–1291.

46. Luster AD. Chemokines-chemotactic cytokines that mediate inflammation. *N Engl J Med* 1998;338:436–445.

47. Kunkel SL, Godessart N. Chemokynes in autoimmunity: from pathology to therapeutics. *Autoimmun Rev* 2002;1:313–320.

48. Rotondi M, Falorni A, De Bellis AM, Laureti S, Ferruzzi P, Romagnani P, Buonamano A, Lazzeri E, Crescioli C, Mannelli M, Santeusanio F, Bellastella A, Serio M. Elevated serum interferon-gamma-inducible chemokine-10/CXC chemokine ligand-10 in autoimmune primary adrenal insufficiency and in vitro expression in human adrenal cells primary cultures after stimulation with proinflammatory cytokines. *J Clin Endocrinol Metab* 2005;90:2357–2363.

49. Colover J, Glynn LE. Experimental iso-immune adrenalitis. *Immunology* 1958;2:172–178.

50. Milcou SM, Pop AI, Lupulescu A, Taga M. L'autoimmunisation experimentale de la surrènale chez le lapin. *An Endocrinol* 1959;20:799–804.

51. Steiner JW, Langer B, Schatz DL, Volpé R. Experimental immunologic adrenal injury: a response to injections of autologous and homologous adrenal antigens in adjuvant. *J Exp Med* 1960; 112:187.

52. Witebsky E, Milgrom F. Immunological studies on adrenal glands: II. Immunization with adrenals of the same species. *Immunology* 1962;5:67–78.

53. Barnett EV, Dumonde DC, Glynn LE. Induction of autoimmunity to adrenal gland. *Immunology* 1963;6:382–402.

54. Andrada JA, Skelton FR, Andrada EC, Milgrom F. Witebsky E. Experimental autoimmune adrenalitis in rats. *Lab Invest* 1968;19;460–465.

55. Irino T, Grollman A. Induction of adrenal insufficiency in the rat by sensitization with homologous tissue. *Metabolism* 1968;17:717–724.

56. Levine S, Wenk EJ. The production and passive transfer of allergic adrenalitis. *Am J Pathol* 1968;52:41–53.

57. Harlton BW. Addison's disease in a dog. *Vet Med Small Anim Clin* 1976;71:285–288.

58. Kaufman J. Diseases of the adrenal cortex of dogs and cats. *Mod Vet Pract* 1984;65:513–516.

59. Little C, Marshall C, Downs J. Addison's disease in the dog. *Vet Rec* 1989;124:469–470.

60. Kintzer PP, Peterson ME. Diagnosis and management of primary spontaneous hypoadrenocorticism (Addison's disease) in dogs. *Sem Vet Med Surg* 1994;9:148–152.

61. Sadek D, Schaer M. Atypical Addison's disease in the dog: a retrospective survey of 14 cases. *J Am Anim Hosp Assoc* 1996;32:159–163.

62. Dunn KJ, Herrtage ME. Hypocortisolaemia in a Labrador retriever. *J Small Anim Pract* 1998;39: 90–93.

63. Peterson ME, Greco DS, Orth DN. Primary hypoadrenocorticism in ten cats. *J Vet Intern Med* 1989;3:55–58

64. Tasker S, MacKay AD, Sparkes AH. Case report. A case of feline primary hypoadrenocorticism. *J Feline Med Surg* 1999;1:257–260.

65. Stonehewer J, Tasker S. Hypoadrenocroticism in a cat. *J Small Anim Pract* 2001;42:186–190.

66. Beales PE, Castri F, Valiani A, Rosignoli G, Buckley L, Pozzilli P. Adrenalitis in the non-obese diabetic mouse. *Autoimmunity* 2002;35:329–333.

67. Anderson JR, Goudie RB, Gray KG, Timbury GC. Autoantibodies in Addison's disease. *Lancet* 1957;1:1123–1124.

68. Betterle C. Addison's disease and autoimmune polyglandular syndromes. In: Geenen V, Chrosus G (eds), *Immunoendocrinology in health and disease*. New York: Marcel Dekker Inc. Publisher, 2004:491–536.

69. Blizzard RM, Kyle M. Studies on adrenal antigens and autoantibodies in Addison's disease. *J Clin Invest* 1963;42:1653–1660.

70. Irvine WJ, Barnes EW. Addison's disease, ovarian failure and hypoparathyroidism. *Clin Endocrinol Metab* 1975;4:379–434.

71. Sotsiu F, Bottazzo GF, Doniach D. Immunofluorescence studies on autoantibodies to steroid-producing cells, and to germline cells in endocrine disease and infertility. *Clin Exp Immunol* 1980;39:97–111.

72. Khoury EL, Hammond L, Bottazzo GF, Doniach D. Surface-reactive antibodies to human adrenal cells in Addison's disease. *Clin Exp Immunol* 1981;45:48–55.

73. Baumann-Antczak A, Wedlock N, Bednarek J, Kiso Y, Krishnan H, Fowler S, Rees Smith B, Furmaniak J. Autoimmune Addison's disease and 21-hydroxylase. *Lancet* 1992; 340:429–430.

74. Bednarek J, Furmaniak J, Wedlock N, Kiso Y, Baumann-Antczak A, Fowler S, Krishnan H, Craft JA, Rees Smith B. Steroid 21-hydroxylase is a major autoantigen involved in adult onset autoimmune Addison's disease. *FEBS Lett* 1992;309:51–55.

75. Winqvist O, Karlsson FA, Kampe O. 21-hydroxylase, a major autoantigen in idiopathic Addison's disease. *Lancet* 1992;339:1559–1562.

76. Colls J, Betterle C, Volpato M, Rees Smith B, Furmaniak J. A new immunoprecipitation assay for autoantibodies to steroid 21-hydroxylase in Addison's disease. *Clin Chem* 1995;41:375–380.

77. Falorni A, Nikoshokov A, Laureti S, Grenbäck E, Hulting AL, Casucci G. High diagnostic accuracy for idiopathic Addison's disease with a sensitive radiobinding assay for autoantibodies against recombinant human 21-hydroxylase. *J Clin Endocrinol Metab* 1995;80:2752–2755.

78. Chen S, Sawicka J, Betterle C, Powell M, Prentice L, Volpato M, Rees Smith B, Furmaniak J. Autoantibodies to steroidogenic enzymes in autoimmune polyglandular syndrome, Addison's disease, and premature ovarian failure. *J Clin Endocrinol Metab* 1996; 83:2977–2986.

79. Tanaka H, Perez MS, Powell M, Sandres JF, Sawicka J, Chen S, Prentice L, Asawa T, Betterle C, Volpato M, Rees Smith B, Furmaniak J. Steroid 21-hydroxylase autoantibodies: measurements with a new immunoprecipations assay. *J Clin Endocrinol Metab* 1997;82:1440–1446.

80. Anderson JR, Goudie RB, Gray K, Stuart-Smith DA. Immunological features of idiopathic Addison's disease: an antibody to cells producing steroid hormones. *Clin Exp Immunol* 1968;3:107–117.

81. Hoek A, Schoemaker J, Drexhage HA. Premature ovarian failure and ovarian autoimmunity. *Endocr Rev* 1997;18:107–134.

82. Krohn K, Uibo R, Aavik E, Peterson P, Savilhati K. Identification by molecular cloning of an autoantigen associated with Addison's disease as steroid 17-a-hydroxylase. *Lancet* 1992;339: 770–773.

83. Winqvist O, Gustafsson J, Rorsman F, Karlsson FA, Kampe O. Two different cytochrome P450 enzymes are the adrenal antigens in autoimmune polyendocrine syndrome type I and Addison's disease. *J Clin Invest* 1993;92:2377–2385.

84. Peterson P, Krohn KJE. Mapping of B cell epitopes on steroid 17-α-hydroxylase, an autoantigen in autoimmune polyglandular syndrome type 1. *Clin Exp Immunol* 1994; 98:104–109.

85. Betterle C, Volpato M, Pedini B, Chen S, Rees Smith B, Furmaniak J. Adrenal-cortex autoantibodies and steroid producing cells autoantibodies in patients with Addison's disease: comparison of immunofluorescence and immunoprecipitation assays. *J Clin Endocrinol Metab* 1999;84:2: 618–622.

86. Ahonen P, Miettinen A, Perheentupa J. Adrenal and steroidal cell antibodies in patients with autoimmune polyglandular disease type I and risk of adrenocortical and ovarian failure. *J Clin Endocrinol Metab* 1987;64:494–500.

87. Betterle C, Rossi A, Dalla Pria S, Artifoni L, Pedini B, Gavasso S, Caretto A. Premature ovarian failure: autoimmunity and natural history of the disease. *Clin Endocrinol* 1993;39:35–43.

88. Wilkin TJ. Receptor autoimmunity in endocrine disorders. *N Engl J Med* 1990; 323:1318–1324.

89. Salim YS, Faber V, Wiik A, Andersewn PL, Hoier-Madsen M, Mouritsen S. Anti-corticosteroid antibodies in AIDS patients. *Acta Pathol Microbiol Immunol Scand* 1988;96:889–894.

90. Kendall-Taylor P, Lambert A, Mitchell R, Robertson WR. Antibody that blocks stimulation of cortisol secretion by adrenocorticotrohic hormone in Addison's disease. *BMJ* 1988;296:1489–1491.

91. Wulfraat NM, Drexhage HA, Bottazzo GF, Wiersinga WM, Jeucken P, Van der Gaag R. Immunoglobulins of patients with idiopathic Addison's disease block the in vitro action of adrenocotropin. *J Clin Endocrinol Metab* 1989;69:231–238.

92. Wardle CA, Weetman AP, Mitchell R, Peers N, Robertson WR. Adrenocorticotropic hormone receptor-blocking immunoglobulins in serum from patients with Addison's disease: a re-examination. *J Clin Endocrinol Metab* 1993;77:750–753.

93. Betterle C, Dal Pra C, Mantero F, Zanchetta R. Autoimmune adrenal insufficiency and autoimmune polyendocrine syndromes: autoantibodies, autoantigens, and their applicability in diagnosis and disease prediction. *Endocr Rev* 2002;23:327–364.

94. Furmaniak J, Talbot D, Reinwein D, Benker G, Creag FM, Smith B. Immunoprecipitation of human adrenal microsomal antigen. *FEBS Lett* 1988;232:25–28.

95. Morgan J, Betterle C, Zanchetta R, Dal Pra C, Chen S, Rees Smith B, Furmaniak J Direct evidence that steroid 21-hydroxylase (21-OH) is the major antigen recognized by adrenal cortex autontibodies (ACA). *J Endocrinol* 2000;167 (Suppl): OC19.

96. Furmaniak J, Sanders J, Rees Smith B. Autoantigens in the autoimmune endocrinopathies. In: Volpé R (ed.), *Contemporary endocrinology: autoimmune endocrinopathies*. Totowa, NJ: Human Press Inc, 1999:183–216.

97. Furmaniak J, Rees Smith B. Addison's disease. In: Gill RG (ed.), *Immunologically mediated endocrine diseases*. Philadelphia: Lippincott Williams & Williams, 2002:431–451.

98. Wedlock N, Asawa T, Baumann-Antczak A, Rees Smith B, Furmaniak J. Autoimmune Addison's disease. Analysis of autoantibody sites on human steroid 21-hydroxylase. *FEBS Lett* 1993;332: 123–126.

99. Asawa T. Wedlock N, Baumann-Antczak A, Rees Smith B, Furmaniak J. Naturally occurring mutations in human steroid 21-hydroxylase influence adrenal autoantibody binding. *J Clin Endcorinol Metab* 1994;79:372–376

100. Song Y, Connor EL, Muir A, She JX, Zorovich B, Derovanesian D, Maclaren N. Autoantibody epitope mapping of the 21-hydroxylase antigen in autoimmune Addison's disease. *J Clin Endocrinol Metab* 1994;78:1108–1112.

101. Volpato M., Prentice L., Chen S., Betterle C., Rees Smith B., Furmaniak J. A study of the epitopes on steroid 21-hydroxylase recognized by autoantibodies in patients with or without Addison's disease. *Clin Exp Immunol* 1998;111:422–428.

102. Neufeld M, Blizzard RM. Polyglandular autoimmune diseases. In: Pinchera A, Doniach D, Fenzi GF, Baschieri L (eds), *Symposium on autoimmune aspects of endocrine disorders*. New York: Academic Press, 1980:357–365.

103. Neufeld M, MacLaren NK, Blizzard RM. Two types of autoimmune Addison's disease associated with different polyglandular autoimmune (PGA) syndromes. *Medicine* 1981; 60:355–362.

104. Betterle C, Lazzarotto F, Presotto F. Autoimmune polyglandular syndrome Type 2: the tip of an iceberg? *Clin Exp Immunol* 2004;137:225–233.

105. Nagamine K, Peterson P, Scott HS, Kudoh J, Minoshima S, Heino M, Krohn KJE, Lalioti MD, Mullis PE, Antonarakis SE, Kawasaki K, Asakawa S, Ito F, Shimizu N. Positional cloning of the APECED gene. *Nat Genet* 1997;17:393–398.

106. The Finnish-German APECED Consortium. An autoimmune disease, APECED, caused by mutations in a novel gene featuring two PHD-type zinc-finger domains. *Nat Genet* 1997;17: 399–403.

107. Peterson P, Pitkanen J, Sillanpaa N, Krohn K. Autoimmune polyendocrinopathy candidiasis ectodermal dystrophy (APECED): a model disease to study molecular aspects of endocrine autoimmunity. *Clin Exp Immunol* 2004;137:225–233.

108. Shapiro MS, Zmir R, Weiss E, Radnay J, Sherkman I. The polyglandular deficiency syndrome: a new variant in Persian Jews. *J Clin Invest* 1998;10:1–7.

109. Betterle C, Greggio NA, Volpato M. Autoimmune polyglandular disease Type 1. *J Clin Endocrinol Metab* 1998;83:1049–1055.

110. Kemp EH, Ajjan RA, Husebye ES, Peterson P, Uibo R, Imrie H, Pearce SH, Watson PF, Weetman AP. A cytotoxic T lymphocytic antigen-4 (CTLA-4) gene polymorphism is associated with autoimmune Addison's disease in English patients. *Clin Endocrinol* 1998; 49:609–613.

111. Blomhoff A, Lie BA, Myhre AG, Kemp EH, Weetman AP, Akselsen HE, Huseby ES, Undlien DE. Polymorphisms in the cytotoxic T lymphocyte antigen-4 gene region confer susceptibility to Addison's disease. *J Clin Endocrinol Metab* 2004; 89:3474–3476.

112. Betterle C, Coco G, Zanchetta R. Adrenal cortex autoantoantibodies in subjects with normal adrenal function. *Best Pract Res Clin Endocrinol Metab* 2005;19:85–99.

113. Blizzard RM, Chee D, Davis W. The incidence of parathyroid and other antibodies in the sera of patients with idiopatic hypoparathyroidism. *Clin Exp Immunol* 1966;1:119–128.

114. Betterle C, Volpato M, Rees Smith B, Furmaniak J, Chen S, Greggio NA, Sanzari M, Tedesco F, Pedini B, Boscaro M, Presotto F. I. Adrenal cortex and steroid 21-hydroxylase autoantibodies in adult patients with organ-specific autoimmune diseases: markers of low progression to clinical Addison's disease. *J Clin Endocrinol Metab* 1997;82:932–938.

115. Betterle C, Volpato M, Rees Smith B, Furmaniak J, Chen S, Zanchetta R, Greggio NA, Pedini B, Boscaro M, Presotto F. II. Adrenal cortex and steroid 21-hydroxylase autoantibodies in children with organ-specific autoimmune diseases: markers of high progression to clinical Addison's disease. *J Clin Endocrinol Metab* 1997;82:939–942.

116. Dal Pra C, Chen S, Furmaniak J, Rees Smith B, Pedini B, Moscon A, Zanchetta R, Betterle C. Autoantibodies to steroidogenic enzymes in patients with premature ovarian failure with and without Addison's disease. *Eur J Endocrinol* 2003;148:565–570.

117. Anderson JR. Auto-antibodies in diseases of man. *Br Med Bull* 1963;19:251–256.

118. Riley JW, Maclaren N, Neufeld M. Adrenal antibodies and Addison's disease in insulin-dependent diabetes mellitus. *J Pediatr* 1980;97:191–195.

119. Scherbaum WA, Berg PA. Development of adrenocortical failure in non-addisonian patients with antibodies to adrenal cortex. *Clin Endocrinol* 1982;16:345–352.

120. Betterle C, Zanchetta R, Trevisan A, Zanette F, Pedini B, Mantero F, Rigon F. Complement-fixing adrenal autoantibodies as a marker for predicting onset of idiopathic Addison's disease. *Lancet* 1983;1:1238–1240.

121. Betterle C, Scalici C, Presotto F, Pedini B, Moro L, Rigon F, Mantero F. The natural history of adrenal function in autoimmune patients with adrenal autoantibodies. *J Endocrinol* 1988;117:467–475.

122. De Bellis A, Bizzarro A, Rossi R, Paglionico VA, Criscuolo T, Lombardi G, Bellastella A. Remission of subclinical adrenocortical failure in subjects with adrenal autoantibodies. *J Clin Endorinol Metab* 1993;76:1002–1007.

123. Peterson P, Uibo R, Peranen J, Krohn KJE. Immunoprecipitation of steroidogenic enzyme autoantigens with autoimmune polyglandular syndrome type 1 (APS I) sera; further evidence for independent humoral immunity to P450 c17 and P450c21. *Clin Exp Immunol* 1997;107:335–340.

124. Laureti S, De Bellis AM, Muccitelli VI, Calcinaro F, Bizzaro A, Rossi R, Bellastella A, Santeusanio F, Falorni A. Levels of adrenocortical autoantibodies correlate with the degree of adrenal dysfunction in subjects in subjects with preclinical Addison's disease. *J Clin Endocrinol Metab* 1998;83:3507–3511.

125. Yu L, Brewer KW, Gates S, Wu A, Wang T, Babu SR, Gottlieb PA, Freed BM, Noble J, Erlich HA, Rewers MJ, Eisenbarth GS. DRB1*04 and DQ alleles: expression of 21-hydroxylase autoantibodies and risk of progression to Addison's disease. *J Clin Endocrinol Metab* 1999;84:328–335.

126. Wesche B, Jaeckel E, Trautwein C, Wedemeyer H, Falorni A, Frank H, von zurMuhlen A, Manns MP, Brabant G. Induction of autoantibodies to the adrenal cortex and pancreatic islet cells by interferon alpha therapy for chronic hepatitis C. *Gut* 2001;48:378–383.

127. Barker JM, Ide A, Hostetler C, Yu L, Miao D, Fain PR, Eisenbarth GS, Gottlieb PA. Endocrine and immunogenetic testing in individuals with type 1 diabetes and 21-hydroxylase autoantibodies: Addison's disease in a high-risk population. *J Clin Endocrinol Metab* 2005;90:28–34.

128. Laureti S, Arvat E, Candeloro P, Di Vito L, Ghigo E, Santeusanio F, Falorni A. Low dose (1 μg) ACTH test in the evaluation of adrenal dysfunction in pre-clinical Addison's disease. *Clin Endocrinol* 2000;53:107–115.

129. De Bellis A, Falorni A, Laureti S, Perrino S, Coronella C, Forini F, Bizzarro E, Bizzarro A, Abbate G, Bellastella A. Time course of 21-hydroxylase autoantibodies and long term remission of subclinical autoimmune adrenalitis after corticosteroid therapy: case report. *J Clin Endocrinol Metab* 2001;86:675–678.

130. Coco G, Dal Pra C, Presotto F, Albergoni MP, Canova C, Pedini B, Zanchetta R, Chen S, Furmaniak J, Rees Smith B, Mantero F, Betterle C. Estimated risk for developing autoimmune Addison's disease in patients with adrenal cortex autoantibodies. *J Clin Endocrinol Metal.* 2006;91:1637–1645.

131. Kamradt T, Mitchinson NA. Tolerance and autoimmunity. *N Engl J Med* 2001;344:655–664.

132. McNatty KP, Short RV. The cytotoxic effect of the serum from patients with Addison's disease and autoimmune ovarian failure on human granulosa cells in culture. *Clin Exp Immunol* 1975;22: 378–384.

133. Bottazzo GF, Dean B, Gorsuch AN, Cudworth AG, Doniach D. Complement-fixing islet-cell antibodies in Type 1 diabetes: possible monitors of active beta-cell damage. *Lancet* 1980;1:668–672.

134. Betterle C. Presotto F, Magrin L, Pedini B, Moro L, Caretto A, Zanchetta R. The natural history of pre-Type 1 (insulin-dependent) diabetes mellitus in patients with autoimmune diseases. *Diabetologia* 1994;37:95–103.

135. Furmaniak J, Kominani S, Asawa T, Wedlock N, Colls J, Rees Smith B. Autoimmune Addison's disease. Evidence for a role of steroid 21-hydroxylase autoantibodies in adrenal insufficiency. *J Clin Endocrinol Metab* 1994;79:1517–1521.

136. Boscaro M, Betterle C, Volpato M, Fallo F, Furmaniak J, Rees Smith B, Sonino N. Hormonal responses during various phases of autoimmune adrenal failure: no evidence for 21-hydroxylase enzyme activity inhibition in vivo. *J Clin Endocrinol Metab* 1996;81:2801–2804.

137. Betterle C, Dal Pra C, Pedini B, Zanchetta R., Chen S, Furmaniak J, Rees Smith B. Assessment of adrenal function and adrenal autoantibodies in a baby of a mother with autoimmune polyglandular syndrome type 2. *J Endocrinol Invest* 2004;27:618–621.

138. Espinosa G, Cervera R, Font J, Asherson RA. Adrenal involvement in the antiphospholipid syndrome. *Lupus* 2003;12(7):569–572.

139. Presotto F, Fornasini F, Betterle C, Federspil G, Rossato M. Acute adrenal failure as the heralding symptom of primary antiphospholipid syndrome: report of a case and review of the literature. *Eur J Endocrinol* 2005;153:507–514.

140. Vaidya B, Pearce S. The emerging role of the CTLA-4 gene in autoimmune endocrinopathies. *Eur J Endocrinol* 2004;150:619–626.

141. Walunas TL, Lenschow DJ, Bakker CY, Linsley PS, Freeman GJ, Green JM, Thompson CB, Bluestone JA. CTLA-4 can function as a negative regulator of T cell activation. *Immunity* 1994;1:405–413.

142. Fisher GH, Rosenberg FJ, Straus SE, Dale JK, Middleton LA, Lin AY, Strober W, Lenardo MJ, Puck JM. Dominant interfering Fas gene mutations impair apoptosis in a human autoimmune lymphoproliferative syndrome. *Cell* 1995;16(81):935–946.

143. Tivol EA, Boriello F, Schweitzer AN, Lynch WP, Bluestone JA, Sharpe AH. Loss of CTLA-4 leads to a massive lymphoproliferation and fatal multiorgan tissue destruction, revealing a critical negative role of CTLA-4. *Immunity* 1995;3:541–547.

144. Okazaki T, Iwai Y, Honjo T. New regulatory co-receptors: inducible co-stimulator and PD-1. *Curr Opin Immunol* 2002;14:779–782.

145. Watanabe N, Gavrieli M, Sedy JR, Yang J, Fallarino F, Loftin SK, Hurchla MA, Zimmerman N, Sim J, Zang X, Murphy TL, Russell JH, Allison JP, Murphy KM. BTLA is a lymphocyte inhibitory receptor with similarities to CTLA-4 and PD-1. *Nat Immunol* 2003;4:670–679.

146. Williams GH, Dluhy RG. Disease of the adrenal cortex. In: Fauci AS, Braunwald E, Isselbacher KJ, Wilson JD, Martin JB, Kasper DL, Hauser SL, Longo DL (eds), *Harrison's Principles of Internal medicine*, 14th edition. McGraw-Hill, New York 1998:2040–2042.

147. Oelkers W, Diederich S, Bahr V. Diagnosis and therapy surveillance in Addison's disease: rapid adrenocorticotropin (ACTH) test and measurement of plasma ACTH, renin activity and aldosterone. *J Clin Endocrinol Metab* 1992;75:259–164.

148. Arlt W, Allolio B. Adrenal insufficiency. *Lancet* 2003;361:1881–1893.

149. Orth DN, Kavacs WJ. The adrenal cortex. In: Wilson JD, Foster DW, Kronenberg HM, Larse PR (eds), *Williams textbook of endocrinology*, 9th edition. Philadelphia: WB Saunders, 1998:517–664.

150. Doppman JL. Adrenal Imaging. In: De Groot LJ, Jameson JL (eds), *Endocrinology*, 4th edition. Philadelphia: WB Saunders Co., 2001:1747–1766.

151. Groves RW, Toms GC, Houghton BJ, Monson JP. Corticosteroid replacement therapy: twice or thrice daily? *J R Soc Med* 1988;81:514–516.

152. Burch WM. Urine free-cortisol determination: a useful tool in the management of chronic hypoadrenal states. *JAMA* 1982;247:2002–2004.

153. Howlett TA. An assessment of optimal hydrocortisone replacement therapy. *Clin Endocrinol (Oxf)* 1997;46:263–268.

14 Premature Ovarian Failure

Victoria Sundblad, PhD,
Violeta A. Chiauzzi, PhD,
and Eduardo H. Charreau, PhD

CONTENTS

Summary

Premature ovarian failure (POF) is defined as hypergonadotropic amenorrhea before the age of 40 years. Resistant ovary syndrome (ROS) is proposed as a follicular form of POF, characterized by the presence of numerous primordial follicles in the ovary. An autoimmune mechanism could be involved in the etiology of idiopathic POF. Several pieces of evidence support the concept that POF in the presence of adrenal autoimmunity (2–10% of cases) is almost certainly an endocrine autoimmune disorder. However, the question whether an eventual true autoimmune POF occurs in the absence of adrenal autoimmunity is controversial; data need to be confirmed and their relevance investigated. Finally, ROS may represent a rare case of autoimmune POF characterized by the presence of antibodies directed to the follicle-stimulating hormone (FSH) receptor (Ig-FSHR).

Diagnosis of an autoimmune etiology remains difficult. Indeed, ovarian biopsy is not currently in use as a diagnostic tool in POF cases. The specificity and diagnostic significance of antiovarian antibodies need to be unanimously established. Determination of adrenal cortex antibodies (ACA) and/or steroid cell antibodies (SCA) should be evaluated as possible research markers to select POF women with autoimmune oophoritis—potential responders to immunosuppressive therapy—with reasonable certainty. Determination of Ig-FSHR by radio-receptor assay could be instrumental in diagnosing ROS, mainly on the basis of serological findings. Young women with POF need hormone replacement therapy. Regarding infertility-related therapy, immunosuppression through corticosteroids has long been used on an empirical basis; however, there is no definite proof of its efficacy in POF treatment. To date, oocyte donation is the only proven therapy for such patients.

Key Words: Premature ovarian failure, resistant ovary syndrome, ovarian autoimmunity, autoimmune oophoritis, antiovarian antibodies.

From: *Contemporary Endocrinology: Autoimmune Diseases in Endocrinology*
Edited by: A. P. Weetman © Humana Press, Totowa, NJ

INTRODUCTION

The prevalence of amenorrhea not because of pregnancy, lactation, or menopause is approximately 3–4% *(1,2)*. Excluding disorders of congenital sexual ambiguity, the list of potential causes of amenorrhea is long. Most cases, however, are grounded on just four conditions: polycystic ovary syndrome, hypothalamic amenorrhea, hyper-prolactinemia, and premature ovarian failure (POF) *(3)*. POF is defined as the cessation of menses before the age of 40 years. It is characterized by primary or secondary amenorrhea, hypoestrogenism, and elevated gonadotropin serum levels *(4)*. An elevated follicle-stimulating hormone (FSH) level (>40 mUI/ml) is the hallmark for diagnosis *(5)*.

POF presents itself not as an all-or-none phenomenon, and the precise time of onset is often impossible to determine. There is no characteristic menstrual record preceding the development of this syndrome. Approximately 50% of patients have a record of oligomenorrhea or dysfunctional uterine bleeding (prodromal POF), 25% have sudden amenorrhea, some postpartum, and others after stopping oral contraceptives *(6)*. In general, women with POF have normal fertility before the onset of the disorder *(7,8)*.

POF was first considered an irreversible condition and was therefore described as premature menopause; however, while normal menopause is indeed an irreversible condition, POF is characterized by intermittent ovarian follicle function in nearly 50% of young women *(9)*. Even though the follicles in these patients are probably not functioning normally, women with POF may exhibit sporadic ovulatory cycles in as many as 16% of cases *(9)*. Moreover, several authors have reported pregnancies after the diagnosis of POF, even in women with no follicles in their ovarian biopsy *(7,10–12)*. However, despite these isolated cases, patients with POF are troubled mainly by infertility because of cessation of their ovarian function.

As previously explained, POF may present itself as either primary or secondary amenorrhea. While primary amenorrhea is not associated with symptoms of estrogen deficiency, in cases of secondary amenorrhea, symptoms may include hot flashes, night sweats, fatigue, and mood changes. Prodromal POF may present itself with hot flashes even when patients are menstruating regularly. Women with primary amenorrhea may present with incomplete development of secondary sex characteristics, whereas these characteristics are usually normal in women with secondary amenorrhea *(6)*. In addition, young women with POF sustain sex steroid deficiency for more years than naturally menopausal women, which results in a significantly higher risk of osteoporosis and cardiovascular disease.

Histopathological Classification of Premature Ovarian Failure

Kinch et al. *(13)* were the first to identify two histopathological types of POF: the afollicular and the follicular forms. In the afollicular form, there may be total depletion of ovarian follicles and a presumed consequent permanent loss of ovarian function; in the follicular form, follicular structures are still preserved, with the consequent possibility of either induced or spontaneous return of ovarian function. The so-called resistant ovary syndrome (ROS) has been proposed as a follicular form of POF *(14)*.

First described by Jones and de Moraes-Ruehsen *(15)*, who called it "Savage Syndrome," ROS is characterized by the presence of numerous primordial follicles in the ovarian examination. Patients with ROS have primary or secondary amenorrhea, usually with normal development of secondary sexual characteristics, and hypergonadotropinemia in the presence of numerous morphologically normal ovarian primordial follicles *(16)*. As in ROS the follicular structures are preserved, there is a likelihood of either spontaneous or induced return to ovarian function.

Etiology of Premature Ovarian Failure

POF is a heterogeneous disorder with a multi-causal pathogenesis. Although the phenotypic expression of POF is similar to that of age-appropriate natural menopause, the underlying pathophysiological mechanisms are diverse and usually unclear. In most cases, the etiology remains unknown; these forms are referred to as idiopathic.

Genetic causes of POF probably comprise about one-third to one-half of all cases. Nevertheless, only 15–20% of these genetic cases are most likely identifiable by current clinical techniques; they are usually due to large chromosomal defects (i.e., Turner syndrome), which can only be diagnosed by karyotype with high-resolution banding. In addition, some regions and genes localized on the X-chromosome (POF-1, POF-2, FMR), are known to cosegregate with POF. Regarding autosomes, the autoimmune regulator (*AIRE*) gene, located in chromosome 21, the *FSH*β gene and the Ataxia Telangiectasia (*ATM*) gene, both in chromosome 11, the *FOXL-2* gene (chromosome 3) linked to blepharophimosis-ptosis epicanthus syndrome (BPES), and the FSH receptor (*FSHR*) gene, on chromosome 2, are Fragile Mental Retard gene (FMR1) most recognized to cosegregrate with, among others, some ovarian failure *(17)*.

In addition, enzyme deficiencies, such as 17α-hydroxylase (17-OH) and 17–20 desmolase deficiencies *(18)*, metabolic disorders, such as galactosemia *(19)*, infectious agents, such as varicella, malaria, and shigellosis *(7)*, and iatrogenic causes, such as chemotherapy, radiotherapy, or ovarian surgery *(18)*, may be some of the alternative etiologic agents involved in POF development.

Finally, autoimmune ovarian failure is another large, generic category that requires some better definition and characterization. The usual occurrence of POF in patients with two or more associated autoimmune diseases *(14,20–22)*, the frequent detection of circulating antibodies to human ovarian tissue in sera from patients with POF *(20,23–25)*, and the presence of a lymphocytic infiltrate in ovarian specimens of some POF patients *(22,26,27)* originally added to the concept that autoimmune mechanisms could be involved in idiopathic POF etiology. This accumulative evidence would place some POF cases in the group of autoimmune diseases that affect hormone-producing glands, the so-called "autoimmune endocrinopathies," such as thyroiditis, type 1 diabetes mellitus (T1D), and Addison's disease *(14)*.

It is the purpose of this chapter to summarize the existing data supporting the concept of autoimmunity as a cause of POF, to discuss possible mechanisms of such autoimmune response and to review proposed treatments of patients with this disorder.

EPIDEMIOLOGY

It is common knowledge that the average or median menopause age is around 50 years, but the probability of menopause at earlier ages has been somewhat disregarded. Little information is available on the incidence and prevalence of POF in population at large. The first and most quoted work on this subject was developed by Coulam et al. in 1986 *(28)*. By following a birth cohort of 1858 women born between 1928 and 1932, identified as Rochester, Minnesota residents in 1950, the authors were able to define a young population and follow them until menopause to determine age-specific incidence rates of menopause. The risk of POF or menopause before the age of 40 years turned out to be of 0.009 (95% confidence interval [CI], 0.003–0.015), whereas the risk of menopause before the age of 45 years was of 0.051 (95% CI, 0.034–0.067). Thus, the study indicated that almost 1% of women can be expected to experience POF. These findings were similar to those reported by Krailo and Pike *(29)*, who found that the fit prevalence of menopause at ages 39 and 40 years was 0.012. In addition, the annual incidence rates of natural menopause per 100,000 person-years were 10 for ages 15–29 years and 76 for ages 30–39 years. In the age group 40–44 years, the incidence of natural menopause increased greatly to 881 per 100,000 person-years at risk *(28)*.

Likewise, applying lifetable methods or logistic models to a perimenopausal population to estimate the probability of menopause by age, Cramer and Xu *(30)* found that the probability of menopause before age 40 years is about 1%, and the probability of menopause before age 45 years is about 5%. The authors also studied other risk factors, besides age, that could influence risk of earlier menopause, including various medical, demographic, reproductive, environmental, and genetic factors. They developed a logistic model and proposed the use of these risk variables to obtain the estimated probabilities of menopause for various age-risk profiles. By means of this model, the authors found that heavy smokers, women estimated to have had >300 ovulatory cycles, women with a history of depression, women losing one ovary at an early age, and women with a family history of early menopause, all had earlier menopause. In addition, the highest probability of menopause was found to occur in women with multiple risk factors.

A more recent study on the transition to menopause in a multi-ethnic population suggested that the prevalence of POF may vary according to ethnicity *(31)*. In a prospective, multi-ethnic longitudinal study of the natural history of menopausal transition (The Study of Women Across the Nation, SWAN), conducted at seven sites in the United States, POF was reported in 1.1% (126/11,652) of women. As per ethnicity, 1.0% (95% CI, 0.7–1.4) Caucasian, 1.4% (95% CI, 1.0–2.1) African-American, 1.4% (95% CI, 0.8–2.5) Hispanic, 0.5% (95% CI, 0.1–1.9) Chinese, and 0.1% (95% CI, 0.02–1.1) Japanese women experienced POF. Differences in frequency across ethnic groups were statistically significant ($p = 0.01$).

Prevalence of Autoimmune Premature Ovarian Failure

As will be discussed later in this chapter, diagnosis of autoimmune POF remains difficult. Cases of POF associated with anti-adrenal autoimmunity may represent a homogeneous and well-characterized subgroup of ovarian failure. About 2–10% of POF cases are associated with Addison's disease and/or adrenal autoimmunity *(14,32)*. In other forms of POF, there is a large diversity in clinical, immunological, and histological features. Therefore, the overall proportion of autoimmune forms of POF has been estimated in between 20% *(33)* and 70% *(34)*.

IMMUNOPATHOGENESIS

The human ovary can be the target of an autoimmune attack under various circumstances, including several organ-specific or systemic autoimmune diseases. Clinically, the ensuing ovarian dysfunction often results in POF, but other pathologies involving ovaries, such as unexplained infertility, polycystic ovary syndrome (PCOS), and endometriosis, have been associated with anti-ovarian autoimmunity *(34)*.

It was the association of POF with autoimmune disorders, together with the findings of circulating antibodies to normal ovarian tissue in sera from patients with POF, which originally suggested an autoimmune mechanism in the pathophysiology of POF. Additional evidence was brought forward with the histological documentation of a lymphocytic infiltrate in the ovaries of some patients with this disorder *(26)*.

It has long been recognized that POF could be associated with nearly all organ-specific as well as some systemic autoimmune diseases. The association best known, although not the most frequent, is with adrenal autoimmunity. The relationship between adrenal disease and ovarian failure has been established in several clinical case reports since the early 1950s *(32)*. Autoimmune Addison's disease, a well-known manifestation of adrenal autoimmunity, seldom develops in isolation; in most cases, several other endocrine glands or organs are also affected, leading to an autoimmune polyglandular syndrome type I (APS-I) or type II (APS-II) as described in Chap. 16 and 17. The prevalence of POF in APS-I is estimated to be 39% at the age of 15 years and 72% at the age of 40 years, whereas the prevalence of ovarian failure in APS-II is only approximately 10% at the age of 40 years. On the contrary, about 2–10% of POF cases are associated with Addison's disease and/or adrenal autoimmunity *(14,32)*.

Several studies have evaluated the prevalence of an associated autoimmune disease in POF patients, yielding different results: 10–20% in some studies *(22,35,36)*, nearly 40% in others *(37,38)*, and up to 55% in yet another *(39)*. Among all autoimmune diseases associated with POF, thyroid disorders are definitely the most common; they can be detected in 12–33% of POF patients *(37–40)*. The second most frequent autoimmune associations in POF patients are APS-I and APS-II. POF may be detected before, after, or simultaneously with the onset of the other autoimmune disorders. However, as far as Addison's disease is concerned, POF frequently precedes the adrenal disease *(32)*. Indeed, ovarian failure could precede the onset of Addison's disease by 8–14 years *(14)*.

Considering the particular association with Addison's disease and the clinical features previously described, autoimmune POF will be divided into two different groups in this chapter: (1) POF associated with adrenal autoimmunity and (2) POF not associated with adrenal autoimmunity. In addition, ROS will be discussed as a separate immunological entity.

POF Associated with Adrenal Autoimmunity

DETECTION OF AUTOANTIBODIES

Patients with idiopathic Addison's disease have antibodies reacting with the adrenal cortex (ACA) as detailed in Chaps. 14–17. If Addison's disease is associated with other endocrine autoimmune diseases, leading to APS-I or APS-II, the antibodies may recognize all steroid-producing cells *(41)*. Since the first reports on patients with

POF and an associated adrenal autoimmune disease, these antibodies that recognize several types of steroid-producing cells of the adrenal cortex, testis, placenta, and ovary have been called "steroid cell antibodies" (SCA) *(42,43)*. In patients with adrenal autoimmunity, SCA generally correlate with the presence of gonadal failure (hypergonadotropic hypogonadism) *(38,44)*. SCA can be detected in 60–80% of APS-I patients and in 25–40% of APS-II patients *(14)*, but the highest prevalence is in patients with both Addison's disease and POF *(38,43)*. In two long-term studies, it has been shown that 33–43% of normally cycling women with APS and SCA develop POF within 8–15 years *(38,45)*, suggesting that, in patients with adrenal failure, the presence of these antibodies constitutes a risk factor for POF. In addition, there is an absolute association between the presence of SCA and that of ACA, the former being detected only when the latter is also present *(14)*. These SCA are of the immunoglobulin (Ig)G type and localize within the ovary to the hilar cells, the cells of the developing follicle, such as theca and granulosa cells, and the corpus luteum cells *(43,46)*. They are associated with histological evidence of an oophoritis (*see* Ovarian Histology).

The finding that sera of patients with ovarian failure and Addison's disease, with high titers of SCA and ACA, are cytotoxic for cultured granulosa cells in the presence of complement *(47)* suggests that complement-dependent cytotoxicity might be one of the mechanism of SCA leading to destruction of steroid-producing cells and, consequently, to ovarian failure.

The particular localization of SCA has led to the hypothesis that they could recognize some steroidogenic enzymes. Three different steroidogenic enzymes, including P450-side chain cleavage (SCC), P450-17-OH, and 3β-hydroxysteroid-dehydrogenase (3-HSD) have been identified as possible antigens *(48–51)*. At present, most authors agree with the interpretation that 17-OH and SCC are the main molecular targets of SCA *(52,53) (14,54,55)*. Nevertheless, in about 10% of SCA-positive patients, neither 17-OH nor SCC antibodies were detected, suggesting that other autoantigens might be recognized by SCA (Table 1). Another steroidogenic enzyme, 3-HSD, could also be an autoimmune target. Antibodies to 3-HSD were first detected in 21% of 48 patients with idiopathic POF *(51)*. However, the rare occurrence of these antibodies in POF patients was initially suggested by Peterson et al. *(53)* and subsequently confirmed by other groups *(54,56)* (Table 1). Despite this low incidence, 3-HSD might also be one of the targets of SCA, given that in these two recent studies, patients with anti-3-HSD antibodies were also positive for SCA. Nevertheless, these findings should be confirmed. The reported high prevalence of SCA in patients whose POF is associated with adrenal autoimmunity suggests the existence of one specific form of POF associated with steroidogenic cell autoimmunity.

OVARIAN HISTOLOGY

In cases where POF is associated with adrenal autoimmunity, histological examination almost always confirms the persistence of ovarian follicles and shows clear signs of an autoimmune oophoritis *(14,32,57,58)*. The ovaries from women with autoimmune oophoritis may be enlarged, sometimes with cystic change, or of normal size. Histological examination shows a mononuclear chronic inflammatory cell infiltrate around developing and atretic follicles, with complete sparing of primordial follicles. In the earlier lesions, the infiltrate is principally in the thecal layer, but in more advanced

Table 1

Prevalence of SCA Detected by Indirect Immunofluoresce and of Autoantibodies to Cytochromes P450-SCC, P450c17, and to 3-HSD Detected by Immunoblotting or Immunoprecipitation of Recombinant Autoantigens in POF Patients

Authors	Patients	SCA	anti-17-OH	anti-SCC	anti-3-HSD
Winqvist et al., 1995 (86)	3 POF with AA	3/3	0/3	2/3	n.a.
Chen et al., 1996 (52)	12 POF with AA	12/12	11/12 positive for 17-OH and/or SCC	11/12 positive for 17-OH and/or SCC	n.a.
	17 isolated POF	0/17	1/17	0/17	n.a.
Arif et al., 1996 (51)	48 isolated POF	1/48	n.a.	n.a.	10/48[a]
Peterson et al., 1997 (53)	11 POF with AA	n.a.	11/11 positive for 17-OH and/or SCC	11/11 positive for 17-OH and/or SCC	0/11
Reimand et al., 2000 (56)	6 POF with AA	2/6	0/6	0/6	1/6
	5 POF with non-AA	0/5	0/5	0/5	0/5
	30 isolated POF	0/30	0/30	0/30	0/30
Falorni et al., 2002 (54)	24 POF with AA	21/24	12/24	17/24	2/24
	21 non-AA POF	0/21	0/21	0/21	0/21
	36 isolated POF	0/36	0/36	1/36	1/36
Dal Pra et al., 2003 (55)	15 POF with AA	11/15	14/15 positive for 17-OH and/or SCC	14/15 positive for 17-OH and/or SCC	n.a.
	26 POF with non-AA	2/26[b]	3/26[b] positive for 17-OH and/or SCC	3/26[b] positive for 17-OH and/or SCC	n.a.
	31 isolated POF	3/31[b]	3/31[b] positive for 17-OH and/or SCC	3/31[b] positive for 17-OH and/or SCC	n.a.

ACA, adrenal cortex antibodies; POF, premature ovarian failure; AA, adrenal autoimmunity; non-AA, non-adrenal autoimmunity; SCA, steroid-cell antibodies; anti-17-OH, antibodies directed to P450-17α-hydroxylase; anti-SCC, antibodies directed to P450-side chain cleavage; anti-3-HSD, antibodies directed to 3β-hydroxysteroid-dehydrogenase; n.a., data not available.

[a]Three patients had hypothyroidism, two of these three patients presented anti-3-HSD antibodies.

[b]All SCA, anti-17-OH and/or anti-SCC antibody-positive patients were also positive for ACA and anti-21-OH, suggesting the presence of a sub-clinical autoimmune adrenal failure.

lesions, the granulosa cell layer is also infiltrated, and many of the follicular cells show degenerative changes. The inflammatory infiltrate does not extend into the stroma, although a hilar infiltrate, presumably related to the endocrine hilar cells, may be present.

The intensity of the inflammatory infiltrate seems to increase with follicle maturation; preantral follicles are surrounded by small rims of lymphocytes and plasma cells, whereas larger follicles have a progressively denser infiltrate, usually in the external and internal theca. Atretic follicles and, when present, corpora lutea are infiltrated as well (14,57,59). This pattern of infiltration confirms that steroid-producing cells are a main target for the autoimmune attack. Immunocytochemical staining identifies the cells as polyclonal B cells, CD4[+] and CD8[+] lymphocytes (with a predominance of the former), macrophages, and occasional NK cells. The overall appearances are suggestive of an antibody-dependent cell-mediated cytotoxicity (57).

CONCLUSIONS

In view of the previously described observations, it is clear that POF, when associated with Addison's disease and/or adrenal autoimmunity (only 2–10% of cases), is almost certainly an endocrine autoimmune disorder (14,32,58). The histological picture of ovaries of such cases (lymphocytic infiltrate particularly around steroid-producing cells), the presence of autoantibodies to steroid-producing cells in these patients, and the characterization of shared autoantigens between adrenal and ovarian steroid-producing cells, all support the proposed concept. Autoimmune oophoritis associated with autoimmune adrenalitis may be a clear-cut clinical and immunological entity, which can quite legitimately be extended to include patients with polyendocrinopathy with both ovarian and adrenal failure and to cases of POF with circulating antiadrenal antibodies but no clinical evidence of adrenal failure (57).

POF Not Associated with Adrenal Autoimmunity

DETECTION OF AUTOANTIBODIES

Even though steroidogenic enzymes represent autoimmune targets in the ovary, their pathophysiological significance seems to be restricted to patients whose ovarian failure is associated with adrenal autoimmunity. In patients whose POF is associated with autoimmune pathologies other than Addison's disease (38,54,55), as well as in isolated POF (38,39,54,55), SCA are almost undetectable (Table 1).

The presence of circulating antibodies directed toward other ovarian antigens has long been considered a suitable marker to identify the participation of an immunological mechanism in POF. In previous studies from our laboratory, by Western blot using human ovarian cytosolic fraction, we have detected specific reactivity against a ~50 kDa antigen in 19.1% of sera from 110 POF patients (60–62). In an attempt to identify the ovarian antigen, proteins of the human ovary homogenate were separated by ion chromatography and, after concentration and enrichment of the fraction of interest, the possible ovarian antigen was analyzed by mass spectrometry. Our recent results indicate that α-enolase may be the molecular target of these anti-ovarian antibodies. Determination of the pressure of circulating anti-α-enolase antibodies might be instrumental in identifying those patients who may present a putative defect in immunoregulation and therefore a possible autoimmune etiology for POF (63).

Several other investigators have found circulating antibodies directed toward human ovarian tissue in the sera from patients with ovarian infertility *(20,23–25)*. Reported antigenic ovarian structures include the oocyte *(64,65)*, corpus luteum *(43,47,66)*, theca cells *(23,43,66,67)*, granulosa cells *(64,66)*, zona pellucida *(68)*, gonadotropins *(69–71)*, and gonadotropin receptors *(72–76)*. Nevertheless, the pathogenic role of these antibodies remains questionable. Despite considerable scientific work, the detection of antiovarian antibodies still produces conflicting results, and neither their specificity nor their diagnostic significance has so far been unanimously established.

OVARIAN HISTOLOGY

Cases of lymphocytic oophoritis can hardly be found in POF patients in the absence of adrenal autoimmunity/Addison's disease. Indeed, histological oophoritis was documented in only six patients whose POF was not associated with adrenal autoimmunity, among 215 cases of POF from 18 studies published between 1965 and 1991 *(14)*. However, the rarity of inflammatory infiltrates in these patients does not exclude the possibility of an autoimmune mechanism. Even though follicular depletion could be the consequence of non-autoimmune etiologies (i.e., genetic or environmental factors), it might also represent the end stage of an autoimmune process directed against ovarian antigens, after the inflammation has ceased.

Approximately 60% of POF patients without adrenal autoimmunity lack ovarian follicles *(14)*. These ovaries are usually small and without macroscopically visible follicles. Histologically, the cortical stroma is hypercellular and devoid of follicular structures; atretic follicles and corporea albicans may, however, be present *(57)*. Conversely, in about 40% of women with POF in the absence of adrenal autoimmunity, ovarian follicles are detectable, and numbers vary from few to numerous *(14)*. About 10% of such follicular cases have numerous follicles, probably indicating a resistant ovary syndrome.

CONCLUSIONS

The reported frequent occurrence of POF in patients with two or more associated autoimmune diseases has currently been considered positive evidence of POF not associated to adrenal failure representing an endocrine autoimmune disease *(21,77)*. Even though the frequent relationship between POF and different autoimmune disorders might suggest that all of them are different manifestations of a single immunologic disorder, data need to be confirmed and their relevance investigated. In addition, the presence of antibodies to ovarian structures in serum of these patients would support an autoimmune etiology for isolated POF. However, the major conclusion drawn from several investigations is that although antibodies to ovarian antigens are common in POF, their pathophysiological significance remains obscure; it is yet to be determined whether they are related to, associated with, or a consequence of the processes leading to POF *(27)*.

Additional positive evidence is given by the fact that isolated cases of POF show cellular immune abnormalities similar to other endocrine autoimmune diseases such as T1D, Graves' disease, and Addison's disease. These cellular immune abnormalities include abnormalities in number and/or function of peripheral monocytes, monocyte-derived DC, and subsets of T cells and B cells *(14)*. In conclusion, there is evidence which, although debateable, indicates that some cases of idiopathic POF, in the absence of adrenal autoimmunity, may belong to the group of endocrine autoimmune diseases. However, the pathogenic mechanism underlying the suspected immunological disorder that results in abnormal ovarian function in such cases is still unknown. In view of the evidence available to date, the label "autoimmune endocrinopathy" in cases of POF not associated to adrenal autoimmunity should be deferred until a clear mechanism of autoimmunity has been characterized. Thus, it is suggested that the diagnosis of autoimmune ovarian failure might be restricted to cases with antiadrenal steroid cells antibodies, except in the rare cases of ROS that are discussed below.

Resistant Ovary Syndrome

DETECTION OF AUTOANTIBODIES

In previous studies from our laboratory, we demonstrated the presence of circulating immunoglobulins that inhibited FSH binding to its receptor (Ig-FSHR), by blocking either the FSHR itself or a receptor-related membrane domain, in patients with ROS *(75,78–80)*. Recently, we developed a retrospective study on a group of 247 POF patients who were referred to our laboratory over the course of 20 years: we found that only 23 of them who had been previously diagnosed as ROS had such Ig-FSHR *(76)*. We therefore suggest that Ig-FSHR may be present in ROS patients. When we analyzed the variation of Ig-FSHR titer over time, we found that, although the serum samples maintained anti-FSH-receptor activity throughout the study, their titers waxed and waned with time, showing a fluctuating course of the disease (Fig. 1). Analysis of the antibody titers over time in each patient might be useful to select the best moment to start treatment.

The Scatchard plots obtained from the inhibition data of FSH ligand-binding experiments clearly demonstrated that the inhibitory activity of immunoglobulin fractions can be classified into two groups. One with "irreversible" inhibitory effect (with an apparent Ki a thousand times higher than the affinity constant for FSHR-binding interaction) that

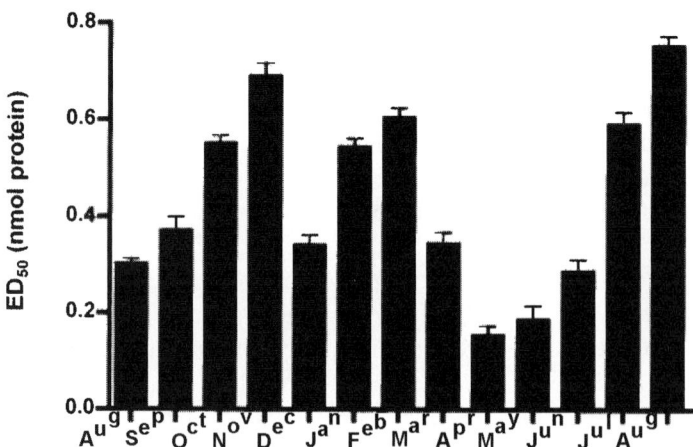

Fig. 1. Monthly profile of Ig-FSHR titer corresponding to ROS patient O. Ig-FSHR levels were determined by radio-receptor assay. Data are expressed as mean of $ED_{50} \pm$ SEM, where ED_{50} is the amount of immunoglobulin (Ig)G fraction (in nmoles) needed to reduce FSH binding by 50%.

could explain the ovary resistance in these patients, even to the elevated endogenous bioactive gonadotropin secretion as well as to exogenous administration. Another group of patients presented a "reversible" mechanism of inhibitory action (with an apparent Ki similar to the affinity constant for FSHR-binding interaction), suggesting that the administration of a high dose of gonadotropin may, at least temporarily, reverse ovarian resistance.

The presence of antibodies directed to the FSHR itself or to a receptor-related membrane domain in these patients is consistent with the clinical and histopathological manifestations of ROS and could therefore explain the failure of follicles to respond to FSH.

Previous evidence of autoantibodies that block the effects of FSH in patients with ROS was provided by van Weissenbruch et al. (72). In addition, reference to a serum antibody specifically directed against the FSHR in a patient with systemic lupus erythematosus and ROS had been previously made in a case report (74). Antibodies to the FSHR were also detected in the serum from a male patient with primary gonadal failure, using bovine testis membranes (81).

OVARIAN HISTOLOGY

At histological examination, the cortical stroma of the so-called "resistant ovaries" appear dense and fibrotic, with numerous follicles. Most follicles show no evidence of development, although a few will have attained the pre-antral stage, whereas occasional follicles will have developed into, but not surpassed, the antral stage. In cases of secondary amenorrhea, stigmata of previous ovulation are usually present (57). The stromal cells appear stimulated: hyperplastic in some areas and luteinized in others, with numerous clumps of well-differentiated hilus cells, probably indicative of high LH stimulation. The histological appearance of the ovaries suggests that the patients are not exposed to FSH stimulation (15).

CONCLUSIONS

The presence of antibodies directed to the FSHR may explain the ovarian resistance to high levels of endogenous FSH in ROS patients. ROS may therefore represent a rare case of autoimmune PDF, in which autoimmune may be directed aganist a cell-membrane receptor. Identification of ROS patients among other POF cases appears important, given that the presence of numerous follicular structures in these patients suggests that recovery of ovarian function, either spontaneously or induced, might be possible.

DIAGNOSIS

Clinical Examination

The presence of at least 6 months of amenorrhea and two consecutive serum FSH values >40 mIU/ml (obtained at least 1 month apart) in a woman under 40 years of age leads to the diagnosis of POF. A karyotype should be performed in all patients suffering from this syndrome, and a complete history should be recorded regarding prior ovarian surgery, chemotherapy, or radiation. A detailed record should also be obtained regarding autoimmune disorders. Diagnosis of an autoimmune etiology remains difficult and relies on several clinical, immunological, and histological features that should be investigated in these patients. It should include tests to diagnose possible concurrent autoimmune disorders, such as hypothyroidism, T1D, and Addison's disease. Particular attention should be paid to symptoms of adrenal failure, which may have a long insidious course before the disease becomes life-threatening.

Ovarian Examination

As previously explained, two subsets of POF patients can be identified: one with a total depletion of follicular structures, another with the presence of follicular structures, which suggest a clear possibility of return of ovarian functional activity *(14,57)*. A distinction into follicular and afollicular histological types seems therefore logical. Identification of autoimmune oophoritis would also be relevant as these patients may be potential responders to corticosteroid or immunosuppressive therapy. A striking characteristic of this specific form of autoimmune oophoritis is the well-established sparing of primordial follicles, despite the presence of intense lymphocytic infiltration in the theca of developing follicles *(57,59,82)*. This distinctive pathophysiological process presents the theoretical possibility of developing immunosuppressive treatments that could restore fertility.

However, ovarian biopsy is not currently indicated in clinical practice, because laparotomy introduces the hazard of future mechanical infertility, and biopsies have proved to be uninformative for either diagnosis or prognosis in as much as pregnancies have occurred after failure of follicle identification in biopsy *(36,57)*. The histological sections from an average ovarian biopsy comprise only 0.1% of a normal size ovary, and absence of follicles in this tissue does not necessarily mean that the ovary is totally depleted of primordial follicles. Ovarian biopsy can be argued to be necessary to identify cases of POF because of autoimmune oophoritis, for these patients may respond well to corticosteroid or other immunosuppressive therapy with a return of normal ovarian function. Diagnosis of POF should, however, rest mainly on serological findings, as in the case with autoimmune organ disease elsewhere in the body, for example, autoimmune adrenalitis.

Even though ovarian biopsy was claimed in a recent study as a reliable tool to evaluate patients with POF *(83)*, ultrasonography (US) remains the most current diagnostic tool in clinical practice. The advent of high-resolution US and the development of the transvaginal transducer have enhanced the ability to visualize the ovaries in fine detail. The presence of follicles on US may allow us to infer the likelihood of follicular activity, thus obviating the need for invasive diagnostic procedures *(36,84,85)*.

In patients with autoimmune POF, US examination may reveal ovarian enlargement because of autoimmune oophoritis *(14,58)*. Moreover, in a recent compilation of data from previous case reports, ovaries were described as normal sized in one-third of reported histologically confirmed cases of autoimmune oophoritis (10 of 29, 34%) and as enlarged in over one-half (17/29, 59%) *(58)*.

Determination of Autoantibodies

STEROID CELL ANTIBODIES

As already explained, patients with POF plus an associated adrenal autoimmune disease have antibodies that recognize several types of steroid-producing cells of the adrenal cortex, testis, placenta, and ovary, the so-called SCA. For many years, the indirect immunofluorescence technique (IIT) on cryostat sections of human and animal adrenal glands, ovary, testis, and placenta has represented the most reliable method for detection of SCA (38,42,43,50–52,55,56,86). Even though this technique is still currently in use, new assays have been developed since different steroidogenic enzymes were identified as possible targets of SCA. Thus, the prevalence of antibodies directed toward the different steroidogenic enzymes was first determined using bacterially expressed proteins in immunoblotting (50,86). The use of in vitro translated recombinant ^{35}S-labeled autoantigens in immunoprecipitation assays rapidly has replaced the former method (52,54–56).

The relationship between the autoantibodies detected by IIT and those detected by the new assays using recombinant autoantigens was investigated in a recent study (87). The authors studied 143 patients with autoimmune Addison's disease, 21 of them with APS-I and 55 with APS-II. ACA and SCA were measured by IIT, and autoantibodies to 21-OH, 17-OH, and SCC, by immunoprecipitation assay using ^{35}S-labeled recombinant proteins. They concluded that provided that a high standard of immunofluorescence is maintained, measurement of ACA or SCA by either IIT or immunoprecipitation assay is essentially equivalent.

ADRENAL CORTEX ANTIBODIES

A possible association between adrenal cortex autoantibodies (detected by ITT on cryostat sections of human and animal adrenal cortex glands) and histologically confirmed autoimmune oophoritis was suggested in several case reports. In a recent study, Bakalov et al. (58) reviewed several reported cases with histological diagnosis of autoimmune oophoritis and found that adrenal cortex autoantibodies, when tested, were present in all 24 reported cases. Moreover, the authors studied four additional POF cases and found a clear association between the two previously mentioned conditions (58), thereby reinforcing previous findings. They suggest that adrenal tissue would be significantly more sensitive as substrate than ovarian tissue in IIT to detect histologically confirmed autoimmune oophoritis. Thus, the presence of adrenal autoimmunity is proposed as a reasonable research marker for identifying POF women with autoimmune oophoritis as prospects for treatments aimed at restoring ovarian function and fertility.

ANTIOVARIAN ANTIBODIES

Several antiovarian antibodies (AOA) other than SCA have been detected in cases of POF not associated with adrenal autoimmunity, and numerous publications have been dealing with this subject since the early 1970s. Nevertheless, neither their specificity nor their diagnostic significance have so far been unanimously established. One of the reasons for these discordances is the diversity of the detection methods as well as the heterogeneity of patient and control groups in the different studies.

The first-described method used for the detection of AOA in serum from POF patients was a radioimmunoassay (RIA) using iodinated proteins from ovaries of normal women (20,88). Nevertheless, the IIT has become the most common method used for the detection of such antibodies (64,89–91). Frozen sections of ovaries are usually used as an antigen source. The method shows the localization of the antibodies in the various histological compartments of the ovary. However, the diverse origin of the tissue sections that include human, primate, bovine, porcine, rat, guinea-pig, and rabbit ovaries may explain the variations in the results of the prevalence, localization, and specificity of the detected antibodies *(32)*. Even with immunofluorescence on human ovary sections, the prevalence of AOA in the serum of POF patients may vary between 2 *(89)* and 50% (64) (Table 2).

Alternatively, homogenized human or animal ovarian tissues are used as a source of ovarian antigens in immunoenzymatic methods, such as enzyme-linked immunoabsorbent assays (ELISA) *(27,33,71,91,92)* (Table 2). Mixing ovarian tissues from different women at various ages and periods of their menstrual cycle provides a large panel of ovarian antigens, yielding more homogeneous results than immunofluorescence studies. Even though these ELISA-detected antibodies are detected in 30–67% of POF patients as compared with only 0–5% of healthy control subjects, their specificity remains questionable because of a degree of cross-reaction with tubal or even muscular antigens *(27,33,71,91)*. Indeed, they have also been detected in patients with iatrogenic POF or Turner syndrome *(33)*.

The comparison of results obtained by ELISA with those obtained by ITT suggested that neither is a robust test for the presence of AOA. Although some authors *(93)* described agreement between positivity in IIT and ELISA (94%), others found that despite some overlap between the two techniques, there were clear discrepancies *(91)*. Characterization of the target antigen or group of antigens involved in autoimmune POF would enable the development of a more reliable diagnostic test.

ELISA and IIT are able to detect one or several antibodies raised against one or several non-specific antigens. By Western blotting, on the contrary, it is possible to identify antibodies raised against a specific antigen. Nevertheless, while focusing on one specific antigen, antibodies directed to other molecular targets may not be detected by this technique. Western blotting utilizing human ovarian preparations has previously been used by Winqvist et al. *(86)* who identified a novel autoantigen of ∼51 kDa. In our laboratory, we developed a Western blot assay using human ovarian cytosolic fraction to detect specific reactivity against a ∼50-kDa antigen, recently identified as α-enolase. Antibodies to this enzyme were found in 19.1% of sera from 110 POF patients and in none of 60 normally menstruating women *(60–63)*. More studies would be necessary to further understand the clinical relevance and the pathological role played by these antibodies in POF disease.

Resistant Ovary Syndrome

Diagnosis of ROS was first supported by high gonadotropin levels in the presence of ovaries filled with numerous primordial follicles *(94)*. In the first patients reported with this disease, further evidence of ovarian resistance was revealed by the fact that attempts to stimulate ovulation with high doses of exogenous gonadotropins produced little or no response *(15,95,96)*. However, not only the response to stimulation with exogenous gonadotropin but also ovarian biopsy are investigative procedures not currently in use as diagnostic tools in cases of POF. Given that ovarian biopsy may give misleading results, US is currently used to tell ROS from other cases of POF. In patients with ROS, ovaries are usually macroscopically normal, although some are small *(57,85)*. US examination shows a hyperechogenic stroma and numerous small follicular images (<3 mm) at the periphery *(76,85)*.

Table 2
Detection of Antiovarian Antibodies by Different Assay Systems

Authors	Assay system	Substrate	AOA in POF	AOA in controls
Coulam et al., 1979 (20)	RIA	Human ovary homogenate	14/15	1/10 ncc
				3/12 pmc
Coulam et al., 1985 (88)	RIA	Human ovary homogenate	30/110	n.a.
Damewood et al., 1986 (64)	IIT	Human ovary sections	14/27	0/24 ncc
				1/22 pmc
Ho et al., 1988 (89)	IIT	Human ovary sections	1/45	0/45
Luborsky et al., 1990 (71)	ELISA	Human ovary homogenate/human oocytes	21/45	0/10 ncc
Kirsop et al., 1991 (90)	IIT	Monkey ovary sections	1/30	0/19 pmc
Wheatcroft et al., 1994 (33)	ELISA	Homogenates from two human ovaries	6/32 (ovary 1)	2/33 (ovary 1)
			18/32 (ovary 2)	2/41 (ovary 2)
Wheatcroft et al., 1997 (91)	IIT	Monkey ovary sections	5/42	0/10
Wheatcroft et al., 1997 (91)	ELISA	Human ovary homogenate	13/42	0/38
Fenichel et al., 1997 (27)	ELISA	Human ovary homogenate	27/46	4/23 ncc
Luborsky et al., 1999 (92)	ELISA	Human ovary homogenate	16/30	n.a.
Sundblad et al., 2003 (62, 63)	Western blot	Human ovary homogenate	21/110	0/60 ncc

AOA, antiovarian antibodies; RIA, radioimmunoassay; IIT, immunofluorescence technique; ELISA, enzyme-linked immunoabsorbent assay; ncc, normally clycing controls; pmc, post-menopausal controls; n.a., data not available; POF, premature ovarian failure.

Even though the advent of high-resolution US has enhanced the ability to visualize the ovaries in fine detail, the presence of primordial follicles can be inferred but not confirmed in ultrasonography examination; US allows visualization of follicles as small as 2 mm diameter *(84)*, but primordial follicle normal size is 30 μm. Consequently, the characterization of a clear mechanism of hormone resistance in these patients, namely the presence of antibodies directed to FSHR *(76)*, provides an important additional diagnostic tool needed for distinction between ROS and other POF cases. Our results obtained throughout a 20-year study suggest the determination of the presence of Ig–FSH by radio-receptor could be an instrument in diagnosing ROS mainly upon the basis of serological findings.

TREATMENT

Hormone Replacement Therapy

Young women with POF sustain sex steroid deficiency for a longer period than naturally menopausal women. Consequently, they need exogenous sex steroids to compensate for the decreased production by their ovaries, considering that these patients present a significantly higher risk of osteoporosis and cardiovascular disease. However, despite a regimen of standard hormone replacement therapy, about 33% of young patients have a significantly reduced Bone Mineral Density (BMD) *(97)*. Several reasons may explain this finding. On one hand, a significant bone loss may occur in the years preceding the development of ovarian failure (prodromal POF). In regularly menstruating women, the normal midcycle rise in free testosterone is markedly diminished in the decade preceding natural menopause, which is significantly related to the bone loss observed during this period. A similar prodrome of reduced testosterone production may underlie the bone loss associated with POF. Consequently, it is suggested that prodrome POF should be included in the differential diagnosis of menstrual irregularities, and early institution of sex hormone replacement, including estrogen and progesterone and probably also testosterone, may be indicated in these patients *(97)*. On the other hand, estrogen "under dosing" of women with POF may be a significant contributing factor to a reduced BMD. In women affected by this syndrome, estrogen should be administrated at a dose greater than the standard given to older women experiencing natural menopause, in an attempt to maintain bone mass as effectively as the normally functioning ovary *(6)*. Finally, another important factor that may contribute to bone loss in association with POF is a delay in diagnosis, which results in several years of amenorrhea without sex hormone replacement *(6)*.

Whether the patient has primary or secondary amenorrhea is determinant for optimal institutions of therapy. Young women with primary amenorrhea in whom secondary sex characteristics have failed to develop should initially be exposed to very low-dose estrogen in an attempt to mimic a gradual pubertal maturation process, with gradual incremental doses until the required maintenance dose. In patients with secondary amenorrhea, the important factor is the duration of estrogen deficiency. Women who have been estrogen-deficient for a year or more should also initially be given low-dose estrogen replacement to avoid unwanted side effects; however, they can be titrated up to the maintenance dose over a shorter period than those with primary amenorrhea. Conversely, women with a brief history of amenorrhea are less likely to experience unwanted side effects with hormone replacement and can therefore be titrated up to the maintenance dose over an even shorter period *(6)*.

Given that estrogens provided in usual replacement doses are not contraceptive and will not suppress spontaneous follicular activity in ovulation and that a progestin should be given each month to prevent endometria hyperplasia, the hormone replacement therapy should produce regular predictable menstrual flow patterns. Moreover, considering that women with POF can have spontaneous pregnancies, if an expected menses is missed, the patient should be tested for pregnancy.

In women experiencing persistent fatigue, poor well being, and low libido despite adequate estrogen replacement, androgen replacement should also be considered. Appropriate androgen replacement does not result in virilization or unwanted metabolic effects *(98)*. In addition, testosterone replacement may be important for preservation of bone mineral content *(99)*. Hormone replacement therapy should be continued at least until the average age of natural menopause (approximately 50 years old) with an appropriate long-term follow-up of the patient's condition.

Infertility-Related Therapy

There is a 5–10% chance for spontaneous pregnancy in women with POF. Indeed, hormone replacement therapy does not prevent conception *(10–12)*; POF patients may even conceive while taking oral contraceptives *(100)*. Even though there is no known immunomodulating therapy for autoimmune POF that has been proven safe and effective by prospective randomized placebo-controlled study, immunosuppression using corticosteroids has long been used on an empirical basis for this condition (Table 3). In two patients with hypergonadotropic secondary amenorrhea and perifollicular lymphocytic infiltrate, menses resumed after only 1 month of corticosteroid therapy, but no pregnancy could be achieved *(26,101)*. A patient with APS who had first documented ovarian failure at age 28 years and had been therefore treated with estrogen replacement therapy for >15 years, resumed menses after 1 year of corticosteroid therapy for Addisonian crisis, conceived, and delivered a normal infant *(102)*. In another report, two patients with POF became pregnant and delivered a healthy infant after high-dose corticotherapy; however, POF resumed after delivery in both cases *(71)*. More recently, a patient with histologically proven autoimmune oophoritis was treated with alternate day glucocorticoid treatment and resumed menstrual bleeding six times and ovulated four times over a 16-week period, but did not get pregnant *(103)*. In addition, a pregnancy and delivery has also been obtained after IVF under corticosteroid treatment in a patient with antiovarian autoimmunity *(104)*. Regarding our own experience, a POF patient with 6 years of amenorrhea and high levels of AOA received high-dose, short-term immunosupressing therapy with Deltisona B. She resumed menstrual bleeding and became pregnant, coincidentally with a decrease in serum AOA concentration (Fig. 2) (unpublished data).

Even though identifying patients with autoimmune POF presents the opportunity to restore ovarian function, treating these patients with the proper immune modulation therapy can have major complications *(103)*. Corticosteroid therapy for autoimmune POF should be used in placebo-controlled trials designed to evaluate the safety and efficacy of such treatment. The only randomized, placebo-controlled trial using corticosteroids and hMG in 36 idiopathic POF patients for 2 weeks failed to show any positive effect as none of these patients became pregnant and did not even ovulate under the treatment *(105)*. However, the presence of specific AOA had not been assessed in these patients.

Table 3
Immunomodulating Theraphy with Corticosteroids in POF Patients

Authors	Patients	Possible evidence of autoimmune etiology			Main outcome
		OB	AAD	AOA	
Coulam et al., 1981 *(26)*	1	Oophoritis	Adrenal	+	RM, 2 menstrual cycles, no pregnancy
Rabinowe et al., 1986 *(101)*	1	Oophoritis	None	+	RM, 10 menstrual cycles, no pregnancy
Cowchock et al., 1988 *(102)*	1	n.a.	Adrenal	n.a.	RM, normal pregnancy and delivery
Luborsky et al., 1990 *(71)*	2	n.a.	Diabetes, Graves'	+	RM, normal pregnancy and delivery
		n.a.	None	+	RM, normal pregnancy and delivery
Barbarino-Monnier et al., 1995 *(104)*	1	n.a.	None	+	Pregnancy by IVF and normal delivery
Kalantaridou et al., 1999 *(103)*	2	Oophoritis	n.a.	n.a.	RM, 6 cycles, no pregnancy
		n.a.	Thyroid	n.a.	No RM, knee osteonecrosis
Corenblum et al., 1993 *(106)*	11	n.a.	RA (1) Thyroid (4)	n.a.	RM and normal pregnancy in 2/11
Blumenfeld et al., 1993 *(107)*	15	n.a.	ITC (1) Thyroid (6)	n.a.	14 pregnancies in 8 patients, 12 healthy babies
Van Kasteren et al., 1999 *(105)*	36	n.a.	None	n.a.	No ovulation, no pregnancy in anyone
Charreau et al., unpublished data -	1	n.a.	None	+	RM and normal pregnancy

OB, ovarian biopsy; AAD, autoimmune associated disease; AOA, anti-ovarian antibodies; RA, rheumatoid arthritis; ITC, idiopathic thrombocytopenia; RM, regular menses; n.a., data not available.

Besides this placebo-controlled trial, two uncontrolled trials have been carried out among chromosomally normal POF patients. In one study, two of 11 idiopathic POF patients receiving high-dose, short-term treatment with corticosteroids for 2 weeks resumed ovarian function and became pregnant *(106)*. In the other trial, 15 POF patients with various autoimmune markers—which suggested an autoimmune etiology to the ovarian failure—were treated with combinations of hMG/hCG and glucocorticosteroids. Fourteen pregnancies were achieved in eight patients, and 12 healthy babies were generated by 10 gestations *(107)*.

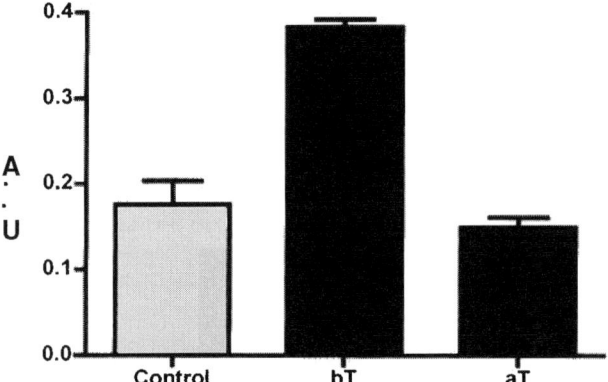

Fig. 2. Circulating antiovarian antibodies (AOA) and immunosuppressive therapy. Premature ovarian failure (POF) patient T received immunosupressing therapy with Deltisona B. AOA were determined by immunoblotting using human ovary homogenate and signal amplification by biotin-extravidin-peroxidase system. Intensity was quantified with a gel scan densitometer. An acute decrease in serum AOA concentration was observed after treatment. bT, levels of AOA before treatment; aT, levels of AOA after treatment; Control, levels of AOA in normally menstruating women. A. U. Absorbance units data are expressed as mean ± SEM.

In addition, there are only few reports on successful ovulation-inducing treatments of selected POF patients (those with concomitant autoimmune phenomena) with other immunomodulating therapies, such as plasmapheresis and/or thymectomy *(108,109)*. In our laboratory, we studied a patient with ROS and high levels of Ig-FSHR who had myasthenia gravis and autoimmune thyroiditis associated to ROS condition. She underwent thymectomy after 5 years of amenorrhea. Interestingly, 2 years after surgery, she showed an acute reduction in Ig-FSHR titer (Fig. 3) and resumed menses (unpublished data).

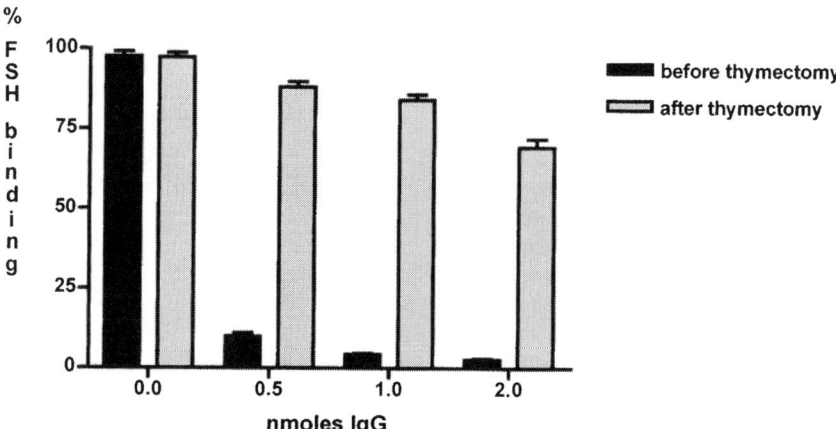

Fig. 3. Determination of Ig-FSHR in a ROS patient who underwent thymectomy. Ig-FSHR were determined by radio-receptor assay. Two years after surgery, the patient showed an acute reduction in Ig-FSHR titer and resumed menses. Data are expressed as mean ± SEM.

Patients with POF wishing to get pregnant are best served by assisted reproductive technology utilizing donor oocytes. To date, oocyte donation is the only proven therapy for such patients; pregnancy rates have been quite high, ranging from 25 to 35% *(8,110)* However, patients should be informed that, in some cases, spontaneous pregnancy may occur and that, if they choose to wait for a while before proceeding, oocyte donation is as successful in older as in younger women *(6)*. In a recent retrospective study, sisters of women with POF have shown to be inappropriate donors, because they presented elevated day 3 FSH levels and poor ovarian response to gonadotropin stimulation *(110)*.

FUTURE DEVELOPMENTS

POF in the presence of Addison's disease and/or adrenal autoimmunity is almost certainly an endocrine autoimmune disorder. However, the question whether a true autoimmune POF occurs which is independent of antiadrenal antibodies is controversial. Several circulating antibodies directed toward different antigenic ovarian structures have been described in POF patients without adrenal autoimmunity. Although these antibodies are common, their pathogenic role remains questionable; neither their specificity nor their diagnostic significance has been unanimously established. Thus, no currently available validated serum antibody marker can confirm a clinical diagnosis of autoimmune POF in such cases. Further investigation into these ovarian targets may lead not only to a better understanding of the pathogenic mechanism that may result in ovarian injury but also to the development of more accurate diagnostic tools to determine the real prevalence of autoimmune etiology in ovarian disease. A precocious and reliable diagnosis of an autoimmune etiology is required to select the patients in whom immune-modulating therapy may, a least temporarily, restore ovarian function and fertility.

Several pieces of evidence suggest that POF associated with steroidogenic cell autoimmunity is a potentially reversible cause of ovarian failure. A research test that could select POF women with this specific form of autoimmune oophoritis with reasonable certainty, thus avoiding the need of ovarian biopsy, would facilitate clinical research toward developing a therapy. Even though the presence of adrenal autoimmunity by IIT is proposed as a reasonable research marker for identifying POF women with autoimmune oophoritis, these results should be confirmed. If so, a validated serum antibody marker to achieve a clinical diagnosis of autoimmune POF in the presence of adrenal autoimmunity would be available.

Treatment with glucocorticoids and replacement therapy with estrogen and progesterone have resulted in resumption of menses and made pregnancy possible in isolated instances. Nevertheless, at this time, no immune modulation therapy for infertile patients with autoimmune ovarian failure has proven effective in a prospective controlled study. Accurate diagnostic tools are needed to analyze the effect of corticosteroids in a selected population of well-defined autoimmune POF patients. In addition, other forms of treatment may be found to be effective after further knowledge can be had about the pathophysiological mechanisms of this autoimmune disorder.

REFERENCES

1. Pettersson F, Fries H, Nillius SJ. Epidemiology of secondary amenorrhea. I. Incidence and prevalence rates. *Am J Obstet Gynecol* 1973; 117:80–86.

2. Bachmann GA, Kemmann E. Prevalence of oligomenorrhea and amenorrhea in a college population. *Am J Obstet Gynecol* 1982; 144:98–102.

3. Current evaluation of amenorrhea. *Fertil Steril* 2004; 82:266–272.

4. Moraes-Ruehsen M, Jones GS. Premature ovarian failure. *Fertil Steril* 1967; 18:440–461.

5. Yen SS, Tsai CC, Vandenberg G, Rebar R. Gonadotropin dynamics in patients with gonadal dysgenesis: a model for the study of gonadotropin regulation. *J Clin Endocrinol Metab* 1972; 35:897–904.

6. Kalantaridou SN, Davis SR, Nelson LM. Premature ovarian failure. *Endocrinol Metab Clin North Am* 1998; 27:989–1006.

7. Rebar RW, Connolly HV. Clinical features of young women with hypergonadotropic amenorrhea. *Fertil Steril* 1990; 53:804–810.

8. Rebar RW, Cedars MI. Hypergonadotropic forms of amenorrhea in young women. *Endocrinol Metab Clin North Am* 1992; 21:173–191.

9. Nelson LM, Anasti JN, Kimzey LM, et al. Development of luteinized graafian follicles in patients with karyotypically normal spontaneous premature ovarian failure. *J Clin Endocrinol Metab* 1994; 79:1470–1475.

10. Alper MM, Jolly EE, Garner PR. Pregnancies after premature ovarian failure. *Obstet Gynecol* 1986; 67:59S–62S.

11. Kreiner D, Droesch K, Navot D, Scott R, Rosenwaks Z. Spontaneous and pharmacologically induced remissions in patients with premature ovarian failure. *Obstet Gynecol* 1988; 72:926–928.

12. Ohsawa M, Wu MC, Masahashi T, Asai M, Narita O. Cyclic therapy resulted in pregnancy in premature ovarian failure. *Obstet Gynecol* 1985; 66:64S–67S.

13. Kinch RA, Plunkett ER, Smout MS, Carr DH. Primary ovarian failure; a clinicopathological and cytogenetic study. *Am J Obstet Gynecol* 1965; 91:630–644.

14. Hoek A, Schoemaker J, Drexhage HA. Premature ovarian failure and ovarian autoimmunity. *Endocr Rev* 1997; 18:107–134.

15. Jones GS, Moraes-Ruehsen M. A new syndrome of amenorrhae in association with hypergonadotropism and apparently normal ovarian follicular apparatus. *Am J Obstet Gynecol* 1969; 104:597–600.

16. Koninckx PR, Brosens IA. The "gonadotropin-resistant ovary" syndrome as a cause of secondary amenorrhea and infertility. *Fertil Steril* 1977; 28:926–931.

17. Christin-Maitre S, Vasseur C, Portnoi MF, Bouchard P. Genes and premature ovarian failure. *Mol Cell Endocrinol* 1998; 145:75–80.

18. Anasti JN. Premature ovarian failure: an update. *Fertil Steril* 1998; 70:1–15.

19. Waggoner DD, Buist NR, Donnell GN. Long-term prognosis in galactosaemia: results of a survey of 350 cases. *J Inherit Metab Dis* 1990; 13:802–818.

20. Coulam CB, Ryan RJ. Premature menopause. I. Etiology. *Am J Obstet Gynecol* 1979; 133:639–643.

21. LaBarbera AR, Miller MM, Ober C, Rebar RW. Autoimmune etiology in premature ovarian failure. *Am J Reprod Immunol Microbiol* 1988; 16:115–122.

22. Coulam CB. The prevalence of autoimmune disorders among patients with primary ovarian failure. *Am J Reprod Immunol* 1983; 4:63–66.

23. Kamp P, Platz P, Nerup J. "Steroid-cell" antibody in endocrine diseases. *Acta Endocrinol (Copenh)* 1974; 76:729–740.

24. Board JA, Redwine FO, Moncure CW, Frable WJ, Taylor JR. Identification of differing etiologies of clinically diagnosed premature menopause. *Am J Obstet Gynecol* 1979; 134:936–944.

25. Elder M, Maclaren N, Riley W. Gonadal autoantibodies in patients with hypogonadism and/or Addison's disease. *J Clin Endocrinol Metab* 1981; 52:1137–1142.

26. Coulam CB, Kempers RD, Randall RV. Premature ovarian failure: evidence for the autoimmune mechanism. *Fertil Steril* 1981; 36:238–240.

27. Fenichel P, Sosset C, Barbarino-Monnier P et al. Prevalence, specificity and significance of ovarian antibodies during spontaneous premature ovarian failure. *Hum Reprod* 1997; 12:2623–2628.

28. Coulam CB, Adamson SC, Annegers JF. Incidence of premature ovarian failure. *Obstet Gynecol* 1986; 67:604–606.

29. Krailo MD, Pike MC. Estimation of the distribution of age at natural menopause from prevalence data. *Am J Epidemiol* 1983; 117:356–361.

30. Cramer DW, Xu H. Predicting age at menopause. *Maturitas* 1996; 23:319–326.

31. Luborsky JL, Meyer P, Sowers MF, Gold EB, Santoro N. Premature menopause in a multi-ethnic population study of the menopause transition. *Hum Reprod* 2003; 18:199–206.

32. Forges T, Monnier-Barbarino P, Faure GC, Bene MC. Autoimmunity and antigenic targets in ovarian pathology. *Hum Reprod Update* 2004; 10:163–175.

33. Wheatcroft NJ, Toogood AA, Li TC, Cooke ID, Weetman AP. Detection of antibodies to ovarian antigens in women with premature ovarian failure. *Clin Exp Immunol* 1994; 96:122–128.

34. Luborsky J. Ovarian autoimmune disease and ovarian autoantibodies. *J Womens Health Gend Based Med* 2002; 11:585–599.

35. Aiman J, Smentek C. Premature ovarian failure. *Obstet Gynecol* 1985; 66:9–14.

36. Conway GS, Kaltsas G, Patel A, Davies MC, Jacobs HS. Characterization of idiopathic premature ovarian failure. *Fertil Steril* 1996; 65:337–341.

37. Alper MM, Garner PR. Premature failure: its relationship to autoimmune disease. *Obstet Gynecol* 1985; 66:27–30.

38. Betterle C, Rossi A, Dalla PS, et al. Premature ovarian failure: autoimmunity and natural history. *Clin Endocrinol (Oxf)* 1993; 39:35–43.

39. de Moraes RM, Blizzard RM, Garcia-Bunuel R, Jones GS. Autoimmunity and ovarian failure. *Am J Obstet Gynecol* 1972; 112:693–703.

40. Rebar RW, Erickson GF, Yen SS. Idiopathic premature ovarian failure: clinical and endocrine characteristics. *Fertil Steril* 1982; 37:35–41.

41. Uibo R, Perheentupa J, Ovod V, Krohn KJ. Characterization of adrenal autoantigens recognized by sera from patients with autoimmune polyglandular syndrome (APS) type I. *J Autoimmun* 1994; 7:399–411.

42. Irvine WJ, Chan MM, Scarth L, et al. Immunological aspects of premature ovarian failure associated with idiopathic Addison's disease. *Lancet* 1968; 2:883–887.

43. Sotsiou F, Bottazzo GF, Doniach D. Immunofluorescence studies on autoantibodies to steroid-producing cells, and to germline cells in endocrine disease and infertility. *Clin Exp Immunol* 1980; 39:97–111.

44. Betterle C, Volpato M. Adrenal and ovarian autoimmunity. *Eur J Endocrinol* 1998; 138:16–25.

45. Ahonen P, Miettinen A, Perheentupa J. Adrenal and steroidal cell antibodies in patients with autoimmune polyglandular disease type I and risk of adrenocortical and ovarian failure. *J Clin Endocrinol Metab* 1987; 64:494–500.

46. Irvine WJ, Chan MM, Scarth L. The further characterization of autoantibodies reactive with extra-adrenal steroid-producing cells in patients with adrenal disorders. *Clin Exp Immunol* 1969; 4:489–503.

47. McNatty KP, Short RV, Barnes EW, Irvine WJ. The cytotoxic effect of serum from patients with Addison's disease and autoimmune ovarian failure on human granulosa cells in culture. *Clin Exp Immunol* 1975; 22:378–384.

48. Krohn K, Uibo R, Aavik E, Peterson P, Savilahti K. Identification by molecular cloning of an autoantigen associated with Addison's disease as steroid 17 alpha-hydroxylase. *Lancet* 1992; 339:770–773.

49. Winqvist O, Gustafsson J, Rorsman F, Karlsson FA, Kampe O. Two different cytochrome P450 enzymes are the adrenal antigens in autoimmune polyendocrine syndrome type I and Addison's disease. *J Clin Invest* 1993; 92:2377–2385.

50. Uibo R, Aavik E, Peterson P, et al. Autoantibodies to cytochrome P450 enzymes P450scc, P450c17, and P450c21 in autoimmune polyglandular disease types I and II and in isolated Addison's disease. *J Clin Endocrinol Metab* 1994; 78:323–328.

51. Arif S, Vallian S, Farzaneh F, et al. Identification of 3 beta-hydroxysteroid dehydrogenase as a novel target of steroid cell autoantibodies: association of autoantibodies with endocrine autoimmune disease. *J Clin Endocrinol Metab* 1996; 81:4439–4445.

52. Chen S, Sawicka J, Betterle C, et al. Autoantibodies to steroidogenic enzymes in autoimmune polyglandular syndrome, Addison's disease, and premature ovarian failure. *J Clin Endocrinol Metab* 1996; 81:1871–1876.

53. Peterson P, Uibo R, Peranen J, Krohn K. Immunoprecipitation of steroidogenic enzyme autoantigens with autoimmune polyglandular syndrome type I (APS I) sera; further evidence for independent humoral immunity to P450c17 and P450c21. *Clin Exp Immunol* 1997; 107: 335–340.

54. Falorni A, Laureti S, Candeloro P, et al. Steroid-cell autoantibodies are preferentially expressed in women with premature ovarian failure who have adrenal autoimmunity. *Fertil Steril* 2002; 78:270–279.

55. Dal Pra C, Chen S, Furmaniak J, et al. Autoantibodies to steroidogenic enzymes in patients with premature ovarian failure with and without Addison's disease. *Eur J Endocrinol* 2003; 148: 565–570.

56. Reimand K, Peterson P, Hyoty H, et al. 3beta-hydroxysteroid dehydrogenase autoantibodies are rare in premature ovarian failure. *J Clin Endocrinol Metab* 2000; 85:2324–2326.

57. Fox H. The pathology of premature ovarian failure. *J Pathol* 1992; 167:357–363.

58. Bakalov VK, Anasti JN, Calis KA, et al. Autoimmune oophoritis as a mechanism of follicular dysfunction in women with 46,XX spontaneous premature ovarian failure. *Fertil Steril* 2005; 84:958–965.

59. Gloor E, Hurlimann J. Autoimmune oophoritis. *Am J Clin Pathol* 1984; 81:105–109.

60. Bussmann L, Chiauzzi V, Cortelezzi M, Comparato M, Charreau EH. Autoinmunidad y Falla Ovárica. *Medicina (Buenos Aires)* 1991; 51:471.

61. Bussmann L, Chiauzzi VA, Charreau EH. Anticuerpos antiovario y falla ovárica prematura. *Medicina (Buenos Aires)* 1998; 58:608.

62. Sundblad V, Chiauzzi V, Bussmann L, Charreau E. Identificación de un autoantígeno ovárico en pacientes con falla ovárica prematura (POF). *Medicina (Buenos Aires)* 2003; 63:633.

63. Damewood MD, Zacur HA, Hoffman GJ, Rock JA. Circulating antiovarian antibodies in premature ovarian failure. *Obstet Gynecol* 1986; 68:850–854.

64. Vallotton MB, Forbes AP. Antibodies to cytoplasm of ova. *Lancet* 1966; 2:264–265.

65. Drury MI, Keelan DM, Timoney FJ, Irvine WJ. Juvenile familial endocrinopathy. *Clin Exp Immunol* 1970; 7:125–132.

66. Williamson HO, Phansey SA, Mathur S, et al. Myasthenia gravis, premature menopause, and thyroid autoimmunity. *Am J Obstet Gynecol* 1980; 137:893–901.

67. Kamada M, Daitoh T, Mori K, et al. Etiological implication of autoantibodies to zona pellucida in human female infertility. *Am J Reprod Immunol* 1992; 28:104–109.

68. Gobert B, Jolivet-Reynaud C, Dalbon P, et al. An immunoreactive peptide of the FSH involved in autoimmune infertility. *Biochem Biophys Res Commun* 2001; 289:819–824.

69. Meyer WR, Lavy G, DeCherney AH, et al. Evidence of gonadal and gonadotropin antibodies in women with a suboptimal ovarian response to exogenous gonadotropin. *Obstet Gynecol* 1990; 75:795–799.

70. Luborsky JL, Visintin I, Boyers S, et al. Ovarian antibodies detected by immobilized antigen immunoassay in patients with premature ovarian failure. *J Clin Endocrinol Metab* 1990; 70:69–75.

71. Van Weissenbruch MM, Hoek A, Vliet-Bleeker I, Schoemaker J, Drexhage H. Evidence for existence of immunoglobulins that block ovarian granulosa cell growth in vitro. A putative role in resistant ovary syndrome? *J Clin Endocrinol Metab* 1991; 73:360–367.

72. Tang VW, Faiman C. Premature ovarian failure: a search for circulating factors against gonadotropin receptors. *Am J Obstet Gynecol* 1983; 146:816–821.

73. Case records of the Massachusetts General Hospital. Weekly clinicopathological exercises. Case 46-1986. A 26-year-old woman with secondary amenorrhea. *N Engl J Med* 1986; 315:1336–1343.

74. Chiauzzi V, Cigorraga S, Escobar ME, Rivarola MA, Charreau EH. Inhibition of follicle-stimulating hormone receptor binding by circulating immunoglobulins. *J Clin Endocrinol Metab* 1982; 54: 1221–1228.

75. Chiauzzi VA, Bussmann L, Calvo JC, Sundblad V, Charreau EH. Circulating immunoglobulins that inhibit the binding of follicle-stimulating hormone to its receptor: a putative diagnostic role in resistant ovary syndrome? *Clin Endocrinol (Oxf)* 2004; 61:46–54.

76. Austin GE, Coulam CB, Ryan RJ. A search for antibodies to luteinizing hormone receptors in premature ovarian failure. *Mayo Clin Proc* 1979; 54:394–400.

77. Escobar ME, Cigorraga SB, Chiauzzi VA, Charreau EH, Rivarola MA. Development of the gonadotrophic resistant ovary syndrome in myasthenia gravis: suggestion of similar autoimmune mechanisms. *Acta Endocrinol (Copenh)* 1982; 99:431–436.

78. Charreau EH, Cigorraga S, Chiauzzi V, Escobar ME, Barañao JL, Rivarola MA. Receptors and antireceptors of the ovary. In: Tozzini RI, Reeves G, Pineda RL, editors. *Endocrine Physiopathology of the Ovary*. Elsevier/North Holland, Biomedical Press, 1980: 191–205.

79. Charreau EH, Chiauzzi V, Cigorraga S, Escobar ME, Rivarola M. Immunoglobulin anti FSH receptor in the resistant ovary syndrome. In: Thomas G. Muldoon, Virendra B. Mahesh and Bautista Palrez- Baltester, editors. Recent Advances in Fertility Research, Part A. Alan R. Liss, Inc. 150 Fifth Avenue, New York.

80. Dias JA, Gates SA, Reichert LE Jr. Evidence for the presence of follicle-stimulating hormone receptor antibody in human serum. *Fertil Steril* 1982; 38:330–338.

81. Bannatyne P, Russell P, Shearman RP. Autoimmune oophoritis: a clinicopathologic assessment of 12 cases. *Int J Gynecol Pathol* 1990; 9:191–207.

82. Massin N, Gougeon A, Meduri G, et al. Significance of ovarian histology in the management of patients presenting a premature ovarian failure. *Hum Reprod* 2004; 19:2555–2560.

83. Pache TD, Wladimiroff JW, de Jong FH, Hop WC, Fauser BC. Growth patterns of nondominant ovarian follicles during the normal menstrual cycle. *Fertil Steril* 1990; 54:638–642.

84. Mehta AE, Matwijiw I, Lyons EA, Faiman C. Noninvasive diagnosis of resistant ovary syndrome by ultrasonography. *Fertil Steril* 1992; 57:56–61.

85. Winqvist O, Gebre-Medhin G, Gustafsson J, et al. Identification of the main gonadal autoantigens in patients with adrenal insufficiency and associated ovarian failure. *J Clin Endocrinol Metab* 1995; 80:1717–1723.

86. Betterle C, Volpato M, Pedini B, et al. Adrenal-cortex autoantibodies and steroid-producing cells autoantibodies in patients with Addison's disease: comparison of immunofluorescence and immuno-precipitation assays. *J Clin Endocrinol Metab* 1999; 84:618–622.

87. Coulam CB, Ryan RJ. Prevalence of circulating antibodies directed toward ovaries among women with premature ovarian failure. *Am J Reprod Immunol Microbiol* 1985; 9:23–24.

88. Ho PC, Tang GW, Fu KH, Fan MC, Lawton JW. Immunologic studies in patients with premature ovarian failure. *Obstet Gynecol* 1988; 71:622–626.

89. Kirsop R, Brock CR, Robinson BG, et al. Detection of anti-ovarian antibodies by indirect immunofluorescence in patients with premature ovarian failure. *Reprod Fertil Dev* 1991; 3:537–541.

90. Wheatcroft NJ, Salt C, Milford-Ward A, Cooke ID, Weetman AP. Identification of ovarian antibodies by immunofluorescence, enzyme-linked immunosorbent assay or immunoblotting in premature ovarian failure. *Hum Reprod* 1997; 12:2617–2622.

91. Luborsky J, Llanes B, Davies S, et al. Ovarian autoimmunity: greater frequency of autoantibodies in premature menopause and unexplained infertility than in the general population. *Clin Immunol* 1999; 90:368–374.

92. Gobert B, Barabarino-Monnier P, Guillet-Rosso F, Bene MC, Faure GC. Ovary antibodies after IVF. *Lancet* 1990; 335:723.

93. Dewhurst CJ, de Koos EB, Ferreira HP. The resistant ovary syndrome. *Br J Obstet Gynaecol* 1975; 82:341–345.

94. Starup J, Sele V, Henriksen B. Amenorrhoea associated with increased production of gonadotrophins and a morphologically normal ovarian follicular apparatus. *Acta Endocrinol (Copenh)* 1971; 66: 248–256.

95. Van Campenhout J, Vauclair R, Maraghi K. Gonadotropin–resistant ovaries in primary amenorrhea. *Obstet Gynecol* 1972; 40:6–12.

96. Anasti JN, Kalantaridou SN, Kimzey LM, Defensor RA, Nelson LM. Bone loss in young women with karyotypically normal spontaneous premature ovarian failure. *Obstet Gynecol* 1998; 91:12–15.

97. Davis SR, Burger HG. The rationale for physiological testosterone replacement in women. *Baillieres Clin Endocrinol Metab* 1998; 12:391–405.

98. Davis SR, McCloud P, Strauss BJ, Burger H. Testosterone enhances estradiol's effects on postmenopausal bone density and sexuality. *Maturitas* 1995; 21:227–236.

99. Wright CS, Jacobs HS. Spontaneous pregnancy in a patient with hypergonadotrophic ovarian failure. *Br J Obstet Gynaecol* 1979; 86:389–392.

100. Rabinowe SL, Berger MJ, Welch WR, Dluhy RG. Lymphocyte dysfunction in autoimmune oophoritis. Resumption of menses with corticosteroids. *Am J Med* 1986; 81:347–350.

101. Cowchock FS, McCabe JL, Montgomery BB. Pregnancy after corticosteroid administration in premature ovarian failure (polyglandular endocrinopathy syndrome). *Am J Obstet Gynecol* 1988; 158:118–119.

102. Kalantaridou SN, Braddock DT, Patronas NJ, Nelson LM. Treatment of autoimmune premature ovarian failure. *Hum Reprod* 1999; 14:1777–1782.

103. Barbarino-Monnier P, Gobert B, Guillet-May F, et al. Ovarian autoimmunity and corticotherapy in an in-vitro fertilization attempt. *Hum Reprod* 1995; 10:2006–2007.

104. van Kasteren YM, Braat DD, Hemrika DJ, et al. Corticosteroids do not influence ovarian responsiveness to gonadotropins in patients with premature ovarian failure: a randomized, placebo-controlled trial. *Fertil Steril* 1999; 71:90–95.

105. Corenblum B, Rowe T, Taylor PJ. High-dose, short-term glucocorticoids for the treatment of infertility resulting from premature ovarian failure. *Fertil Steril* 1993; 59:988–991.

106. Blumenfeld Z, Halachmi S, Peretz BA, et al. Premature ovarian failure–the prognostic application of autoimmunity on conception after ovulation induction. *Fertil Steril* 1993; 59:750–755.

107. Bateman BG, Nunley WC Jr, Kitchin JD III. Reversal of apparent premature ovarian failure in a patient with myasthenia gravis. *Fertil Steril* 1983; 39:108–110.

108. Lundberg PO, Persson BH. Disappearance of amenorrhea after thymectomy. A case report. *Acta Soc Med Ups* 1969; 74:206–208.

109. Sauer MV, Paulson RJ, Ary BA, Lobo RA. Three hundred cycles of oocyte donation at the University of Southern California: assessing the effect of age and infertility diagnosis on pregnancy and implantation rates. *J Assist Reprod Genet* 1994; 11:92–96.

110. Sung L, Bustillo M, Mukherjee T, et al. Sisters of women with premature ovarian failure may not be ideal ovum donors. *Fertil Steril* 1997; 67:912–916.

15 Autoimmune Hypophysitis

Patrician Anne Crock, MBBS, FRACP, Sophie Bensing, MD, PhD, Casey Jo Anne Smith, BBiomedSc (Hons), Christine Burns, BSc, Grad. Dip. Med. Lab. Sci. and Phillip J. Robinson, BSc, PhD

Contents

Summary

Autoimmune hypophysitis or pituitary autoimmune disease is now considered to be part of the organ-specific spectrum of endocrine autoimmunity. It is predominantly seen in women, often in association with pregnancy. The most common presentation in the acute phase mimics that of a pituitary adenoma with a mass and hypopituitarism. There is a predilection for adrenocorticotrophin (ACTH) and thyrotrophin deficiencies, in contrast to tumors and radiation-induced hypopituitarism where these are usually the last axes to be lost. Extension of the inflammatory process into the infundibulum causes diabetes insipidus and is termed infundibuloneurohypophysitis. Sub-acute cases classically present in the peripartum period, and the pituitary mass may resolve spontaneously. Chronic cases should be considered in patients with isolated ACTH deficiency or idiopathic hypopituitarism in the context of other autoimmune diseases and the empty sella syndrome (also with hypopituitarism). Magnetic resonance imaging usually shows a symmetrical pituitary mass with bright, homogeneous contrast enhancement. Biopsy is still considered the gold standard for diagnosis. Serological tests for pituitary autoantibodies are reviewed. Immunoblotting has identified a number of target autoantigens. The latest assay, based on the in vitro transcription translation of pituitary gland-specific proteins followed by an immunoprecipitation step, has identified pituitary gland-specific protein factor (PGSF) 1a and PGSF2 as probable target autoantigens. Management of potentially life-threatening adrenal insufficiency is of the utmost importance.

From: *Contemporary Endocrinology: Autoimmune Diseases in Endocrinology*
Edited by: A. P. Weetman © Humana Press, Totowa, NJ

A conservative approach has been recommended except in those patients with sight-threatening lesions or in those with recurrent disease despite a course of immunosuppression. Future directions are discussed.

Key Words: Lymphocytic hypophysitis, pituitary autoantibodies, pituitary autoimmunity, target autoantigens.

INTRODUCTION

Autoimmune endocrinopathies are classified as organ specific in the spectrum of autoimmune diseases. The classic example is autoimmune thyroiditis that was first described by Dr. Hakaru Hashimoto in 1912 *(1)* and still bears his name. Pituitary autoimmunity was not described until 50 years later by Goudie and Pinkerton *(2)* as "anterior hypophysitis." Interestingly, it was the association with Hashimoto's thyroiditis in this index case that led the pathologist and physician to make the etiological link. They also noted the link with pregnancy and the postpartum period that continues to hold true in over 50% of cases in the literature.

HISTORICAL PERSPECTIVE

It is tempting to surmise that there were some cases of end-stage hypophysitis among Sheehan's original series of patients who died of chronic hypopituitarism in the early 1900's *(3)*. Close examination of Carpenter's review of Schmidt's syndrome in 1964 *(4)* identified at least two cases of Addison's disease from the 1930s with lymphoid infiltration not just of the thyroid but also of the hypophysis *(5,6)*. However, the original case reported by Goudie and Pinkerton in 1962 *(2)* was the first time that the distinct entity of anterior hypophysitis or pituitary autoimmunity was formally enunciated.

Since then, autoimmune pituitary disease has seen a range of terminology, but the most common terms are currently lymphocytic hypophysitis and lymphocytic infundibuloneurohypophysitis, when there is associated diabetes insipidus (DI). The clinical spectrum of disease is increasingly recognized although the gold standard for diagnosis remains pituitary biopsy. The ability to detect pituitary autoantibodies, whether they are pathological or epiphenomena in the autoimmune process, would obviate the need for pituitary surgery in some cases. By analogy with Addison's disease *(7)* and type 1 diabetes *(8)*, autoantibodies could one day also be used to predict the risk of gland failure, in this case of hypopituitarism.

EPIDEMIOLOGY

The incidence and prevalence of lymphocytic hypophysitis are not known exactly, and population-based data are scarce. The nature and clinical course of cases that proceed to surgery ("biopsy proven") are quite different to those of cases that are "suspected" or represent the sub-acute and chronic ends of the spectrum *(9–14)*. These latter cases have become better defined by new imaging techniques and will be further defined as new, more specific and sensitive pituitary autoantibody assays evolve.

In the early histopathology literature, there was considerable discussion about what constitutes a "normal" pattern of lymphocytic infiltration and its significance. Simmonds and Brandes *(15)* described four types of lymphocytic infiltration in 200 unselected autopsy cases. Only two cases were found in "Group III," defined as having diffuse lymphocytic infiltration of the anterior hypophysis, which would now be regarded as pathological. Shanklin's series of 100 autopsies *(16)* found no cases with lymphocytes in the anterior pituitary.

Sheehan and Summers *(3)* reviewed the pathology and clinical correlates of 95 autopsy cases of hypopituitarism. Some cases with end-stage fibrosis and scarring of the pituitary were clearly because of postpartum necrosis, named eponymously after Sheehan, but some may have been because of end-stage lymphocytic hypophysitis. Scheithauer et al. *(17)* examined the pituitary glands of 69 autopsies of women who had died in the peripartum period (during and after pregnancy or following abortion) on the assumption that undiagnosed cases of lymphocytic hypophysitis may be more common in this scenario. They found five pituitaries that had areas of lymphocytic infiltration on histopathology.

The incidence determined from large surgical series ranges from 0.24 to 0.88% *(18,19)* but, again, may only represent those cases that presented more acutely. In addition, neurosurgeons and their neuroendocrine teams who specialize in pituitary surgery may be more likely to suspect the diagnosis preoperatively and avoid surgery where possible. The largest series of 2500 surgical pituitary pathology cases, collected in Hamburg, Germany, between 1970 and 1996, were reported by Sautner et al. *(19)* and Fehn et al. *(20)*. Six cases (0.24%) of lymphocytic hypophysitis were identified. In another large German series from Erlangen, Honegger et al. *(21)* found 7 cases of hypophysitis among 2362 pituitary cases (0.3%). A review of 2000 case records from Charlottesville, Virginia, identified 16 patients, 13 of whom underwent surgery (0.65%), 10 with lymphocytic hypophysitis, and 3 with granulomatous hypophysitis *(22)*. The series of 5 patients from Nottingham in the United Kingdom, based on 619 consecutive cases, had a calculated incidence of 0.8% *(23)*. The preference of this surgical unit was for surgical decompression. The Johns Hopkins Hospital review of 905 pituitary surgical cases from the archives found 8 cases (0.88%) *(18)*.

GENETIC AND ENVIRONMENTAL FACTORS

Autoimmune diseases are often associated with particular major histocompatibility complex (MHC) alleles. A number of patients with hypophysitis have had haplotype analysis performed *(10,24–33)*. The first two cases studied were black, female patients, both with the allele Bw35 *(24,27)*. This allele is associated with type 1 diabetes in non-Caucasians *(34)*. The two patients in Pestell et al.'s report *(30)* shared a number of human leukocyte antigen (HLA) alleles that have been associated with Hashimoto's thyroiditis and type 1 diabetes. As the number of patients investigated is small, no firm conclusions can be drawn *(9,10)*.

There are no known environmental triggers for hypophysitis, but the association with viral infections, particularly meningoencephalitis, may be relevant. Pituitary autantibody testing, once sensitive and specific enough, would be helpful to answer this question.

DIAGNOSIS

Clinical Presentation

The diagnosis of lymphocytic hypophysitis should be entertained in a range of clinical scenarios that depend on the rapidity or otherwise of the disease process. It has a striking female preponderance with a female to male ratio of 6:1 *(18)*, and its strong association with pregnancy should not be forgotten. It has been increasingly recognized in male patients *(14,18,26,30)*, but the recent preponderance of male cases probably reflects some reporting bias. Females tend to present at a younger age (34.5 years) than males (44.7 years) *(9)*. At the acute end of the spectrum, hypophysitis mimics the effects of a non-secretory pituitary tumor with adrenocorticotrophin (ACTH) deficiency predominating, and sub-acute cases have frequently been described as a resolving pituitary mass in the peripartum setting. The chronic spectrum is believed to include idiopathic hypopituitarism, sometimes in the context of other autoimmune endocrinopathies, and the empty sella syndrome.

ACUTE PRESENTATIONS

Apart from some of the original autopsy cases *(11)*, the most dramatic, acute presentation was a case report of sudden death in labor of a young woman who presumably had undiagnosed adrenal insufficiency *(35)*. Another case involving sudden death was reported as recently as 1992 *(36)*. The first case to be diagnosed premortem was in 1980 by Mayfield et al. *(27)*, and the clinical presentation was indistinguishable from that of a pituitary adenoma. The symptoms are those of a pituitary mass lesion with or without suprasellar extension, including headaches, visual impairment with loss of visual acuity and field defects, and hypopituitarism *(14)*.

The predilection for corticotroph involvement and thus secondary adrenal insufficiency is unexplained. ACTH deficiency is usually the last component to develop in patients with hypopituitarism because of tumors, and yet in hypophysitis, it may be the first and only element of hypopituitarism *(12,37,38)*. Thyrotrophin (TSH) deficiency is also frequently seen *(13)*. There have been cases that presented with symptoms of pituitary apoplexy *(39)*, including three from our original Australian series *(40)* and one further Australian case *(41)*, but apoplexy is unusual and more suggestive of an underlying tumor or granulomatous or necrotizing hypophysitis. Hypercalcemia is another unusual manifestation of acute adrenal insufficiency that has been seen in a number of cases of hypophysitis *(14,38,42–48)*.

SUB-ACUTE PRESENTATIONS

The classical sub-acute scenario is a young pregnant or postpartum woman who presents with symptoms and signs of a pituitary mass lesion that resolves with time *(25,40,49)*. Hypophysitis usually presents in the second or third trimester rather than the first, and a typical magnetic resonance imaging (MRI) scan is shown in Fig. 1. In the peripartum setting, some cases may be incorrectly attributed to Sheehan's syndrome even though there was no history of obstetric hemorrhage. Interestingly, the development of lymphocytic hypophysitis does not necessarily imply secondary infertility, and a number of cases of subsequent pregnancies have been reported *(50–53)*.

Prolactin levels may be high, low, or normal in approximately equal proportions *(18,54)*. High levels are normal in pregnancy and breast-feeding but may also suggest a prolactinoma. Alternatively, hyperprolactinemia may be because of stalk pressure, hypothyroidism, or in theory, autoantibodies that stimulate lactotrophs directly *(55)* or that cross-react in the prolactin assay, simulating macroprolactinemia. There is recent evidence that prolactin may have an immunomodulatory role *(56)*. Data on growth

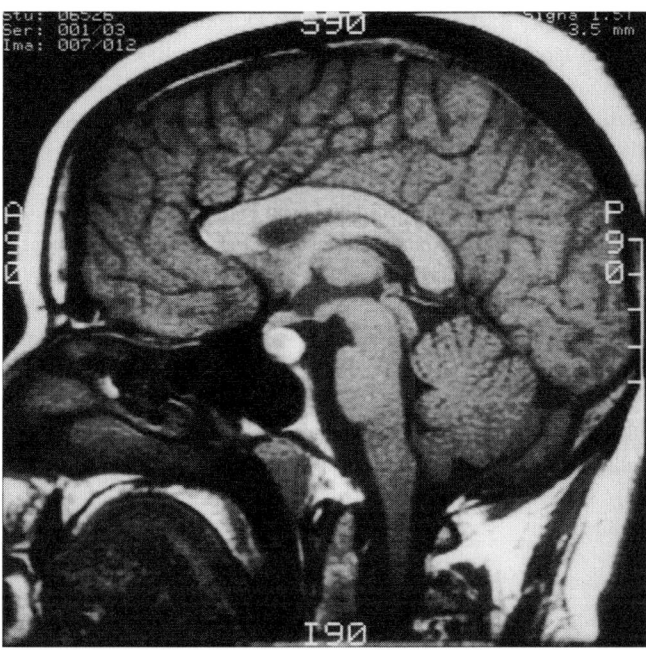

Fig. 1. Magnetic resonance imaging (MRI) scan of a classic case of lymphocytic hypophysitis in a 24-year-old woman who presented with symptoms of a pituitary tumor. Note the uniform enhancement with contrast with extension to the hypothalamus.

hormone (GH) status are less robust as this axis does not appear to be regularly assessed in adult patients *(11,13,18)*. In other causes of hypopituitarism such as traumatic brain injury *(57)* and cranial irradiation *(58)*, GH deficiency (GHD) is usually the first deficit detected, whereas in hypophysitis, it is the last or is even spared.

EXTENSION OF THE INFLAMMATORY PROCESS

In both acute and sub-acute presentations, there may be extension of the inflammatory process into surrounding structures. This was evident as early as the original case (original histopathological sections reviewed by Prof. Goudie, personal communication). Involvement of the cavernous sinus has been reported, with patients complaining of persistent headaches and then developing diplopia with third, fourth, or sixth cranial nerve palsies *(32,59,60)*. The inflammation can even extend to cause bilateral internal carotid artery occlusion *(61)*.

Dural involvement is often seen on computed tomography (CT) or MRI scans *(62)* and can progress to the point that the diagnosis of hypertrophic cranial pachymeningitis is made *(63)*. It is likely that the association of aseptic meningitis with lymphocytic hypophysitis is part of this phenomenon of extension to surrounding structures *(59,64–67)*, although the alternative explanation is that the hypophysitis was triggered by viral meningitis. In their series of nine patients that were treated prospectively with high-dose methylprednisolone therapy, Kristof et al. *(68)* performed cerebrospinal fluid (CSF) analysis showing a significantly higher lympho-monocytic pleocytosis in patients with presumed lymphocytic hypophysitis [72 (SD = 64) cells/mm^3] compared with patients with pituitary adenomas [14 (SD 11) cells/mm^3].

INFUNDIBULONEUROHYPOPHYSITIS

Extension of the inflammatory process into the posterior pituitary and up into the neurohypophysis will lead to DI. Imura et al. *(69)* described the first cases in 1993 and coined the term infundibuloneurohypophysitis. Since then, an increasing number of cases of DI in the context of hypophysitis have been reported, particularly by Japanese colleagues *(13,60,66,70–78)*. In the review by Hashimoto et al. *(13)*, they found 30 of 152 cases (19.7%) with DI. Interestingly, this presentation appears to be more common in male patients.

Recently, the term lymphocytic panhypophysitis has been used to indicate that posterior pituitary dysfunction co-exists with anterior dysfunction *(18,79)*. It is extremely rare for pituitary adenomata to cause DI preoperatively, and so this is an important clue to an underlying inflammatory process and the chance to manage the patient conservatively *(14)*. The major concern is not to miss a dysgerminoma or Langerhans' cell histiocytosis *(80)* as well as the gamut of granulomatous conditions. Rathke's cysts can also present with DI but tend to have a characteristic appearance on T2-weighted MRI. A pericystic lymphocytic infiltrate in this situation is more likely to represent secondary hypophysitis than a primary event *(19)*.

CHRONIC PRESENTATIONS

A sensitive and specific assay for pituitary autoantibodies is needed to delineate the chronic spectrum of the disease. This group of patients are far less likely to undergo pituitary biopsy unless there is a large fibrotic mass that resembles a tumor. In general, postinflammatory fibrosis leads to pituitary gland atrophy and an empty sella on CT or MRI scan. An example of this sequence of events is shown in Fig. 2.

The empty sella syndrome is almost certainly a heterogenous condition *(81)*. In a Swedish study of empty sella patients, we were unable to demonstrate a higher rate of pituitary autoantibodies by immunoblotting than in control patients *(81)*, but only 4 of 30 patients had pituitary dysfunction. Isolated ACTH and TSH deficiencies have been reported in association with autoimmune endocrinopathies and the empty sella syndrome. In the former, pituitary autoantibodies have been demonstrated by both immunofluorescence (IF) *(82–84)* and IB *(37,40)*. In contrast, pituitary tumors initially tend to cause GH or gonadotroph dysfunction.

Association with Other Autoimmune and Inflammatory Diseases

Autoimmune diseases have a tendency to cluster, and lymphocytic hypophysitis has been reported with both organ-specific and systemic autoimmunity in 25–50% of cases *(11,13,14,18,40)*. The most common association is Hashimoto's thyroiditis *(2,11,49,85)*. Other associations have included Addison's disease *(86,87)*, type 1 diabetes mellitus *(13,40)*, Graves' disease *(40,88)*, atrophic gastritis *(40,89)*, autoimmune polyendocrinopathy–candidiasis–ectodermal dystrophy (APECED) *(90)*, systemic lupus erythematosus *(72,91–93)*, Sjögren's syndrome *(63)*, autoimmune hepatitis *(94)*, and primary biliary cirrhosis *(95)*.

In the neurological and ophthalmological literature, there are a number of localized inflammatory conditions that seem to overlap with lymphocytic hypophysitis. Tolosa Hunt syndrome describes patients with painful ocular inflammation *(62,96,97)*. On closer examination of one case report, the patient was noted coincidentally to have

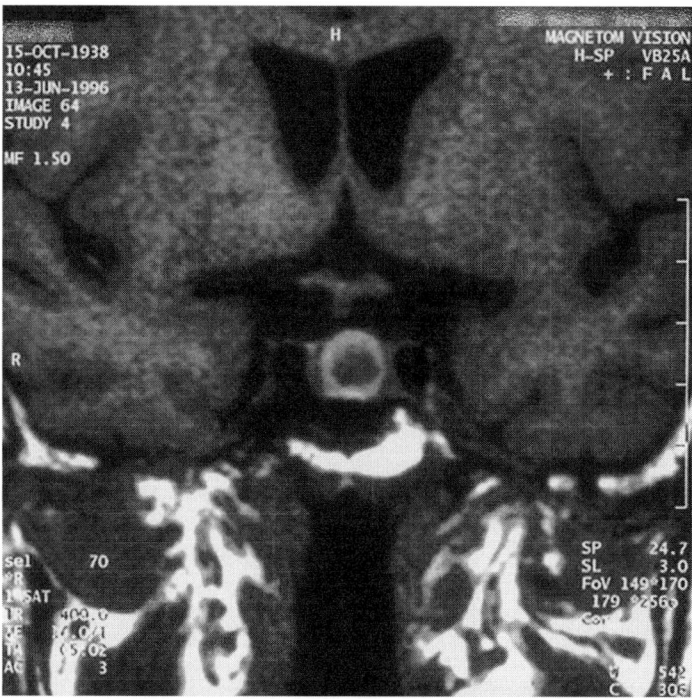

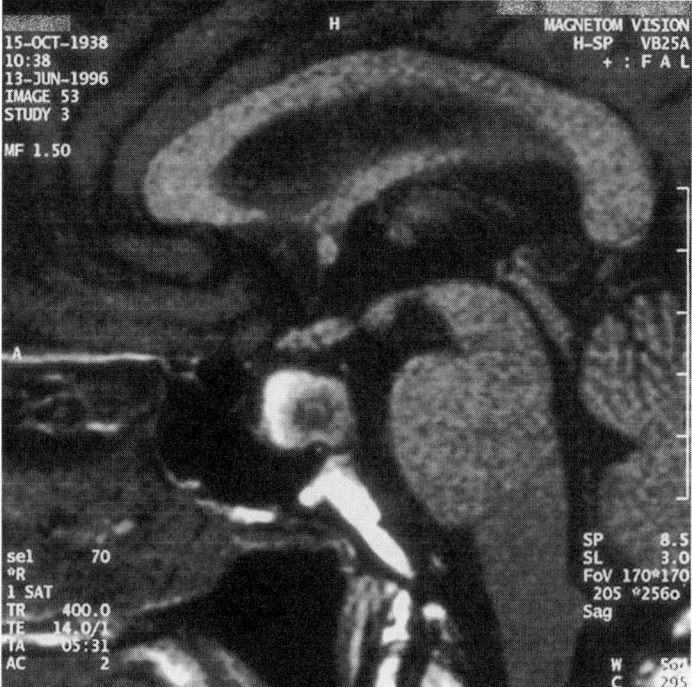

Fig. 2. *(Continued).*

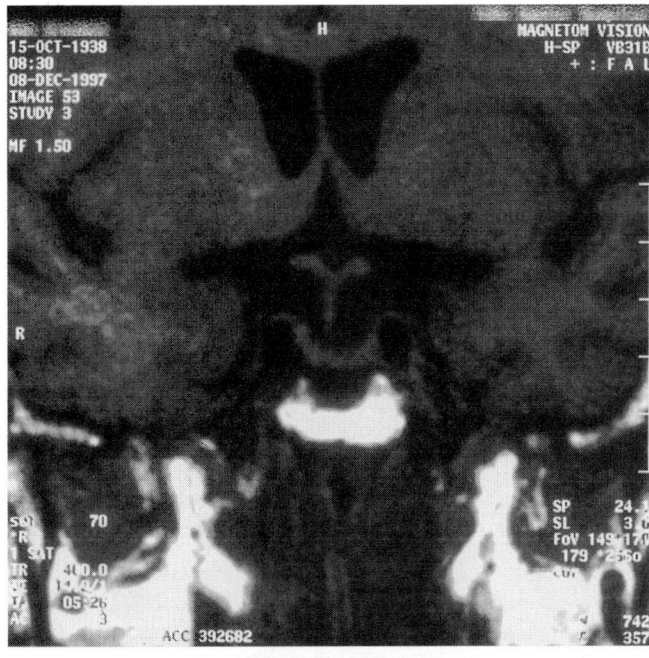

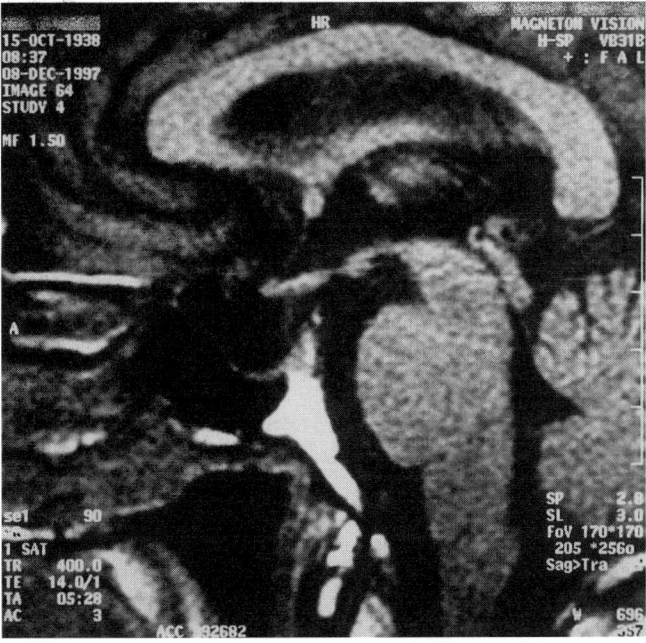

Fig. 2. Sequential magnetic resonance imaging (MRI) scans in a 57-year-old man who presented with hypopituitarism and diabetes insipidus (DI) presumed to be due to lymphocytic hypophysitis. Scans 1 (coronal section) and 2 (sagittal section) show a pituitary mass with ring enhancement. This appearance could also be sagittal granulomatous hypophysitis. Subsequent scans 3 (coronal section) and 4 (sagittal section), taken 18 months later, show progression to an empty sella.

an enlarged pituitary that resolved with steroid therapy for the ocular inflammation. Similarly, fibrosing pseudotumor *(22,98)*, inflammatory pseudotumor *(99)*, dacryoadenitis *(100)*, temporal arteritis *(22)*, and lymphocytic lacrimal and salivary gland involvement with Hashimoto's thyroiditis *(101)* have all been reported in association with hypophysitis, and some have been treated successfully with intravenous steroids. The conditions previously described are local, but lymphocytic hypophysitis has also been reported in patients with generalized inflammatory pathologies such as retroperitoneal fibrosis *(87,102)*. There is no unifying hypothesis to explain these associations other than some infectious trigger or the tendency for autoimmune conditions to cluster *(103)*.

As with other autoimmune conditions, there may be a relapsing and remitting course *(65)*. The longest time to full disease expression has been 8 years in two instances *(72,104)*. Spontaneous recovery has also been widely reported *(25,31,49,105–108)*.

APECED

Autoimmune polyendocrinopathy–candidiasis–ectodermal dystrophy (OMIM 240300), also known as polyglandular autoimmune disease type 1, is a rare, autosomal recessive disorder caused by mutations in the autoimmune regulator (*AIRE*) gene (*see* Chap. 17). *AIRE* has an important role in central tolerance by promoting the expression of organ-specific antigens in the thymus *(109,110)*. Hypopituitarism is an uncommon feature. There has been one convincing case of clinical hypophysitis *(90)* in a French-Canadian patient with a severe phenotype where virtually no endocrine gland was spared. Autoantibodies to pituitary membrane proteins were demonstrated by IB but have not been further characterized *(90)*. Isolated GHD has been documented in another nine patients, isolated secondary hypogonadism in one case, and central DI in three *(111–113)*. Finally, three siblings with partial ACTH deficiency *(114)* and one patient with selective hypopituitarism *(115)* have been reported. Pituitary autoantibodies have been studied in the cohort of APECED patients from Scandinavia *(116)*, but their clinical significance is uncertain.

Special Case Scenarios

Pregnant Women with Type 1 Diabetes

A particularly interesting group of patients are pregnant women with type 1 diabetes *(40)*. The Australian prevalence study of postpartum thyroid dysfunction from Perth showed that 11.5% of normal women had evidence of hypothyroidism or hyperthyroidism 6 months postpartum *(117)*. It is well recognized that diabetic patients are at an even higher risk of postpartum thyroiditis (*see* Chap. 8). Therefore, these women may also be at higher risk of peripartum hypophysitis, which should be suspected in patients with peripartum headache and rapidly falling insulin requirements. In our experience, these patients can be easily overlooked and fatigue attributed to psychosocial factors and to the stress of caring for a new baby. Finally, hypopituitarism, presenting as the Houssay phenomenon (hypoglycemia because of hypopituitarism), has been attributed to microvascular disease because of the diabetes itself. In fact, some of these cases may have been autoimmune in etiology *(40)*.

SHEEHAN'S SYNDROME

The other interesting group of patients are those given a diagnosis of Sheehan's syndrome as a cause of their hypopituitarism when there was no history of postpartum hemorrhage or other obstetric calamity. Goswami et al. *(118)* used the IB method to study a large cohort of Indian women with severe peripartum hemorrhage leading to Sheehan's syndrome up to 8 years later. They found that 63.1% (12 of 19) developed anti-enolase antibodies compared with 17.8% (5 of 28) women with normal pregnancies and 14.2% (4 of 28) women who had never conceived. Despite near catastrophic hemorrhage at the time of delivery in all patients, some had a significant delay in the development of hypopituitarism. This delay supported the theory that an autoimmune process was triggered by the obstetric event.

PEDIATRIC CASES

Pediatric cases of lymphocytic hypophysitis outside of APECED can be counted on one hand *(119–122)*. It is interesting that the third of the original three cases of xanthomatous hypophysitis was an adolescent female *(123)*. Granulomatous lesions have also been seen in adolescence *(124,125)*.

PATIENTS WITH CANCER TREATED WITH CYTOTOXIC T-LYMPHOCYTE-ASSOCIATED ANTIGEN-4 BLOCKADE

Cytotoxic T-lymphocyte-associated antigen (CTLA)-4 is a receptor expressed on activated T cells and a subset of regulatory T cells. It inhibits T-cell responses and is therefore important in the maintenance of peripheral tolerance against self-antigens *(126,127)*. Many malignant tumors are known to express self-antigens on their surfaces. Recent reports have established that administration of CTLA-4 blocking antibodies in patients with advanced melanoma mediates cancer regression *(128,129)*. Unfortunately, this kind of immunotherapy may also induce autoimmune manifestations such as enterocolitis, dermatitis, and hypophysitis *(128,130)*.

Blansfield et al. *(131)* reported six patients with melanoma and two patients with renal cell carcinoma that all developed hypophysitis during treatment with CTLA-4 antibodies. Before the immunotherapy was started, all patients had normal pituitary function and normal pituitary imaging on MRI, except for one patient who had an empty sella but no hypopituitarism. After CTLA-4 blockade, seven of eight patients had an evident increase in pituitary size, and all eight patients developed clinical signs of hypopituitarism. Low levels of cortisol and TSH were detected in the patients, and in seven of them, testosterone was also low. Once the immunotherapy was interrupted and hormonal replacement therapy started, all patients had resolution of their clinical symptoms. Based on these findings, it is recommended that patients treated with CTLA-4 antibodies be closely monitored for clinical and laboratory signs of hypopituitarism. Reversible hypopituitarism has also been reported after alpha-interferon therapy *(132)*.

INVESTIGATIONS

Imaging

Computed tomography scanning performed on the first case of hypophysitis diagnosed in a living patient *(27)* could not differentiate the mass from that of an adenoma. MRI is now the preferred technology.

The MRI findings of lymphocytic hypophysitis vary depending on the stage and extent of the inflammatory process. On T1-weighted precontrast images, lymphocytic hypophysitis appears isointense relative to gray matter. The sellar floor regularly appears flat and intact, whereas erosion that can be unilateral is more often seen in pituitary adenomata *(9)*. Postcontrast, acute cases often present as a symmetric homogeneous contrast-enhancing sellar mass with suprasellar extension *(133)*. Rarely, a heterogeneous cystic appearance can be found *(134–136)*. The intense enhancement may be confined to the periphery of the lesion as "ring enhancement" *(71)* or extend along the dura mater as a "dural tail" *(137)*. Interpretation of scans can be difficult in pregnant women as pregnancy itself leads to hyperintensity of the anterior pituitary on MRI *(138)*.

Dynamic MRI has displayed delayed contrast enhancement of the pituitary mass as a sign of abnormal hypophyseal vasculature *(139)*. A striking finding is that the pituitary stalk often is thickened and enhanced but rarely displaced *(70)*. If the inflammatory process involves the posterior pituitary lobe, its precontrast hyperintense bright spot may be lost *(69)*. Involvement of the cavernous sinus resulting in cranial nerve palsies as well as occlusion of one or both internal carotid arteries have been described *(32,61, 140)*. In its sub-acute and chronic presentations, lymphocytic hypophysitis may show a normal pituitary on MRI or signs of pituitary atrophy and empty sella *(141)*. Figure 2 shows the progression of hypophysitis from a mass with ring enhancement and stalk involvement causing DI to an empty sella over 18 months.

Features such as a homogeneous symmetrical mass, marked contrast enhancement, and stalk thickening with no deviation speak in favor of lymphocytic hypophysitis but can also be seen with other pituitary lesions. Therefore, it may be very hard to predict hypophysitis on MRI, and histopathological examination remains the definitive arbiter.

Immunopathogenesis

GROSS PATHOLOGY

Inspection of the pituitary gland in the autopsy cases showed significant atrophy *(14)*, together with secondary atrophy of the adrenals in nearly all cases. The tissue at neurosurgery is often described as looking white-gray to yellowish with a consistency that may be soft but is more often firm, fibrous, and adherent to surrounding structures such as the dura mater. In occasional cases, a cystic appearance with yellow liquid is described, which raises the possibilities of a Rathke's cyst with secondary hypophysitis or of necrotizing or xanthomatous hypophysitis.

HISTOPATHOLOGY

Lymphocytic hypophysitis is characterized by extensive, diffuse lympho-plasmacytic infiltration of the anterior pituitary as seen in Fig. 3. As in Hashimoto's thyroiditis, the lymphocytes can aggregate to form lymphoid follicles with germinal centers. The inflammatory infiltrate consists mainly of a polyclonal mixture of T and B lymphocytes with an admixture of plasma cells and occasional eosinophils, macrophages, and histiocytes *(19,20) (142–144)*. Recently, mast cells have been described *(145)* and also activation of the supporting dendritic-like pituitary folliculo-stellate cells *(146)*.

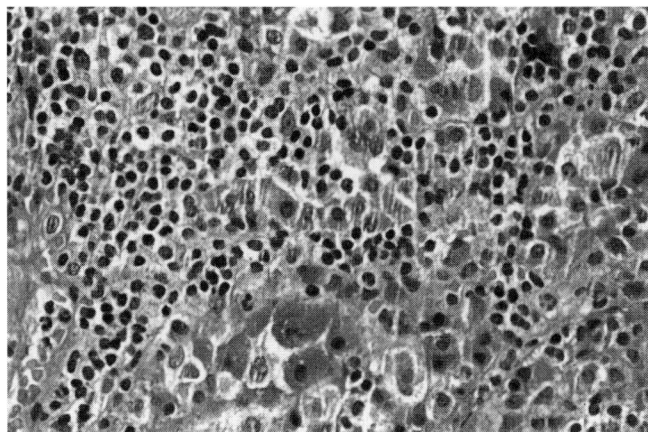

Fig. 3. Histological section of a classic peripartum case of lymphocytic hypophysitis stained with hematoxylin and eosin, showing the diffuse lymphocytic infiltrate with scattered plasma cells and eosinophils and islands of remnant pituitary cells.

In acute cases with large numbers of lymphocytes, it is important to exclude clonality, which would indicate an underlying lymphoma *(147)* or leukemia. In cases where the surgeon has found firm tissue, there is a correlation with significant fibrosis on light microscopy. Occasional neutrophils may be seen, but significant areas of necrosis or granuloma formation indicate other entities such as necrotizing infundibuloneuro-hypophysitis and granulomatous hypophysitis discussed under Differential Diagnosis.

IMMUNOHISTOCHEMISTRY

Characterization of the T-cell and B-cell infiltrates has shown that the former predominate except in areas with lymphoid follicles. The tissue ratio of T-helper (CD4+) to T-suppressor (CD8+) cells has been described as 2:1 or greater in the majority of cases *(12,20,38,66,140,143,148)*. Gutenberg et al. *(143)* showed that the highest numbers of activated CD8+ T cells were observed in cases presenting in pregnancy and with a shorter duration of clinical symptoms.

ELECTRON MICROSCOPY

The first description of changes seen on electron microscopy (EM), by Asa et al. *(24)*, was of pituitary cells interdigitating with activated lymphocytes in those areas of the most dense inflammatory cell infiltration. Some pituitary cells were intact *(24,149)*, whereas others showed signs of oncocytic transformation or enlarged lysosomal bodies *(20)*. No immune complex deposits were seen. Jensen et al. *(38)* also noted phagocytosis of organelles from degenerating adenohypophyseal cells. In their case, isolated corticotropin deficiency was confirmed on EM by the selective loss of corticotrophs. Isolated loss of prolactin cells has also been shown *(146)*. Professor Ross McD. Anderson, an eminent neuropathologist in Melbourne, captured an exquisite example of an activated lymphocyte interacting with an adenohypophyseal cell in peripartum hypophysitis, and this is shown in Fig. 4 *(12)*.

Differential Diagnosis

In patients presenting acutely, the immediate concern is to treat the underlying hypopituitarism, to preserve vision, and then to exclude a pituitary tumor. If clinical

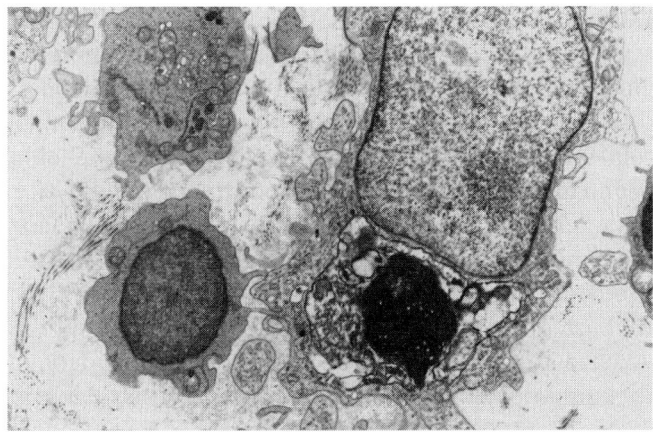

Fig. 4. Electron microscopy (EM) study of the case shown in Fig. 3. Note the lymphocyte "embracing" a degenerating adenohypophyseal cell. (Photograph reproduced with the kind permission of *Current Opinion in Endocrinology and Diabetes*.).

findings or imaging are suggestive of an inflammatory process, then there are a number of ancillary investigations, which help to narrow the diagnostic possibilities. However, biopsy may be needed to differentiate the types of hypophysitis.

PRIMARY HYPOPHYSITIS

Hypophysitis can be classified as primary or secondary. Broadly, the primary inflammatory processes are lymphocytic hypophysitis, granulomatous hypophysitis, and the recently described xanthomatous hypophysitis. However, there are cases described as lympho-granulomatous hypophysitis *(21,29,150)*, necrotizing infundibuloneurohypophysitis *(151)*, and xantho-granulomatous hypophysitis *(144)*. It is unclear whether these are separate entities. Cheung et al. *(142)* illustrated the three major sub-types with classical case reports, as did Flanagan et al. *(135)*. Neither granulomatous and xanthomatous hypophysitis appear to have an autoimmune basis. They do not have a preponderance of female patients and are not usually associated with other autoimmune diseases *(143)*.

GRANULOMATOUS HYPOPHYSITIS

Granulomatous inflammation of the pituitary may be primary or secondary to an underlying systemic granulomatous disease (*see* Secondary Hypophysitis). Idiopathic primary granulomatous hypophysitis mainly affects the anterior pituitary but may also involve the neurohypophysis and infundibulum, particularly in male patients. Headache and visual disturbances are common, as are varying degrees of hypopituitarism with or without DI. The diagnosis is rarely made on clinical grounds but rather on the histological findings of granulomas with epithelioid histiocytes and multinucleated giant cells *(142)*. A variable number of lymphocytes and plasma cells may also be present. On radiological examination, an intrasellar mass, sometimes with parasellar extension, is seen *(21)*. There may also be stalk thickening and loss of the posterior pituitary bright spot on MRI *(152)* in those patients with DI.

Xanthomatous Hypophysitis

Xanthomatous hypophysitis is a recently described entity *(123)*, with less than 10 cases in the literature *(142–144,153,154)*. The mass lesions often appear cystic on MRI. The anterior pituitary is infiltrated with lipid-rich, foamy histiocytes strongly reactive to CD68 antibody (indicating monocyte–macrophage lineage), and some lymphocytes. There may be foci of liquefaction. The pathogenesis is not understood but felt to be infective.

Secondary Hypophysitis

It is important to consider whether there is an underlying treatable systemic condition that may manifest as primary hypophysitis. As intimated in the discussion on primary hypophysitis, this can be difficult when the two can co-exist. The list of conditions that can affect the pituitary is extensive *(155)*.

It was the observation of lymphocytic infiltration around craniopharyngiomas that led Puchner et al. *(19,156)* to coin the term "secondary hypophysitis." Hypophysitis secondary to tumors has been seen also with both GH-secreting *(157)* and prolactin-secreting *(158)* adenomata and in association with Rathke's cysts *(135,159–162)*.

In patients with DI, the entity of infundibuloneurohypophysitis needs to be differentiated from two major conditions—dysgerminoma and Langerhans' cell histiocytosis, especially in children and adolescents *(80)*. Even biopsy of pituitary stalk lesions can be misleading, as there may be a secondary lymphocytic infiltrate around a dysgerminoma *(163)*. This phenomenon was best illustrated by the case of a young patient from Germany whose initial biopsy suggested lymphocytic hypophysitis, but whose subsequent course was that of an aggressive dysgerminoma *(164,165)*. Langerhans' cell histiocytosis is S100 positive on biopsy, but preoperatively, the diagnosis can be suspected when there is a characteristic rash (more common in pediatric patients), an ear discharge, or a positive bone scan *(166)*.

Neurosarcoidosis can involve the infundibulum and extend into the pituitary. Serum angiotensin-converting enzyme (ACE) levels may be raised, and a chest radiograph may show the classical infiltrate. There has been a case report of pulmonary sarcoidosis being associated with biopsy-proven lymphocytic hypophysitis *(167)*. Granulomatous diseases including Wegener's disease *(168)*, sarcoidosis *(169)*, tuberculosis *(170,171)*, Takayasu's disease *(172)*, and Crohn's disease *(173)* have all presented with pituitary manifestations.

Tuberculosis of the sella turcica *(174)* was not uncommon in the early 1900's and features in Sheehan's series of cases. It is also still a consideration in regions that have a high prevalence of tuberculosis, especially as HIV/AIDS is contributing to its resurgence. A tuberculin test and antigen polymerase chain reaction (PCR) of CSF are informative *(170)*. Alternatively, new sensitive and specific tests of lymphocyte interferon-gamma responses to tuberculous antigens are increasingly being used. Syphilis was also more common last century but is a consideration in patients with other manifestations who are *treponema pallidum* hemagglutination positive.

Pituitary Autoantibodies

Pituitary autoantibodies and their relation to lymphocytic hypophysitis have recently been reviewed *(175)*. The other autoimmune endocrinopathies, such as Hashimoto's thyroiditis, Addison's disease, type 1 diabetes mellitus, and Graves' disease, have been traditionally considered as organ-specific processes. Their respective target autoantigens are tissue-specific or cell-specific enzymes *(7,176,177)*, hormones *(178)*, or receptors *(179)*. Yet, islet cell antibodies (ICA) detected by IF in patients with type 1 diabetes recognize not only insulin-secreting beta cells but multiple pituitary cells *(180)* as well as islet alpha cells, delta cells, and those making pancreatic polypeptide *(181)*. This ICA reactivity is not completely preabsorbed by glutamic acid decarboxylase (GAD) 65 and islet antigen (IA) 2, suggesting that there are other relevant islet cell autoantigens *(182)*. Patients with Graves' disease can also have autoantibodies that cross-react with the pituitary *(183)*, and those with Hashimoto's thyroiditis can develop an encephalopathy that is related to their thyroid autoantibody status and not some concurrent neurological condition *(184,185)*. One interpretation has been that pituitary autoantibody reactivity is therefore non-specific, but this is partly contradicted by recent data on autoantibodies to type 2 iodothyronine deiodinase (D2) *(186)*. This enzyme is expressed in both the pituitary and the thyroid.

The pituitary contains at least five different hormone-secreting cell types. If there are cell-specific or enzyme-specific targets, then pituitary autoantibodies in a patient with lymphocytic hypophysitis and isolated ACTH deficiency are probably going to be different to those from a patient with isolated TSH deficiency or panhypopituitarism. A number of techniques have been used to look for pituitary autoantibodies as summarized in Table 1. Some methods, such as IF, identify the target cell type and sub-cellular localization but not the target protein. Others, such as IB, identify the molecular weight of the target protein but not the cell of origin. Finding a pituitary-specific autoantigen is not so simple, as the enzymes in the pituitary are also present in the hypothalamus and neuroendocrine tissues including the placenta—for example, neuron-specific enolase (NSE) *(187)*, prohormone convertase (PC) *(188)*, and the family of carboxypeptidases (CPs) *(189)*. Using a candidate autoantigen approach, Tanaka et al. looked at the expression profile of active genes in the human pituitary gland and found two pituitary gland-specific factor (PGSF) 1a and PGSF2. These factors have been recognized by sera from patients with rheumatoid arthritis, which intuitively would exclude them as specific autoantigens. However, there is preliminary evidence that rheumatoid patients may have subtle pituitary dysfunction *(190)*.

COMPLEMENT CONSUMPTION ASSAYS

Pituitary autoantibodies were first sought using a complement consumption assay and crude autopsy pituitary gland homogenate *(191)*. This type of assay works on the basis of the interaction of antigen-antibody complexes with complement and is particularly neither sensitive nor specific. The results in 128 normal peripartum women linked the development of positive antibody status 5–7 days postpartum (seen in 18%) with symptoms suggestive of pituitary dysfunction 6–12 months later, but hormonal data were lacking.

INDIRECT IF ASSAYS

The first study was by Goudie *(192)*, who was unable to find positive anti-pituitary reactivity. In 1969, Nerup et al. *(193)* also unsuccessfully attempted to demon-

Table 1
Techniques and Substrates Used for the Detection of Pituitary Autoantibodies

Technique	Pituitary substrate		References
Complement consumption	Human	Autopsy material	Engelberth and Jezkova, 1965 (191)
Indirect immuno-fluorescence	Human	Autopsy material	Bottazzo et al., 1975 (55)
			Pouplard et al., 1985 (202)
		Fresh material from surgery	Bottazzo et al., 1975 (55)
			Mirakian et al., 1982 (180)
			Gluck et al., 1993 (193)
		Fetal glands	Scherbaum et al., 1987 (197)
			Gluck and Scherbaum, 1990 (200)
			Gluck et al., 1993
	Primate	Cymologous monkey	Gluck and Scherbaum, 1990 (200)
		Rhesus monkey	Maghnie et al., 1994 (196)
			Maghnie et al., 1995 (197)
		Baboon	Gluck and Scherbaum, 1990 (200)
			De Bellis et al., 2003 (198)
			De Bellis et al., 2005 (201)
	Non-primate	Rat	Bottazzo et al., 1975 (55)
			Pouplard et al., 1980 (200)
			Hansen et al., 1989 (183)
			Møller et al., 1985 (201)
			Sugiura et al., 1986 (203)
			Kobayashi et al., 1988 (203)
			Gluck and Scherbaum, 1990 (200)
			Kajita et al., 1991 (82)
			Fetissov et al., 2002 (223)
		Bovine	Bottazzo et al., 1975 (55)
			Gluck and Scherbaum, 1990 (200)
		Guinea pig	Pouplard, 1982 (196)
			Pouplard et al., 1985 (202)
		Porcine	Hansen et al., 1989 (183)
			Gluck and Scherbaum, 1990 (200)
		Sheep	Gluck and Scherbaum, 1990 (200)
	Cell lines	Murine AtT_{20} and Rat GH_3	Sugiura et al., 1987 (84)
			Komatsu et al., 1988 (204)
			Kajita et al., 1991 (82)
Immunoblotting	Human		Crock et al., 1993 (205)
			Crock, 1998 (40)
			Strömberg et al., 1998 (208)
			Nishiki et al., 2001 (206)

			Takao et al., 2001 *(210)*
			Goswami et al., 2002 *(118)*
			O'Dwyer et al., 2002 *(207)*
			O'Dwyer et al., 2002 *(187)*
			Bensing et al., 2004 *(81)*
			Bensing et al., 2005 *(37)*
	Primate	Rhesus monkey	Crock et al., 1993 *(205)*
	Non-primate	Rat	Yabe et al., 1995 *(212)*
			Yabe et al., 1998 *(213)*
			Kikuchi et al., 2000 *(215)*
			Nishino et al., 2001 *(214)*
		Porcine	Kobayashi et al., 1997 *(212)*
			Kobayashi et al., 1998 *(211)*
Enzyme-linked immunosorbent assay	Human	Adenoma cells	Keda et al., 2002 *(216)*
	Non-primate	Rat	Yabe et al., 1998 *(213)*
			Kikuchi et al., 2000 *(215)*
			Nishino et al., 2001 *(214)*
			Keda et al., 2002 *(216)*
		Porcine	Kobayashi et al., 1998 *(211)*
In vitro transcription translation and immunoprecipitation of pituitary proteins	Human		Tanaka et al., 2002 *(219)*
			Tanaka et al., 2003 *(190)*
			Tanaka et al., 2003 *(220)*
			Tatsumi et al., 2003 *(188)*

strate pituitary autoantibodies in 16 patients with idiopathic hypopituitarism (and 232 controls) using IF on fresh human surgical pituitary tissue from breast cancer sufferers as well as monkey and rabbit pituitaries. None of the 16 had other autoimmune conditions except one with thyroglobulin antibodies. In 1975, Bottazzo et al. *(55)* first described autoantibodies to pituitary prolactin-secreting cells using indirect IF in 287 patients with endocrine autoimmunity, but none had clinical hypopituitarism.

The IF assay is still widely used, but it has rarely identified pituitary autoantibodies in patients with biopsy-proven or suspected lymphocytic hypophysis *(27,194)*. This method recognizes the conformational structure of antigens, their sub-cellular localization, and the pituitary cell type targeted. In general, the titer of pituitary autoantibodies found by IF is low. The choice of pituitary substrate is problematic in terms of species specificity issues, ethical issues, and limited supply.

Human Tissues as Substrate. Bottazzo et al. *(55)* used a four-layer double-fluorochrome method on fresh, human pituitaries from women whom had undergone hypophysectomy for breast cancer. These glands did not have entirely normal histology, as they had prolactin cell and GH cell hypertrophy and a reduced number of basophils. Prior treatment with stilbestrol and prednisone may have accounted for these changes. Sera from 10 patients with autoimmune polyendocrinopathy and 9 patients with a single endocrine autoimmune disease gave a diffuse, finely granular cytoplasmic IF on pituitary cells. None had hypopituitarism. Conversely, none of the 13 patients with idiopathic panhypopituitarism gave positive results.

Subsequently, using undiluted serum, antibodies to "multiple pituitary cell types" were shown in patients with newly diagnosed diabetes and their high-risk first-degree relatives (180). There was a striking correlation between pituitary cell antibodies and positive ICA. The authors speculated that this may have indicated a viral trigger for diabetes that simultaneously involved the pituitary. The idea is supported by the work of Onodera et al. (195) discussed in "Animal Models."

Pouplard (196) had shown in 1982 that immunoglobulins from normal sera bind through Fc receptors to the surface of corticotrophs but not those in fetal pituitary glands. Thus, pituitary antibodies against corticotrophs need to be interpreted with caution. Scherbaum et al. (197) have shown that pituitary autoantibodies to corticotrophs in Cushing's disease patients are associated with an unfavorable outcome after microsurgical resection. They have not published results on patients with lymphocytic hypophysitis.

Other cell types targeted have included thyrotrophs, gonadotrophs in patients with cryptorchidism and their mothers (198), and somatotrophs (199). Again, no patients with hypophysitis were studied.

Non-Human Tissues as Substrate.   Although fresh human tissue would be ideal, the ethical issues of using fetal glands and the limited supply of surgical tissue make this untenable. Non-human tissues raise the problems of species specificity because of heterophile antibodies as outlined by the study from Gluck and Scherbaum (200).

Bottazzo's original publications concluded that baboon pituitary was the optimal non-human tissue substrate. Recently, De Bellis and colleagues (201) have revisited IF using young baboon pituitary glands in patients with idiopathic GHD and autoimmune endocrine diseases. Specific staining of somatotrophs alone was typical of isolated GHD; however, more diffuse staining of other cells was seen in patients with GHD and other autoimmune diseases.

A range of other pituitary tissues has been used including guinea pig (202), rat (203), porcine (183), and a murine AtT20 cell line (84). Positive reactivity has been seen in patients with cryptorchidism (202), isolated ACTH deficiency (203), the empty sella syndrome (204), and Graves' disease (183).

Immunoblotting Assays

The IB (or Western) assay was developed to overcome the problems with IF (205). The preparation of whole pituitary glands by homogenization means that the immunoreactivity detected by patient sera is to proteins of a particular molecular size rather than a specific pituitary cell type. In addition, the initial centrifugation step gives a pellet containing nuclei and mitochondria. If this fraction contains any potential autoantigens, they will be discarded at this step. Proteins from the membrane or cytosolic fractions are then denatured, separated electrophoretically by size and transferred to a membrane. The assay method is outlined in Fig. 5. In contrast to IF, patient sera react with linear epitopes rather than a three-dimensional structure.

In the original IB article *(205)*, both membrane and cytosolic pituitary fractions were probed with sera from pediatric patients with GHD and normal pediatric control sera. Autoantibodies were identified to a 45-kDa pituitary-specific membrane protein in 1 of 19 patients with idiopathic GHD and the empty sella syndrome. One other patient with idiopathic GHD and 1 of 14 patients with secondary GHD had autoantibodies to a 43-kDa membrane protein, found in both pituitary and brain. None of 27 control subjects had these autoantibodies. In light of recent IF data in an adult cohort of Italian patients with GHD *(201)*, it will be of great interest to identify the protein(s) seen by IF and to see whether they have the same molecular weights as those in our IB study. Nishiki et al. *(206)* also identified pituitary-specific antibodies to 43-kDa, 49-kDa, or 68-kDa membrane proteins in 5 of 13 patients with lymphocytic hypophysitis, 1 of 12 patients with infundibuloneurohypophysis, but none of 4 patients with isolated ACTH deficiency. These proteins are of great interest but have yet to be further characterized. No other membrane studies have been published.

Subsequent IB studies using pituitary cytosolic preparations in a series of 10 patients with biopsy-proven hypophysitis and 22 patients with suspected disease showed autoantibodies to a 49-kDa protein in 70% patients with biopsy-proven hypophysitis, 50% with suspected disease, and 9.8% normal controls. A number of other autoantigens were identified, particularly a 40-kDa protein. Titers as high as >1:1000 were seen in contrast to IF studies that have consistently used undiluted sera or dilutions up to 1:8. Species specificity experiments using IB demonstrated that the 49-kDa protein was conserved across species *(40)* but also demonstrated the extent of tissue cross-reactivity that can confound IF results.

The 49-kDa protein was purified using column chromatography, sequenced, and identified as alpha-enolase *(207)*. Enolase has three isoforms, one of which is found

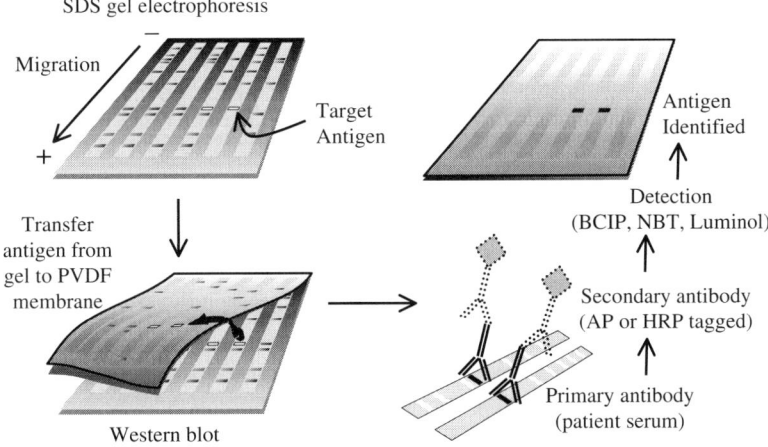

Fig. 5. Schematic representation of the immunoblotting (IB) assay for pituitary autoantibodies.

in neuroendocrine tissues (NSE). A study using two-dimensional gel electrophoresis showed that serum from a peripartum woman with lymphocytic hypophysitis recognized NSE in both the placenta and the pituitary *(187)*. It was hypothesized that the sharing of placental and pituitary antigens may explain the association of lymphocytic hypophysitis with pregnancy. The study by Goswami et al. *(118)* of Indian women with true Sheehan's syndrome who developed hypopituitarism up to 8 years later also hints at this link.

Anti-enolase antibodies have been found in a wide range of patients with classical non-organ-specific autoimmunity *(40)* but also in up to 20% of patients with pituitary adenoma and 5–10% of control subjects using IB. Using another method (in vitro transcription translation [ITT]; *see* In Vitro Transcription Translation or Immunoprecipitate of Pituitary Proteins), the incidence of these antibodies in tumor patients was even higher (46%), suggesting that they may not be a reliable discriminator of an autoimmune condition.

Isolated ACTH deficiency has been reported in association with autoimmune diseases *(83,208)*, including lymphocytic hypophysitis *(38,209)*. In a large Polish series of patients with ACTH deficiency (isolated in 61 of 65), 51% (33 of 65) had another autoimmune disease and 85% (55 of 65) had positive thyroid autoantibodies. IB identified a novel 36-kDa pituitary cytosolic autoantigen in 12 patients (18.5%) compared with 2 of 57 healthy controls (3.5%, $p < 0.021$) *(37)*. Patients with autoantibodies to the 36-kDa protein had a higher frequency of thyroglobulin autoantibodies than the patients whose sera were not immunoreactive. This target autoantigen has not been further characterized as yet. A Japanese study of nine patients with isolated ACTH deficiency demonstrated that seven (77.8%) had autoantibodies to a 22-kDa human pituitary cytosolic protein, subsequently identified as GH *(210)*. The same study found these autoantibodies in 11 of 15 (73%) patients with lymphocytic hypophysitis. GHD was found on testing in 9 of 11 patients with autoantibodies. GH reactivity was lost by preabsorption with pancreatic antigens *(211)*, a finding that mirrors Bottazzo's earlier observations in patients with diabetes and ICA cross-reactivity with the pituitary.

The empty sella syndrome almost certainly has a heterogenous etiology with one component being end-stage hypophysitis. Bensing et al. *(81)* studied a group of 30 patients with empty sella syndrome, 15 of whom had type 2 diabetes or impaired glucose tolerance and a body phenotype of central obesity. They did not have evidence of high-titer pituitary autoantibodies compared with controls, but only four patients (13%) had pituitary dysfunction. Therefore, it appears that patients with an empty sella syndrome and normal pituitary function are very unlikely to have had hypophysitis.

ENZYME-LINKED IMMUNOSORBENT ASSAY

The first group to investigate an enzyme-linked immunosorbent assay (ELISA) was Yabe et al. *(211–213)*. Rat or porcine pituitary antigens from tissue preparations were used. A typical ELISA procedure was developed using the cytosolic fraction of homogenized rat pituitary glands, coated onto the ELISA plate at alkaline pH. Serum reactivity to bound antigens was detected using a peroxidase-conjugated second antibody and a colored substrate. Measurement of absorbance at an appropriate wavelength related to the concentration of pituitary autoantibodies present. This approach presents a cocktail of potential autoantigens and preserves the three-dimensional structure of the antigens. However, the advantage may be nullified if a low level of target autoantigen

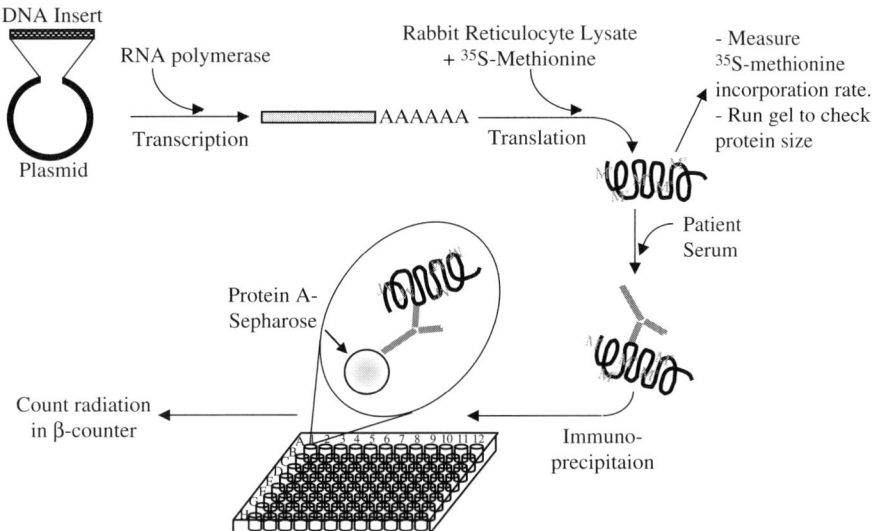

Fig. 6. Schematic representation of the immunoprecipitation (in vitro transcription translation [ITT]) assay for pituitary autoantibodies.

(cytosolic or membrane) is masked by other proteins or if there is significant species cross-reactivity. Pituitary autoantibodies were detected by this method in patients with non-insulin-dependent diabetes mellitus *(212)* and autoimmune thyroiditis *(214)* as well as various pituitary disorders *(215)*. This research group has also found the prevalence of pituitary autoantibodies to be significantly higher in type 2 diabetes patients than in control subjects using porcine instead of rat pituitary as antigen *(211)*.

Keda et al. *(216)* modified the ELISA by using human pituitary adenoma cells to develop a cellular variant. Serum from patients with idiopathic hyperprolactinemia or idiopathic-isolated GHD had autoantibodies more frequently to prolactin-secreting cells and GH-secreting cells, respectively, than patients with other forms of pituitary diseases.

Evaluation of these ELISA techniques using sera from biopsy-proven lymphocytic hypophysitis patients has yet to be performed.

IN VITRO TRANSCRIPTION TRANSLATION AND IMMUNOPRECIPITATION OF PITUITARY PROTEINS

The latest assay uses rabbit reticulocyte lysate to produce recombinant pituitary proteins in vitro. Methionine residues on these proteins are labeled with ^{35}S, and the proteins then mixed with patient sera and protein-A sepharose in an immunoprecipitation step *(217)*. The method is outlined schematically in Fig. 6. A number of potential pituitary autoantigens have been tested in this system. Tanaka et al. *(218)* tested two novel PGSFs, PGSF1a and PGSF2, isolated from a hypothalamic cDNA expression library. Other candidates studied included enolase; GH; the prohormone-processing enzymes, PC, PC1/3, and PC2; CPE; and PC2-regulatory protein, 7B2 *(188)*. None of these enzymes is pituitary specific.

Positive antibody indices to PGSF1a were found in 1 of 3 (33%) patients with biopsy-proven hypophysitis and 2 of 10 (20%) patients with isolated ACTH deficiency *(219)*. Reactivity to PGSF2 was seen in 2 of 14 (14%) patients with suspected hypophysitis or infundibuloneurohypophysitis and 3 of 14 (21%) patients with hypopituitarism. Anti-GH antibodies were detected in 2 of 8 (25%) patients with hypophysitis (1 of whom was biopsy proven), 2 of 14 (14%) with hypopituitarism, and 2 of 31 (6.5%) with other autoimmune diseases. None of the antibody indices was above 2, which implies very low titer reactivity. Patients with pituitary adenomata did not show any reactivity to either PGSF1a or PGSF2 *(219)*, but 5 of 11 (45%) patients had antibodies against PC1/3 *(188)* and 6 of 11 (55%) to 7B2 compared with 2 of 14 (14%) patients with lymphocytic hypophysitis for both antigens *(188)*. PGSF1a antibodies have also been detected in 20 of 26 (77%) rheumatoid arthritis patients *(190)*. Before these latest results are dismissed as non-specific, it will be important to exclude subtle pituitary hormone dysfunction in these patients.

Enolase was tested as an autoantigen in the ITT assay by Tanaka et al. *(220)*. They demonstrated positive autoantibodies in 7 of 17 (41%) patients with lymphocytic hypophysitis, 6 of 30 (20%) with non-functioning pituitary macroadenoma, 4 of 17 (23.5%) with other autoimmune diseases, and 2 of 46 (4.3%) healthy controls. These results are similar to those reported with IB except for the high prevalence in patients with pituitary adenomata. In the ITT system, enolase antibodies appear quite non-specific.

The ITT assay has the potential to test multiple target autoantigens in high-throughput assays that are less labor intensive than IF or IB. However, expression of proteins in this system does not always guarantee that they are in their native conformation required for binding of patient sera *(221)*.

AUTOANTIBODIES TO PITUITARY HORMONES

There are limited studies showing that pituitary hormones can be targets, analogous to insulin as a major target autoantigen in type 1 diabetes. In 1993, Mau et al. *(222)* demonstrated by IB, anti-ACTH and anti-GH antibodies in two of six patients with empty sella syndrome and anti-ACTH and anti-TSH antibodies in three of five patients with pituitary tumors. Six normal controls were negative. Positive antibodies did not correlate with hormonal function *(222)*. A significant subset of sera from patients with anorexia nervosa and bulimia nervosa contains antibodies against MSH and/or ACTH *(223)*. IB studies from Kikuchi et al. *(215)* and Takao et al. *(210)* identified a 22-kD protein as a target autoantigen, subsequently shown to be GH.

Animal Models

Experimental induction of cellular or humoral autoimmunity by sensitizing animals with autologous pituitary antigens is one of the major criteria for organ-specific autoimmunity. In 1967, Levine *(224)* successfully induced "allergic adenohypophysitis" by injecting rat pituitary tissue homogenate emulsified in complete Freund's adjuvant into 14 rats. Six animals (43%) developed focal or diffuse mononuclear cell infiltration of the pituitary within 2–3 weeks of a single injection. The addition of pertussis toxin as a second adjuvant increased disease incidence to 75%. The hypophysitis was more severe in a sub-group of pregnant and postpartum rats, analogous to the human condition. Subsequent experiments *(225)* showed guinea pig pituitary extracts were the most successful inducer of disease in the rat model, whereas human and bovine tissues were poor inducers. Similar experiments in rabbits gave similar results *(226)*. In 2001, Watanabe et al. *(227)* revisited Levine's experiment in female Lewis rats. Although no severe lymphocytic infiltration of the adenohypophysis was seen, they identified GH, TSH, and luteinizing hormone (LH) as major autoantigens. These findings accord with the data from Japanese clinical studies *(210)*.

One of the most interesting experiments in this field was by Beck and Melvin in 1970 *(228)* who induced autoimmune hypophysitis in a female rhesus monkey using repeated exposure to human placental extracts and chorionic gonadotrophins over 3 years. No evidence was presented to show that the lympho-plasmacytic infiltrate had affected pituitary function. The pituitary and placenta share the expression of many molecules, including such autoantigens as NSE *(187)*. Whether this is relevant to the close association of lymphocytic hypophysitis and pregnancy or to Sheehan's syndrome and delayed hypopituitarism with pituitary antibodies *(118)* is intriguing but unclear.

VIRALLY INDUCED HYPOPHYSITIS

Four animal models of virally induced pituitary autoimmunity have been reported. In the first model, mice infected with reovirus type 1 developed autoantibodies against anterior pituitary, islets of Langerhans' and gastric mucosa, as well as to hormones such as insulin and GH *(195)*. This model is consistent with IF data in newly diagnosed type 1 diabetes patients *(180)*. Yoon et al. *(229)* injected male golden Syrian hamsters with rubella virus E1 and E2 glycoproteins and detected pituitary cell autoantibodies by IF within 3 weeks in 95% of animals. All animals had diffuse inflammatory infiltrates in their pituitary glands, but by 8 weeks, only 20% of animals still had autoantibodies. Neonatal thymectomy almost completely prevented the disease, implying that it was T-cell mediated, but it could not be transferred by autoantibodies. T-cell transfer experiments were not conducted.

The other models were part of recent studies into gene therapy for pituitary disease. Adenovirus-mediated gene transfer studies in sheep, using direct stereotaxic injection, showed evidence of a severe inflammatory reaction with lymphocytic infiltration, venulitis, and periglandular fibrosis *(230)*. Expression of influenza nucleoprotein as a transgene under the control of the human GH locus-control region localized this virus to secretory vesicles in pituitary somatotrophs. Activation of monoclonal CD8 T cells specific to the viral protein resulted in spontaneous autoimmune hypophysitis of the pituitary gland targeting somatotrophs. In turn, this resulted in significantly reduced GH levels in adult mice and a dwarf phenotype *(231)*. In a follow-up study, these authors showed that antigen dose, T-cell precursor frequency, the degree of lymphopenia, and the context of target antigen expression are all important modulators of disease expression *(232)*. These studies highlight the potential problems with the use of therapeutic strategies based on vaccination against soluble pituitary proteins. However, they also support the theory that viral infections can trigger hypophysitis and that cases of viral meningoencephalitis preceding hypophysitis are not just coincidental occurrences but pathogenetic.

Treatment

Management of a patient with lymphocytic hypophysitis is dictated by the rapidity of onset, by the severity of symptoms and signs, and by the certainty of the clinical diagnosis. Even when hypophysitis is suspected preoperatively, it is not always possible to avoid surgery. The indications for surgical intervention include visual compromise that cannot be rapidly improved with medical therapy, recurrent mass effects despite immunosuppression, and cases where the diagnosis of a pituitary adenoma or other tumor cannot be excluded *(14)*.

There is now a body of literature on the use of steroids as immunosuppressive agents in lymphocytic hypophysitis *(12,18)*. Prednisolone was first tried successfully in 1980 by Mayfield et al. *(27)*. There has been only one prospective trial of high-dose methylprednisolone therapy (120 mg/day for 2 weeks, then tapering doses over 1 month) *(68)*, where four of nine patients had some improvement in hormonal function and seven had a reduction in size of the mass on MRI scan. Methylprednisolone has been tried up to lymphocytotoxic doses of 1 g *(65,233)*. Dexamethasone has also been used *(11,234)* but can cause severe Cushingoid features *(142)*. Prolonged steroid use can lead to bilateral necrosis of the head of the femur *(59)*, among many other toxicities. Alternative treatments have been used in individual cases including low-dose stereotactic radiotherapy *(164,235)*, methotrexate *(22,60)*, and azathioprine *(64)*.

Conservative management is more likely to be successful in those cases that present in a sub-acute fashion, such as with hypopituitarism and a resolving pituitary mass. As spontaneous remission has been reported *(49,105)*, many endocrinologists and neuro-surgeons now advocate a conservative approach, with or without a trial of immunosuppression. However, it should be stressed that a response to immunosuppressive (rather than replacement) doses of steroids does not necessarily confirm a diagnosis of lymphocytic hypophysitis. A number of conditions can be steroid responsive including dysgerminoma, neurosarcoidosis, Wegener's granulomatosis, and Langerhans' cell histiocytosis.

There is clearly a role for surgical intervention in some patients; however, aggressive resection of inflammatory tissue almost always results in permanent hypopituitarism *(14)*. There are rare cases where recurrence of the inflammatory mass has required a second surgery *(21,22,74,135,235,236)*. In these, surgery was very effective at relieving symptoms, particularly headache and visual field defects.

FUTURE DIRECTIONS

Future directions for lymphocytic hypophysitis research hinge on finding the relevant target autoantigens and identifying reliable autoantibody markers for the disease. Hopefully, these will give us new insights into the underlying autoimmune trigger(s) and mechanisms. New therapeutic approaches with "biologicals" are targeting these mechanisms in other diseases, such as rituximab therapy for thyroid-associated ophthalmopathy *(237)* and CD3 antibody therapy in new-onset type 1 diabetes *(238)*. It is therefore critical to establish the immunopathogenesis of lymphocytic hypophysitis to tailor any future immunotherapies.

ACKNOWLEDGMENTS

We would like to acknowledge the generous support of the Hunter Children's Research Foundation, the Hunter Medical Research Institute, the John Hunter Hospital Charitable Trust, NH&MRC Grant 100952 and the NH&MRC PhD Research Scholarship to CJAS. We would also like to thank Dr. Martin Epstein and Professor Roger Smith for providing the MRI scans of their patients and constructive and Dr. Glenn Reeves for helpful advice.

REFERENCES

1. Hashimoto H. Zur Kenntnsiss der lymphomatosen veranderung def schilddruse (struma lymphomatos). *Arch Klin Chir* 1912;97:219–23.

2. Goudie RB, Pinkerton PH. Anterior hypophysitis and Hashimoto's disease in a young woman. *J Pathol Bacteriol* 1962;83:584–5.

3. Sheehan HL, Summers VK. The syndrome of hypopituitarism. *Q J Med* 1949;18(72):319–78.

4. Carpenter CC, Solomon N, Silverberg SG, et al. Schmidt's syndrome (thyroid and adrenal insufficiency). A review of the literature and a report of fifteen new cases including ten instances of coexistent diabetes mellitus. *Medicine (Baltimore)* 1964;43:153–80.

5. Duff GL, Bernstein C. Five cases of Addison's disease with so-called atrophy of the adrenal gland. *Bull Johns Hopkins Hosp* 1933;52:67–83.

6. Susman W. Atrophy of the adrenals associated with Addison's disease. *J Pathol Bacteriol* 1930;33(3):749–60.

7. Winqvist O, Karlsson FA, Kampe O. 21-Hydroxylase, a major autoantigen in idiopathic Addison's disease. *Lancet* 1992;339(8809):1559–62.

8. Verge CF, Gianani R, Kawasaki E, et al. Number of autoantibodies (against insulin, GAD or ICA512/IA2) rather than particular autoantibody specificities determines risk of type I diabetes. *J Autoimmun* 1996;9(3):379–83.

9. Bellastella A, Bizzarro A, Coronella C, Bellastella G, Sinisi AA, De Bellis A. Lymphocytic hypophysitis: a rare or underestimated disease? *Eur J Endocrinol* 2003;149(5):363–76.

10. Beressi N, Beressi JP, Cohen R, Modigliani E. Lymphocytic hypophysitis. A review of 145 cases. *Ann Med Interne (Paris)* 1999;150(4):327–41.

11. Cosman F, Post KD, Holub DA, Wardlaw SL. Lymphocytic hypophysitis. Report of 3 new cases and review of the literature. *Medicine (Baltimore)* 1989;68(4):240–56.

12. Crock PA. Lymphocytic hypophysitis. *Curr Opin Endocrinol Diabet* 1997;4:115–23.

13. Hashimoto K, Takao T, Makino S. Lymphocytic adenohypophysitis and lymphocytic infundibuloneurohypophysitis. *Endocr J* 1997;44(1):1–10.

14. Thodou E, Asa SL, Kontogeorgos G, Kovacs K, Horvath E, Ezzat S. Clinical case seminar: lymphocytic hypophysitis: clinicopathological findings. *J Clin Endocrinol Metab* 1995;80(8):2302–11.

15. Simmonds JP, Brandes WW. The pathology of the hypophysis. II. Lymphocytic infiltration. *Am J Pathol* 1925;1:273–80.

16. Shanklin WM. Lymphocytes and lymphoid tissue in the human pituitary. *Anat Rec* 1951;111(2):177–91.

17. Scheithauer BW, Sano T, Kovacs KT, Young WF Jr, Ryan N, Randall RV. The pituitary gland in pregnancy: a clinicopathologic and immunohistochemical study of 69 cases. *Mayo Clin Proc* 1990;65(4):461–74.

18. Caturegli P, Newschaffer C, Olivi A, Pomper MG, Burger PC, Rose NR. Autoimmune hypophysitis. *Endocr Rev* 2005;26(5):599–614.

19. Sautner D, Saeger W, Ludecke DK, Jansen V, Puchner MJ. Hypophysitis in surgical and autoptical specimens. *Acta Neuropathol (Berl)* 1995;90(6):637–44.

20. Fehn M, Sommer C, Ludecke DK, Plockinger U, Saeger W. Lymphocytic hypophysitis: light and electron microscopic findings and correlation to clinical appearance. *Endocr Pathol* 1998;9(1):71–8.

21. Honegger J, Fahlbusch R, Bornemann A, et al. Lymphocytic and granulomatous hypophysitis: experience with nine cases. *Neurosurgery* 1997;40(4):713–22, discussion 22–3.

22. Leung GK, Lopes MB, Thorner MO, Vance ML, Laws ER Jr. Primary hypophysitis: a single-center experience in 16 cases. *J Neurosurg* 2004;101(2):262–71.

23. Buxton N, Robertson I. Lymphocytic and granulocytic hypophysitis: a single centre experience. *Br J Neurosurg* 2001;15(3):242–5, discussion 5–6.

24. Asa SL, Bilbao JM, Kovacs K, Josse RG, Kreines K. Lymphocytic hypophysitis of pregnancy resulting in hypopituitarism: a distinct clinicopathologic entity. *Ann Intern Med* 1981;95(2):166–71.

25. Feigenbaum SL, Martin MC, Wilson CB, Jaffe RB. Lymphocytic adenohypophysitis: a pituitary mass lesion occurring in pregnancy. Proposal for medical treatment. *Am J Obstet Gynecol* 1991;164(6 Pt 1):1549–55.

26. Guay AT, Agnello V, Tronic BC, Gresham DG, Freidberg SR. Lymphocytic hypophysitis in a man. *J Clin Endocrinol Metab* 1987;64(3):631–4.

27. Mayfield RK, Levine JH, Gordon L, Powers J, Galbraith RM, Rawe SE. Lymphoid adenohypophysitis presenting as a pituitary tumor. *Am J Med* 1980;69(4):619–23.

28. Meichner RH, Riggio S, Manz HJ, Earll JM. Lymphocytic adenohypophysitis causing pituitary mass. *Neurology* 1987;37(1):158–61.

29. Miyamoto M, Sugawa H, Mori T, Hashimoto N, Imura H. A case of hypopituitarism due to granulomatous and lymphocytic adenohypophysitis with minimal pituitary enlargement: a possible variant of lymphocytic adenohypophysitis. *Endocrinol Jpn* 1988;35(4):607–16.

30. Pestell RG, Best JD, Alford FP. Lymphocytic hypophysitis. The clinical spectrum of the disorder and evidence for an autoimmune pathogenesis. *Clin Endocrinol (Oxf)* 1990;33(4):457–66.

31. Pholsena M, Young J, Couzinet B, Schaison G. Primary adrenal and thyroid insufficiencies associated with hypopituitarism: a diagnostic challenge. *Clin Endocrinol (Oxf)* 1994;40(5):693–5.

32. Supler ML, Mickle JP. Lymphocytic hypophysitis: report of a case in a man with cavernous sinus involvement. *Surg Neurol* 1992;37(6):472–6.

33. Yamaguchi T, Abe H, Matsui T, et al. Lymphocytic hypophysitis, pustulosis palmaris et plantaris and eosinophilia. *Intern Med* 1994;33(3):150–4.

34. Srikanta S, Mehra NK, Vaidya MC, Malaviya AN, Ahuja MM. HLA antigens in type I (insulin-dependent) diabetes mellitus in North India. *Metabolism* 1981;30(10):992–3.

35. Gal R, Schwartz A, Gukovsky-Oren S, Peleg D, Goldman J, Kessler E. Lymphoid hypophysitis associated with sudden maternal death: report of a case review of the literature. *Obstet Gynecol Surv* 1986;41(10):619–21.

36. Blisard KS, Pfalzgraf RR, Balko MG. Sudden death due to lymphoplasmacytic hypophysitis. *Am J Forensic Med Pathol* 1992;13(3):207–10.

37. Bensing S, Kasperlik-Zaluska AA, Czarnocka B, Crock PA, Hulting A. Autoantibodies against pituitary proteins in patients with adrenocorticotropin-deficiency. *Eur J Clin Invest* 2005;35(2):126–32.

38. Jensen MD, Handwerger BS, Scheithauer BW, Carpenter PC, Mirakian R, Banks PM. Lymphocytic hypophysitis with isolated corticotropin deficiency. *Ann Intern Med* 1986;105(2):200–3.

39. Lee MS, Pless M. Apoplectic lymphocytic hypophysitis. Case report. *J Neurosurg* 2003;98(1):183–5.

40. Crock PA. Cytosolic autoantigens in lymphocytic hypophysitis. *J Clin Endocrinol Metab* 1998;83(2):609–18.

41. Dan NG, Feiner RI, Houang MT, Turner JJ. Pituitary apoplexy in association with lymphocytic hypophysitis. *J Clin Neurosci* 2002;9(5):577–80.

42. Halimi D, Benhamou CL, Amor B, Bricaire H, Luton JP. [Osteoarticular pathology, hypercalcemia and adrenal insufficiency. Analysis of 113 cases of adrenal insufficiency]. *Ann Endocrinol (Paris)* 1986;47(6):403–8.

43. Jowsey J, Simons GW. Normocalcaemia in relation to cortisone secretion. *Nature* 1968;217(135):1277–9.

44. Mundy GR, Shapiro JL, Bandelin JG, Canalis EM, Raisz LG. Direct stimulation of bone resorption by thyroid hormones. *J Clin Invest* 1976;58(3):529–34.

45. Novoa-Takara L, Cornford M, Williams C, Tayek JA. Lymphocytic hypophysitis in a man presenting with hypercalcemia. *Am J Med Sci* 2001;321(3):206–8.

46. Richtsmeier AJ, Henry RA, Bloodworth JM Jr, Ehrlich EN. Lymphoid hypophysitis with selective adrenocorticotropic hormone deficiency. *Arch Intern Med* 1980;140(9):1243–5.

47. Strachan MW, Walker JD, Patrick AW. Severe hypercalcaemia secondary to isolated adrenocorticotrophic hormone deficiency and subacute thyroiditis. *Ann Clin Biochem* 2003;40(Pt 3):295–7.

48. Vasikaran SD, Tallis GA, Braund WJ. Secondary hypoadrenalism presenting with hypercalcaemia. *Clin Endocrinol (Oxf)* 1994;41(2):261–4.

49. Patel MC, Guneratne N, Haq N, West TE, Weetman AP, Clayton RN. Peripartum hypopituitarism and lymphocytic hypophysitis. *QJM* 1995;88(8):571–80.

50. Brandes JC, Cerletty JM. Pregnancy in lymphocytic hypophysitis: case report and review. *Wis Med J* 1989;88(11):29–32.

51. Gagneja H, Arafah B, Taylor HC. Histologically proven lymphocytic hypophysitis: spontaneous resolution and subsequent pregnancy. *Mayo Clin Proc* 1999;74(2):150–4.

52. Hayes FJ, McKenna TJ. The occurrence of lymphocytic hypophysitis in a first but not subsequent pregnancy. *J Clin Endocrinol Metab* 1996;81(8):3131–2.

53. Tsur A, Leibowitz G, Samueloff A, Gross DJ. Successful pregnancy in a patient with pre-existing lymphocytic hypophysitis. *Acta Obstet Gynecol Scand* 1996;75(8):772–4.

54. Ezzat S, Josse RG. Autoimmune hypophysitis. *Trends Endocrinol Metab* 1997;8:74–80.

55. Bottazzo GF, Pouplard A, Florin-Christensen A, Doniach D. Autoantibodies to prolactin-secreting cells of human pituitary. *Lancet* 1975;2(7925):97–101.

56. De Bellis A, Bizzarro A, Pivonello R, Lombardi G, Bellastella A. Prolactin and autoimmunity. *Pituitary* 2005;8(1):25–30.

57. Aimaretti G, Ambrosio MR, Di Somma C, et al. Traumatic brain injury and subarachnoid haemorrhage are conditions at high risk for hypopituitarism: screening study at 3 months after the brain injury. *Clin Endocrinol (Oxf)* 2004;61(3):320–6.

58. Darzy KH, Shalet SM. Radiation-induced growth hormone deficiency. *Horm Res* 2003;59(Suppl 1):1–11.

59. Nussbaum CE, Okawara SH, Jacobs LS. Lymphocytic hypophysitis with involvement of the cavernous sinus and hypothalamus. *Neurosurgery* 1991;28(3):440–4.

60. Tubridy N, Saunders D, Thom M, et al. Infundibulohypophysitis in a man presenting with diabetes insipidus and cavernous sinus involvement. *J Neurol Neurosurg Psychiatry* 2001;71(6):798–801.

61. Ikeda J, Kuratsu J, Miura M, Kai Y, Ushio Y. Lymphocytic adenohypophysitis accompanying occlusion of bilateral internal carotid arteries–case report. *Neurol Med Chir (Tokyo)* 1990;30(5):346–9.

62. Nakamura Y, Okada H, Wada Y, Kajiyama K, Koshiyama H. Lymphocytic hypophysitis: its expanding features. *J Endocrinol Invest* 2001;24(4):262–7.

63. Li JY, Lai PH, Lam HC, et al. Hypertrophic cranial pachymeningitis and lymphocytic hypophysitis in Sjogren's syndrome. *Neurology* 1999;52(2):420–3.

64. Lecube A, Francisco G, Rodriguez D, et al. Lymphocytic hypophysitis successfully treated with azathioprine: first case report. *J Neurol Neurosurg Psychiatry* 2003;74(11):1581–3.

65. Matta MP, Kany M, Delisle MB, Lagarrigue J, Caron PH. A relapsing remitting lymphocytic hypophysitis. *Pituitary* 2002;5(1):37–44.

66. Paja M, Estrada J, Ojeda A, Ramon y Cajal S, Garcia-Uria J, Lucas T. Lymphocytic hypophysitis causing hypopituitarism and diabetes insipidus, and associated with autoimmune thyroiditis, in a non-pregnant woman. *Postgrad Med J* 1994;70(821):220–4.

67. Vanneste JA, Kamphorst W. Lymphocytic hypophysitis. *Surg Neurol* 1987;28(2):145–9.

68. Kristof RA, Van Roost D, Klingmuller D, Springer W, Schramm J. Lymphocytic hypophysitis: non-invasive diagnosis and treatment by high dose methylprednisolone pulse therapy? *J Neurol Neurosurg Psychiatry* 1999;67(3):398–402.

69. Imura H, Nakao K, Shimatsu A, et al. Lymphocytic infundibuloneurohypophysitis as a cause of central diabetes insipidus. *N Engl J Med* 1993;329(10):683–9.

70. Abe T, Matsumoto K, Sanno N, Osamura Y. Lymphocytic hypophysitis: case report. *Neurosurgery* 1995;36(5):1016–9.

71. Duran Martinez M, Santonja C, Pavon de Paz I, Monereo Megias S. Lymphocytic hypophysitis: report of an unusual case of a rare disorder. *J Endocrinol Invest* 2001;24(3):190–3.

72. Hashimoto K, Asaba K, Tamura K, Takao T, Nakamura T. A case of lymphocytic infundibuloneurohypophysitis associated with systemic lupus erythematosus. *Endocr J* 2002;49(6):605–10.

73. Iglesias P, Diez JJ. Diabetes insipidus as a primary manifestation of lymphocytic hypophysitis in a post-menopausal woman. *Endocrinologist* 2000;10:127–30.

74. Miyagi K, Shingaki T, Ito K, et al. [Lymphocytic infundibulo-hypophysitis with diabetes insipidus as a new clinical entity: a case report and review of the literature]. *No Shinkei Geka* 1997;25(2):169–75.

75. Nishioka H, Ito H, Sano T, Ito Y. Two cases of lymphocytic hypophysitis presenting with diabetes insipidus: a variant of lymphocytic infundibulo-neurohypophysitis. *Surg Neurol* 1996;46(3):285–90, discussion 90–1.

76. Saito T, Yoshida S, Nakao K, Takanashi R. Chronic hypernatremia associated with inflammation of the neurohypophysis. *J Clin Endocrinol Metab* 1970;31(4):391–6.

77. Shimono T, Yamaoka T, Nishimura K, et al. Lymphocytic hypophysitis presenting with diabetes insipidus: MR findings. *Eur Radiol* 1999;9(7):1397–400.

78. Tamiya A, Saeki N, Kubota M, Oheda T, Yamaura A. Unusual MRI findings in lymphocytic hypophysitis with central diabetes insipidus. *Neuroradiology* 1999;41(12):899–900.

79. Iida M, Takamoto S, Masuo M, Makita K, Saito T. Transient lymphocytic panhypophysitis associated with SIADH leading to diabetes insipidus after glucocorticoid replacement. *Intern Med* 2003;42(10):991–5.

80. Leger J, Velasquez A, Garel C, Hassan M, Czernichow P. Thickened pituitary stalk on magnetic resonance imaging in children with central diabetes insipidus. *J Clin Endocrinol Metab* 1999;84(6):1954–60.

81. Bensing S, Rorsman F, Crock P, et al. No evidence for autoimmunity as a major cause of the empty sella syndrome. *Exp Clin Endocrinol Diabetes* 2004;112(5):231–5.

82. Kajita K, Yasuda K, Yamakita N, et al. Anti-pituitary antibodies in patients with hypopituitarism and their families: longitudinal observation. *Endocrinol Jpn* 1991;38(2):121–9.

83. Sauter NP, Toni R, McLaughlin CD, Dyess EM, Kritzman J, Lechan RM. Isolated adrenocorticotropin deficiency associated with an autoantibody to a corticotroph antigen that is not adrenocorticotropin or other proopiomelanocortin-derived peptides. *J Clin Endocrinol Metab* 1990;70(5):1391–7.

84. Sugiura M, Hashimoto A, Shizawa M, et al. Detection of antibodies to anterior pituitary cell surface membrane with insulin dependent diabetes mellitus and adrenocorticotropic hormone deficiency. *Diabetes Res* 1987;4(2):63–6.

85. Barbaro D, Loni G. Lymphocytic hypophysitis and autoimmune thyroid disease. *J Endocrinol Invest* 2000;23(5):339–40.

86. Ludwig H, Schernthaner G. [Multi-organ specific autoimmunity in idiopathic adrenal insufficiency: autosensitization to steroid hormone-producing cells and antigens of the anterior pituitary gland (author's transl)]. *Wien Klin Wochenschr* 1978;90(20):736–41.

87. Sobrinho-Simoes M, Brandao A, Paiva ME, Vilela B, Fernandes E, Carneiro-Chaves F. Lymphoid hypophysitis in a patient with lymphoid thyroiditis, lymphoid adrenalitis, and idiopathic retroperitoneal fibrosis. *Arch Pathol Lab Med* 1985;109(3):230–3.

88. Bayram F, Kelestimur F, Ozturk F, Selcuklu A, Patiroglu TE, Beyhan Z. Lymphocytic hypophysitis in a patient with Graves' disease. *J Endocrinol Invest* 1998;21(3):193–7.

89. Mazzone T, Kelly W, Ensinck J. Lymphocytic hypophysitis. Associated with antiparietal cell antibodies and vitamin B12 deficiency. *Arch Intern Med* 1983;143(9):1794–5.

90. Ward L, Paquette J, Seidman E, et al. Severe autoimmune polyendocrinopathy-candidiasis-ectodermal dystrophy in an adolescent girl with a novel AIRE mutation: response to immunosuppressive therapy. *J Clin Endocrinol Metab* 1999;84(3):844–52.

91. Hasegawa Y, Matsumoto M, Kamimura A, Yamamoto M. [A case of systematic lupus erythematosus with autoimmune hypophysitis]. *Nippon Naika Gakkai Zasshi* 1993;82(4):582–3.

92. Ji JD, Lee SY, Choi SJ, Lee YH, Song GG. Lymphocytic hypophysitis in a patient with systemic lupus erythematosus. *Clin Exp Rheumatol* 2000;18(1):78–80.

93. Katano H, Umemura A, Kamiya K, Kanai H, Yamada K. Visual disturbance by lymphocytic hypophysitis in a non-pregnant woman with systemic lupus erythematosus. *Lupus* 1998;7(8):554–6.

94. Pinol V, Cubiella J, Navasa M, et al. [Autoimmune hepatitis associated with thyroiditis and hypophysitis. A case report]. *Gastroenterol Hepatol* 2000;23(3):123–5.

95. Nishiki M, Murakami Y, Koshimura K, et al. A case of autoimmune hypophysitis associated with asymptomatic primary biliary cirrhosis. *Endocr J* 1998;45(5):697–700.

96. Hama S, Arita K, Kurisu K, Sumida M, Kurihara K. Parasellar chronic inflammatory disease presenting Tolosa-Hunt syndrome, hypopituitarism and diabetes insipidus: a case report. *Endocr J* 1996;43(5):503–10.

97. Hida C, Yamamoto T, Endo K, Tanno Y, Saito T, Tsukamoto T. Inflammatory involvement of the hypophysis in Tolosa-Hunt syndrome. *Intern Med* 1995;34(11):1093–6.

98. Olmos PR, Falko JM, Rea GL, Boesel CP, Chakeres DW, McGhee DB. Fibrosing pseudotumor of the sella and parasellar area producing hypopituitarism and multiple cranial nerve palsies. *Neurosurgery* 1993;32(6):1015–21, discussion 21.

99. Hansen I, Petrossians P, Thiry A, et al. Extensive inflammatory pseudotumor of the pituitary. *J Clin Endocrinol Metab* 2001;86(10):4603–10.

100. Joussen AM, Sommer C, Flechtenmacher C, Voelcker HE. Lymphocytic hypophysitis associated with dacryoadenitis: an autoimmunologically mediated syndrome. *Arch Ophthalmol* 1999;117(7):959–62.

101. Lidove O, Piette JC, Charlotte F, Cassoux N, Correas JM, Papo T. Lymphocytic hypophysitis with lachrymal, salivary and thyroid gland involvement. *Eur J Intern Med* 2004;15(2):121–4.

102. Alvarez A, Cordido F, Sacristan F. Hypopituitarism due to lymphocytic hypophysitis in a patient with retroperitoneal fibrosis. *Postgrad Med J* 1997;73(865):732–4.

103. Ermann J, Fathman CG. Autoimmune diseases: genes, bugs and failed regulation. *Nat Immunol* 2001;2(9):759–61.

104. Wong RW, Ooi TC, Benoit B, Zackon D, Jansen G, Telner A. Lymphocytic hypophysitis with a long latent period before development of a pituitary mass. *Can J Neurol Sci* 2004;31(3):406–8.

105. Krimholtz MJ, Thomas S, Bingham J, Powrie JK. Lymphocytic hypophysitis: spontaneous resolution on MRI with progression of endocrine defect. *Int J Clin Pract* 2001;55(5):339–40.

106. Ozawa Y, Shishiba Y. Recovery from lymphocytic hypophysitis associated with painless thyroiditis: clinical implications of circulating antipituitary antibodies. *Acta Endocrinol (Copenh)* 1993;128(6):493–8.

107. Parent AD. The course of lymphocytic hypophysitis. *Surg Neurol* 1992;37(1):71.

108. Zeller JR, Cerletty JM, Rabinovitch RA, Daniels D. Spontaneous regression of a postpartum pituitary mass demonstrated by computed tomography. *Arch Intern Med* 1982;142(2):373–4.

109. Anderson MS, Venanzi ES, Klein L, et al. Projection of an immunological self shadow within the thymus by the aire protein. *Science* 2002;298(5597):1395–401.

110. Liston A, Lesage S, Wilson J, Peltonen L, Goodnow CC. Aire regulates negative selection of organ-specific T cells. *Nat Immunol* 2003;4(4):350–4.

111. Clifton-Bligh P, Lee C, Smith H, Posen S. The association of diabetes insipidus with hypoparathyroidism. Addison's disease and mucocutaneous candidiasis. *Aust N Z J Med* 1980;10(5):548–51.

112. Scherbaum WA, Wass JA, Besser GM, Bottazzo GF, Doniach D. Autoimmune cranial diabetes insipidus: its association with other endocrine diseases and with histiocytosis X. *Clin Endocrinol (Oxf)* 1986;25(4):411–20.

113. Hung SO, Patterson A. Ectodermal dysplasia associated with autoimmune disease. *Br J Ophthalmol* 1984;68(5):367–9.

114. Castells S, Inamdar S, Orti E. Familial moniliasis, defective delayed hypersensitivity, and adrenocorticotropic hormone deficiency. *J Pediatr* 1971;79(1):72–9.

115. Arvanitakis C, Knouss RF. Selective hypopituitarism. Impaired cell-mediated immunity and chronic mucocutaneous candidiasis. *JAMA* 1973;225(12):1492–5.

116. O'Dwyer DT, McElduff P, Peterson P, Perheentupa J, Crock PA. Pituitary autoantibodies in autoimmune polyendocrinopathy – candidiasis – ectodermal dystrophy (APECED). *Acta Biomed* 2007;78; Suppl 1:248–254.

117. Kent GN, Stuckey BG, Allen JR, Lambert T, Gee V. Postpartum thyroid dysfunction: clinical assessment and relationship to psychiatric affective morbidity. *Clin Endocrinol (Oxf)* 1999;51(4):429–38.

118. Goswami R, Kochupillai N, Crock PA, Jaleel A, Gupta N. Pituitary autoimmunity in patients with Sheehan's syndrome. *J Clin Endocrinol Metab* 2002;87(9):4137–41.

119. Bastida Eizaguirre M, Arto Urzainqui MJ, Iturbe Ortiz de Urbina R. [Diabetes insipidus and panhypopituitarism in an 8-year-old girl due to probable lymphocytic hypophysitis]. *An Esp Pediatr* 1996;44(4):402–4.

120. Cemeroglu AP, Blaivas M, Muraszko KM, Robertson PL, Vazquez DM. Lymphocytic hypophysitis presenting with diabetes insipidus in a 14-year-old girl: case report and review of the literature. *Eur J Pediatr* 1997;156(9):684–8.

121. Ogawa R. A child with necrotizing infundibulo-neurohypophysitis. *Hormone to Rinsho* 1995;43(Suppl 27):33–6.

122. Younes JS, Secord EA. Panhypopituitarism in a child with common variable immunodeficiency. *Ann Allergy Asthma Immunol* 2002;89(3):322–5.

123. Folkerth RD, Price DL Jr, Schwartz M, Black PM, De Girolami U. Xanthomatous hypophysitis. *Am J Surg Pathol* 1998;22(6):736–41.

124. Heinze HJ, Bercu BB. Acquired hypophysitis in adolescence. *J Pediatr Endocrinol Metab* 1997;10(3):315–21.

125. Mueller B, Burgi U, Seiler R. Lymphocytic and granulomatous hypophysitis: experience with nine cases. *Neurosurgery* 1999;44(2):426–7.

126. Krummel MF, Allison JP. CD28 and CTLA-4 have opposing effects on the response of T cells to stimulation. *J Exp Med* 1995;182(2):459–65.

127. Tivol EA, Borriello F, Schweitzer AN, Lynch WP, Bluestone JA, Sharpe AH. Loss of CTLA-4 leads to massive lymphoproliferation and fatal multiorgan tissue destruction, revealing a critical negative regulatory role of CTLA-4. *Immunity* 1995;3(5):541–7.

128. Phan GQ, Yang JC, Sherry RM, et al. Cancer regression and autoimmunity induced by cytotoxic T lymphocyte-associated antigen 4 blockade in patients with metastatic melanoma. *Proc Natl Acad Sci USA* 2003;100(14):8372–7.

129. Ribas A, Camacho LH, Lopez-Berestein G, et al. Antitumor activity in melanoma and anti-self responses in a phase I trial with the anti-cytotoxic T lymphocyte-associated antigen 4 monoclonal antibody CP-675,206. *J Clin Oncol* 2005;23(35):8968–77.

130. Beck KE, Blansfield JA, Tran KQ, et al. Enterocolitis in patients with cancer after antibody blockade of cytotoxic T-lymphocyte-associated antigen 4. *J Clin Oncol* 2006;24(15):2283–9.

131. Blansfield JA, Beck KE, Tran K, et al. Cytotoxic T-lymphocyte-associated antigen-4 blockage can induce autoimmune hypophysitis in patients with metastatic melanoma and renal cancer. *J Immunother* 2005;28(6):593–8.

132. Sakane N, Yoshida T, Yoshioka K, Umekawa T, Kondo M, Shimatsu A. Reversible hypopituitarism after interferonalfa therapy. *Lancet* 1995;345(8960):1305.

133. Ahmadi J, Meyers GS, Segall HD, Sharma OP, Hinton DR. Lymphocytic adenohypophysitis: contrast-enhanced MR imaging in five cases. *Radiology* 1995;195(1):30–4.

134. Farah JO, Rossi M, Foy PM, MacFarlane IA. Cystic lymphocytic hypophysitis, visual field defects and hypopituitarism. *Int J Clin Pract* 1999;53(8):643–4.

135. Flanagan DE, Ibrahim AE, Ellison DW, Armitage M, Gawne-Cain M, Lees PD. Inflammatory hypophysitis – the spectrum of disease. *Acta Neurochir (Wien)* 2002;144(1):47–56.

136. Lee SJ, Yoo HJ, Park SW, Choi MG. A case of cystic lymphocytic hypophysitis with cacosmia and hypopituitarism. *Endocr J* 2004;51(3):375–80.

137. Saiwai S, Inoue Y, Ishihara T, et al. Lymphocytic adenohypophysitis: skull radiographs and MRI. *Neuroradiology* 1998;40(2):114–20.

138. Miki Y, Asato R, Okumura R, et al. Anterior pituitary gland in pregnancy: hyperintensity at MR. *Radiology* 1993;187(1):229–31.

139. Sato N, Sze G, Endo K. Hypophysitis: endocrinologic and dynamic MR findings. *AJNR Am J Neuroradiol* 1998;19(3):439–44.

140. Hashimoto M, Yanaki T, Nakahara N, Masuzawa T. Lymphocytic adenohypophysitis: an immuno-histochemical study. *Surg Neurol* 1991;36(2):137–44.

141. Mau M, Ratner R, Gindoff P. Antipituitary antibodies in a postpartum woman with partial pituitary deficiency and a normal pituitary MRI scan. *South Med J* 1994;87(2):267–9.

142. Cheung CC, Ezzat S, Smyth HS, Asa SL. The spectrum and significance of primary hypophysitis. *J Clin Endocrinol Metab* 2001;86(3):1048–53.

143. Gutenberg A, Buslei R, Fahlbusch R, Buchfelder M, Bruck W. Immunopathology of primary hypophysitis: implications for pathogenesis. *Am J Surg Pathol* 2005;29(3):329–38.

144. Tashiro T, Sano T, Xu B, et al. Spectrum of different types of hypophysitis: a clinicopathologic study of hypophysitis in 31 cases. *Endocr Pathol* 2002;13(3):183–95.

145. Vidal S, Rotondo F, Horvath E, Kovacs K, Scheithauer BW. Immunocytochemical localization of mast cells in lymphocytic hypophysitis. *Am J Clin Pathol* 2002;117(3):478–83.

146. Horvath E, Vidal S, Syro LV, Kovacs K, Smyth HS, Uribe H. Severe lymphocytic adenohy-pophysitis with selective disappearance of prolactin cells: a histologic, ultrastructural and immuno-electron microscopic study. *Acta Neuropathol (Berl)* 2001;101(6):631–7.

147. Megan Ogilvie C, Payne S, Evanson J, Lister TA, Grossman AB. Lymphoma metastasizing to the pituitary: an unusual presentation of a treatable disease. *Pituitary* 2005;8(2):139–46.

148. McCutcheon IE, Oldfield EH. Lymphocytic adenohypophysitis presenting as infertility. Case report. *J Neurosurg* 1991;74(5):821–6.

149. Levine SN, Benzel EC, Fowler MR, Shroyer JV 3rd, Mirfakhraee M. Lymphocytic adenohy-pophysitis: clinical, radiological, and magnetic resonance imaging characterization. *Neurosurgery* 1988;22(5):937–41.

150. McKeel DW. Common histopathologica and ultrastructural features in granulomatous and lymphoid adenohypophysitis. *Endocrinology* 1983;112(Suppl):190.

151. Ahmed SR, Aiello DP, Page R, Hopper K, Towfighi J, Santen RJ. Necrotizing infundibulo-hypophysitis: a unique syndrome of diabetes insipidus and hypopituitarism. *J Clin Endocrinol Metab* 1993;76(6):1499–504.

152. Bhansali A, Velayutham P, Radotra BD, Pathak A. Idiopathic granulomatous hypophysitis presenting as non-functioning pituitary adenoma: description of six cases and review of literature. *Br J Neurosurg* 2004;18(5):489–94.

153. Burt MG, Morey AL, Turner JJ, Pell M, Sheehy JP, Ho KK. Xanthomatous pituitary lesions: a report of two cases and review of the literature. *Pituitary* 2003;6(3):161–8.

154. Deodhare SS, Bilbao JM, Kovacs K, et al. Xanthomatous hypophysitis: a novel entity of obscure etiology. *Endocr Pathol* 1999;10(3):237–41.

155. Kovacs K, Horvath E. The differential diagnosis of lesions involving the sella turcica. *Endocr Pathol* 2001;12(4):389–95.

156. Puchner MJ, Ludecke DK, Saeger W. The anterior pituitary lobe in patients with cystic craniopharyngiomas: three cases of associated lymphocytic hypophysitis. *Acta Neurochir (Wien)* 1994;126(1):38–43.

157. McConnon JK, Smyth HS, Horvath E. A case of sparsely granulated growth hormone cell adenoma associated with lymphocytic hypophysitis. *J Endocrinol Invest* 1991;14(8):691–6.

158. Holck S, Laursen H. Prolactinoma coexistent with granulomatous hypophysitis. *Acta Neuropathol (Berl)* 1983;61(3–4):253–7.

159. Daikokuya H, Inoue Y, Nemoto Y, Tashiro T, Shakudo M, Ohata K. Rathke's cleft cyst associated with hypophysitis: MRI. *Neuroradiology* 2000;42(7):532–4.

160. Hama S, Arita K, Tominaga A, et al. Symptomatic Rathke's cleft cyst coexisting with central diabetes insipidus and hypophysitis: case report. *Endocr J* 1999;46(1):187–92.

161. Roncaroli F, Bacci A, Frank G, Calbucci F. Granulomatous hypophysitis caused by a ruptured intrasellar Rathke's cleft cyst: report of a case and review of the literature. *Neurosurgery* 1998;43(1):146–9.

162. Wearne MJ, Barber PC, Johnson AP. Symptomatic Rathke's cleft cyst with hypophysitis. *Br J Neurosurg* 1995;9(6):799–803.

163. Houdouin L, Polivka M, Henegar C, Blanquet A, Delalande O, Mikol J. [Pituitary germinoma and lymphocytic hypophysitis: a pitfall. Report of two cases]. *Ann Pathol* 2003;23(4):349–54.

164. Bettendorf M, Fehn M, Grulich-Henn J, et al. Lymphocytic hypophysitis with central diabetes insipidus and consequent panhypopituitarism preceding a multifocal, intracranial germinoma in a prepubertal girl. *Eur J Pediatr* 1999;158(4):288–92.

165. Fehn M, Bettendorf M, Ludecke DK, Sommer C, Saeger W. Lymphocytic hypophysitis masking a suprasellar germinoma in a 12-year-old girl–a case report. *Pituitary* 1999;1(3–4):303–7.

166. Donadieu J, Rolon MA, Thomas C, et al. Endocrine involvement in pediatric-onset Langerhans' cell histiocytosis: a population-based study. *J Pediatr* 2004;144(3):344–50.

167. Hayashi H, Yamada K, Kuroki T, et al. Lymphocytic hypophysitis and pulmonary sarcoidosis. Report of a case. *Am J Clin Pathol* 1991;95(4):506–11.

168. Goyal M, Kucharczyk W, Keystone E. Granulomatous hypophysitis due to Wegener's granulomatosis. *AJNR Am J Neuroradiol* 2000;21(8):1466–9.

169. Bullmann C, Faust M, Hoffmann A, et al. Five cases with central diabetes insipidus and hypogonadism as first presentation of neurosarcoidosis. *Eur J Endocrinol* 2000;142(4):365–72.

170. Basaria S, Ayala AR, Guerin C, Dobs AS. A rare pituitary lesion. *J Endocrinol Invest* 2000;23(3):189–92.

171. Estopinan V, Riobo P, Varona C, Lara JI, Gonzalez F, de la Calle H. [Granulomatous giant-cell hypophysitis. Report of a case and review of the literature]. *Med Clin (Barc)* 1987;89(15):650–2.

172. Toth M, Szabo P, Racz K, et al. Granulomatous hypophysitis associated with Takayasu's disease. *Clin Endocrinol (Oxf)* 1996;45(4):499–503.

173. de Bruin WI, van't Verlaat JW, Graamans K, de Bruin TW. Sellar granulomatous mass in a pregnant woman with active Crohn's disease. *Neth J Med* 1991;39(3–4):136–41.

174. Pereira J, Vaz R, Carvalho D, Cruz C. Thickening of the pituitary stalk: a finding suggestive of intrasellar tuberculoma? Case report. *Neurosurgery* 1995;36(5):1013–5, discussion 5–6.

175. Crock PA, Bensing S, Smith CJA, Burns C, Robinson PJ. Pituitary autoantibodies. *Curr Opin Endocrinol Diabet* 2006;13(4):344–50.

176. Baekkeskov S, Aanstoot HJ, Christgau S, et al. Identification of the 64K autoantigen in insulin-dependent diabetes as the GABA-synthesizing enzyme glutamic acid decarboxylase. *Nature* 1990;347(6289):151–6.

177. Weetman AP. Thyroid peroxidase as an antigen in autoimmune thyroiditis. *Clin Exp Immunol* 1990;80(1):1–3.

178. Palmer JP, Asplin CM, Clemons P, et al. Insulin antibodies in insulin-dependent diabetics before insulin treatment. *Science* 1983;222(4630):1337–9.

179. Furmaniak J, Smith BR. Immunity to the thyroid-stimulating hormone receptor. *Springer Semin Immunopathol* 1993;14(3):309–21.

180. Mirakian R, Cudworth AG, Bottazzo GF, Richardson CA, Doniach D. Autoimmunity to anterior pituitary cells and the pathogenesis of insulin-dependent diabetes mellitus. *Lancet* 1982;1(8275):755–9.

181. Schatz DA, Atkinson MA. Islet cell autoantibodies: a case of a premature obituary. *Pediatr Diabetes* 2005;6(4):181–3.

182. Pietropaolo M, Yu S, Libman IM, et al. Cytoplasmic islet cell antibodies remain valuable in defining risk of progression to type 1 diabetes in subjects with other islet autoantibodies. *Pediatr Diabetes* 2005;6(4):184–92.

183. Hansen BL, Hegedus L, Hansen GN, Hagen C, Hansen JM, Hoier-Madsen M. Pituitary-cell autoantibody diversity in sera from patients with untreated Graves' disease. *Autoimmunity* 1989;5(1–2):49–57.

184. Janes SE, Santosh B, Thomas D, Vyas H. Hashimoto's encephalopathy: an unusual cause of seizures in the intensive care unit. *Pediatr Crit Care Med* 2004;5(6):578–81.

185. Piga M, Serra A, Deiana L, et al. Brain perfusion abnormalities in patients with euthyroid autoimmune thyroiditis. *Eur J Nucl Med Mol Imaging* 2004;31(12):1639–44.

186. Nakahara R, Tsunekawa K, Yabe S, et al. Association of antipituitary antibody and type 2 iodothyronine deiodinase antibody in patients with autoimmune thyroid disease. *Endocr J* 2005;52(6):691–9.

187. O'Dwyer DT, Clifton V, Hall A, Smith R, Robinson PJ, Crock PA. Pituitary autoantibodies in lymphocytic hypophysitis target both gamma- and alpha-enolase – a link with pregnancy? *Arch Physiol Biochem* 2002;110(1–2):94–8.

188. Tatsumi KI, Tanaka S, Takano T, et al. Frequent appearance of autoantibodies against prohormone convertase 1/3 and neuroendocrine protein 7B2 in patients with nonfunctioning pituitary macroadenoma. *Endocrine* 2003;22(3):335–40.

189. Fricker LD, Supattapone S, Snyder SH. Enkephalin convertase: a specific enkephalin synthesizing carboxypeptidase in adrenal chromaffin granules, brain, and pituitary gland. *Life Sci* 1982;31 (16–17):1841–4.

190. Tanaka S, Tatsumi K, Tomita T, et al. Novel autoantibodies to pituitary gland specific factor 1a in patients with rheumatoid arthritis. *Rheumatology (Oxford)* 2003;42(2):353–6.

191. Engelberth O, Jezkova Z. Autoantibodies in Sheehan's syndrome. *Lancet* 1965;1:1075.

192. Goudie RB. Anterior hypophysitis associated with autoimmune disease. *Proc R Coll Med* 1968;61:275.

193. Gluck M, Schrell U, Scherbaum WA. Reactivity and intracellular location of the ACTH cell autoantigen in human fetal and adult anterior pituitary tissue. *Autoimmunity*. 1993;14(4):299–305.

194. Wild RA, Kepley M. Lymphocytic hypophysitis in a patient with amenorrhea and hyperprolactinemia. A case report. *J Reprod Med* 1986;31(3):211–6.

195. Onodera T, Toniolo A, Ray UR, Jenson AB, Knazek RA, Notkins AL. Virus-induced diabetes mellitus. XX. Polyendocrinopathy and autoimmunity. *J Exp Med* 1981;153(6):1457–73.

196. Maghnie M, Lorini R, Severi F. Antipituitary antibodies in patients with pituitary abnormalities and hormonal deficiency. *Clin Endocrinol (Oxf)*. 1994;40(6):809–10.

197. Maghnie M, Lorini R, Vitali L, Mastricci N, Carra AM, Severi F. Organ- and non-organ-specific auto-antibodies in children with hypopituitarism on growth hormone therapy. *Eur J Pediatr.* 1995;154(6):450–3.

198. De Bellis A, Bizzarro A, Conte M, Perrino S, Coronella C, Solimeno S, Sinisi AM, Stile LA, Pisano G, Bellastella A. Antipituitary antibodies in adults with apparently idiopathic growth hormone deficiency and in adults with autoimmune endocrine diseases. *J Clin Endocrinol Metab.* 2003;88(2):650–4.

199. Bottazzo GF, McIntosh C, Stanford W, Preece M. Growth hormone cell antibodies and partial growth hormone deficiency in a girl with Turner's syndrome. *Clin Endocrinol (Oxf)* 1980;12(1):1–9.

200. Pouplard A, Bigorgne JC, Chevalier JM, Rohmer V, Poron MF. Pituitary insufficiency and auto-immunity (author's transl) *Nouv Presse Med.* 1980;9(25):1757–60.

201. Møller A, Hansen BL, Hansen GN, Hagen C. Autoantibodies in sera from patients with multiple sclerosis directed against antigenic determinants in pituitary growth hormone-producing cells and in structures containing vasopressin/oxytocin. *J Neuroimmunol.* 1985;8(2–3):177–84.

202. Pouplard A, Job JC, Luxembourger I, Chaussain JL. Antigonadotropic cell antibodies in the serum of cryptorchid children and infants and of their mothers. *J Pediatr* 1985;107(1):26–30.

203. Kobayashi I, Inukai T, Takahashi M, Ishii A, Ohshima K, Mori M, Shimomura Y, Kobayashi S, Hashimoto A, Sugiura M. Anterior pituitary cell antibodies detected in Hashimoto's thyroiditis and Graves' disease. *Endocrinol Jpn.* 1988;35(5):705–8.

204. Komatsu M, Kondo T, Yamauchi K, et al. Antipituitary antibodies in patients with the primary empty sella syndrome. *J Clin Endocrinol Metab* 1988;67(4):633–8.

205. Crock P, Salvi M, Miller A, Wall J, Guyda H. Detection of anti-pituitary autoantibodies by immunoblotting. *J Immunol Methods* 1993;162(1):31–40.

206. Nishiki M, Murakami Y, Ozawa Y, Kato Y. Serum antibodies to human pituitary membrane antigens in patients with autoimmune lymphocytic hypophysitis and infundibuloneurohypophysitis. *Clin Endocrinol (Oxf)* 2001;54(3):327–33.

207. O'Dwyer DT, Smith AI, Matthew ML, et al. Identification of the 49-kDa autoantigen associated with lymphocytic hypophysitis as alpha-enolase. *J Clin Endocrinol Metab* 2002;87(2):752–7.

208. Kasperlik-Zaluska AA, Czarnocka B, Czech W. Autoimmunity as the most frequent cause of idiopathic secondary adrenal insufficiency: report of 111 cases. *Autoimmunity* 2003;36(3):155–9.

209. Stromberg S, Crock P, Lernmark A, Hulting AL. Pituitary autoantibodies in patients with hypopituitarism and their relatives. *J Endocrinol.* 1998;157(3):475–80.

210. Takao T, Nanamiya W, Matsumoto R, Asaba K, Okabayashi T, Hashimoto K. Antipituitary antibodies in patients with lymphocytic hypophysitis. *Horm Res* 2001;55(6):288–92.

211. Kobayashi T, Yabe S, Kanda T, Kobayashi I. Studies on circulating anti-pituitary antibodies in NIDDM patients. *Endocr J* 1998;45(3):343–50.

212. Yabe S, Murakami M, Maruyama K, Miwa H, Fukumura Y, Ishii S, Sugiura M, Kobayashi I. Western blot analysis of rat pituitary antigens recognized by human antipituitary antibodies. *Endocr J.* 1995;42(1):115–9.

213. Yabe S, Kanda T, Hirokawa M, et al. Determination of antipituitary antibody in patients with endocrine disorders by enzyme-linked immunosorbent assay and Western blot analysis. *J Lab Clin Med* 1998;132(1):25–31.

214. Nishino M, Yabe S, Murakami M, Kanda T, Kobayashi I. Detection of antipituitary antibodies in patients with autoimmune thyroid disease. *Endocr J* 2001;48(2):185–91.

215. Kikuchi T, Yabe S, Kanda T, Kobayashi I. Antipituitary antibodies as pathogenetic factors in patients with pituitary disorders. *Endocr J* 2000;47(4):407–16.

216. Keda YM, Krjukova IV, Ilovaiskaia IA, et al. Antibodies to pituitary surface antigens during various pituitary disease states. *J Endocrinol* 2002;175(2):417–23.

217. Grubin CE, Daniels T, Toivola B, et al. A novel radioligand binding assay to determine diagnostic accuracy of isoform-specific glutamic acid decarboxylase antibodies in childhood IDDM. *Diabetologia* 1994;37(4):344–50.

218. Tanaka S, Tatsumi K, Okubo K, et al. Expression profile of active genes in the human pituitary gland. *J Mol Endocrinol* 2002;28(1):33–44.

219. Tanaka S, Tatsumi KI, Kimura M, et al. Detection of autoantibodies against the pituitary-specific proteins in patients with lymphocytic hypophysis. *Eur J Endocrinol* 2002;147(6):767–75.

220. Tanaka S, Tatsumi KI, Takano T, et al. Anti-alpha-enolase antibodies in pituitary disease. *Endocr J* 2003;50(6):697–702.

221. Prentice L, Sanders JF, Perez M, et al. Thyrotropin (TSH) receptor autoantibodies do not appear to bind to the TSH receptor produced in an in vitro transcription/translation system. *J Clin Endocrinol Metab* 1997;82(4):1288–92.

222. Mau M, Phillips TM, Ratner RE. Presence of anti-pituitary hormone antibodies in patients with empty sella syndrome and pituitary tumours. *Clin Endocrinol (Oxf)* 1993;38(5):495–500.

223. Fetissov SO, Hallman J, Oreland L, et al. Autoantibodies against alpha -MSH, ACTH, and LHRH in anorexia and bulimia nervosa patients. *Proc Natl Acad Sci USA* 2002;99(26):17155–60.

224. Levine S. Allergic adenohypophysis: new experimental disease of the pituitary gland. *Science* 1967;158(805):1190–1.

225. Levine S. Allergic adrenalitis and adenohypophysis: further observations on production and passive transfer. *Endocrinology* 1969;84(3):469–75.

226. Klein I, Kraus KE, Martines AJ, Weber S. Evidence for cellular mediated immunity in an animal model of autoimmune pituitary disease. *Endocr Res Commun* 1982;9(2):145–53.

227. Watanabe K, Tada H, Shimaoka Y, et al. Characteristics of experimental autoimmune hypophysis in rats: major antigens are growth hormone, thyrotropin, and luteinizing hormone in this model. *Autoimmunity* 2001;33(4):265–74.

228. Beck JS, Melvin JM. Chronic adenohypophysis in a rhesus monkey immunised with extracts of human placenta. *J Pathol* 1970;102(3):125–9.

229. Yoon JW, Choi DS, Liang HC, et al. Induction of an organ-specific autoimmune disease, lymphocytic hypophysis, in hamsters by recombinant rubella virus glycoprotein and prevention of disease by neonatal thymectomy. *J Virol* 1992;66(2):1210–4.

230. Davis JR, McMahon RF, Lowenstein PR, Castro MG, Lincoln GA, McNeilly AS. Adenovirus-mediated gene transfer in the ovine pituitary gland is associated with hypophysis. *J Endocrinol* 2002;173(2):265–71.

231. de Jersey J, Carmignac D, Barthlott T, Robinson I, Stockinger B. Activation of CD8 T cells by antigen expressed in the pituitary gland. *J Immunol* 2002;169(12):6753–9.

232. De Jersey J, Carmignac D, Le Tissier P, Barthlott T, Robinson I, Stockinger B. Factors affecting the susceptibility of the mouse pituitary gland to CD8 T-cell-mediated autoimmunity. *Immunology* 2004;111(3):254–61.

233. Yamagami K, Yoshioka K, Sakai H, et al. Treatment of lymphocytic hypophysis by high-dose methylprednisolone pulse therapy. *Intern Med* 2003;42(2):168–73.

234. Reusch JE, Kleinschmidt-DeMasters BK, Lillehei KO, Rappe D, Gutierrez-Hartmann A. Preoperative diagnosis of lymphocytic hypophysis (adenohypophysis) unresponsive to short course dexamethasone: case report. *Neurosurgery* 1992;30(2):268–72.

235. Selch MT, DeSalles AA, Kelly DF, et al. Stereotactic radiotherapy for the treatment of lymphocytic hypophysis. Report of two cases. *J Neurosurg* 2003;99(3):591–6.

236. Virally-Monod ML, Barrou Z, Basin C, Thomopoulos P, Luton JP. [Lymphocytic hypophysis: a reality]. *Presse Med* 1996;25(20):933–8.

237. Salvi M, Vannucchi G, Campi I, et al. Efficacy of rituximab treatment for thyroid-associated ophthalmopathy as a result of intraorbital B-cell depletion in one patient unresponsive to steroid immunosuppression. *Eur J Endocrinol* 2006;154(4):511–7.

238. Keymeulen B, Vandemeulebroucke E, Ziegler AG, et al. Insulin needs after CD3-antibody therapy in new-onset type 1 diabetes. *N Engl J Med* 2005;352(25):2598–608.

16 Autoimmune Polyglandular Syndrome Type 1

Pärt Peterson, PhD

CONTENTS

Summary

Autoimmune polyglandular syndrome type 1 (APS1) is a monogenic autoimmune disease with organ-specific autoimmune destruction of several endocrine tissues. Most common disorders of the syndrome are chronic mucocutaneous candidiasis, hypoparathyoidism, and Addison's disease but the clinical spectrum may vary. The disease is caused by the mutations in autoimmune regulator (AIRE) gene. More than 50 mutations have been described, which are spread over the AIRE gene with two major mutation hotspots, R257X and 967-979del13bp. AIRE protein has several motifs supporting its role in transcriptional control and is highly expressed in thymic medullary epithelial cells. Analysis of AIRE deficient mice have demonstrated its role in transcriptional regulation of tissue specific antigens in medullary thymic epithelial cells, and suggested that AIRE is critical protein responsible for the maintenance of central tolerance. In agreement with mouse model, patients with APS1 have autoantibodies to multiple self-proteins. The data on cell-mediated immune responses and the reason for chronic candidiasis are still elusive. The identification of AIRE mutations and a recent finding of high titer autoantibodies to type 1 interferons should facilitate diagnosis of APS1.

Key Words: Autoimmune polyendocrinopathy, autoimmune regulator, autoantibodies, thymus, mutation.

INTRODUCTION

Autoimmune polyglandular syndrome type 1 (APS1; OMIM 240300) is one of the rare monogenic autoimmune diseases. The syndrome has an alternative name, autoimmune polyendocrine-candidiasis-ectodermal dystrophy (APECED), given by the Finnish physician Jaakko Perheentupa.

From: *Contemporary Endocrinology: Autoimmune Diseases in Endocrinology*
Edited by: A. P. Weetman © Humana Press, Totowa, NJ

The co-occurrence of candidiasis-hypoparathyroidism-Addison's disease, the major clinical features of APS1, was first described in juvenile patients in 1956, and for some time period, the clinical picture was called the Whitaker triad *(1)*. Clinically, APS1 is similar in many features to APS2 (reviewed in Chap. 17), and early reports often described the patients of both syndromes as one clinical entity. The autosomal recessive monogenic inheritance of some cases of the polyendocrinopathy was fully recognized already during the 1970s. In 1981, after studying co-existing clinical pictures in large patient material, two different types of polyendocrinopathy syndromes, APS1 and APS2, were proposed by Neufeld et al. *(2)*. Since that time, the APS1 was considered as a unique model for autoimmunity and tolerance studies. The first comprehensive characterizations of APS1, which were based on large patient cohorts, were given by Neufeld et al. (1981) *(2)*, Brun (1982) *(3)*, and Ahonen et al. (1990) *(4)*.

EPIDEMIOLOGY

Although APS1 is rare with an estimated number of 500 patients worldwide, the syndrome is more common among certain populations. The prevalence is higher among Finns (1:25,000), Sardinians (1:14,000), and Iranian Jews (1:9000). An even higher prevalence (1:4400) has been reported in a small town Bassano del Grappa in Northern Italy *(5)*. It seems that all populations with a high incidence of APS1 have for some time in their history been isolated, which through the genetic bottleneck has resulted in enrichment of APS1 mutations.

GENETIC FACTORS

The defective gene in APS1, autoimmune regulator (*AIRE*) was identified on chromosome 21q22.3 by positional cloning in 1997 *(6,7)*. The protein sequence suggested that AIRE is involved in nuclear transcriptional processes. The most prominent motifs in the AIRE protein are the N-terminal homogenously staninig region (HSR) region, a SAND domain, an LXXLL motif, and two PHD zinc fingers (Fig. 1). The primary sequence and the computer-predicted structure of the protein resemble other nuclear proteins involved in transcription. The closest homologous proteins to AIRE are Sp100 and Sp140 proteins, which share HSR, SAND, and PHD domains.

The AIRE N-terminal region between the amino acids 1 and 96 is called the HSR domain, also present in Sp100 and Sp140 proteins. The HSR domain is predicted to have a four alpha helix bundle structure with helixes linked together by loops of different length. Similarly to Sp100 family proteins, the HSR domain in AIRE has been shown to mediate the protein homodimerization *(8)*.

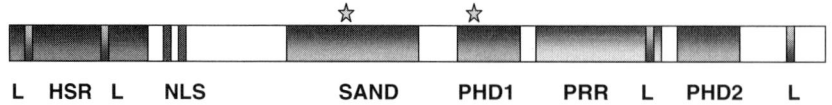

Fig. 1. Schematic picture of AIRE protein domains. HSR, homogenously staining region; NLS, nuclear localization signal; SAND, domain for Sp100, AIRE-1, NucP41/75, and DEAF-1; PHD1 and PHD2, plant homeodomains; PRR, proline rich region; L, LXXLL motifs. Asterisks mark locations of R257X and 967–979del13bp mutations.

The SAND domain (for Sp100, AIRE-1, NucP41/75, and DEAF-1) is located between amino acids 189 and 264. The domain occurs in many nuclear proteins that function in chromatin-dependent transcriptional control and has been proposed to mediate the DNA-binding activity. NMR spectroscopy studies of the Sp100 SAND domain confirmed that the Sp100 SAND domain is DNA-binding region, with the amino acid KDWK motif being essential for DNA recognition (9). Although AIRE lacks the KDWK motif in the SAND domain, DNA binding as homodimer and homotetramer, but not as monomer, takes place suggesting involvement of SAND domain in this process (10).

The PHD zinc fingers are cysteine-rich structures having a consensus of $Cys_4HisCys_3$ (C_4HC_3), and each is bound to two zinc atoms. The PHD finger is similar to the RING finger (C_3HC_4) and LIM domain (C_2HC_5), but the functional role of each finger structure seems to be specific (11). The PHD finger domains are thought to mediate protein–protein interactions and are found in many proteins that are involved in chromatin-mediated transcriptional regulation. AIRE has in addition four LXXLL (where L is leucine and X is any amino acid) nuclear receptor-binding motifs, which are known to mediate the interactions of the nuclear receptors, the proteins involved in transcriptional regulation (12).

At least 56 *AIRE* gene mutations in APS1 patients have been described (Table 1, Fig. 1). The mutations are spread over the cDNA sequence with two major mutation hotspots. The introduction of a stop codon instead of arginine at the amino acid position 257 in exon 6 (R257X) and the deletion of a 13 base pair nucleotide stretch in exon 8 (967-979del13bp) are the two most commonly found mutations. Both the R257X and the 967-979del13bp mutations are widely found in APS1 patients but tend to be more prevalent in certain populations. For example, among a large cohort of the Finnish patients, the R257X mutation is found in 83% of APS1 alleles. In addition to the Finnish APS1 patients, the R257X mutation is often found in patients of Italian, Central and Eastern European origin. The 967-979del13bp mutation is more commonly found among British and American Caucasian patients and accounts for 50–70% of APS1 alleles in these populations. The third population-specific mutation is R139X, which is prevalent among Sardinian APS1 patients. Overall, the majority of the AIRE mutations introduce a stop codon, which truncates the protein before the PHD finger region, and most likely result in a total loss of function. Several missense mutations are concentrated into the HSR region of the protein, particularly in the regions between amino acids 15–29 and 77–95. One of the mutations in this region, Y85C, is typical for APS1 patients from Iranian Jewish population.

Since the first description of diseased patients, it soon became evident that the APS1 phenotype may vary considerably between affected siblings. Considerable clinical variation is found in patients with the R257X or the 967-979del13bp mutation, and several reports describe variation in APS1 siblings with identical mutations. A large proportion of APS1 patients, in particular from non-founder populations, are compound heterozygotes for AIRE mutations, which makes it difficult to assess the phenotype correlations. Although a recent report found a striking gender association with lower and later incidence of hypoparathyroidism in male patients (36), clear correlations between the specific mutations and disease phenotype components have not been found. One potential correlation is between candidiasis and missense mutations in the

Table 1
Autoimmune Regulator Mutations Found in Autoimmune Polyglandular Syndrome Type1 Patients

No.	cDNA change	Exon/intron	Domain	Effect on coding sequence	Ethnic origin	Reference
1	30-52dup23bp	E1	HSR	R15fsX19	Hungarian, Austrian	13
2	43C>T	E1	HSR	R15C	Japanese	14
3	44G>T	E1	HSR	R15L	British	15
4	47C>T	E1	HSR	T16M	Russian	13
5	62C>T	E1	HSR	A21V	Swedish, North American	16
6	64-69del6bp	E1	HSR	V22-D23del	Italian	20
7	83T>C	E1	HSR	L28P	USA Caucasian, British	5,15
8	86T>C	E1	HSR	L29P	Japanese	18
9	IVS1_IVS4	I1	HSR	Deletion of exons 2-4	Azerbaijan, Iranian	13,19
10	191-226del36bp	E2	HSR	del64-75andD76Y	USA Caucasian	17
11	208 209insCAGG	E2	HSR	D70fsX216	Arabian	17
12	230T>C	E2	HSR	F77S	Italian	20
13	232T>A	E2	HSR	W78R	Russian, Italian	13,20
14	238G>T	E2	HSR	V80L	Italian	21
15	247A>G	E2	HSR	K83E	Finnish	6,7,22
16	254A>G	E2	HSR	Y85C	Iranian Jewish	21
17	269A>G	E2	HSR	Y90C	British	15
18	278T>G	E2	HSR	L93R	French-Canadian	23
19	415C>T	E3	before SAND	R139X	Sardinian, Egyptian	13,24
20	IVS3+2T>C	I3		GT>GC	USA Caucasian	25
21	508 509ins13bp	E4	before SAND	A170fsX219	German	21
22	517C>T	E4	before SAND	Q173X	Hispanic, Italian	17,21
23	540delG	E5	before SAND	G180X376	Slovenian	26
24	607C>T	E5	SAND	R203X	North Italian, Italian	21,22
25	653-7_-5delCTC	E5&E6	SAND	G218fsX	Slovenian	26
26	682T>G	E6	SAND	G228W	Italian	27
27	755C>T	E6	SAND	P252L	Italian	20

#	Mutation	Exon	Domain	Protein	Population	Ref
28	769C>T	E6	SAND	R257X	Finnish, North Italian, USA Caucasian, Swiss, British, New Zealander, Swedish, Dutch, German, French, Czech, Hungarian, Austrian, Slovenian, Croatian, Yugoslavian, Russian.	6,7,13,17,21–23,25,28
29	789delC	E6	SAND	A264fsX377	Australian (European origin)	29
30	901G>A	E8	PHD1	V301M	Norwegian	30
31	931delT	E8	PHD1	C311fsX376	French	21
32	932G>A	E8	PHD1	C311Y	Finnish	21
33	967-979del13bp	E8	PHD1	C322fsX370	Finnish, North Italian, American Caucasian, British, New Zealander, Dutch, German, Canadian, Swedish, Hungarian, Russian, Slovenian, Norwegian	7,13,15,17,21,22,23–26,31,32
34	969^970ins CCTG	E8	PHD1	L323fsX370	Italian	21,22
35	977C>A	E8	PHD1	P326Q	Finnish	21
36	977C>T	E8	PHD1	P326L	French	28
37	1064-1068dupCCCGG	E9	PRR	Q358fsX377	Slovenian	26
38	1072C>T	E9	PRR	Q358X	Italian	20
39	1103^1104insC	E10	PRR	P368fsX370	Japanese	33
40	1163^1164insA	E10	PRR	M388fsX422	Finnish	21
41	1189delC	E10	PRR	L397fsX478	French	21
42	1193delC	E10	PRR	P398fsX478	French, Italian	7,21
43	1242^1243insA	E10	LXXLL	H415fsX422	Norwegian	31

(Continued)

Table 1
(Continued)

No.	cDNA change	Exon/intron	Domain	Effect on coding sequence	Ethnic origin	Reference
44	1244^1245insC	E10	LXXLL	L417fsX422	German	21
45	1249delC	E10	LXXLL	L417fsX478	British	15
46	1264delC	E10	PRR	P422fsX478	USA Caucasian	17
47	IVS9-1G>C	I9		AG>AC del exon 10/60aa	Japanese	18
48	IVS9-1G>A	I9		AG>AA del exon 10/60aa	Hispanic	17
49	1295insAC	E11	PHD2	C434fsX479	USA Caucasian	25
50	1296delGinsAC	E11	PHD2	R433fsX502	USA Caucasian	17
51	1344delCinsTT	E11	PHD2	C449fsX502	Japanese	34
52	IVS11+1G>A	I11		GT>AT, X476	Japanese	34
53	1450G>A	E12	C-terminus	V484M	Italian	35
54	1513delG	E13	C-terminus	A502fsX519	Korean	33
55	1616C>T	E14	C-terminus	P539L	Italian	20
56	1638A>T	E14	STOP codon	X564C + 59aa	Finnish	21,22

N-terminal HSR region. For example, Iranian Jewish patients having a Y85C mutation do not seem to have *Candida* infection.

In contrast to complex autoimmune diseases, APS1 has no strict HLA association. The HLA associations with APS1 disease components have been reported in a larger series of patients, for example Addison's disease was found associated with HLA DRB1*03 and alopecia with DRB1*04-DQB1*0302, whereas type 1 diabetes correlated negatively with DRB1*15-DQB1*0602 alleles *(16)*. In another study, no clear association with HLA alleles was found *(36)*. The role of HLA in determining APS1 disease manifestations remains open.

As *AIRE* gene defects clearly influence the outcome of autoimmunity, AIRE mutations have been searched for in patients with complex autoimmune diseases where multiple genes are involved in forming the disease phenotype. It seems that the two most common AIRE mutations (R257X and 967-979del13bp) do not have an influence on complex autoimmune diseases as no contributions to the susceptibility have been found in type 1 diabetes, Graves' disease, autoimmune hepatitis, inflammatory bowel disease, or sporadic idiopathic hypoparathyroidism *(37–43)*. In contrast, an AIRE polymorphism at amino acid S278R has been reported to have association with alopecia universalis *(44)*. The role of this and other AIRE polymorphisms in autoimmune diseases remains to be studied.

The AIRE protein function studies clearly indicate that the protein functions as a transcriptional activator. The transcriptional activation region of AIRE has been mapped to the two C terminal PHD fingers, and mutations in these domains severely decrease the transactivation capacity *(21) (46)*. The activation is further enhanced by AIRE-interacting CREB (cAMP-response element binding)-binding protein (CBP). CBP functions as a transcriptional coactivator for various transcription factors, including nuclear receptors, Jun, Fos, nuclear factor-kB, and STAT protein family members *(46)*. The actual functional significance of AIRE interacting with CBP is unclear. It is possible that CBP forms the link between AIRE and the basal transcriptional machinery by regulating the subcellular location of the transcriptional complex *(47,48)*. The CBP also has an intrinsic histone acetyltransferase activity and is a coactivator that modulates transcription by changing access of chromatin to transcriptional complexes. The transactivation activity and the interaction with the CBP strongly support the role of the AIRE protein as a transcriptional regulator; however, this aspect of AIRE function demands further studies.

Another interesting mechanism by which AIRE might have effects is ubiquitination of target proteins. The addition of ubiquitin molecule to substrate proteins, named ubiquitination, often leads to the protein degradation. The process requires several molecules such as ubiquitin-activating protein (E1) and ubiquitin carrier protein (E2) and also ubiquitin ligase (E3), which determines the specificity of the target protein. Similarly to some other proteins having RING or PHD finger domains that function as E3 ligases, the first PHD finger of AIRE was found to have E3 ligase activity *(49)*. AIRE ubiquitin E3 ligase activity could have a role in several aspects of its function, for example in transcriptional regulation or regulating self-antigen expression levels.

IMMUNOPATHOGENESIS

The Role of AIRE Protein

Autoimmune regulator protein is predominantly expressed in the thymus and at a lower level in spleen, lymph nodes, and fetal liver *(50)*. Immunohistochemistry and *in situ* hybridization revealed a distinct expression pattern in medullary thymic epithelial cells. Inside the medullary epithelial cells, AIRE is located in nuclear body-like structures. Immunofluorescence stainings indicated that almost all AIRE-positive cells costained with cytokeratin markers and some colocalization with costimulatory markers CD80, CD86, and CD40 was observed *(50)*. The expression pattern of mouse AIRE in the thymus is similar to the human counterpart *(51)*. Another type of cell positive for AIRE is the monocyte-dendritic cell *(52,53)*. The restricted expression of AIRE in monocyte-dendritic cell lineages has been shown in CD14+ peripheral blood monocytes and also in differentiated dendritic cells, cultured in medium containing GM-CSF, IL-4, and TNF-alpha *(54)*. Mouse AIRE mRNA was detected in all DC populations with slightly stronger expression in thymic DC populations whereas thymocytes and splenic macrophages were negative *(52)*. The thymic expression in ontogeny has been studied in mouse and AIRE was already present at day E14, at a late organogenesis stage of the thymus influenced by lymphoid progenitors *(51,55)*. At this time point, cortical and medullary epithelial cell subpopulations can be clearly distinguished. More abundant AIRE expression was demonstrated at E16, a time when the first CD4+CD8+ double positive thymocytes appear in the thymus *(51)*.

AIRE expression in the thymus is particularly interesting as the medullary epithelium of thymus has an important role in central tolerance mechanism deleting autoreactive thymocytes. The thymus gland is formed by crosstalk between the bone marrow-derived T-cell progenitors and the non-hematopoietic epithelial cells *(56)*. The developing thymus attracts hematopoietic progenitor cells; epithelial cells together with thymic mesenchymal cells and developing thymocytes finally generate a three-dimensional thymic architecture consisting of inner medulla regions surrounded by cortex areas. Thymocytes are differentiated when they move from cortex to medulla, where the thymic clonal deletion occurs. The thymocytes capable of recognizing self-peptides are eliminated through a negative selection mechanism by interacting with dendritic and medullary epithelial cells. The self-antigens are processed in the medullary epithelial and dendritic cells and presented to the autoreactive T cells, and thus any changes affecting antigen-presenting cell and T-cell interaction can potentially cause defective tolerance.

How does the defect in the *AIRE* gene cause APS1? The essential role of AIRE in central tolerance emerged after AIRE-deficient mouse models were developed. The first AIRE-deficient mouse was reported to have overall normal development of T and B cells but the mice had autoantibodies against several peripheral tissues such as the adrenal cortex, exocrine and endocrine pancreas, spermatogonia in testis, and hepatocytes *(57)*. No apparent autoimmune tissue destruction was observed but several organs had lymphocytic infiltration. In particular, periportal accumulation of lymphocytes in the liver was observed. The mice were also hyperresponsive to foreign antigen immunization. A more recent publication reported an increased number of dendritic cells in spleen and lymph nodes and of monocytes in the blood with upregulated expression of VCAM-1 protein on both AIRE-deficient dendritic cells and on APS1 patient monocytes *(58)*. Similar lymphocyte infiltrates and autoantibodies were seen in other AIRE-targeted mice with slight variations in disrupted gene sequence *(59,60)*. In accordance with the first AIRE-deficient mouse, no changes were observed in the standard functional and histological studies of the immune system apart from increased frequency of activated or memory T cells in the peripheral lymphoid tissues.

To address the mechanism of how AIRE protects from autoimmunity, microarray expression analysis of genes expressed in thymic medullary epithelial cells from normal and AIRE-deficient mice was performed, which showed that the expression of multiple tissue specific genes is decreased or abolished in samples of AIRE-deficient thymic epithelial cells *(59)*. It has been shown, in accordance with the ectopic gene expression model proposed by Kyewski and coworkers, that many tissue-specific self-antigens are expressed in the thymus and that the expression of self-antigen in thymus leads to negative selection, whereas lack of AIRE or low expression allows autoreactive thymocytes to escape clonal deletion *(61)*. Thus, one important defect in AIRE deficiency or APS1 is disturbed thymic deletion of T-cells reactive to self-antigens, which might be caused by defective expression and presentation of self-antigens in thymic epithelial cells *(62)*. It remains to be studied whether the aberrantly expressed self-antigens are APS1 autoantigens bona fide, that is, whether these proteins are the targets of the autoimmune reaction. Furthermore, despite the findings in the thymus it is conceivable that AIRE has also an important role in peripheral immunity.

Autoantibodies in APS1

The characteristic feature of APS1 is the finding of autoantibodies to multiple self-proteins. The first autoantibody targets were reported in 1992 demonstrating autoantibodies to two enzymes involved in adrenal steroidogenesis, steroid 17alpha hydroxylase (P450c17; [*63*]) and steroid 21-hydroxylase (P450c21; [*64*]). Soon after, the third steroidogenic enzyme, side-chain cleavage enzyme (P450scc), was found as the autoantigen in APS1 *(65,66)*. The steroidogenic P450 enzymes are highly expressed in the adrenal cortex, and the presence of the autoantibodies to the steroidogenic P450 protein family members correlates with the Addison's disease in APS1. For example, 75, 68, and 65% of the patients with Addison's disease have autoantibodies to P450c21, P450scc, and P450c17, respectively. Autoantibodies to P450scc are also associated with gonadal dysfunction.

APS1 patients have autoantibodies to many self-proteins (Table 2). Often, these antigens are intracellular enzymes belonging to distinct protein families expressed in a tissue-specific manner. It is unclear what factors determine the antigen as a target of autoimmune reaction and whether the autoantibodies cause tissue damage. Several detected autoantigens in APS1 have some correlation with clinical disease components. APS1 patients have autoantibodies to glutamic acid decarboxylases (GAD65 and GAD67), tyrosine phosphatase-like protein IA-2 (IA-2), and insulin, the major autoantigens in type 1 diabetes *(67–69)*. Structurally related to GAD enzymes are group II pyridoxal phosphate-dependent amino acid decarboxylases, which are also autoimmune targets in APS1, in particular aromatic L-amino acid decarboxylase (AADC), histidine decarboxylase (HDC), and cysteine sulfinic acid decarboxylase (CSAD) *(70–72)*. Another protein family of autoantigens comprises

Table 2
Prevalence of Autoantibodies in Autoimmune Polyglandular
Syndrome Type 1 Patients (Adapted from refs. *71,72,74,* **and 80**)

Autoantigen	Prevalence %
Type1 interferons steroid 21 hydroxylase (P450c21)	100
Side-chain cleavage enzyme (P450scc)	52
Steroid 17 alpha hydroxylase (P450c17)	44
Aromatic L-amino acid decarboxylase (AADC)	51
Glutamic acid decarboxylase (GAD65)	37
Histidine decarboxylase (HDC)	37
Cysteine sulfinic acid decarboxylase (CSAD)	3.6
Tryptophan hydroxylase (TPH)	45
Tyrosine hydroxylase (TH)	44
Thyroglobulin (TG)	36
Thyroid peroxidase (TPO)	36
Transcription factor SOX10	22
Cytochrome P4501A2 (P4501A2)	8
Tyrosine phosphatase-like protein IA-2 (IA-2)	7

tryptophan, tyrosine, and phelylalanine hydroxylases (TPH, TH, and PAH, respectively), forming a group of pteridine-dependent hydroxylases *(73–75)*. In addition to steroidogenic P450 enzymes, several APS1 patients have autoimmune reaction to hepatic P450 cytochromes, P4501A2, and 2A6 *(76)*. Autoantibodies have been detected to intrinsic factors, thyroid-specific thyroid peroxidase, and thyroglobulin *(77)*, and to two transcription factors, SOX9 and SOX10 *(78)*. The calcium-sensing receptor protein was reported as autoantigen in patients with hypoparathyroidism *(79)*, but this finding has been disputed by later studies *(36,80)*. Recently, the autoantibodies to type 1 interferons (interferon alpha, beta, and omega) with remarkably high titers were reported in 100% of APS1 patients *(81)*. This new finding might be useful for the APS1 diagnosis in future.

Response to Candida

In addition to the reactivity to self-antigens, the APS1 patients have strong immunoglobulin-G- and immunoglobulin-A-mediated humoral immune response to *Candida albicans* antigens such as enolase, heat shock protein 90, pyruvate kinase, and alcohol dehydrogenase proteins *(82)*. These proteins have corresponding orthologues in humans, and at least theoretically candidal antigen may trigger an autoimmune reaction but so far no evidence for molecular mimicry between candidal and self-antigens has been reported. We have found that in addition to humoral immunity, APS1 patients have normal cell-mediated immune reaction to candidal antigens as found using peripheral T-cell proliferation assay (Peterson and Krohn, unpublished data). Others have found altered cytokine production in response to *Candida*, in particular finding impaired production of IL-12 in parallel with increased levels of IL-6 and IL-10 suggesting, as one possibility, a monocyte or dendritic cell defect *(83)*. Although rare cases have been reported in literature *(84)*, patients with chronic mucocutaneous candidiasis rarely suffer from invasive candidal infections. Antibodies to heat-shock protein 90 have been proposed as one protective role from systemic infection as the antibodies correlate with the course of the infection, and in patients with fatal cases of systemic infection, low levels or no antibodies have been found *(85)*. However, not all APS1 patients have anti-HSP90 antibodies *(82)*. Interestingly, APS1 patients are often negative for skin tests of reactivity to candidal antigens. Considering that APS1 patients have anti-candidal peripheral T-cell responses with altered function of antigen-presenting cells such as monocytes and dendritic cells, the negative candidal skin tests might be explained by a specific defect in the ability of monocytes or dendritic cells to recruit active T cells to mucosa and skin tissues.

T Cells

The tissues in APS1 patients are destroyed gradually, resulting in atrophy. The functional gland is replaced by fibrotic or fat tissue. Autopsies have revealed tissue infiltrations or nonexisting tissues. Earlier studies have reported that infiltrations often contain lymphocytes and also macrophages. However, specific data on autoimmune T cells in APS1 are rather elusive. An increased number and percentage of CD3+CD4+ and fewer CD8+CD11b+ cells have been reported in APS1 patients, whereas B (CD19) and NK (CD16/CD56) cell numbers were not significantly changed *(86,87)*. One report described significantly lower percentages of CD4+CD25+ cells in patients, including cells positive for GITR, a marker for regulatory T cells *(88)*. In contrast, another study found increased numbers and percentages of CD4+CD25+ positive cells *(88)*. Low production of IFN gamma cytokine was observed in two APS1 patients *(86)*.

DIAGNOSIS

The three most important manifestations of APS1 are chronic mucocutaneous candidiasis, hypoparathyroidism, and Addison's disease (Table 3). The chronic mucocutaneous candidiasis starts within the first years of childhood, usually before the age of 5 years, and is most often seen as oral thrush on the tongue. The infection can spread to the esophagus and intestine and, with time, to the skin of the scalp and hands, especially affecting nails. APS1 is one of the frequent causes of the chronic mucocutaneous candidiasis in children. It is likely that the first reported case of chronic mucocutaneous candidiasis, describing a 4.5-year-old child with chronic superficial candidiasis and hypoparathyroidism by Thorpe and Handley *(89)*, was in fact an APS1 patient *(90)*. Chronic candidiasis is usually followed by hypoparathyroidism before the age of 10 years and Addison's disease before the age of 15 years, but any of the three diseases may also start later in adulthood.

For clinical diagnosis, two of the three disease components should be present. This criterion has been recently repeatedly questioned as with the emergence of gene analysis several patients have been described carrying APS1-causing *AIRE* gene mutation but having only one of the common features *(35)*. For example, in a large cohort of Finnish APS1 patients, only 22% of the patients had two of three clinical entities at the age of 5 years, 65% at the age of 10 years, and 93.5% at the age of 30 years *(91)*. Therefore, it is possible that a significant number of APS1 patients might be overlooked especially in younger patients before the full development of the clinical phenotype. As APS1 is difficult to diagnose in patients with milder or atypical phenotypes, APS1 can be

Table 3
Autoimmune Polyglandular Syndrome Type 1 Clinical
Features (Adapted from refs. *5 and 91*)

Disease components	Percent
Addison's disease	60–100
Hypoparathyroidism	77–100
Chronic candidiasis	73–100
Ectodermal dysplasia	10–77
Autoimmune thyroid disease	8–18
Type 1 diabetes	4–23
Hypogonadism	31–60
Alopecia	27–72
Vitiligo	4–26
Keratopathy	12–35
Autoimmune hepatitis	10–19
Pernicious anemia	12–15
Chronic gastritis	6

suspected even in patients having only one of the three diseases, in particular in children with chronic candidiasis or hypoparathyroidism. If possible, *AIRE* gene analysis and autoantibody screening, in particular against type 1 interferons, should be performed to support the diagnosis.

The spectrum of other clinical features in APS1 is broad and variable, including several, often endocrine, autoimmune disorders (Table 3). These are premature gonadal failure, hypothyroidism, hypophysitis, pernicious anemia, malabsorption, type 1 diabetes, autoimmune hepatitis, and gastritis but also autoimmune skin diseases such as alopecia, vitiligo, and urticaria-like erythema *(91)*. Premature ovarian failure is more common than primary testicular failure. In addition to polyendocrinopathies, cholelithiasis, hypo- or asplenism and ectodermal dystrophies such as enamel and nail dysplasia and keratoconjuctivitis are often present. The variable clinical picture of APS1 contains also many diseases that have been less commonly found in patients; primary pulmonary hypertension, growth failure, metaphyseal dysplasia, progressive muscular atrophy, lupus-like panniculitis, vasculitis, idiopathic giant cell myocarditis, retrobulbar neuritis, extrapontine myelinolysis, intracranial calcification, toxic epidermal necrolysis, erythropoietin-deficient anemia, and mild mental retardation. It is worth of special note that, in early APS1 patient descriptions, where the mortality was high because of late diagnosis and lack of treatment, several reports mentioned hypoplasia or total atrophy of the thymus in young APS1 patients (reviewed in ref. *3*).

TREATMENT

In the treatment of the candidiasis, anticandidal drugs such as amphotericin B, ketoconazole, or fluconazole are often used. Itraconazole has been reported to be effective for nail candidiasis; however, 4–6-month treatment is needed to eliminate the infection *(91)*. The long-term use of ketoconazole and fluconazole often leads to drug resistance; instead, it is preferential to use local short-term pulse treatments of amphotericin B or nystatin. Clinical follow-up of oral candidal infection is needed at least once or twice per year, and, because of the high risk of cancer, attention should be paid to suppression of the oral infection. For example, 10% of Finnish APS1 patients over 25-years of age develop squamous cell carcinoma of mouth or esophagus *(91)*.

Replacement therapy with hormones has been efficiently used for Addison's disease and hypoparathyroidism. Patients with Addison's disease are treated with hydrocortisone or prednisolone at the smallest dose that relieves symptoms, and, as a substitute for aldosterone, the patients should also receive fludrocortisone. For dehydroepiandrosterone (DHEA) deficiency, DHEA-containing tablets can be used. The therapy of hypoparathyroidism is aimed at maintaining a normal calcium plasma level, and serum calcium and phosphate levels should be monitored regularly. Therapies are calciferol sterols (vitamin D hydroxylated forms, often calcitriol, or dihydrotachysterol) and calcium salt preparations, preferably calcium carbonate, but these, however, do not efficiently substitute for parathyroid hormone and are difficult to regulate. As the calcium levels may vary significantly over a short time, there is significant risk of both hypo- and hypercalcemia. The patients should receive advice and written information about the symptoms complications and risk elements of the disease *(91)*.

REFERENCES

1. Esselborn VM, Landing BH, Whitaker J, Williams RR. (1956) The syndrome of familial juvenile hypoadrenocorticism, hypoparathyroidism and superficial moniliasis. *J Clin Endocrinol Metab* 16: 1374–1387.
2. Neufeld M, Maclaren NK, Blizzard RM. (1981) Two types of autoimmune Addison's disease associated with different polyglandular autoimmune (PGA) syndromes. *Medicine* 60: 355–362.
3. Brun JM. (1982) Juvenile autoimmune polyendocrinopathy. *Horm Res* 16: 308–316.
4. Ahonen P, Myllärniemi S, Sipilä I, Perheentupa J. (1990) Clinical variation of autoimmune polyendocrinopathy-candidiasis-ectodermal dystrophy (APECED) in a series of 68 patients. *N Engl J Med* 322: 1829–1836.
5. Betterle C, Dal Pra C, Mantero F, Zanchetta R. (2002) Autoimmune adrenal insufficiency and autoimmune polyendocrine syndromes: autoantibodies, autoantigens, and their applicability in diagnosis and disease prediction. *Endocr Rev* 23, 327–364.
6. Nagamine K, Peterson P, Scott HS, Kudoh J, Minoshima S, Heino M, Krohn KJ, Lalioti MD, Mullis PE, Antonarakis SE, Kawasaki K, Asakawa S, Ito F, and Shimizu N. (1997) Positional cloning of the APECED gene. *Nat Genet* 17: 393–398.
7. Finnish-German APECED Consortium. (1997) An autoimmune disease, APECED, caused by mutations in a novel gene featuring two PHD-type zinc-finger domains. *Nat Genet* 17: 399–403.
8. Pitkänen J, Doucas V, Stemsdorf T, Nakajima T, Aratani S, Jensen K, Will H, Vähämurto P, Ollila J, Vihinen M, Scott HS, Antonarakis SE, Kudoh J, Shimizu N, Krohn K, Peterson P. (2000) The autoimmune regulator protein has transcriptional transactivating properties and interacts with the common coactivator CREB-binding protein. *J Biol Chem* 275: 16802–16809.
9. Bottomley MJ, Collard MW, Huggenvik JI, Liu Z, Gibson TJ, Sattler M. (2001) The SAND domain structure defines a novel DNA-binding fold in transcriptional regulation. *Nat Struct Biol* 8: 626–633.
10. Kumar PG, Laloraya M, Wang CY, Ruan QG, Davoodi-Semiromi A, Kao KJ, She JX. (2001) The autoimmune regulator (AIRE) is a DNA-binding protein. *J Biol Chem* 276: 41357–41364.
11. Bienz M. (2006) The PHD finger, a nuclear protein-interaction domain. *Trends Biochem Sci* 31: 35–40.
12. Savkur RS, Burris TP. (2004) The coactivator LXXLL nuclear receptor recognition motif. *J Pept Res* 63: 207–212.

13. Cihakova D, Trebusak K, Heino M, Fadeyev V, Tiulpakov A, Battelino T, Tar A, Halasz Z, Blumel P, Tawfik S, Krohn K, Lebl J, Peterson P. (2001) Novel AIRE mutations and P450 cytochrome autoantibodies in Central and Eastern European patients with APECED. *Hum Mutat* 18, 225–232.

14. Sato K, Nakajima K, Imamura H, Deguchi T, Horinouchi S, Yamazaki K, Yamada E, Kanaji Y, Takano K. (2002) A novel missense mutation of AIRE gene in a patient with autoimmune polyendocrinopathy, candidiasis and ectodermal dystrophy (APECED), accompanied with progressive muscular atrophy: case report and review of the literature in Japan. *Endocr J* 49: 625–633.

15. Pearce SH, Cheetham T, Imrie H, Vaidya B, Barnes ND, Bilous RW, Carr D, Meeran K, Shaw NJ, Smith CS, Toft AD, Williams G, Kendall-Taylor P. (1998) A common and recurrent 13-bp deletion in the autoimmune regulator gene in British kindreds with autoimmune polyendocrinopathy type 1. *Am J Hum Genet* 63: 1675–1684.

16. Halonen M, Eskelin P, Myhre AG, Perheentupa J, Husebye ES, Kämpe O, Rorsman F, Peltonen L, Ulmanen I, Partanen J. (2002) AIRE mutations and human leukocyte antigen genotypes as determinants of the autoimmune polyendocrinopathy-candidiasis-ectodermal dystrophy phenotype. *J Clin Endocrinol Metab* 87: 2568–2574.

17. Heino M, Scott HS, Chen Q, Peterson P, Mäenpää U, Papasavvas MP, Mittaz L, Barras C, Rossier C, Chrousos GP, Stratakis CA, Nagamine K, Kudoh J, Shimizu N, Maclaren N, Antonarakis SE, Krohn K. (1999) Mutation analyses of North American APS-1 patients. *Hum Mutat* 13: 69–74.

18. Kogawa K, Kudoh J, Nagafuchi S, Ohga S, Katsuta H, Ishibashi H, Harada M, Hara T, Shimizu N. (2002) Distinct clinical phenotype and immunoreactivity in Japanese siblings with autoimmune polyglandular syndrome type 1 (APS-1) associated with compound heterozygous novel AIRE gene mutations. *Clin Immunol* 103: 277–283.

19. Ulinski T, Perrin L, Morris M, Houang M, Cabrol S, Grapin C, Chabbert-Buffet N, Bensman A, Deschenes G, Giurgea I. (2006) Autoimmune polyendocrinopathy-candidiasis-ectodermal dystrophy syndrome with renal failure: impact of posttransplant immunosuppression on disease activity. *J Clin Endocrinol Metab* 91: 192–195.

20. Meloni A, Perniola R, Faa V, Corvaglia E, Cao A, Rosatelli MC. (2002) Delineation of the molecular defects in the AIRE gene in autoimmune polyendocrinopathy-candidiasis-ectodermal dystrophy patients from Southern Italy. *J Clin Endocrinol Metab* 87: 841–846.

21. Björses P, Halonen M, Palvimo JJ, Kolmer M, Aaltonen J, Ellonen P, Perheentupa J, Ulmanen I, Peltonen L. (2000) Mutations in the AIRE gene: effects on subcellular location and transactivation function of the autoimmune polyendocrinopathy-candidiasis-ectodermal dystrophy protein. *Am J Hum Genet* 66: 378–392.

22. Scott HS, Heino M, Peterson P, Mittaz L, Lalioti MD, Betterle C, Cohen A, Seri M, Lerone M, Romeo G, Collin P, Salo M, Metcalfe R, Weetman A, Papasavvas MP, Rossier C, Nagamine K, Kudoh J, Shimizu N, Krohn KJ, Antonarakis SE. (1998) Common mutations in autoimmune polyendocrinopathy-candidiasis ectodermal dystrophy patients of different origins. *Mol Endocrinol* 12: 1112–1119.

23. Ward L, Paquette J, Seidman E, Huot C, Alvarez F, Crock P, Delvin E, Kampe O, Deal C. (1999) Severe autoimmune polyendocrinopathy-candidiasis-ectodermal dystrophy in an adolescent girl with a novel AIRE mutation: response to immunosuppressive therapy. *J Clin Endocrinol Metab* 84: 844–852.

24. Rosatelli MC, Meloni A, Meloni A, Devoto M, Cao A, Scott HS, Peterson P, Heino M, Krohn KJ, Nagamine K, Kudoh J, Shimizu N, Antonarakis SE. (1998) A common mutation in Sardinian autoimmune polyendocrinopathy-candidiasis-ectodermal dystrophy patients. *Hum Genet* 103: 428–434.

25. Wang CY, Davoodi-Semiromi A, Huang W, Connor E, Shi JD, She JX. (1998) Characterization of mutations in patients with autoimmune polyglandular syndrome type 1 (APS1). *Hum Genet* 103: 681–685.

26. Podkrajsek KT, Bratanic N, Krzisnik C, Battelino T. (2005) Autoimmune regulator-1 messenger ribonucleic acid analysis in a novel intronic mutation and two additional novel AIRE gene mutations

in a cohort of autoimmune polyendocrinopathy-candidiasis-ectodermal dystrophy patients. *J Clin Endocrinol Metab* 90: 4930–4935.

27. Cetani F, Barbesino G, Borsari S, Pardi E, Cianferotti L, Pinchera A, Marcocci C. (2001) A novel mutation of the autoimmune regulator gene in an Italian kindred with autoimmune polyendocrinopathy-candidiasis-ectodermal dystrophy, acting in a dominant fashion and strongly cosegregating with hypothyroid autoimmune thyroiditis. *J Clin Endocrinol Metab* 86: 4747–4752.

28. Saugier-Veber P, Drouot N, Wolf LM, Kuhn JM, Frebourg T, Lefebvre H. (2001) Identification of a novel mutation in the autoimmune regulator (AIRE-1) gene in a French family with autoimmune polyendocrinopathy-candidiasis-ectodermal dystrophy. *Eur J Endocrinol* 144: 347–351.

29. Harris M, Kecha O, Deal C, Howlett CR, Deiss D, Tobias V, Simoneau-Roy J, Walker J. (2003) Reversible metaphyseal dysplasia, a novel bone phenotype, in two unrelated children with autoimmunepolyendocrinopathy-candidiasis-ectodermal dystrophy: clinical and molecular studies. *J Clin Endocrinol Metab* 88: 4576–4585.

30. Söderbergh A, Rorsman F, Halonen M, Ekwall O, Björses P, Kämpe O, Husebye ES. (2000) Autoantibodies against aromatic L-amino acid decarboxylase identifies a subgroup of patients with Addison's disease. *J Clin Endocrinol Metab* 85: 460–463.

31. Myhre AG, Halonen M, Eskelin P, Ekwall O, Hedstrand H, Rorsman F, Kämpe O, Husebye ES. (2001) Autoimmune polyendocrine syndrome type 1 (APS I) in Norway. *Clin Endocrinol (Oxf)* 54: 211–217.

32. Vogel A, Strassburg CP, Deiss D, Manns MP. (2003) A novel AIRE mutation in an APECED patient with candidiasis, adrenal failure, hepatitis, diabetes mellitus and osteosclerosis. *Exp Clin Endocrinol Diabetes* 111: 174–176.

33. Ishii T, Suzuki Y, Ando N, Matsuo N, Ogata T. (2000) Novel mutations of the autoimmune regulator gene in two siblings with autoimmune polyendocrinopathy-candidiasis-ectodermal dystrophy. *J Clin Endocrinol Metab* 85: 2922–2926.

34. Sato U, Horikawa R, Katsumata N, Asakura Y, Kitanaka S, Tanaka T. (2004) Novel compound heterozygous AIRE mutations in a Japanese patient with APECED. *J Pediatr Endocrinol Metab* 17: 917–921.

35. Buzi F, Badolato R, Mazza C, Giliani S, Notarangelo LD, Radetti G, Plebani A, Notarangelo LD. (2003) Autoimmune polyendocrinopathy-candidiasis-ectodermal dystrophy syndrome: time to review diagnostic criteria? *J Clin Endocrinol Metab* 88: 3146–3148.

36. Gylling M, Kääriainen E, Väisanen R, Kerosuo L, Solin ML, Halme L, Saari S, Halonen M, Kämpe O, Perheentupa J, Miettinen A. (2003) The hypoparathyroidism of autoimmune polyendocrinopathy-candidiasis-ectodermal dystrophy protective effect of male sex. *J Clin Endocrinol Metab* 88: 4602–4608.

37. Vaidya B, Imrie H, Geatch DR, Perros P, Ball SG, Baylis PH, Carr D, Hurel SJ, James RA, Kelly WF, Kemp EH, Young ET, Weetman AP, Kendall-Taylor P, Pearce SH. (2000). Association analysis of the cytotoxic T lymphocyte antigen-4 (CTLA-4) and autoimmune regulator-1 (AIRE-1) genes in sporadic autoimmune Addison's disease. *J Clin Endocrinol Metab* 85: 688–691.

38. Nithiyananthan R, Heward JM, Allahabadia A, Barnett AH, Franklyn JA, Gough SCL. (2000). A heterozygous deletion of the autoimmune regulator (AIRE1) gene, autoimmune thyroid disease, and type 1 diabetes: no evidence for association. *J Clin Endocrinol Metab* 85: 1320–1322.

39. Meyer G, Donner H, Herwig J, Bohles H, Usadel KH, Badenhoop K. (2001) Screening for an AIRE-1 mutation in patients with Addison's disease, type 1 diabetes, Graves' disease and Hashimoto's thyroiditis as well as in APECED syndrome. *Clin Endocrinol (Oxf)* 54: 335–338.

40. Djilali-Saiah I, Renous R, Caillat-Zucman S, Debray D, Alvarez F. (2004) Linkage disequilibrium between HLA class II region and autoimmune hepatitis in pediatric patients. *J Hepatol* 40: 904–909.

41. Torok HP, Tonenchi L, Glas J, Schiemann U, Folwaczny C. (2004) No significant association between mutations in exons 6 and 8 of the autoimmune regulator (AIRE) gene and inflammatory bowel disease. *Eur J Immunogenet* 31: 83–86.

42. Goswami R, Gupta N, Ray D, Rani R, Tomar N, Sarin R, Vupputuri MR. (2005) Polymorphisms at +49A/G and CT60 sites in the 3' UTR of the CTLA-4 gene and APECED-related AIRE gene mutations analysis in sporadic idiopathic hypoparathyroidism. *Int J Immunogenet* 32: 393–400.

43. Turunen JA, Wessman M, Forsblom C, Kilpikari R, Parkkonen M, Pontynen N, Ilmarinen T, Ulmanen I, Peltonen L, Groop PH. (2006) Association analysis of the AIRE and insulin genes in Finnish type 1 diabetic patients. *Immunogenetics* 58: 5–6.

44. Tazi-Ahnini R, Cork MJ, Gawkrodger DJ, Birch MP, Wengraf D, McDonagh AJ, Messenger AG. (2002) Role of the autoimmune regulator (AIRE) gene in alopecia areata: strong association of a potentially functional AIRE polymorphism with alopecia universalis. *Tissue Antigens* 60: 489–495.

45. Pitkänen J, Vähämurto P, Krohn K, Peterson P. (2001) Subcellular localization of the autoimmune regulator protein. Characterization of nuclear targeting and transcriptional activation domain. *J Biol Chem* 276: 19597–195602.

46. Kalkhoven E. (2004) CBP and p300: HATs for different occasions. *Biochem Pharmacol* 68: 1145–1155.

47. Akiyoshi H, Hatakeyama S, Pitkänen J, Mouri Y, Doucas V, Kudoh J, Tsurugaya K, Uchida D, Matsushima A, Oshikawa K, Nakayama KI, Shimizu N, Peterson P, Matsumoto M. (2004) Subcellular expression of autoimmune regulator is organized in a spatiotemporal manner. *J Biol Chem* 279: 33984–33991.

48. Pitkänen J, Rebane A, Rowell J, Murumagi A, Ströbel P, Möll K, Saare M, Heikkilä J, Doucas V, Marx A, Peterson P. (2005) Cooperative activation of transcription by autoimmune regulator AIRE and CBP. *Biochem Biophys Res Commun* 333: 944–953.

49. Uchida D, Hatakeyama S, Matsushima A, Han H, Ishido S, Hotta H, Kudoh J, Shimizu N, Doucas V, Nakayama KI, Kuroda N, Matsumoto M. (2004) AIRE functions as an E3 ubiquitin ligase. *J Exp Med* 199:167–172.

50. Heino M, Peterson P, Kudoh J, Nagamine K, Lagerstedt A, Ovod V, Ranki A, Rantala I, Nieminen M, Tuukkanen J, Scott HS, Antonarakis SE, Shimizu N, Krohn K. (1999) Autoimmune regulator is expressed in the cells regulating immune tolerance in thymus medulla. *Biochem Biophys Res Commun* 257: 821–825.

51. Zuklys S, Balciunaite G, Agarwal A, Fasler-Kan E, Palmer E, Hollander GA. (2000) Normal thymic architecture and negative selection are associated with Aire expression, the gene defective in the autoimmune-polyendocrinopathy-candidiasis-ectodermal dystrophy (APECED). *J Immunol* 165: 1976–1983.

52. Heino M, Peterson P, Sillanpää N, Guerin S, Wu L, Anderson G, Scott HS, Antonarakis SE, Kudoh J, Shimizu N, Jenkinson EJ, Naquet P, Krohn KJ. (2000) RNA and protein expression of the murine autoimmune regulator gene (Aire) in normal, RelB-deficient and in NOD mouse. *Eur J Immunol* 30:1884–1893.

53. Sillanpää N, Magureanu CG, Murumägi A, Reinikainen A, West A, Manninen A, Lahti M, Ranki A, Saksela K, Krohn K, Lahesmaa R, Peterson P. (2004) Autoimmune regulator induced changes in the gene expression profile of human monocyte-dendritic cell-lineage. *Mol Immunol* 41: 1185–1198.

54. Kogawa K, Nagafuchi S, Katsuta H, Kudoh J, Tamiya S, Sakai Y, Shimizu N, Harada M. (2002) Expression of AIRE gene in peripheral monocyte/dendritic cell lineage. *Immunol Lett* 80: 195–198.

55. Blechschmidt K, Schweiger M, Wertz K, Poulson R, Christensen HM, Rosenthal A, Lehrach H, Yaspo ML. (1999) The mouse Aire gene: comparative genomic sequencing, gene organization, and expression. *Genome Res* 9:158–166.

56. Anderson G, Jenkinson WE, Jones T, Parnell SM, Kinsella FA, White AJ, Pongrac'z JE, Rossi SW, Jenkinson EJ. (2006) Establishment and functioning of intrathymic microenvironments. *Immunol Rev* 209: 10–27.

57. Ramsey C, Winqvist O, Puhakka L, Halonen M, Moro A, Kampe O, Eskelin P, Pelto-Huikko M, Peltonen L. 2002. Aire deficient mice develop multiple features of APECED phenotype and show altered immune response. *Hum Mol Genet.* 11: 397–409.

58. Ramsey C, Hassler S, Marits P, Kampe O, Surth CD, Peltonen L, Winqvist O. 2006 Increased antigen presenting cell-mediated T cell activation in mice and patients without the autoimmune regulator. *Eur J Immunol*. 36: 305–317.

59. Anderson MS, Venanzi ES, Klein L, Chen Z, Berzins SP, Turley SJ, von Boehmer H, Bronson R, Dierich A, Benoist C, Mathis D. (2002) Projection of an immunological self shadow within the thymus by the aire protein. *Science* 298: 1395–1401.

60. Kuroda N, Mitani T, Takeda N, Ishimaru N, Arakaki R, Hayashi Y, Bando Y, Izumi K, Takahashi T, Nomura T, Sakaguchi S, Ueno T, Takahama Y, Uchida D, Sun S, Kajiura F, Mouri Y, Han H, Matsushima A, Yamada G, Matsumoto M. (2005) Development of autoimmunity against transcriptionally unrepressed target antigen in the thymus of Aire-deficient mice. *J Immunol* 174: 1862–1870.

61. Kyewski B, Klein L. (2006) A central role for central tolerance. *Annu Rev Immunol* 24: 571–606.

62. Villasenor J, Benoist C, Mathis D. (2005) AIRE and APECED: molecular insights into an autoimmune disease. *Immunol Rev* 204: 156–164.

63. Krohn K, Uibo R, Aavik E, Peterson P, Savilahti K. (1992) Identification by molecular cloning of an autoantigen associated with Addison's disease as steroid 17 alpha-hydroxylase. *Lancet* 339: 770–773.

64. Winqvist O, Karlsson FA, Kämpe O. (1992) 21-Hydroxylase, a major autoantigen in idiopathic Addison's disease. *Lancet* 339: 1559–1562.

65. Winqvist O, Gustafsson J, Rorsman F, Karlsson FA, Kämpe O. (1993) Two different cytochrome P450 enzymes are the adrenal antigens in autoimmune polyendocrine syndrome type I and Addison's disease. *J Clin Invest* 92: 2377–2385.

66. Uibo R, Aavik E, Peterson P, Perheentupa J, Aranko S, Pelkonen R, Krohn KJ. (1994) Autoantibodies to cytochrome P450 enzymes P450scc, P450c17, and P450c21 in autoimmune polyglandular disease types I and II and in isolated Addison's disease. *J Clin Endocrinol Metab* 78: 323–328.

67. Björk E, Velloso LA, Kämpe O, Karlsson FA. (1994) GAD autoantibodies in IDDM, stiff-man syndrome, and autoimmune polyendocrine syndrome type I recognize different epitopes. *Diabetes* 43, 161–165.

68. Velloso LA, Winqvist O, Gustafsson J, Kämpe O, Karlsson FA. (1994) Autoantibodies against a novel 51 kDa islet antigen and glutamate decarboxylase isoforms in autoimmune polyendocrine syndrome type I. *Diabetologia* 37: 61–69.

69. Gylling M, Tuomi T, Björses P, Kontiainen S, Partanen J, Christie MR, Knip M, Perheentupa J, Miettinen A. (2000) ss-Cell autoantibodies, human leukocyte antigen II alleles, and type 1 diabetes in autoimmune polyendocrinopathy-candidiasis-ectodermal dystrophy. *J Clin Endocrinol Metab* 85: 4434–4440.

70. Husebye ES, Gebre-Medhin G, Tuomi T, Perheentupa J, Landin-Olsson M, Gustafsson J, Rorsman F, Kämpe O. (1997) Autoantibodies against aromatic L-amino acid decarboxylase in autoimmune polyendocrine syndrome type I. *J Clin Endocrinol Metab* 82: 147–150.

71. Sköldberg F, Portela-Gomes GM, Grimelius L, Nilsson G, Perheentupa J, Betterle C, Husebye ES, Gustafsson J, Rönnblom A, Rorsman F, Kämpe O. (2003) Histidine decarboxylase, a pyridoxal phosphate-dependent enzyme, is an autoantigen of gastric enterochromaffin-like cells. *J Clin Endocrinol Metab* 88: 1445–1452.

72. Sköldberg F, Rorsman F, Perheentupa J, Landin-Olsson M, Husebye ES, Gustafsson J, Kämpe O. (2004) Analysis of antibody reactivity against cysteine sulfinic acid decarboxylase, a pyridoxal phosphate-dependent enzyme, in endocrine autoimmune disease. *J Clin Endocrinol Metab* 89: 1636–1640.

73. Ekwall O, Hedstrand H, Grimelius L, Haavik J, Perheentupa J, Gustafsson J, Husebye E, Kämpe O, Rorsman F. (1998) Identification of tryptophan hydroxylase as an intestinal autoantigen. *Lancet* 352: 279–283.

74. Ekwall O, Hedstrand H, Haavik J, Perheentupa J, Betterle C, Gustafsson J, Husebye E, Rorsman F, Kämpe O. (2000) Pteridin-dependent hydroxylases as autoantigens in autoimmune polyendocrine syndrome type I. *J Clin Endocrinol Metab* 85: 2944–2950.

75. Hedstrand H, Ekwall O, Haavik J, Landgren E, Betterle C, Perheentupa J, Gustafsson J, Husebye E, Rorsman F, Kämpe O. (2000) Identification of tyrosine hydroxylase as an autoantigen in autoimmune polyendocrine syndrome type I. *Biochem Biophys Res Commun* 267: 456–461.

76. Clemente MG, Meloni A, Obermayer-Straub P, Frau F, Manns MP, De Virgiliis S. (1998) Two cytochromes P450 are major hepatocellular autoantigens in autoimmune polyglandular syndrome type 1. *Gastroenterology* 114: 324–328.

77. Perniola R, Falorni A, Clemente MG, Forini F, Accogli E, Lobreglio G. (2000). Organ-specific and non-organ-specific autoantibodies in children and young adults with autoimmune polyendocrinopathy-candidiasis-ectodermal dystrophy (APECED). *Eur J Endocrinol* 143: 497–503.

78. Hedstrand H, Ekwall O, Olsson MJ, Landgren E, Kemp EH, Weetman AP, Perheentupa J, Husebye E, Gustafsson J, Betterle C, Kämpe O, Rorsman F. (2001) The transcription factors SOX9 and SOX10 are vitiligo autoantigens in autoimmune polyendocrine syndrome type I. *J Biol Chem* 276: 35390–35395.

79. Li Y, Song YH, Rais N, Connor E, Schatz D, Muir A, Maclaren N. (1996) Autoantibodies to the extracellular domain of the calcium sensing receptor in patients with acquired hypoparathyroidism. *J Clin Invest* 97: 910–914.

80. Söderbergh A, Myhre AG, Ekwall O, Gebre-Medhin G, Hedstrand H, Landgren E, Miettinen A, Eskelin P, Halonen M, Tuomi T, Gustafsson J, Husebye ES, Perheentupa J, Gylling M, Manns MP, Rorsman F, Kämpe O, Nilsson T. (2004). Prevalence and clinical associations of 10 defined autoantibodies in autoimmune polyendocrine syndrome type I. *J Clin Endocrinol Metab* 89: 557–562.

81. Meager A, Visvalingam K, Peterson P, Moll K, Murumagi A, Krohn K, Eskelin P, Perheentupa J, Husebye E, Kadota Y, Willcox N. (2006) Anti-interferon autoantibodies in autoimmune polyen-docrinopathy syndrome type 1. PLoS Med. 3: e289

82. Peterson P, Perheentupa J, Krohn KJ. (1996) Detection of candidal antigens in autoimmune polyg-landular syndrome type I. *Clin Diagn Lab Immunol* 3: 290–294.

83. Lilic D, Gravenor I, Robson N, Lammas DA, Drysdale P, Calvert JE, Cant AJ, Abinun M. (2003) Deregulated production of protective cytokines in response to Candida albicans infection in patients with chronic mucocutaneous candidiasis. *Infect Immun* 71: 5690–5609.

84. Germain M, Gourdeau M, Hebert J. (1994) Case report: familial chronic mucocutaneous candidiasis complicated by deep candida infection. *Am J Med Sci* 307: 282–283.

85. Matthews R, Burnie J. (1992) The role of hsp90 in fungal infection. *Immunol Today* 13: 345–348.

86. Sediva A, Cihakova D, Lebl J. (2002) Immunological findings in patients with autoimmune polyendocrinopathy-candidiasis-ectodermal dystrophy (APECED) and their family members: are heterozygotes subclinically affected? *J Pediatr Endocrinol Metab* 15: 1491–1496

87. Perniola R, Lobreglio G, Rosatelli MC, Pitotti E, Accogli E, De Rinaldis C. (2005) Immunophenotypic characterisation of peripheral blood lymphocytes in autoimmune polyglandular syndrome type 1: clinical study and review of the literature. *J Pediatr Endocrinol Metab* 18: 155–164.

88. Ryan KR, Lawson CA, Lorenzi AR, Arkwright PD, Isaacs JD, Lilic D. (2005) CD4+CD25+ T-regulatory cells are decreased in patients with autoimmune polyendocrinopathy candidiasis ectodermal dystrophy. *J Allergy Clin Immunol* 116: 1158–1159.

89. Thorpe ES, Handley HE. (1929) Chronic tetany and chronic mycelial stomatitis in a child aged four and one-half years. *Am J Dis Child* 38: 228–238.

90. Kirkpatrick CH. (2001) Chronic mucocutaneous candidiasis. *Pediatr Infect Dis J* 20: 197–206.

91. Perheentupa J. (2002) APS-I/APECED: the clinical disease and therapy. *Endocrinol Metab Clin North Am* 31: 295–320.

17 Autoimmune Polyglandular Syndrome Type 2

George J. Kahaly, Prof
and Manuela Dittmar, Prof

Contents

Summary

The nature of autoimmune polyglandular syndrome type 2 (APS-2) has been based on the presence of lymphocyte infiltration in the affected gland, organ-specific antibodies (Abs) in the serum, cellular immune defects, and an association with the human leukocyte antigen (HLA)-DR/DQ genes or immune-response genes. Autoantibodies to the various endocrine and non-endocrine tissues not only offer a diagnostic clue to the autoimmune nature of diseases but also can be used to identify asymptomatic individuals who are at risk of developing other component diseases of the syndrome. Although target tissues or glands differ, several common threads link the diseases of the APS. The autoimmune destruction of most target glands appears to be a slow process with a long preclinical prodrome that may last for years. During this period, autoantibodies, lymphocyte abnormalities, and subclinical endocrine defects are usually present. As knowledge of target antigens has progressed, it appears that despite polyendocrine disease, within each gland, specific antigens are the targets of the autoimmune process. A defect resides in one of the genes of the HLA locus, which, in concert with other gene(s), results in susceptibility. Genetic susceptibility is necessary but not sufficient to produce the disorder. This is illustrated by the lack of 100% concordance of disease in identical twins. When the genetic defects and environmental influences of organ-specific autoimmunity are better understood, it may be possible to devise specific replacement or corrective therapies. Given the similar features of many of the organ-specific autoimmune disorders, it is likely that if immunotherapeutic modalities are successful in one disease, they may be of benefit in related disorders. With respect to the significant morbidity and potential mortality of the disease, the main diagnostic objective is to detect APS-2 at an early stage, with the advantage of less frequent complications, effective therapy, and better prognosis. This requires that patients at risk be regularly

From: *Contemporary Endocrinology: Autoimmune Diseases in Endocrinology*
Edited by: A. P. Weetman © Humana Press, Totowa, NJ

screened for subclinical endocrinopathies before clinical manifestation occurs. Regarding the possible large time interval between manifestation of the first and further endocrinopathies, regular and long-term follow-up of patients with endocrine autoimmune disorders is warranted. Considering the high incidence of one or more endocrinopathies in first-degree relatives of patients with APS-2, family members of patients should be regularly screened, because they may develop autoimmune endocrinopathies in the future.

Key Words: Autoimmune polyglandular syndrome type 2, polyglandular autoimmunity, epidemiology, diagnosis, genetics, pathogenesis.

INTRODUCTION

The autoimmune polyglandular syndromes (APS) (also polyglandular autoimmune syndromes (PGA)] may be divided in a primarily juvenile type 1 (*see* Chap. 17) and a more common adult type 2 *(1)*. They form different clusters of autoimmune disorders *(2,3)*. APS-2 is often defined by the occurrence of two or more autoimmune endocrine disorders in the same individual including Graves' disease, primary hypothyroidism, type 1 diabetes mellitus, Addison's disease, and premature hypogonadism. Several non-endocrine disorders such as myasthenia gravis, celiac disease, pernicious anemia, vitiligo, and alopecia also occur in these patients. The coexistence of adrenal failure with either autoimmune thyroid disease or type 1 diabetes mellitus also is defined as Schmidt's syndrome or Carpenter's syndrome (Fig. 1). Type 2 APS is more varied in its manifestations than type 1, also called autoimmune polyendocrinopathy-candidiasis-ectodermal dystrophy (APECED). The latter is characterized by three specific disorders, that is chronic mucocutaneous candidiasis, autoimmune hypoparathyroidism, and Addison's disease *(4,5)*. Other endocrine and non-endocrine autoimmune disorders either may be present or will develop later. APS-1 manifests in infancy or early childhood. It is a monogenic disease with autosomal recessive inheritance caused by mutations in the autoimmune regulatory (*AIRE*) gene on chromosome 21. In contrast, APS-2 shows a complex inheritance pattern.

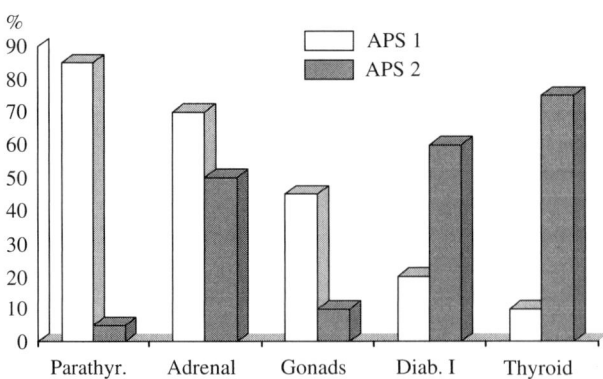

Fig. 1. Prevalence of most frequent autoimmune endocrine component diseases in APS-1 and APS-2. parathyr., hypoparathyroidism; adrenal, Addison's disease; gonads, hypogonadism; diab 1, type 1 diabetes mellitus; thyroid, autoimmune thyroid disease.

EPIDEMIOLOGY

Autoimmune polyglandular syndrome type 2 is a rare disease. Its prevalence is 1:20,000 *(6)*. It is more frequently encountered in women, and the male-to-female ratio is 1:3 *(7)*. This syndrome has a peak incidence at ages 20–60 years, mostly in the 30–40 years, and it is common for multiple generations to be affected by one or more component diseases. There is familial clustering, and family members of patients are often affected *(2)*. Although there is some correlation between the ages of onset of one polyglandular syndrome illness with another, many years may separate the onset of different diseases *(7)*. There are many common themes linking each of these individual illnesses. All the disorders resulting in tissue destruction appear to have a prolonged phase of cellular loss preceding overt autoimmune glandular disease.

GENETIC AND ENVIRONMENTAL FACTORS

The inheritance of the type 2 APS is complex, with genes on chromosome 6 playing a predominant role. In man, this chromosome contains the major histocompatibility loci. Many of the diseases of the type 2 syndrome are associated with human leukocyte antigen (HLA) alleles B8 and DR3. The DR antigen has two glycoprotein chains coded for by the DR loci of chromosome 6. The alleles HLA-B8 and DR3, which are coded for by separate genes, are more often found together on the same chromosome than one would predict from their frequency in the general population. Such associations are common for alleles of different genes in the histocompatibility region (linkage disequilibrium). The allele DR3 is most closely associated with autoimmune endocrine disease. Within some families, autoimmune endocrine disease susceptibility appears to be inherited as an autosomal-dominant form associated with a specific HLA haplotype. Nevertheless, family members may manifest different diseases, although the more common the disease in the general population, the higher its prevalence in affected families.

Although genetic factors determine disease susceptibility, there is <100% concordance in monozygotic twins for the respective diseases. This suggests that other factors may be involved in disease pathogenesis. Environmental factors that can trigger DR3-associated autoimmunity include iodine and the wheat protein gliadin for celiac disease. Thus, both genetic and environmental factors contribute to the loss of immune self-tolerance. On the basis of a genetic predisposition, epigenetic external factors, such as viral or bacterial infections *(8)*, and psychosocial factors might induce an autoimmune cascade. Environmental factors may have an important influence on the development of autoimmune diseases, but the exposure to environmental pathogens does not always lead to disease. With respect to genetics, APS-2 is supposed to be a polygenic disease with autosomal-dominant inheritance and incomplete penetrance. Also, familial clustering provided evidence for a genetic predisposition.

Type 2 APS is associated with HLA-DR3 and -DR4 antigens, and interestingly, frequencies for DQA1*0301 and *0501 were increased in patients with APS-2 compared with controls *(9)*. The genotype DR3/4, DQ2/DQ8 with DRB1*0404 has been found to be the highest HLA genotype risk for Addison's disease, either as a single disease or within APS-2 *(10)*. An association of APS-2 with HLA-B8 has been observed in three generations of a family, whereas 10 unaffected subjects did not show B8 *(11)*. HLA associations have also been described for APS-2 component diseases type 1 diabetes (DR4-DQB1*0302) and Graves' disease (B8). Type 1 diabetes locus 1 contains the MHC region (6p21) and in whites revealed a positive association with HLA DRB1*04-DQA1*0301-DQB1*0302 (DR4-DQ8) or DRB1*03-DQA1*0501-DQB1*0201 (DR3-DQ2) and a negative association with DRB1*15-DQA1*0102-DQB1*0602 *(12,13)*. Other studies appear to indicate that heterozygosis for tumor necrosis factor (TNF)-α increased the risk for type 1 diabetes in DQA1*0501-DQB1*0201/DQA1*0301-DQB1*0302-positive individuals, but this may also be the result of a linkage disequilibrium with HLA class 2 genes *(14)*. Tandon et al. *(15)* identified a significant association between Hashimoto's thyroiditis and HLA-DR3, whereas Roman et al. *(16)* found an increase in HLA-DR5 in affected family members with Hashimoto's thyroiditis.

Tomer et al. *(17)* performed a whole genome linkage study on a data set of 56 multiplex, multigenerational autoimmune thyroid disease families, using 387 microsatellite markers. Only one locus on chromosome 6 was linked with both Graves' disease and Hashimoto's thyroiditis. This locus was close to, but distinct from, the region. Finally, the cytotoxic T lymphocyte-associated antigen *(CTLA)-4* gene, or a gene closely associated with it, confers susceptibility to Hashimoto's thyroiditis as reported in other autoimmune diseases *(18)*.

The MHC class I-related gene A (*MICA*) is an additional locus associated within the HLA region because the frequency of the MICA 5.1 allele was increased in patients with APS-2 compared with healthy controls *(19)*. Recently, Gambelunghe et al. *(20)* suggested that the combination of MICA 5 and HLA-DR3-DQ2 and/or HLA-DR4-DQ8 represents a strong genetic marker for type 1 diabetes with or without APS. Furthermore, there is evidence that MHC class III genes are associated with APS type 2, most specifically the gene encoding TNF-α, a multifunctional proinflammatory cytokine, which mediates inflammatory and immune functions. Within the *TNF*-α gene, the −308*A allele of an A/G single-nucleotide dimorphism occurred more frequently in patients with APS-2 than in healthy control subjects *(21)*.

Of great interest is the recent finding that the protein tyrosine phosphatase nonreceptor 22 (*PTPN22*) gene might contribute to susceptibility to APS-2 *(22)*. This gene encodes an intracellular phosphatase with negative regulatory effects on T-cell activation. A functional single-nucleotide polymorphism (C1858T) in the *PTPN22* gene is associated with several autoimmune diseases, that is type 1 diabetes, Graves' disease, systemic lupus erythematosus, rheumatoid arthritis, and primary Sjogren's syndrome *(23–26)*. Finally and in contrast to type 2, APS 1 is a monogenic disease with autosomal recessive inheritance. Type 1 is caused by mutations in the *AIRE* gene on chromosome 21 *(27–36)*.

IMMUNOPATHOGENESIS

Cell-mediated immune processes are important in APS-2. Lymphocyte infiltrations of the various glands are associated with functional loss of epithelial cells with scarring. The cellular defect in the APS-2 may be associated with abnormal balances in cytokine production by T cells. The subgroups of T-helper cells—Th1 and Th2, and natural killer cells—produce different profiles of cytokines. Th1 cells secrete interferon-γ, interleukin (IL)-2, and TNF-α, whereas Th2 cells secrete IL-4, IL-5, and IL-10.

A polarized Th2 response is associated with Graves' disease and Th1 with type 1 diabetes. In contrast, APS-1 results from biased Th2 immune responses to self-antigens and defective protective Th1 responses against invasion of yeast *Candida albicans (37, 38)*. Table 1 summarizes the localization of various autoantigens and corresponding component diseases of APS-2. A viral or bacterial etiology for autoimmunity has been supposed *(8)*. A dominance of T-helper cells and a deficiency of T-suppressor cells have been demonstrated for endocrine autoimmunity *(39)*. Also, a hypothesis for the pathogenesis of APS-2 has been recently presented by Canbay et al. *(40)*. Accordingly, a genetically predisposed person might develop an autoimmune process after initiation by an infectious agent. This might initiate through cross-reactivity in the area of antigen-presenting MHC molecules, a Th 2-dependent immune process, which is primarily of humoral origin and partly local. This immune process probably progresses because of deficient T-suppressor cell activity.

In APS, several organ-specific autoimmune diseases are clustered. Although APS type 1 is caused by loss of central tolerance, the etiology of APS type 2 is currently unknown. Further evidence refers to regulatory cells that are implicated in self-tolerance and autoimmunity. The adaptive immune system not only consists of immune-stimulatory CD4+ helper or effector T cells and cytotoxic CD8+ T cells but also is regulated by immunosuppressive T cells. Three classes of immunosuppressive CD4+ T cells are known to date: induced Th3 and Tr1 cells, as well as the naturally present CD4+CD25+FoxP3+ regulatory T cells (Treg) *(41)*. Treg are generated in the thymus and are present in all healthy animals and humans. Because the FOXP3-encoded scurfin protein interferes with *IL-2* gene activation, Treg do not secrete IL-2 and do not proliferate on T-cell receptor (TCR)-stimulation. Treg suppress the activation of CD4+ and CD8+ cells in vitro and in vivo. They thereby prevent autoimmune disease, although the exact mechanism of suppression is unknown, and cell contact is crucial at least in vitro. Depletion of Treg leads to autoimmunity in mice *(42)*, and dysfunction of Treg has been linked to autoimmune diseases *(43)*. Defects in survival or the suppressive

Table 1
Localization of the Different Autoantigen(s) and the Corresponding Diseases

Disease	Autoantigen	Tissue/cells
Graves' disease	TSH receptor	Thyrocytes
Hashimoto's thyroiditis	TPO/TG	Enzyme/protein
Type 1 diabetes	GAD_{65}, IA-2, insulin	ß-cells
Addison's disease	21-OH, 17-OH, P450scc	Enzyme
Hypogonadism	17-OH, CYP450scc	Leydig/Theca cells
Hypoparathyroidism	Ca^{2+}-sensitive receptor	Parathyroid
Immungastritis	H^+, K^+-ATPase	Parietal cells
Pernicious anemia	Intrinsic factor	Chief cells (stomach)
Celiac disease	Transglutaminase, Gliadin	Small intestine
Vitiligo	Tyrosinase	Melanocytes
Alopecia areata	Tyrosine hydroxylase	Hair follicles

GAD, glutamic acid decarboxylase; OH, hydroxylase; TG, thyroglobulin; TPO, thyroid peroxidase; TSH, thyroid-stimulating hormone.

function of Treg may contribute to uncontrolled expansion of autoaggressive lymphocytes. Reduced numbers of Treg are observed in myasthenia gravis, and a reduction of suppressive Treg function has been reported in multiple sclerosis, rheumatoid arthritis, and other autoimmune diseases *(44–46)*.

In a murine model, depletion of thymically derived CD4(+) CD25(+)Treg, which exert suppression in a contact-dependent manner, resulted in a syndrome that is similar to human APS-2 with multiple endocrinopathies *(47)*. On the basis of these findings, Kriegel et al. *(43)* recently hypothesized that loss of active suppression in the periphery could be a hallmark of APS-2. Treg from peripheral blood of APS-2, control patients with single-autoimmune endocrinopathies, and normal healthy donors showed no differences in quantity, except for patients with isolated autoimmune diseases, in functionally important surface markers, or in apoptosis induced by growth factor withdrawal. Strikingly, APS-2 Treg were defective in their suppressive capacity. The defect was persistent and not because of responder cell resistance, whereas overt quantitative or phenotypic abnormalities in Treg from these patients were not observed. Also samples of FOXP3 messenger RNA from APS-2 Treg were semi-quantified and showed similar levels of FOXP3 transcripts compared with normal donor Treg despite defective suppressor function, clearly indicating that true Treg were dysfunctional.

Defective Treg function in humans with APS-2 has wide implications for autoimmunity in general. The results indicate that, once molecular mechanisms of suppressor function are better delineated, manipulations of human Treg may eventually allow improvement of immunomodulatory strategies in diseases with impaired suppressor function. Another important category of immunosuppressive cells are the Treg Tr1/Th3, and knowledge of the development and regulatory functions of such immunoregulatory cells may elucidate the etiology for developing autoimmunity *(48)*.

Another factor is related to the activity of the enzyme DNase 1. This glycoprotein is ubiquitously expressed in human tissues and plays a role in the regulation of apoptosis. It catalyzes DNA hydrolysis by cleaving double-stranded DNA. The activity of this enzyme was lowered in patients with APS-2 compared with healthy subjects *(49)*. Such a deficiency in DNase 1 may result in reduced or delayed removal of DNA from nuclear antigens and, thereby, may promote disease susceptibility to autoimmune disorders.

DIAGNOSIS AND CLINICAL SPECTRUM

APS-2 mostly occurs in adulthood during the 30–40 years. APS-2 presenting in childhood is extremely rare; a case with hypothyroidism, followed by diabetic ketoacidosis, and adrenal insufficiency has recently been reported *(50)*. In adults, the presence of one autoimmune endocrine disease is associated with an increased risk of developing autoimmunity to other tissues. Each of these disorders is characterized by several stages beginning with active autoimmunity and followed by metabolic abnormalities with overt disease. Type 1 diabetes is one of the most frequent component disorders of APS-2 and is often its first symptom. At the Gutenberg University Endocrine Department, Mainz, screening in the early 1990s of 471 patients with type 1 diabetes, aged 39 ± 16 years, disease duration 15 ± 10 years, showed in 127 cases (85 females) or 27% a multiple glandular involvement or APS-2. Additionally, 19 (4%) and 8 (2%) had vitiligo and immune gastritis, respectively.

Subsequent screening, at the same institution, of 15,000 consecutive subjects with endocrine disorders revealed a high prevalence (1%) of patients with APS-2 ($n = 151$, 75% females, Table 2, ref. *51*). These 151 subjects with APS-2 have been followed since then. There is often a long time interval between the manifestation of the first and second component disease of APS-2, which often comprises years to decades *(51)*. Most frequent disease combinations are type 1 diabetes/autoimmune thyroid disease (41%), followed by thyroid disease/Addison's disease (14.6%), type 1 diabetes/vitiligo (9.9%), thyroid disease/vitiligo (9.9%), type 1 diabetes/thyroid disease/pernicious anemia (5.3%), hypogonadism/alopecia (5.3%), and type 1 diabetes/Addison's disease (3.3%) *(51)*. Therefore, patients with monoglandular autoimmune disease should be functionally screened for APS-2 every 3 years until the age of 75 years. If positive, subsequent serological screening is recommended.

The simultaneous occurrence of hypothyroidism (Hashimoto's thyroiditis) and type 1 diabetes is often accompanied by hypoglycemia because of decreased insulin request and increased insulin sensitivity. Hypothyroid children show growth disorders caused by chronic hypoglycemia and decreased food intake. Substitution therapy with levothyroxine leads to increased insulin dosage. In contrast, hyperthyroidism is accompanied in 50% of the cases by glucose intolerance and in 3% of the cases by overt diabetes. Impaired glucose tolerance is because of decreased insulin sensitivity and hepatic storage of glycogen, whereas both secretion of glucagon and intestinal glucose absorption are enhanced. Similarly, concomitant presence of Addison's disease and type 1 diabetes also leads to frequent hypoglycemia because of decreased gluconeogenesis and increased insulin sensitivity.

Table 2
Screening of 15,000 Consecutive Subjects in the Specialized Endocrine Outpatient Clinic of the Gutenberg University Hospital Revealed a High Prevalence (1%) of Patients with APS-2 ($n = 151$, 75% Females)

Disease	*N (%)*
Type 1 diabetes	92 (61)
Graves' disease	50 (33)
Immune thyroiditis	49 (32.5)
Vitiligo	30 (20)
Addison's disease	28 (18.5)
Alopecia	9 (6)
Hypogonadism	8 (5.3)
Pernicious anemia	8 (5.3)

These APS-2 patients have been followed meanwhile for >15 years. The distribution of the various autoimmune endocrine diseases is shown *(51)*.

Circulating organ-specific autoantibodies are present in each of the component diseases of APS-2 (Table 3). Occasionally, as in anti-gonadal and anti-adrenal Abs, a given group of Abs will cross-react with more than one gland (e.g., all steroid-producing cells). Abs may bind to a cell surface without functional effects or may be blocking or stimulatory. Examples of blocking Abs include those directed at the acetylcholine receptor in myasthenia gravis. Other autoantibodies such as anti-microsomal and anti-parietal cell Abs are prevalent in healthy relatives of patients with APS-2. The presence of such Abs may precede clinical disease by many years, but in contrast to anti-islet Abs, anti-thyroid Abs can be present for decades without progression to overt disease.

Antibodies against steroidal enzymes (e.g., 21-hydroxylase [21-OH]) are of high prognostic value and will help identify patients at risk for developing Addison's disease *(52,53)*. This might prevent delayed diagnosis of adrenal failure. With respect to type 1 diabetes, it has been demonstrated that anti-idiotope reagents were able to distinguish between childhood-onset type 1 diabetes and adult-onset type 1 diabetes with polyendocrine susceptibility *(54)*. Childhood-onset type 1 diabetes-IAA differed from adult-onset type 1 diabetes-IAA in their specifity for human insulin and from their anti-idiotope amino acid sequence. Based on improved immuno-genetic understanding and autoantibody screening assays, type 1 diabetes is now predictable *(38)*.

At our institution, the autoantibody profile in 60 patients with APS-2, 54 with mono-glandular and non-glandular autoimmune diseases (MGA2), 14 with monoglandular autoimmunity (MGA), 15 with non-glandular autoimmunity (NGA), and 82 clinically healthy relatives has been analyzed. Subjects were screened for Abs against alpha-fodrin-immunoglobulin (Ig)A/IgG, SS-A/SS-B, thyroid peroxidase (TPO), gliadin-IgA/IgG, transglutaminase (TG)-IgA/IgG, ASCA-IgA/IgG, anti-nuclear Abs (ANA), and anti-neutrophil cytoplasmic Abs (ANCA) using ELISA and/or radioimmunoassay. The overall antibody prevalence in patients with APS-2, MGA2, relatives with MGA, NGA, and healthy relatives was 92, 87, 79, 67, and 56%, respectively (Fig. 2A). Prevalences for TPO were different between APS2, MGA2, MGA, NGA, and healthy relatives amounting 50, 54, 50, 13 (2/15), and 12%, respectively, ($p < 0.0001$, Fig. 2B).

Table 3
**Prevalence of Frequent Organ-Specific Autoantibodies in
Patients with APS Type 2 *(51)***

Antibodies	Prevalence (%)
Thyroid peroxidase (TPO)	77.2
Parietal cells (PCA)	53.9
Thyroglobulin (Tg)	49.5
TSH receptor	46.7
Insulin (IAA)	41.8
Glutamic acid decarboxylase (GAD)	30.3
Adrenal cortex	26.0
Islet cells (ICA)	21.1

APS, autoimmune polyglandular syndrome type; TSH, thyroid-stimulating hormone.

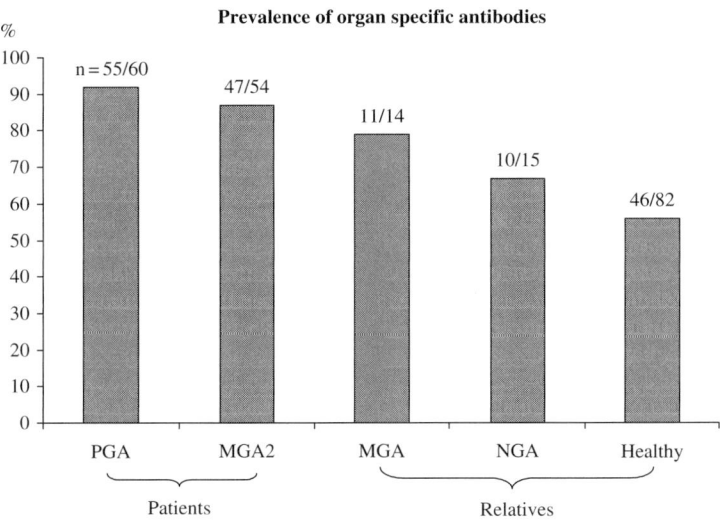

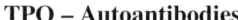

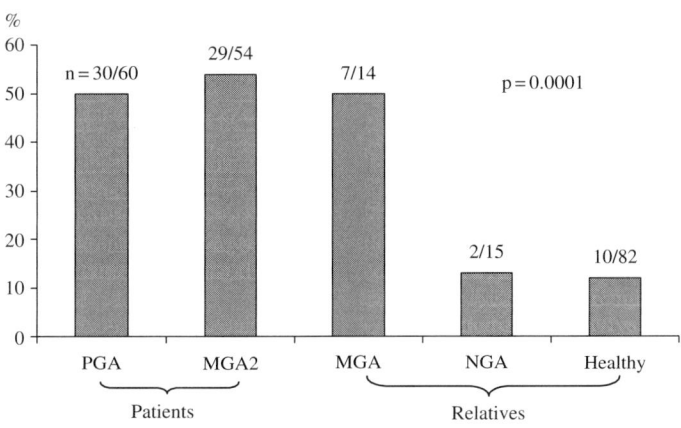

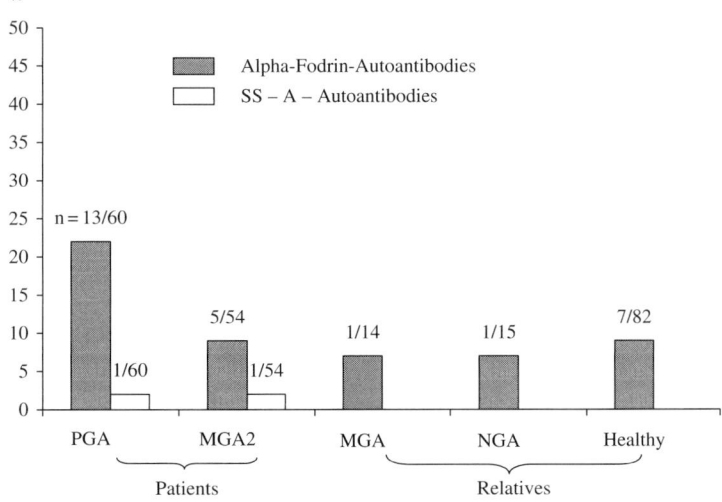

Fig. 2. *(Continued).*

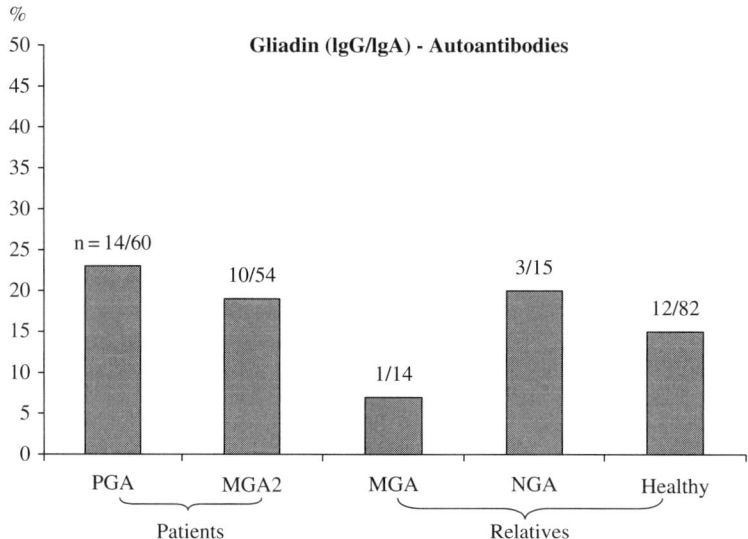

Fig. 2. Prevalence of organ specific (**A**), thyroid peroxidase (TPO, **B**), alpha-fodrin and SS-A (**C**), as well as gliadin (IgG/IgA, **D**) autoantibodies, respectively in patients with APS-2 or PGA, MGA2, and their relatives. PGA, autoimmune polyglandular syndrome type 2; MGA, monoglandular autoimmunity; NGA, non-glandular autoimmunity; MGA2, monoglandular autoimmunity with non-endocrine or non-glandular autoimmune disease, MGA + NGA.

Also, prevalence of glutamic acid decarboxylase (GAD) autoantibodies was increased in patients with APS-2 (8/10) compared with healthy persons (1/300, 0.3%) *(55)*. There were no statistically significant group differences with respect to the other autoanti-bodies (Fig. 2C,D). In summary, silent autoantibodies were highly prevalent in families with APS-2, and the prevalence of these Abs was associated with the number of involved glands. Thus, these Abs may be predictive for the development of future autoimmune endocrine diseases.

SCREENING FOR APS, FUNCTIONAL TESTING, AND TREATMENT

Approximately one in seven first-degree relatives of patients with the type 2 syndrome has an unrecognized endocrine disorder, usually the relatively common autoimmune thyroiditis, and we recommend routine screening of thyroid function in this high-risk population. In contrast and most specifically, in subjects with either monog-landular type 1 diabetes or relatively rare autoimmune adrenal failure, organ-specific autoantibody screening and functional testing will help identify both patients at risk for developing APS-2 as well as an already present subclinical polyglandular syndrome. In the presence of a patient with clinical and biochemical signs of primary adrenal failure, the determination of 21-OH Abs enables the unequivocal demonstration of the autoimmune origin of the disease. In subjects with autoimmune Addison's disease, screening for other endocrine disorders is required, given the frequent association of autoimmune adrenal insufficiency with thyroid diseases, type 1 diabetes, or other immune-mediated diseases. Thus, in any patient with Addison's disease, determination of TPO, thyroglobulin, GAD 65, and islet Abs should be performed and if negative, repeated every few years.

As most APS-2 patients are adults, determination of insulin or IA2 Abs is not strictly necessary, given the low diagnostic sensitivity of these markers for adult-onset type 1 diabetes. In the case of positivity for GAD65 and islet cell Abs, an oral glucose tolerance is needed to demonstrate glucose intolerance not revealed by fasting blood glucose. Although type 1 diabetes develops frequently before Addison's disease, GAD65 Abs are detected in 5–7% Addison patients without type 1 diabetes and a proper follow-up should be performed in islet-cell antibody-positive patients. The determination of 17-OH and P450scc Abs will enable the identification of subjects at high risk for primary hypogonadism, with a high positive predictive value in women. Furthermore, determination of TG Abs could be included in the screening of APS-2 children with type 1 diabetes.

Also, determination of 21-OH Abs should be performed in all patients with type 1 diabetes and thyroid autoimmune diseases, as the identification of subjects positive for adrenal autoantibodies is highly predictive for future adrenal insufficiency. In subjects with 21-OH Abs and normal cortisol levels, an ACTH stimulation test will enable the identification of subjects with pre-clinical adrenal dysfunction. Subjects with normal cortisol response could simply be followed-up, with re-evaluation of adrenal antibody levels, basal and adrenotropin ACTH-stimulated cortisol on a yearly basis.

Many of the endocrine disorders of the APS type 2 are adequately treated with hormonal replacement therapy if the disease is recognized early. Subjects with pathological ACTH test and increased levels of basal plasma ACTH require close clinical follow-up with repetition of the test every 6 months. Replacement therapy with hydrocortisone or cortisone acetate should be considered in the case of undercurrent stressful events. Hypoglycemic episodes and a decreasing insulin requirement in a type 1 diabetic can be one of the earliest signs of the development of adrenal failure. Replacement of levothyroxine without simultaneous adrenal steroid replacement in a hypothyroid patient with Addison's disease can precipitate an adrenal crisis (56). Replacement of thyroxine increases the cortisol turnover rate in the liver, and this may tax a failing adrenal gland.

FUTURE DEVELOPMENTS

In type 2 APS, genetic associations with HLA haplotypes and polymorphisms of genes encoding immunologically relevant gene products have been reported. The associations of autoimmune endocrinopathies with polymorphisms of these particular genes support the hypotheses that they may function to influence general predisposition, increase susceptibility, or influence the clinical presentation of autoimmune diseases. Other factors such as environmental triggers and yet unidentified genetic loci may modulate disease or target tissue phenotype. Therefore, future research is required to identify the other players in the process of regulating immune tolerance and the process of defining the tissue targets of autoimmune diseases. As actual immunogenetic data are scarce, further studies are necessary to elucidate the specific and general immunologic mechanisms, which underlie the development of APS-2. Nowadays, genetic screening is useful for the monogenic APS-1, but not for the polygenic type 2. Continuing research is warranted to further clarify the genetic background of APS-2, to identify susceptibility genes, and to understand their interactions. Potential susceptibility genes to APS-2—besides the *HLA* and *MICA* genes—are the *CTLA-4* and cytokine-related genes *(57)*, in particular, IL-10 and TNF-α, as well as the *PTPN22* gene. Additional knowledge regarding these genes will allow genetic screening of patients at risk. Advances in genetics and in pathogenesis of the type 2 APS and its component diseases may be valuable in the prevention of morbidity and mortality of the subjects involved. Future research should also focus on family studies with a large number of samples from different population groups. This might offer further knowledge on the inheritance of APS-2 as well as on the familial risk to develop APS-2.

REFERENCES

1. Eisenbarth GS, Gottlieb PA. Autoimmune polyendocrine syndromes. *N Engl J Med* 2004;350: 2068–2079.
2. Neufeld M, MacLaren N, Blizzard R. Autoimmune polyglandular syndromes. *Pediatr Ann* 1980;9: 154–162.
3. Jenkins RC, Weetman AP. Disease associations with autoimmune thyroid disease. *Thyroid* 2002;12: 977–988.
4. Betterle C, Greggio NA, Volpato M. Clinical review 93: autoimmune polyglandular syndrome type 1. *J Clin Endocrinol Metab* 1998;83:1049–1055.
5. Obermayer-Straub P, Strassburg CP, Manns MP. Autoimmune polyglandular syndrome type 1. *Clin Rev Allergy Immunol* 2000;18:167–183.
6. Ten S, New M, MacLaren N. Clinical review 130: Addison's disease 2001. *J Clin Endocrinol Metab* 2000; 86:2909–2922.
7. Förster G, Krummenauer F, Kühn I, Beyer J, Kahaly G. Polyglandular autoimmune syndrome type II: epidemiology and forms of manifestation; in German. *Dtsch Med Wschr* 199;124:1476–1481.
8. Gianani R, Sarvetnick N. Viruses, cytokines, antigens, and autoimmunity. *Proc Natl Acad Sci USA* 1996;93:2257–2259.
9. Wallaschofski H, Meyer A, Tuschy U, Lohmann T. HLA-DQA1*0301-associated susceptibility for autoimmune polyglandular syndrome type II and III. *Horm Metab Res* 2003;35:120–124.
10. Robles DT, Fain PR, Gottlieb PA, Eisenbarth GS. The genetics of autoimmune polyendocrine syndrome type II. *Endocrinol Metab Clin North Am* 2002; 31:353–368.
11. Eisenbarth GS, Wilson P, Ward F, Lebovita H. HLA type and occurrence of disease in familial polyglandular failure. *N Engl J Med* 1978; 298:92–94.
12. Tisch R, McDevitt H. Insulin-dependent diabetes mellitus. *Cell* 1996; 85:291–297.
13. Sanjeevi CB, Lybrand TP, DeWeese C, Landin-Olsson M, Kockum I, Dahlquist G, Sundkvist G, Stenger D, Lernmark A. Polymorphic amino acid variations in HLA-DQ are associated with systematic physical property changes and occurrence of IDDM. Members of the Swedish Childhood Diabetes Study. *Diabetes* 1995;44:125–131.
14. Moghaddam PH, Zwinderman AH, de Knijff P, Roep BO, Schipper RF, Van der Auwera B, Naipal A, Gorus F, Schuit F, Giphart MJ. TNFa microsatellite polymorphism modulates the risk of IDDM in Caucasians with the high-risk genotype HLA DQA1*0501-DQB1*0201/DQA1*0301-DQB1*0302. Belgian Diabetes Registry. *Diabetes* 1997;46:1514–1515.
15. Tandon N, Zhang L, Weetman AP. HLA associations with Hashimoto's thyroiditis. *Clin Endocrinol (Oxf)* 1991;34:383–386.
16. Roman SH, Greenberg D, Rubinstein P, Wallenstein S, Davies TF. Genetics of autoimmune thyroid disease: lack of evidence for linkage to HLA within families. *J Clin Endocrinol Metab* 1992;74:496–503.

17. Tomer Y, Barbesino G, Greenberg DA, Concepcion E, Davies TF. Mapping the major susceptibility loci for familial Graves' and Hashimoto's diseases: evidence for genetic heterogeneity and gene interactions. *J Clin Endocrinol Metab* 1999;84:4656–4664.

18. Kotsa K, Watson PF, Weetman AP. A CTLA-4 gene polymorphism is associated with both Graves disease and autoimmune hypothyroidism. *Clin Endocrinol (Oxf)* 1997;46:551–554.

19. Kahaly GJ, Dittmar M. Immunoregulatory genes in thyroid and polyglandular autoimmunity. Abstract band 11th International Symposium on Molecular Thyroidology, Okinawa, Japan, 2004, p. 33.

20. Gambelunghe G, Ghaderi M, Cosentino A, Falorni A, Brunetti P, Falorni A, Sanjeevi CB. Association of MHC Class I chain-related A (MIC-A) gene polymorphism with type I diabetes. *Diabetologia* 2000;43:507–514.

21. Dittmar M, Höhler T, Schneider PM, Adams P, Antunes C, Weber M, Kahaly GJ. Cytokine gene promoter polymorphisms in polyglandular autoimmunity. *Exp Clin Endocrinol Diabetes (Heidelberg)* 2004;112 (Suppl 1):S14 (Abstract).

22. Siminovitch KA. *PTPN22* and autoimmune disease. *Nat Genet* 2004;36:1248–1249.

23. Bottini N, Musumeci L, Alonso A, Rahmouni S, Nika K, Rostamkhani M, MacMurray J, Meloni GF, Lucarelli P, Pellecchia M, Eisenbarth GS, Comings D, Mustelin T. A functional variant of lymphoid tyrosine phosphatase is associated with type I diabetes. *Nat Genet* 2004;36:337–338.

24. Begovich AB, Carlton VE, Honigberg LA, Schrodi SJ, Chokkalingam AP, Alexander HC, Ardlie KG, Huang Q, Smith AM, Spoerke JM, Conn MT, Chang M, Chang SY, Saiki RK, Catanese JJ, Leong DU, Garcia VE, Mc McAllister LB, Jeffery DA, Lee AT, Batliwalla F, Remmers E, Criswell LA, Seldin MF, Kastner DL, Amos CI, Sninsky JJ, Gregersen PK. A missense single-nucleotide polymorphism in a gene encoding a protein tyrosine phosphatase (PTPN22) is associated with rheumatoid arthritis. *Am J Hum Genet* 2004;75:330–337.

25. Kyogoku C, Langefeld CD, Ortmann WA, Lee A, Selby S, Carlton VE, Chang M, Ramos P, Baechler EC, Batliwalla FM, Novitzke J, Williams AH, Gillett C, Rodine P, Graham RR, Ardlie KG, Gaffney PM, Moser KL, Petri M, Begovich AB, Gregersen PK, Behrens TW. Genetic association of the R620W polymorphism of protein tyrosine phosphatase PTPN22 with human SLE. *Am J Hum Genet* 2004;75:504–507.

26. Gomez LM, Anaya JM, Gonzalez CI, Pineda-Tamayo R, Otero W, Arango A, Martin J. PTPN22 C1858T polymorphism in Colombian patients with autoimmune diseases. *Genes Immun* 2005;6:628–631.

27. Aaltonen J, Bjorses P, Sandkuijl L, Perheentupa J, Peltonen L. An autosomal locus causing autoimmune disease: autoimmune polyglandular disease type I assigned to chromosome 21. *Nat Genet* 1994;8:83–87.

28. Bjorses P, Aaltonen J, Vikman A, Perheentupa J, Ben-Zion G, Chiumello G, Dahl N, Heideman P, Hoorweg-Nijman JJ, Mathivon L, Mullis PE, Pohl M, Ritzen M, Romeo G, Shapiro MS, Smith CS, Solyom J, Zlotogora J, Peltonen L. Genetic homogeneity of autoimmune polyglandular disease type I. *Am J Hum Genet* 1996;59:879–886.

29. Nagamine K, Peterson P, Scott HS, Kudoh J, Minoshima S, Heino M, Krohn KJ, Lalioti MD, Mullis PE, Antonarakis SE, Kawasaki K, Asakawa S, Ito F, Shimizu N. Positional cloning of the APECED gene. *Nat Genet* 1997;17:393–398.

30. Pearce SH, Cheetham T, Imrie H, Vaidya B, Barnes ND, Bilous RW, Carr D, Meeran K, Shaw NJ, Smith CS, Toft AD, Williams G, Kendall-Taylor P. A common and recurrent 13-bp deletion in the autoimmune regulator gene in British kindreds with autoimmune polyendocrinopathy type 1. *Am J Hum Genet* 1998;63:1675–1684.

31. Wang CY, Davoodi-Semiromi A, Huang W, Connor E, Shi JD, She JX. Characterization of mutations in patients with autoimmune polyglandular syndrome type 1 (APS1). *Hum Genet* 1998;103:681–685.

32. Chen QY, Lan MS, She JX, Maclaren NK. The gene responsible for autoimmune polyglandular syndrome type 1 maps to chromosome 21q22.3 in US patients. *J Autoimmun* 1998;11:177–183.

33. Heino M, Peterson P, Kudoh J, Shimizu N, Antonarakis SE, Scott HS, Krohn K. APECED mutations in the autoimmue regulator (AIRE) gene. *Hum Mutat* 2001;18:205–211.

34. Halonen M, Eskelin P, Myhre AG, Perheentupa J, Husebye ES, Kampe O, Rorsman F, Peltonen L, Ulmanen I, Partanen J. AIRE Mutations and Human Leukocyte Antigen Genotypes as Determinants of the Autoimmune Polyendocrinopathy-Candidiasis-Ectodermal Dystrophy Phenotype. *J Clin Endocrinol Metab* 2002;87:2568–2574.

35. Skorka A, Bednarczuk T, Bar-Andziak E, Nauman J, Ploski R. Lymphoid tyrosine phosphatase (PTPN22/LYP) variant and Graves' disease in a Polish population: association and gene dose-dependent correlation with age of onset. *Clin Endocrinol (Oxf)* 2005;62:679–682.

36. Vogel A, Strassburg CP, Obermayer-Straub P, Brabant G, Manns MP. The genetic background of autoimmune polyendocrinopathy-candidiasis-ectodermal dystrophy and its autoimmune disease components. *J Mol Med* 2002;80:201–211.

37. Anderson MS Autoimmune endocrine diseases. *Curr Opin Immunol* 2002;14:760–764.

38. Devendra D, Eisenbarth GS. Immunologic endocrine disorders. *J Allergy Clin Immunol* 2003;111:S624–S636.

39. Topliss D, How J, Lewis M, Row V, Volpe R. Evidence for cell-mediated immunity and specific suppressor T lymphocyte dysfunction in Graves' disease and diabetes mellitus. *J Clin Endocrinol Metab* 1983;57:700–705.

40. Canbay A, Gieseler R, Ella R, Fink H, Saller B, Mann K. Manifestation of adrenal insufficiency after administration of levothyroxine in a patient with polyglandular autoimmune syndrome type II (Schmidt-syndrome); in German. *Internist (Berlin)* 2000;41:588–591.

41. Sakaguchi S. Naturally arising CD4+ regulatory t cells for immunologic self-tolerance and negative control of immune responses. *Annu Rev Immunol* 2004;22:531–562.

42. Shevach EM. Regulatory T cells in autoimmmunity*. *Annu Rev Immunol* 2000;18:423–449.

43. Kriegel MA, Lohmann T, Gabler C, Blank N, Kalden JR, Lorenz HM. Defective suppressor function of human CD4+ CD25+ regulatory T cells in autoimmune polyglandular syndrome type II. *J Exp Med* 2004;199:1285–1291.

44. Luther C, Poeschel S, Varga M, Melms A, Tolosa E. Decreased frequency of intrathymic regulatory T cells in patients with myasthenia-associated thymoma. *J Neuroimmunol* 2005;164:124–128.

45. Suda T, Takahashi T, Golstein P, Nagata S. Molecular cloning and expression of the Fas ligand, a novel member of the tumor necrosis factor family. *Cell* 1993;75:1169–1178.

46. Viglietta V, Baecher-Allan C, Weiner HL, Hafler DA. Loss of functional suppression by CD4+CD25+ regulatory T cells in patients with multiple sclerosis. *J Exp Med* 2004;199:971–979.

47. Sakaguchi S, Sakaguchi N, Asano M, Itoh M, Toda M. Immunologic self-tolerance maintained by activated T cells expression IL-2 receptor alpha-chains (CD25). Breakdown of a single mechanism of self-tolerance causes various autoimmune diseases. *J Immunol* 1995;155:1151–1164.

48. Lan RY, Ansari AA, Lian ZX, Gershwin ME. Regulatory T cells: development, function and role in autoimmunity. *Autoimmun Rev* 2005;4:351–363.

49. Dittmar M, Tietz S, Poppe R, Fredenhagen G, Weber M, Kahaly GJ. Impaired DNase activity in patients with endocrine autoimmunity and their healthy relatives. *Exp Clin Endocrinol Diabetes* 2004;112(Suppl 1):S75 (Abstract).

50. Kumar R, Reddy DV, Unnikrishnan AG, Bhadada SK, Agrawal NK, Singh SK. Polyglandular autoimmune endocrinopathy in type 2 diabetes. *J Assoc Physicians India* 2004;52:999–1000.

51. Dittmar M, Kahaly GJ. Polyglandular autoimmune syndromes: Immunogenetics and long-term follow-up. *J Clin Endocrinol Metab* 2003;88:2983–2992.

52. Chen S, Sawicka J, Betterle C, Powell M, Prentice L, Volpato M, Smith BR, Furmaniak J. Autoantibodies to steroidogenic enzymes in autoimmune polyglandular syndrome, Addison's disease, and premature ovarian failure. *J Clin Endocrinol Metab* 1996;81:1871–1876.

53. Hrdá P, Sterzl I, Matucha P, Korioth F, Kromminga A. HLA antigen expression in autoimmune endocrinopathies. *Physiol Res* 2004;53:191–197.

54. Devendra D, Franke B, Galloway TS, Horton SJ, Knip M, Wilkin TJ. Distinct idiotypes of insulin autoantibody in autoimmune polyendocrine syndrome type 2 and childhood onset type 1 diabetes. *J Clin Endocrinol Metab* 2004;89:5266–5270.

55. Kahaly GJ, Förster G, Otto E, Hansen C, Schulz G. Diabetes mellitus Typ I als Teil des polyglandulären Autoimmunsyndroms. *Diabetes Stoffwechsel* 1997;6:19–27.

56. Betterle C, Lazzarotto F, Presotto F. Autoimmune polyglandular syndrome Type 2: the tip of an iceberg? *Clin Exp Immunol* 2004;137:225–233.

57. Dittmar M, Kahaly GJ. Immunoregulatory and susceptibility genes in thyroid and polyglandular autoimmunity. *Thyroid* 2005;15:239–250.

INDEX